1999
YEAR BOOK OF
SURGERY®

Statement of Purpose

The YEAR BOOK Service

The YEAR BOOK series was devised in 1901 by practicing health professionals who observed that the literature of medicine and related disciplines had become so voluminous that no one individual could read and place in perspective every potential advance in a major specialty. In the final decade of the 20th century, this recognition is more acutely true than it was in 1901.

More than merely a series of books, YEAR BOOK volumes are the tangible results of a unique service designed to accomplish the following:

- to *survey* a wide range of journals of proven value
- to *select* from those journals papers representing significant advances and statements of important clinical principles
- to provide *abstracts* of those articles that are readable, convenient summaries of their key points
- to provide *commentary* about those articles to place them in perspective

These publications grow out of a unique process that calls on the talents of outstanding authorities in clinical and fundamental disciplines, trained literature specialists, and professional writers, all supported by the resources of Mosby, the world's preeminent publisher for the health professions.

The Literature Base

Mosby and its editors survey approximately 500 journals published worldwide, covering the full range of the health professions. On an annual basis, the publisher examines usage patterns and polls its expert authorities to add new journals to the literature base and to delete journals that are no longer useful as potential YEAR BOOK sources.

The Literature Survey

The publisher's team of literature specialists, all of whom are trained and experienced health professionals, examines every original, peer-reviewed article in each journal issue. More than 250,000 articles per year are scanned systematically, including title, text, illustrations, tables, and references. Each scan is compared, article by article, to the search strategies that the publisher has developed in consultation with the 270 outside experts who form the pool of YEAR BOOK editors. A given article may be reviewed by any number of editors, from one to a dozen or more, regardless of the discipline for which the paper was originally published. In turn, each editor who receives the article reviews it to determine whether the article should be included in the YEAR BOOK. This decision is based on the article's inherent quality, its probable usefulness to readers of that YEAR BOOK, and the editor's goal to represent a balanced picture of a given field in each volume of the YEAR BOOK. In addition, the editor indicates when to include figures and tables from the article to help the YEAR BOOK reader better understand the information.

Of the quarter million articles scanned each year, only 5% are selected for detailed analysis within the YEAR BOOK series, thereby assuring readers of the high value of every selection.

The Abstract

The publisher's abstracting staff is headed by a seasoned medical professional and includes individuals with training in the life sciences, medicine, and other areas, plus extensive experience in writing for the health professions and related industries. Each selected article is assigned to a specific writer on this abstracting staff. The abstracter, guided in many cases by notations supplied by the expert editor, writes a structured, condensed summary designed so that the reader can rapidly acquire the essential information contained in the article.

The Commentary

The YEAR BOOK editorial boards, sometimes assisted by guest commentators, write comments that place each article in perspective for the reader. This provides the reader with the equivalent of a personal consultation with a leading international authority—an opportunity to better understand the value of the article and to benefit from the authority's thought processes in assessing the article.

Additional Editorial Features

The editorial boards of each YEAR BOOK organize the abstracts and comments to provide a logical and satisfying sequence of information. To enhance the organization, editors also provide introductions to sections or individual chapters, comments linking a number of abstracts, citations to additional literature, and other features.

The published YEAR BOOK contains enhanced bibliographic citations for each selected article, including extended listings of multiple authors and identification of author affiliations. Each YEAR BOOK contains a Table of Contents specific to that year's volume. From year to year, the Table of Contents for a given YEAR BOOK will vary depending on developments within the field.

Every YEAR BOOK contains a list of the journals from which papers have been selected. This list represents a subset of approximately 500 journals surveyed by the publisher and occasionally reflects a particularly pertinent article from a journal that is not surveyed on a routine basis.

Finally, each volume contains a comprehensive subject index and an index to authors of each selected paper.

The 1999 Year Book Series

Year Book of Allergy, Asthma, and Clinical Immunology: Drs. Rosenwasser, Boguniewicz, Borish, Routes, Spahn, and Weber

Year Book of Anesthesiology and Pain Management®: Drs. Tinker, Abram, Chestnut, Roizen, Rothenberg, and Wood

Year Book of Cardiology®: Drs. Schlant, Collins, Gersh, Graham, Kaplan, and Waldo

Year Book of Chiropractic®: Dr. Lawrence

Year Book of Critical Care Medicine®: Drs. Parrillo, Balk, Calvin, Franklin, and Shapiro

Year Book of Dentistry®: Drs. Meskin, Berry, Jeffcoat, Leinfelder, Roser, Summitt, and Zakariasen

Year Book of Dermatology and Dermatologic Surgery™: Drs. Thiers and Lang

Year Book of Diagnostic Radiology®: Drs. Osborn, Birdwell, Dalinka, Groskin, Maynard, Pentecost, Ros, Smirniotopoulos, and Young

Year Book of Emergency Medicine®: Drs. Wagner, Dronen, Davidson, King, Niemann, and Hamilton

Year Book of Endocrinology®: Drs. Bagdade, Braverman, Fitzpatrick, Horton, Kannan, Landsberg, Molitch, Morley, Odell, Poehlman, and Rogol

Year Book of Family Practice®: Drs. Berg, Bowman, Davidson, Dexter, and Scherger

Year Book of Gastroenterology: Drs. Aliperti and Fleshman

Year Book of Hand Surgery®: Drs. Amadio and Hentz

Year Book of Medicine®: Drs. Klahr, Frishman, Malawista, Mandell, Jett, Young, Barkin, and Bagdade

Year Book of Neonatal and Perinatal Medicine®: Drs. Fanaroff, Maisels, and Stevenson

Year Book of Nephrology, Hypertension, and Mineral Metabolism: Drs. Schwab, Bennett, Emmett, Hostetter, and Moe

Year Book of Neurology and Neurosurgery®: Drs. Bradley and Gibbs

Year Book of Nuclear Medicine®: Drs. Gottschalk, Blaufox, Coleman, Strauss, and Zubal

Year Book of Obstetrics, Gynecology, and Women's Health®: Drs. Mishell, Herbst, and Kirschbaum

Year Book of Oncology®: Drs. Ozols, Eisenberg, Glatstein, Loehrer, and Urba

Year Book of Ophthalmology®: Drs. Wilson, Augsburger, Cohen, Eagle, Grossman, Laibson, Maguire, Nelson, Penne, Rapuano, Sergott, Spaeth, Tipperman, Ms. Gosfield, and Ms. Salmon

Year Book of Orthopedics®: Drs. Morrey, Beauchamp, Currier, Tolo, Trigg, and Swiontkowski

Year Book of Otolaryngology–Head and Neck Surgery®: Drs. Paparella, Holt, and Otto

Year Book of Pathology and Laboratory Medicine®: Drs. Raab, Cohen, Dabbs, Olson, and Stanley

Year Book of Pediatrics®: Dr. Stockman

Year Book of Plastic, Reconstructive, and Aesthetic Surgery®: Drs. Miller, Bartlett, Garner, McKinney, Ruberg, Salisbury, and Smith

Year Book of Psychiatry and Applied Mental Health®: Drs. Talbott, Ballenger, Frances, Lydiard, Meltzer, Jensen, and Tasman

Year Book of Pulmonary Disease®: Drs. Jett, Castro, Maurer, Peters, Phillips, and Ryu

Year Book of Rheumatology, Arthritis, and Musculoskeletal Disease™: Drs. Panush, Hadler, Hellmann, LeRoy, Pisetsky, and Simon

Year Book of Sports Medicine®: Drs. Shephard, Drinkwater, Eichner, Torg, Alexander, and Mr. George

Year Book of Surgery®: Drs. Copeland, Bland, Deitch, Eberlein, Howard, Luce, Seeger, Souba, and Sugarbaker

Year Book of Urology®: Drs. Andriole and Coplen

Year Book of Vascular Surgery®: Dr. Porter

1999

The Year Book of SURGERY®

Editor-in-Chief

Edward M. Copeland III, M.D.

The Edward R. Woodward Professor and Chairman, Department of Surgery, University of Florida College of Medicine, Gainesville, Florida

Mosby

St. Louis Baltimore Boston Carlsbad Naples New York Philadelphia Portland London Madrid Mexico City Singapore Sydney Tokyo Toronto Wiesbaden

Mosby
Dedicated to Publishing Excellence

Associate Publisher: Cynthia Baudendistel
Developmental Editor: Sarah A. Zagarri
Manager, Periodical Editing: Kirk Swearingen
Production Editor: Pat Costigan
Project Supervisor, Production: Joy Moore
Production Assistant: Karie House
Manager, Literature Services: Idelle L. Winer
Illustrations and Permissions Specialist: Steve Ramay

1999 EDITION

Printed in the United States of America
Composition by Reed Technology and Information Services, Inc.
Printing/binding by Maple-Vail

Mosby, Inc.
11830 Westline Industrial Drive
St. Louis, MO 63146

International Standard Serial Number: 0090-3671
International Standard Book Number: 0–8151-9744-6

Editors

Editorial Board

Kirby I. Bland, M.D.

J. Murray Beardsley Professor and Chairman, Department of Surgery, Professor of Medical Sciences, Brown University School of Medicine; Surgeon-in-Chief, Rhode Island Hospital; Executive Surgeon-in-Chief, Brown University Affiliated Hospitals, Providence, Rhode Island

Edwin A. Deitch, M.D.

Professor and Chairman, Department of Surgery, UMD-New Jersey Medical School; Chairman, Department of Surgery, University of Medicine and Dentistry, Newark, New Jersey

Timothy J. Eberlein, M.D.

Bixby Professor and Chairman, Department of Surgery, Washington University School of Medicine; Surgeon-in-Chief, Barnes-Jewish Hospital, St. Louis Children's Hospital, Veterans Administration Hospital, St. Louis, Missouri

Richard J. Howard, M.D., Ph.D.

Robert H. and Kathleen M. Axline Professor of Surgery, University of Florida College of Medicine, Shands Hospital at the University of Florida, Gainesville, Florida

Edward A. Luce, M.D.

Kiehn-Desprez Professor, Case Western Reserve University; Chief, Division of Plastic Surgery, University Hospitals of Cleveland, Cleveland, Ohio

James M. Seeger, M.D.

Professor and Chief, Section of Vascular Surgery, Department of Surgery, University of Florida College of Medicine, Gainesville, Florida

Wiley W. Souba, M.D., Sc.D.

Professor of Surgery, Harvard Medical School; Professor of Nutrition, Harvard School of Public Health; Chief, Division of Surgical Oncology, Director, Surgical Oncology Research Laboratories, Director, Nutritional Support Service, Massachusetts General Hospital; Deputy Director, Massachusetts General Hospital Cancer Center, Boston, Massachusetts

David J. Sugarbaker, M.D.

Associate Professor of Surgery, Harvard Medical School; Chief, Division of Thoracic Surgery, Brigham and Women's Hospital, Chief of Surgical Services, Dana Farber Cancer Institute, Boston, Massachusetts

Contributing Editors

Joseph F. Amaral, M.D.

Associate Professor of Surgery, Brown University School of Medicine; Director of Laparoscopic Surgery, Rhode Island Hospital, Providence, Rhode Island

William G. Cioffi, M.D.
Professor of Surgery, Brown University School of Medicine; Chief of Trauma and Burns, Rhode Island Hospital, Providence, Rhode Island

Francois I. Luks, M.D.
Associate Professor of Surgery and Pediatrics, Brown University School of Medicine; Attending Pediatric Surgeon, Hasbro Children's Hospital and Rhode Island Hospital, Providence, Rhode Island

Victor E. Pricolo, M.D.
Professor of Surgery, Brown University School of Medicine; Director, Division of Colon and Rectal Surgery, Rhode Island Hospital, Providence, Rhode Island

H. Hank Simms, M.D.
Associate Professor of Surgery, Brown University School of Medicine; Chief, Division of Surgical Critical Care, Department of Surgery, Rhode Island Hospital, Providence, Rhode Island

Thomas F. Tracy, M.D., M.S.
Professor of Surgery and Pediatrics, Brown University School of Medicine; Pediatric Surgeon-in-Chief, Hasbro Children's Hospital, Providence, Rhode Island

Table of Contents

Journals Represented

Mosby and its editors survey approximately 500 U.S. and foreign medical and allied health journals. From these journals, the editors select the articles to be abstracted. Journals represented in this YEAR BOOK are listed below.

American Journal of Clinical Nutrition
American Journal of Gastroenterology
American Journal of Medicine
American Journal of Otolaryngology
American Journal of Respiratory and Critical Care Medicine
American Journal of Roentgenology
American Journal of Surgery
American Journal of Surgical Pathology
American Journal of the Medical Sciences
American Surgeon
Anaesthesia
Anaesthesia and Intensive Care
Anesthesia and Analgesia
Annals of Internal Medicine
Annals of Otology, Rhinology and Laryngology
Annals of Plastic Surgery
Annals of Surgery
Annals of Surgical Oncology
Annals of Thoracic Surgery
Annals of the Royal College of Surgeons of England
Archives of Otolaryngology-Head and Neck Surgery
Archives of Physical Medicine and Rehabilitation
Archives of Surgery
Breast Journal
British Journal of Surgery
Burns
Cancer
Cancer Research
Chest
Clinical Cancer Research
Clinical Infectious Diseases
Clinical Journal of Pain
Critical Care Medicine
Digestive Diseases and Sciences
Diseases of the Colon and Rectum
Endoscopy
European Journal of Plastic Surgery
European Journal of Surgery
European Respiratory Journal
Gastroenterology
Head and Neck
Human Reproduction
Infection Control and Hospital Epidemiology
International Journal of Cancer
International Journal of Radiation, Oncology, Biology, and Physics
Journal of Burn Care and Rehabilitation

Journal of Clinical Investigation
Journal of Clinical Oncology
Journal of Computer Assisted Tomography
Journal of Hand Surgery (British)
Journal of Pediatric Surgery
Journal of Surgical Oncology
Journal of Surgical Research
Journal of Thoracic and Cardiovascular Surgery
Journal of Trauma: Injury, Infection, and Critical Care
Journal of Vascular Surgery
Journal of the American College of Surgeons
Journal of the American Medical Association
Journal of the National Cancer Institute
Lancet
New England Journal of Medicine
Plastic and Reconstructive Surgery
Radiology
Respiratory Medicine
Southern Medical Journal
Surgery
The Laryngoscope Journal
Transplantation
World Journal of Surgery

STANDARD ABBREVIATIONS

The following terms are abbreviated in this edition: acquired immunodeficiency syndrome (AIDS), cardiopulmonary resuscitation (CPR), central nervous system (CNS), cerebrospinal fluid (CSF), computed tomography (CT), deoxyribonucleic acid (DNA), electrocardiography (ECG), health maintenance organization (HMO), human immunodeficiency virus (HIV), intensive care unit (ICU), intramuscular (IM), intravenous (IV), magnetic resonance (MR) imaging (MRI), and ribonucleic acid (RNA).

NOTE

The YEAR BOOK OF SURGERY is a literature survey service providing abstracts of articles published in the professional literature. Every effort is made to assure the accuracy of the information presented in these pages. Neither the editor nor the publisher of the YEAR BOOK OF SURGERY can be responsible for errors in the original materials. The editors' comments are their own opinions. Mention of specific products within this publication does not constitute endorsement.

To facilitate the use of the YEAR BOOK OF SURGERY as a reference tool, all illustrations and tables included in this publication are now identified as they appear in the original article. This change is meant to help the reader recognize that any illustration or table appearing in the YEAR BOOK OF SURGERY may be only one of many in the original article. For this reason, figure and table numbers appear to be out of sequence within the YEAR BOOK OF SURGERY.

1 General Considerations

Introduction

The workforce of clinical nonphysicians is enlarging and becoming somewhat autonomous. These groups are an important component of patient care in this country and are lobbying to have laws passed to give them even more responsibility not supervised by a physician. The inability to limit the physician workforce in this country has been aimed, at times, at the inability to limit the influx of international medical graduates. In fact, these international medical graduates represent 10% of the surgical faculty in the United States, and 14 have been or are department chairpersons. It would seem that they are making a positive contribution to medical education in this country in the same proportion to U.S. medical graduates. The stimulus to enter the discipline of surgery for women is, no doubt, the same as it is for men; therefore, the comparison of female surgeons to women in other specialties uncovers differences not dissimilar to those that would be expected when comparing male surgeons to men in other specialties (the categories are just different).

Canada has a mature national health care system where comparable costs for surgical procedures are much less than in the United States. The amenities of medical care, such as waiting time for a procedure, appear to be better in this country. To some degree, you still get what you pay for. Yet, much of the data collected for comparison purposes among U.S. hospitals is derived from the study of the healthiest patient populations. Thus, the patient with multiple co-morbid conditions is put at risk for being an undesirable customer in our new reimbursement system. Likewise, as a shift to outpatient care has occurred, there has been a dramatic increase in deaths secondary to medication errors. Adverse drug reactions in hospitalized patients also remain a national health care hazard. Evidence continues to mount that operative morbidity and mortality are correlated to the volume of more difficult surgical procedures done within a hospital or by an individual surgeon. One wonders, however, if the bias of the authors (usually all from high-volume institutions) might be a factor in these analyses. Competency skills, especially for simple but often lifesaving procedures (e.g., endotracheal intubation, venous cut-down, and chest tube insertion), can be taught to and maintained by all surgical residents with almost no failures. At the other end of the medical care spectrum, decisions made by physicians vary widely, such as when to withdraw life-support systems.

The value of some time-honored tests and medical treatments continues to be challenged. There is evidence that a preoperative bleeding time lacks clinical benefit in a patient without a bleeding disorder. Vena caval filters do prevent acute pulmonary emboli but result in significant long-term sequelae from deep venous thrombosis. Venous thrombosis in surgical patients can be significantly reduced by the combined use of heparin and compression stockings.

With the use of CT, highly specialized radiologists can diagnose appendicitis with 98% accuracy and, therefore, reduce unnecessary appendectomy. The question is whether this diagnostic success with CT technology can be extrapolated to community hospitals accross the country. Should a few highly skilled physicians in an institution with the latest technology set the standards of care for the remainder of the nation? Or should these results be the ones to which all of us strive, assuming the costs are not prohibitive?

Edward M. Copeland III, M.D.

Current and Projected Workforce of Nonphysician Clinicians

Cooper RA, Laud P, Dietrich CL (Med College of Wisconsin, Milwaukee)

JAMA 280:788-794, 1998 1–1

Objective.—The number of nonphysician clinicians (NPCs) is increasing, but the effect on demand for physicians in the future is not known. The supply and distribution of NPCs and the supply of physicians were examined.

Methods.—The numbers of NPCs in 10 disciplines (nurse practitioners, physician assistants, nurse-midwives, chiropractors, acupuncturists, naturopaths, optometrists, podiatrists, nurse anesthetists, and clinical nurse specialists) and the current and past numbers of physicians were obtained from professional organizations and associations.

Results.—Between 1992 and 1997, the number of nurse practitioners grew by a factor of 4, physician assistants by 2, certified nurse-midwives by 4, chiropractors by 2.5, acupuncturists by 1.7, naturopaths by 2.5, podiatrists by 1.25, and certified registered nurse anesthetists by 2.4. The numbers of optometrists increased by only 5%, and the numbers of clinical nurse specialists actually declined by 20%. The ages of graduates and practitioners ranged from the late 20s to the early 40s. Most of these areas are expected to grow by 20% by the year 2001. Most of the growth is expected to occur with primary care providers. The growth of the supply of NPCs and physicians is expected to be greatest in those states that now have the largest number of NPCs and physicians. Growth is anticipated to be lower among NPCs who provide specialty care. The growth in NPCs by

2005 is expected to outstrip the growth of physicians by a factor of 2. The impact of this growth has not been studied.

Conclusion.—The growth in the NPC and physician supply should be studies to determine the impact on physician demand.

Roles of Nonphysician Clinicians as Autonomous Providers of Patient Care

Cooper RA, Henderson T, Dietrich CL (Med College of Wisconsin, Milwaukee; Natl Conference of State Legislatures, Washington, DC)

JAMA 280:795-802, 1998 1–2

Objective.—The practice prerogative accorded to nonphysician clinicians (NPCs), including nurse practitioners (NPs), certified nurse-midwives, physician assistants, chiropractors, naturopaths, practitioners of acupuncture and herbal medicine, optometrists, podiatrists, certified registered nurse anesthetists (CRNAs), and clinical nurse specialists, depends on regulations and state statutes and varies considerably. The status of NPC regulation as of July 1, 1998 was reported.

Methods.—Data from professional organizations, the Health Policy Tracking System at the National Conference of State Legislature, state Internet Web sites, telephone interviews with professional organizations, and legislation were summarized.

Results.—Most NPCs hold graduate degrees at the master's level and are trained in primary care with emphasis on specialties, principally in a clinical setting. Most NPs can perform a wide variety of diagnostic activities, can order and interpret tests, and can prescribe in 60% of states, sometimes independent of physician involvement. Alternative NPCs such as chiropractors are trained to be primary care providers, acupuncturists and herbalists are trained as clinicians of first encounter, and naturopaths are trained as outpatient clinicians. Chiropractors are licensed in all 50 states and the District of Columbia and are board-regulated. They have broad latitude to treat disease or dysfunction by physical treatments or natural remedies. Optometrists and podiatrists are licensed in all 51 jurisdictions and have wide privileges. CRNAs are recognized or licensed in most states and have privileges depending on the level of their training, certification, and experience. The NPC field is growing and is creating, in some states, overlapping services with physicians. Because this emerging pluralism has no unifying theme, it has the potential for fragmenting the health care system.

Conclusion.—Interdisciplinary regulation and clinician integration must be pursued to stabilize and strengthen the health care system.

▶ I don't think there is any question that NPCs can provide medical care to patients who are currently in the purview of physicians. In fact, many physicians employ NPCs to do so. There is an ever-increasing ability of these individuals to function independently as care-givers, and in many states they can be reimbursed for doing so. They represent a "windfall profit" for managed care organizations because as primary caregivers, they will, at least initially, cost less. We can all talk about diminishing quality of care, but in reality, will quality of basic medical care be any less? Probably not. There is still enormous emphasis (and money) in medical schools aimed at producing primary care physicians. Both the students interested in this field and deans of medical schools might possibly want to rethink their priorities in view of the data contained in Abstracts 1–1 and 1–2.

E.M. Copeland III, M.D.

Characteristics of Women Surgeons in the United States

Frank E, Brownstein M, Ephgrave K, et al (Emory Univ, Atlanta, Ga)

Am J Surg 176:244-250, 1998 1–3

Objective.—Data from the Women Physicians' Health Study, a national questionnaire-based study of 716 characteristics of 4,501 U.S. women physicians, were used to compare the characteristics of women surgeons in the United States with those of other U.S. female physicians.

Methods.—Stratified by decade of graduation from medical school, the sample selected 2,500 women from each of the last 4 decades' graduating classes (1950-1989) The women were aged 30 to 70 years and the sample was based on the American Medical Association's Physician Masterfile. Older physicians were oversampled to avoid underrepresentation. The response rate was 59% of eligible physicians.

Results.—Compared with other physicians, surgeons were younger, more likely to be born in the United States, more likely to be white, less likely to be Asian, and more likely to practice in a medical school setting and spend more time on continuing medical education. Surgeons were more likely to be single, never married, less likely to be married now, not significantly more likely to be divorced, less likely to have stress at home, less likely to have had children than other physicians, reported better health, reported higher personal and household incomes, and worked significantly more clinic hours and call nights. Surgeons were no more likely to report feeling overworked or having less control over their environment than other physicians. Surgeons' politics, partners' educational levels, and percentages that were the primary preschool caretakers of their children were similar to those of other physicians'. Surgeons board certified in another specialty were also board certified in surgery. Age and marital status did not change these results. Surgeons' career satisfaction was similar to that of other physicians. Satisfaction with their specialty was higher for surgeons than for other physicians.

Conclusion.—This first national study comparing personal characteristics among women surgeons and other women physicians show that women surgeons differ in many important ways from other women physicians.

▶ My observations are that women applicants to surgical residencies are often more motivated as a group than are the men. The range of desire to be a surgeon is more narrow for women because women make a conscious decision to commit to an arduous training program and to delay their more traditional roles. This study, however, compares women surgeons to women in other specialties. I wonder whether a commitment to a surgical career early in their medical maturation and having attained their goal are reasons for their job satisfaction?

E.M. Copeland III, M.D.

The International Medical Graduate in US Academic General Surgery

Aranha GV (Loyola Univ, Chicago; Hines Veterans Affairs Hosp, Ill)

Arch Surg 133:130-133, 1998 1–4

Objective.—The percentage of international medical graduates (IMGs) in the physician workforce has increased from 10% in 1963 to 18% in 1970 to almost 24% today. The contributions of IMGs to surgery were assessed.

Methods.—A questionnaire was sent to the chairpersons of the departments of general surgery in all 128 U.S. medical schools to identify IMGs in training and on faculties between 1959 and 1995.

Results.—Of 122 responders, 108 (88.5%) had at least 1 IMG on their faculty, and 14 had none. Countries with at least 10 IMGs on U.S. academic surgical faculties included India (88), Canada (62), South Africa (28), the United Kingdom (28), China (25), Lebanon (22), Argentina (19), Italy (15), Egypt (14), Japan (14), Iran (13), the Philippines (13), Peru (13), Germany (13), Ireland (12), South Korea (11), Mexico (11), and Israel (11). There were 142 IMGs in the Midwest, 133 in the mid-Atlantic states, 96 in the South, 84 in the Pacific Coast states, 53 in New England, 31 in the Southwest, 22 in Hawaii, 6 in the Rocky Mountain states, and 5 in Washington, DC. California, New York, and Illinois had the most IMGs with 78, 75, and 42, respectively. There were 182 professors, 142 associate professors, 216 assistant professors, 19 instructors, and 13 research associates. Surgical appointments increased from 1 in 1959 to 35 between 1960 and 1969, to 114 between 1970 and 1979, to 221 between 1980 and 1989, and to 190 between 1990 and 1995. The number of IMG faculty appointments is increasing even though the number of IMGs in training programs is decreasing. Of the 43,199 active fellows in the American College of Surgeons in 1993, 6,527 (15%) were surgeons with degrees from foreign schools, and 572 (8.8%) of these IMGs held 10.6% of the 5,399 U.S. academic surgery faculty positions. Ten percent of surgical residents in the United States are IMGs.

Conclusions.—IMGs represent 10% of U.S. surgical faculty. Fourteen have been or are department chairpersons. The number of IMG faculty appointments is increasing even though the number of IMGs in training programs is decreasing. The U.S. experience with IMGs appears to be favorable.

▶ From its origin, the success of the United States has been dependent upon immigration of individuals from other countries seeking to improve their political, socioeconomic, and/or educational situation. Recent evidence of this phenomenon is the success of many Vietnamese immigrants. If a reliable database ever does indicate too many physicians in this country, the solution should not necessarily be to limit foreign medical graduate access to medical education or to further restrict immigration laws, for to do so would violate the principles upon which the United States was originally founded.

E.M. Copeland III, M.D.

Shopping Around for Hospital Services: A Comparison of the United States and Canada

Bell CM, Crystal M, Detsky AS, et al (Univ of Toronto; Sunnybrook Health Science Ctr, Toronto; Mount Sinai Hosp, Toronto; et al)

JAMA 279:1015-1017, 1998 1–5

Objective.—Health care costs in the United States are one third higher than those in Canada. Because the U.S. health care system has changed substantially in recent years, historical comparisons are difficult. The price and convenience of 7 generally available, elective, standardized diagnostic and therapeutic services were determined by a cross-sectional telephone survey.

Methods.—Eighteen Canadian and 48 U.S. acute care hospitals in cities with a population of more than 500,000 were telephoned and asked about out-of-pocket prices and waiting times for MRI of the head without gadolinium, a screening mammogram, a 12-lead ECG, a prothrombin time measurement, 1 hemodialysis session, a screening colonoscopy, and total knee replacement. Callers constructed a scenario when talking with hospital personnel to avoid cueing them or creating carryover effects.

Results.—Waiting times in American hospitals were the same as or significantly shorter than in Canadian hospitals. The wait for MRI of the head was 3 days in the United States and 150 days in Canada. Only single-session hemodialysis was less expensive in the United States. The prices of all other services were significantly higher in the United States than in Canada, particularly for total knee replacement, which was priced at $26,805 in the United States and at $10,651 in Canada. None of the hospitals negotiated either price or waiting times. Whereas differences in prices were related to differences in waiting times, there was no association between waiting time and price for any service in either country.

Conclusion.—Hospitals in the United States provide faster service at higher prices for patients who pay out-of-pocket.

▶ Prices are fixed in Canada and are flexible (depending on the purchaser) in the United States. The hospital charge data in the United States, no doubt, reflect the maximum charges. However, the waiting time in the 2 countries should be directly comparable. As managed care contracts become more widespread throughout the United States, my prediction is that Canadian and U.S. costs for hospitalization will equalize and that waiting time will remain much shorter in the United States.

E.M. Copeland III, M.D.

An Analysis of 25 Milliman & Robertson Guidelines for Surgery: Data-driven Versus Consensus-derived Clinical Practice Guidelines

Rutledge R (Univ of North Carolina, Chapel Hill)

Ann Surg 228:579-587, 1998 1–6

Objective.—There is a lot of interest in the development of clinical practice guidelines, based on sound clinical and scientific evidence, for monitoring the quality and cost of health care. Because guidelines should clearly demonstrate that they promote improved patient outcomes and do not harm patients, the actuarial firm of Milliman & Robertson (M&R), which analyzes the major issues in health care, has prepared guidelines to assist in delivering efficient health care. A large-scale database of inpatients was used to assess the actual length of stay (LOS) for a variety of illnesses to determine the appropriateness of the guidelines and to investigate the accuracy, reasonableness, and applicability of the guidelines.

Methods.—North Carolina hospital discharge data for 1996 from the HCIA hospital discharge database, that included demographic, diagnostic, treatment, LOS, and charge data, were used. HCIA is a leading health care information company that develops and markets clinical and financial decision support systems. Patients used to evaluate 25 M&R guidelines were defined as those between 16 and 65 years who lived, who were not transferred from another hospital, and who had an LOS of 21 days or less.

Results.—There were 74,538 patients in 25 categories varying from 22 patients in the esophagectomy category to 10,546 in the abdominal hysterectomy category. LOS data varied considerably among North Carolina hospital discharge data, American College of Surgeons survey results, and M&R guidelines, particularly for high-risk procedures such as esophagectomy (Table 3). Good guidelines can have a major beneficial impact on costs and quality of care, as this study shows. Good scientific research allows the makers of guidelines to target and design cost-reduction efforts but maintain quality. Poorly framed guidelines can be misused and misinterpreted and can lead to inferior patient care or even patient harm; they can also alienate physicians. Guidelines must accurately assess the resources required to provide care for particular patients so that underre-

TABLE 3.—A Comparison of Milliman & Robertson, American College of Surgeons, and North Carolina Hospital Length of Stay Sorted in Order of the Difference Between the Milliman & Robertson and the Actual Length of Stay

Operative Procedure	ACS Mean	MR LOS	NC Mean	NC Median	NC Mode	# of NC Patients	MR vs. ACS Mean	MR vs. NC Mean
Esophagectomy	13	5	12.9	12	14	22	−8	−7.9
ORIF femur Fx	6	1	7.4	6	6	4,553	−5	−6.4
MVR	7	4	9.7	9	7	354	−3	−5.7
Radical cystectomy	8.5	5	10.5	10	8	162	−4	−5.5
CABG	5	3	8.3	8	6	10,138	−2	−5.3
Thoracotomy (lung, lobe)	7	3	8.3	7	7	883	−4	−5.3
AVR	5.5	4	9.1	8	6	611	−2	−5.1
Partial colectomy	6	4	9.1	8	7	4,739	−2	−5.1
V-P shunt	2	1	5.3	4	3	159	−1	−4.3
Chole + CBDE	3.5	3	7.1	6	5	508	−1	−4.1
Craniotomy	8	3	7	6	4	2,587	−5	−4
Radical hysterectomy	9	2	5.9	5	4	190	−7	−3.9
Nephrectomy	5	3	6.3	5	5	1,046	−2	−3.3
Mastectomy	2.5	0	2.7	2	2	2,286	−3	−2.7
Small bowel obstruction	7.5	4	6.6	5	3	3,895	−4	−2.6
Appendectomy	5	1	3.5	3	2	3,746	−4	−2.5
Total hip replacement	4.5	3	5.5	5	4	3,584	−2	−2.5
Radical prostatectomy	4	2	4.4	4	4	1,859	−2	−2.4
TURP	3	1	3.4	3	2	2,908	−2	−2.4
Total knee replacement	4.5	3	5.3	5	4	5,942	−2	−2.3
Cervical fusion	4	1	2.9	2	2	1,534	−3	−1.9
Cystocele	2	1	2.8	2	2	865	−1	−1.8
Total hysterectomy	3.5	2	3.5	3	3	10,546	−2	−1.5
Vaginal hysterectomy	3	1	2.2	2	2	7,081	−2	−1.2
ORIF tibial Fx	4	4	4.8	4	2	44	0	−0.8

Abbreviations: ACS, American College of Surgeons, *MR*, Milliman & Robertson; *NC*, North Carolina; *LOS*, length of stay; *ORIF*, open reduction internal fixation; *MVR*, mitral valve replacement; *CABG*, coronary artery bypass graft; *AVR*, aortic valve replacement; *V-P*, ventriculoperitoneal; *CBDE*, common bile duct exploration; *TURP*, transurethral resection of the prostate.

(Courtesy of Rutledge R: An analysis of 25 Milliman & Robertson guidelines for surgery: Data-driven versus consensus-derived clinical practice guidelines. *Ann Surg* 228:579-587, 1998.)

imbursement for services does not lead to patient harm. LOS predicted by the American College of Surgeons survey jibed with those found in North Carolina. Nonetheless, M&R guidelines proposed a lower standard of care than was found in general practice in North Carolina in all cases.

Conclusion.—Managed care guidelines should not be too aggressive, thus providing underreimbursement and perhaps compromising patient care. Many of the M&R guidelines were at variance with those practiced in North Carolina. Rigid application of these guidelines to some patients who need longer hospital stays may be harmful.

► M&R data are for the healthy patient who undergoes an uncomplicated operation and may be discharged at the earliest possible date. Thus, M&R present data to the far left of the bell-shaped distribution curve. The American College of Surgeons and North Carolina hospital data are closer to the mean LOS for the stated procedures. Reimbursement cannot be based on M&R data. If it is, 1 of 2 things will occur: Either the patient will suffer or the health care system will go broke. LOS targets should be a blend of the American College of Surgeons, North Carolina, and M&R data. A realistic LOS target would be embraced by the surgical community just as practice guidelines have been (especially those developed by surgeons).

E.M. Copeland III, M.D.

Increases in US Medication-Error Deaths Between 1983 and 1993

Phillips DP, Christenfeld N, Glynn LM (Univ of California at San Diego, La Jolla)

Lancet 351:643-644, 1998 1–7

Introduction.—With the decrease in inpatient visits and the increase in outpatient visits between 1983 and 1993, quality control of medications is increasingly becoming the responsibility of the patient. That raises the potential for an increasing number of medication errors (MEs), which can result in accidental poisonings from errors by patients or medical personnel. MEs in hospital settings have been investigated, but little information is available on nationwide trends. Death certificates in the United States between 1983 and 1993 were examined for cause of death, race, sex, and inpatient/outpatient status.

Results.—In 1983, 2,876 individuals died from MEs, whereas in 1993, the number of deaths from MEs (n = 7,391) had risen by a significant 2.57-fold (Figure). Undetermined poisonings, which probably include ME poisonings, rose by 2.24-fold during the same period. The fact that outpatient ME deaths rose 8.48 times while inpatient deaths rose 2.37 times indicates a significant relationship between the increase in ME deaths and the shift to outpatient care. In 1983, the proportion of ME deaths was 3.0 times greater for outpatients than for inpatients; in 1993, the proportion of ME deaths was 6.5 times greater for outpatients, an increase that cannot be accounted for by an increased number of prescriptions. The increase in

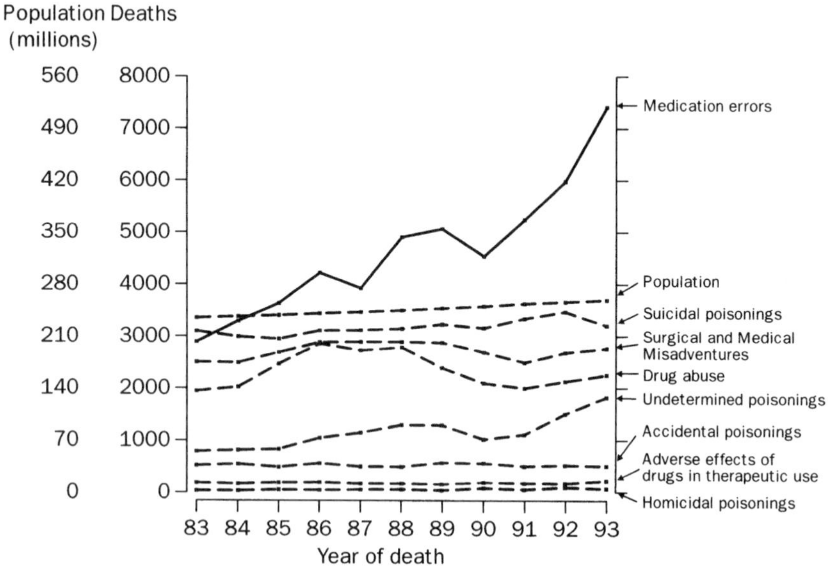

FIGURE.—Trends in U.S. deaths from medication errors and for related causes, 1983-1993. The causes plotted (with their International Classification of Disease Codes) are: medication errors (E850-858); homicidal poisoning (E962); suicidal poisoning (E950); poisonings undetermined whether accidental or purposeful (E980); dependent and nondependent abuse of drugs (304-305); misadventures during medical care (E870-879); accidental poisonings by nonmedicinal substances (E860-866); drugs causing adverse effects in therapeutic use (E930-949—this contains deaths from the correct drug properly administered and explicitly excludes deaths for errors by patients or medical personnel). (Courtesy of Phillips DP, Christenfeld N, Glynn LM: Increases in US medication-error deaths between 1983 and 1993. *Lancet* 351:643-644. Copyright 1998, The Lancet Ltd.)

ME deaths varied by drug category but was largest for opiate and "unspecified" drugs (Table). The largest increase was seen in black males (5.23-fold), followed by white males (2.80-fold), black females (2.27-fold), and white females (1.53-fold).

TABLE

	1983	1993	Ratio
Analgesics, antipyretics, and antirheumatics	851	2098	2·47
Barbiturates	75	18	0·24
Other sedatives and hypnotics	43	17	0·40
Tranquillisers	95	65	0·68
Other psychotropics	156	315	2·02
Other central and autonomic nervous system drugs	289	1184	4·10
Antibiotics	56	43	0·77
Anti-infectives	9	9	1·00
Other drugs	1302	3642	2·80

(Courtesy of Phillips DP, Christenfeld N, Glynn LM: Increases in US medication-error deaths between 1983 and 1993. *Lancet* 351:643-644. Copyright 1998, The Lancet Ltd.)

Conclusions.—The increase in ME deaths suggests that increased vigilance by medical personnel of the delivery and monitoring of prescription drugs is important, particularly for outpatients.

▶ As health care entities (e.g., hospitals, HMOs) keep "score" of patients' length of stay in hospitals and "grade" physicians accordingly, earlier discharge from the hospital and an increased hesitancy by some physicians to admit patients will continue. Because this "grade" may determine financial remuneration from a contractor or employer, length of stay may continue to decline. If a decrease in length of stay is, in fact, correlated with MEs and misdiagnoses, then each will continue to escalate and the welfare of the public will deteriorate. Such a situation will eventually become intolerable to the public, who will begin to reform the system by their ability to vote for legislators who will curb "organized" medicine.

E.M. Copeland III, M.D.

Incidence of Adverse Drug Reactions in Hospitalized Patients: A Meta-analysis of Prospective Studies

Lazarou J, Pomeranz BH, Corey PN (Univ of Toronto)
JAMA 279:1200-1205, 1998 1–8

Introduction.—Now that a recent bill passed by the U.S. Senate requires pharmaceutical companies to provide adverse drug reaction (ADR) information to consumers, public attention is focused on ADRs. A meta-analysis of prospective studies, from which ADR incidences were obtained, was conducted. Serious and fatal ADRs were evaluated, because they represent the greatest impact of drug therapy.

Methods.—Thirty-nine prospective studies of ADRs were conducted over 32 years, and these studies were included in the meta-analysis. The incidence of ADRs occurring in the hospital and the incidence of ADRs causing admission to hospital were combined to obtain the overall incidence of ADRs in hospitalized patients. Errors in drug administration, overdose, noncompliance, therapeutic failures, drug abuse, and possible adverse reactions were excluded. Reactions that required hospitalization, were permanently disabling, or resulted in death were defined as serious.

Results.—There was a 6.7% overall incidence of serious ADRs, with a 0.32% incidence of fatal ADRs in hospitalized patients. Serious ADRs were estimated to number 2,216,000 in 1994, with fatal ADRs estimated to number 106,000; making ADRs between the 4th and 6th leading cause of death, ranking below heart disease, cancer, stroke, pulmonary disease, and accidents, and above pneumonia and diabetes.

Conclusion.—There was an extremely high incidence of serious and fatal ADRs in U.S. hospitals. These data suggest that ADRs are clinically important, although these results must be viewed with caution because of heterogeneity among studies and small biases in the samples.

▶ These ADRs were not necessarily medication errors: they were adverse reactions to indicated drugs. The ranking of ADRs as the fourth- to sixth-leading cause of death in the United States is sobering. How many of these ADRs are preventable is, of course, the question. Likewise, was the potential benefit of the drug worth the risk of the ADR? Preventive medicine specialists would be well advised to consider ADRs a major health risk, and to study them accordingly.

E.M. Copeland III, M.D.

Impact of Hospital Volume on Operative Mortality for Major Cancer Surgery

Begg CB, Cramer LD, Hoskins WJ, et al (Mem Sloan-Kettering Cancer Ctr, New York)

JAMA 280:1747-1751, 1998 1–9

Objective.—All U.S. population-based studies using state discharge databases and in-hospital mortality as the end point have found a significantly lower mortality rate in high-volume hospitals. In-hospital mortality data are affected by length of stay. Information about disease severity is limited by the availability and quality of data. Identification of individual patients and time since diagnosis is difficult. Using the Surveillance, Epidemiology, and End Results (SEER)–Medicare linked database allowed the creation of a population-based census of cancer incidence between 1984 and 1993. Postoperative 30-day mortality rates were compared for hospitals with high-volume and low-volume surgical oncology procedures, after adjusting for case mix, in a retrospective cohort study.

Methods.—The SEER database comprises about 10% of the U.S. population, and the Medicare database contains data on 97% of individuals aged 65 years and older. There were 5,013 patients in the SEER Registry who underwent pancreatectomy, esophagectomy, pneumonectomy, liver resection, or pelvic exenteration. Mortality within 30 days, based on hospital volume, was adjusted for age, cancer stage, and co-morbidity.

Results.—Co-morbidity was not related to volume except for pancreatectomy; there the association was significant. Cancer stage and patient age were not related to volume, with the exception of an increased frequency of unstaged cancers in low-volume institutions. High volume significantly decreased mortality for all procedures except pneumonectomy. The effect of volume was particularly evident with esophagectomy; there the mortality rate was 17.3% in low-volume hospitals vs. 3.4% in high-volume hospitals. This difference also held for pancreatectomy in which the rates were 12.9% vs. 5.8%. Case-mix adjustments and other confounding factors did not alter the results. Discharge before death within 30 days did not affect results.

Conclusion.—Thirty-day mortality rates for hospitals with high-volume surgical oncology procedures are significantly lower than for hospitals with low-volume surgical oncology procedures.

▶ The authors have shown, in a Medicare patient population, that hospitals with a high volume of technically challenging oncologic procedures have an improved mortality rate. They make the assumption that a few highly skilled, technically experienced surgeons within the high-volume hospitals do the procedures. What if many surgeons in a high-volume hospital did only 1 procedure each? Then the care provided for the patients in the hospital, not the expertise of the surgeons, would be the reason for the lower mortality. We know from distribution data recently compiled by the American Board of Surgery (unpublished) that the majority of the procedures studied here are done by 10% of the surgeons. Therefore, high-volume hospitals probably do compare with high-volume surgeons, but this direct correlation is missing from this and most studies evaluating the effect of hospital volume on operative mortality.

E.M. Copeland III, M.D.

Competency-based Instruction in Critical Invasive Skills Improves Both Resident Performance and Patient Safety

Martin M, Vashisht B, Frezza E, et al (Staten Island Univ Hosp, NY; State Univ of New York Health Science Ctr, Brooklyn)

Surgery 124:313-317, 1998 1–10

Introduction.—Instruction in invasive skills such as endotracheal intubation, chest-tube insertion, and venous cutdown are included in residency training in surgery. Often one resident teaches these skills to another resident, and faulty habits may be perpetuated. Life-threatening consequences can follow incorrect performance of these invasive skills. A cadaver laboratory approach was used to help residents to achieve mastery.

Methods.—A competency-based approach was used to instruct 8 postgraduate first-year residents in the cadaver laboratory. Each resident had been evaluated before the laboratory. Individual pretesting and hands-on teaching followed group instruction in endotracheal tube insertion, venous cutdown, and chest-tube insertion. The goal was 100% competency. An inability to perform the task correctly or within 120 seconds was considered a failure. An assessment was made of the number of complications produced and of the impact of training on the overall time required for resuscitation for level I trauma patients.

Results.—There were 7 endotracheal tube failures, 5 chest-tube insertion failures, and 7 venous cutdown failures in the prelaboratory section (Table 1). There were no failures in the postlaboratory section. Complications in the prelaboratory testing were 3.3±1.1 in endotracheal tube insertions, 1.9±1.0 in chest-tube insertions, and 3±1.0 in venous cutdowns. There were no complications in the postlaboratory testing. The

TABLE 1.—Pass/Fail Rates Before and After Instruction

	ET Pre	Post Immed	Post 3 wk	CT Pre	Post Immed	Post 3 wk	VC Pre	Post Immed	Post 3 wk
1	F	P	P	F	P	P	F	P	P
2	F	P	P	F	P	P	F	P	P
3	F	P	F	F	P	P	F	P	P
4	F	P	P	P	P	P	F	P	P
5	P	P	P	P	P	P	P	P	P
6	F	P	P	P	P	P	F	P	P
7	F	P	F	F	P	P	F	P	P
8	F	P	P	F	P	P	F	P	P
# Fail	7	0	2	5	0	0	7	0	0
% Fail	88	13	29	63	0	0	88	0	0

Abbreviations: ET, endotracheal tube; *Pre,* before instruction; *Post immed,* immediately after instruction; *Post 3 wk,* 3 weeks after instruction; *CT,* chest tube; *VC,* venous cutdown; *P,* pass; *F,* fail; *Fail,* failures.

(Courtesy of Martin M, Vashisht B, Frezza E, et al: Competency-based instruction in critical invasive skills improves both resident performance and patient safety. *Surgery* 124:313-317, 1998.)

prelaboratory times were 66.5±30.8 seconds in the endotracheal tube insertions, 104±4.1 seconds in the chest-tube insertion, and 116.3±0.7 seconds in the venous cutdowns. The postlaboratory times were 25±7 seconds in endotracheal tube insertions, 65.5±10.7 seconds in the chest-tube insertion, and 81.3±2.5 seconds in the venous cutdowns. For all groups, changes were statistically significant. There was a decrease in time required for initial trauma resuscitation (25 minutes to 10 minutes). At 3-week follow-up, residents performed 20 chest-tube insertions with 1 pneumothorax, 80 endotracheal tube insertions with 2 failures, and 20 venous cutdowns with no complications.

Conclusion.—The competency-based approach resulted in residents' skills improving rapidly. The skills learned in the laboratory with the competency-based approach can be translated to and sustained in the clinical setting. Competency-based instruction produces competent residents who perform skills rapidly and with minimal complications.

▶ I am intrigued by the use of fresh cadavers to teach simple but sometimes difficult technical skills. Medical schools no longer have animal surgery courses and now include little to no laboratory experience that requires animal preparation. The reasons range from cost to animal rights. Medical students thus arrive at the resident level ill prepared for lifesaving technical maneuvers required in multiple different medical specialties. The experimental model, therefore, becomes a human being—in this study, a corpse, but more frequently a patient. Fresh cadavers are not readily available in most medical schools, but manikins could be used to simulate the technical procedures, probably with the same improved results achieved by the use of fresh cadavers.

E.M. Copeland III, M.D.

Confidence in Life-Support Decisions in the Intensive Care Unit: A Survey of Healthcare Workers

Walter SD, for the Canadian Critical Care Trials Group (McMaster Univ, Hamilton, Ont; et al)

Crit Care Med 26:44-49, 1998 1–11

Objective.—Although medical science has provided advanced life-support techniques that can restore health and prolong life, when measures become extreme, life support can be withdrawn. A previously reported survey by the authors demonstrated that there is extreme variability among Canadian health care workers about withdrawal of life support in the same patient care scenarios. Whether this variability is the result of lack of confidence about the right course of action, and resolves when clinicians are confident about their decisions, was explored in a cross-sectional survey of Canadian intensivists, ICU staff, and bedside nurses.

Methods.—The instrument, developed from a literature review and semistructured interviews with ICU physicians and nurses, included item generation, item reduction, and scenario generation. The scenarios included 4 primary variables—patient age, premorbid cognitive function, likelihood of surviving current episode, and likelihood of long-term survival—and 5 fixed factors—socioeconomic status, premorbid physical function, premorbid emotional function, sex, and employment status. In the scenarios, the patient, family, and friends were unable to help with the decision. Respondents could choose from 5 management options: discontinue supportive measures but continue comfort measures; discontinue all supportive measures except mechanical ventilation but continue comfort measures; continue with current management; continue with current management but add more inotropes, change antibiotics, etc., but don't start dialysis; or continue with current aggressive management and plan for dialysis. Respondents reported their level of confidence on a 5-point scale. The pattern of disagreement for highly confident decisions was investigated.

Results.—Participants included 37 of 39 university-affiliated hospitals and 1,361 (76%) ICU workers. Data from 1,306 respondents were used. Respondents were highly confident only 19% to 48% of the time depending on the scenario, and were more likely to be highly confident when they chose extremes. When full aggressive therapy was selected, 36% were highly confident of their decision. Similarly, when comfort only was chosen, 48% were highly confident. By contrast, intermediate levels of care were selected highly confidently only 29%, 20%, and 19% of the time. Intensivists were very confident 40% of the time, nurses 29% of the time, and house staff 23% of the time. Intensivists were least aggressive in their care choices, and ICU house staff were most aggressive. Whereas high confidence levels were associated with extremes of care, there was considerable disagreement among health care workers even when they were highly confident.

Conclusions.—Health care workers were more confident when selecting extreme care options but frequently made opposite choices. In reality, such decisions are rarely made by individuals. Wishes of family and friends would probably minimize the impact of contradictory physician choices. Nonetheless, physician choices have a significant influence on end-of-life decisions, and physicians need to understand patient preferences.

► In this study, the ethical, family structure, and hospital resource issues necessary to make life-support decisions have been eliminated as variables in the clinical scenarios presented to the health care workers. Responses were widely divergent when only clinical parameters were presented. Medicine remains both an art and a science. Clinical pathways for management are important, but "humanism" remains an important ingredient in the art of medicine.

E.M. Copeland III, M.D.

The Preoperative Bleeding Time Test Lacks Clinical Benefit: College of American Pathologists' and American Society of Clinical Pathologists' Position Article

Peterson P, Hayes TE, Arkin CF, et al (Cornell Univ, New York; Maine Med Ctr, Portland; Univ of Vermont, Burlington; et al)

Arch Surg 133:134-139, 1998 1–12

Background.—Prolonged bleeding time is indicative of platelet disorders or abnormalities of vascular wall integrity. The mechanism of formation of a platelet plug is not well understood. Although bleeding time is one of the most widely used tests of hemostasis, it is not a reliable estimate of platelet count because the relationship between the two is variable, and it should not be used to predict risk of hemorrhage. Studies have found no relationship between preoperative bleeding time and blood loss during cardiopulmonary surgery. Bleeding time is not able to detect patients who have taken aspirin, a drug that is known to interfere with platelet function and to increase blood loss in open-heart surgery, hip surgery, childbirth, and gastrointestinal bleeding. The correlation between bleeding and prolongation of the bleeding time in patients taking aspirin is poor. Furthermore, bleeding time does not appear to predict increased blood loss in these patients during hip surgery.

Conclusions.—Absent a history of a bleeding disorder, bleeding time is not a predictor of risk of hemorrhage during surgery, and a normal bleeding time does not preclude excessive hemorrhage. Bleeding times cannot identify patients who have taken aspirin or nonsteroidal anti-inflammatory drugs. A detailed and complete clinical history, rather than a bleeding time, is the best way to detect a possible bleeding problem.

► I will admit to ordering an occasional bleeding time test in a patient who is ingesting aspirin or nonsteroidals. I have also had an occasional patient who has had excessive bleeding at the time of operation secondary to the ingestion of these compounds. As I recall, most of these patients had a preoperative positive clinical history such as bleeding into a hepatic adenoma. This article gives me some comfort because aspirin and nonsteroidal medication ingestion is almost ubiquitous. Nevertheless, the article emphasizes the importance of a careful history to detect a potential bleeding disorder preoperatively.

E.M. Copeland III, M.D.

A Clinical Trial of Vena Caval Filters in the Prevention of Pulmonary Embolism in Patients With Proximal Deep-Vein Thrombosis

Decousus H, for the Prévention du Risque d'Embolie Pulmonaire par Interruption Cave Study Group (Bellevue Hosp, Saint-Etienne, France; et al)

N Engl J Med 338:409-415, 1998 1–13

Background.—The safety and efficacy of vena caval filters in preventing pulmonary embolism in patients with proximal deep-vein thrombosis have not been definitively established. These issues were further investigated.

Methods.—In a 2-by-2 factorial design, 400 patients with proximal deep-vein thrombosis at risk for pulmonary embolism were randomly assigned to receive a vena caval filter or no filter and to receive low–molecular weight heparin or unfractionated heparin. On day 12 and at 2 years, the rates of recurrent venous thromboembolism, death, and major bleeding were determined.

Findings.—By day 12, symptomatic or asymptomatic pulmonary embolism had occurred in 1.1% of the patients with filters and in 4.8% of those with no filters. By 2 years, 20.8% and 11.6%, respectively, had had recurrent deep-vein thrombosis. Mortality and other outcomes did not differ significantly between groups. By day 12, 1.6% of the patients receiving low–molecular weight heparin and 4.2% given unfractionated heparin had had symptomatic or asymptomatic pulmonary embolism.

Conclusions.—The initial benefits of vena caval filter use for preventing pulmonary embolism in high-risk patients with proximal deep-vein thrombosis are counterbalanced by an excess of recurrent deep-vein thrombosis, with no difference in mortality. Low–molecular weight heparin is as safe and effective as unfractionated heparin for preventing pulmonary embolism.

▶ This important study demonstrates that the immediate beneficial effect of vena caval filters is counteracted by an increase in long-term deep venous thrombosis. Although these results might have been anticipated, they were confirmed in a randomized trial, very tightly controlled, for the detection of pulmonary emboli. Yes, vena caval filters may be lifesaving acutely, but they should only be used with the knowledge of the long-term complications to which the patient will be exposed.

E.M. Copeland III, M.D.

Enoxaparin Plus Compression Stockings Compared With Compression Stockings Alone in the Prevention of Venous Thromboembolism After Elective Neurosurgery

Agnelli G, Piovella F, Buoncristiani P, et al (Università di Perugia, Italy; Università di Pavia, Italy; Ospedale Galliera, Genoa, Italy; et al)
N Engl J Med 339:80-85, 1998 1–14

Objective.—The efficacy and safety of compression stockings alone were compared with compression stockings plus the low–molecular weight heparin enoxaparin for prevention of venous thromboembolism in patients undergoing neurosurgery in a multicenter, randomized, double-blind trial.

Methods.—Either enoxaparin (40 mg) (n = 153) or placebo (n = 154) was administered subcutaneously once daily to 307 patients for at least 7 days after neurosurgery. Patients were assessed daily in the hospital and followed up by telephone or hospital visits for 60 days after surgery. Venous thromboembolism, bleeding, and death were recorded. The end point was symptomatic, venous thromboembolism or deep-vein thrombosis.

Results.—Clinically overt thromboembolic events occurred in 9 patients who were taking placebo (6%) and 1 patient who was taking enoxaparin (1%). Four patients in each group had major bleeding events. Thrombocytopenia developed in 1 patient receiving placebo and 2 patients receiving enoxaparin. Enoxaparin and compression stockings reduced the venous thromboembolism rate to 17% from 33%. The 17% venous thromboembolism rate was probably due to thrombogenic stimuli resulting from brain or spinal tumors present in 97% of the patients and to the delay between surgery and the onset of prophylaxis. Whereas beginning prophylaxis before surgery or increasing the dose might decrease the thromboembolism rate, it would also probably increase bleeding side effects. The relative safety and efficacy of enoxaparin and unfractionated heparin have not been compared in a clinical trial. No thromboembolic events were detected at follow-up, probably because most late-developing thrombi probably become symptomatic only after discharge, raising the issue of optimum duration of prophylaxis. Whereas patients in this study underwent venography before discharge, most patients do not.

Conclusion.—Enoxaparin and compression stockings reduced the venous thromboembolism rate to 17% from 33%.

► This is an important study for two reasons. One, it justifies the use of both compression stockings and an anticoagulant to prevent thromboembolism postoperatively (thereby satisfying Resource Utilization Committees). Two, it demonstrates that, even when begun postoperatively, anticoagulation effectively reduces thromboembolic events. I use low-dose heparin preoperatively, but occasionally patients fail to receive it. In such patients, I will begin administration of low-dose heparin intraoperatively or postoperatively, now that there is more scientific evidence to justify its use under these circumstances.

E.M. Copeland III, M.D.

Effect of Computed Tomography of the Appendix on Treatment of Patients and Use of Hospital Resources

Rao PM, Rhea JT, Novelline RA, et al (Massachusetts Gen Hosp, Boston)
N Engl J Med 338:141-146, 1998 1–15

Objective.—Approximately half of the patients hospitalized for suspected appendicitis ultimately have some other condition diagnosed. About 20% of appendicitis cases are missed, and 15% to 40% of patients undergo appendectomies unnecessarily. The accuracy of CT in helping diagnose or rule out appendicitis was evaluated.

Methods.—Appendiceal CT was performed on 100 consecutive patients (43 male), aged 6 to 75 years, admitted for suspected appendicitis. The CT results were compared with surgical findings, and final results were evaluated by clinical follow-up at 2 months in 41 patients. Treatment plans before CT were compared with actual treatment after CT. Utilization of hospital resources was analyzed retrospectively.

Results.—At surgery for appendicitis or other conditions, 53 patients had appendicitis and 47 did not. The CT results were positive in 53 patients, negative in 45, false positive in 1, and false negative in 1, yielding a sensitivity, specificity, positive predictive value, negative predictive value, and an overall accuracy rate of 98%. The CT results changed treatment strategies for 59 patients, including prevention of unnecessary appendectomy in 13, admission for observation in 18, admission for observation before appendectomy in 21, and admission for observation before diagnosis by CT of other medical conditions in 11. Prevention of unnecessary appendectomy in 13 patients resulted in a savings of $47,281 in surgical and allied costs and in a savings of 50 hospitalization days ($20,250). After deducting the cost of 100 CT scans ($22,800), the resulting savings per patient was $447.

Conclusions.—Routine appendiceal CT in patients with suspected appendicitis decreases unnecessary surgery and reduces the use of hospital resources, resulting in a $447 per patient savings.

▶ In the hands of radiologists at the Massachusetts General Hospital, appendiceal CT may be 98% accurate. I would, however, hesitate to recommend this diagnostic test to replace changes in physical examination findings over time (as is obtained by 24-hour observation) as a nationwide gold standard. Reports such as this from experts in a medical teaching institution are too often extrapolated to community hospitals where the same level of expertise and technology do not always exist.

E.M. Copeland III, M.D.

2 Critical Care

Introduction

The first article chosen for this chapter addresses the question "Has the mortality of septic shock significantly improved with time?" Unfortunately, the answer is a sobering no. On the other hand, the prospective study by Schröder (Abstract 2–2) documents that the prognosis of sepsis is better in women than men, confirming animal studies indicating that gender differences can effect survival. Additionally, there is a body of emerging data based on prospective randomized trials that steroids might have a place in the treatment of the ICU patient. Two such studies (Abstract 2–3 and 2–4) were chosen. One documents that the institution of a prolonged course of low-dose steroids improves survival in patients who develop pressor-resistant septic shock, and the other indicates that the administration of steroids improves survival in patients with unresolving acute respiratory distress syndrome (ARDS). What these 2 studies have in common is that the steroids are given for prolonged periods of time and are used therapeutically only in patients failing conventional therapy. Another approach getting increased attention is the use of the aerosolized route for drug administration. Three studies (Abstracts 2–5 to 2–7) illustrating the spectrum of the approach were chosen. These include a phase II clinical trial of nitric oxide and a phase I trial of prostaglandin E_1 in patients with ARDS as well as a study testing the efficacy of aerosolized antibiotics in patients with ventilator-associated pneumonia. The nitric oxide study was chosen to illustrate how the authors' biases can lead to a positive clinical spin of a negative study.

Did you know that approximately 5% (150,000) of the 3 million short-term unimpregnated central venous catheters implanted each year lead to bloodstream infections with an associated mortality rate in excess of 10%? Well, the pharmaceutical industry sure did. The net result comprises 2 competing brands of antibiotic-impregnated central line catheters, which are promoted as being effective in reducing line sepsis. Are these catheters like Pepsi and Coke and should we just take a taste test and use whichever one we like best, or is there an advantage to one over the other? Based on a prospective randomized multi-institutional clinical trial, it appears that the colonization and infection rate is lower in the catheters impregnated with minocycline and rifampin than in those impregnated with chlorhexidine and silver sulfadiazine (Abstract 2–8). A number of other articles also were chosen because of their direct clinical relevance.

The first of these (Abstract 2–9) is a set of practice parameters for evaluating a new-onset fever in ICU patients that was generated from a consensus conference supported by several societies. The second (Abstract 2–10) deals with the topic of unplanned extubation and provides criteria to be used in considering which of these patients should be immediately reintubated. Another article (Abstract 2–11) illustrates the important, practical, and clinically relevant physiologic principle that the blood pressure recorded from radial artery lines can be falsely low in patients receiving vasopressor agents.

A series of articles dealing with nutrition or the gut were chosen because of the importance of enteral nutrition in the critically ill. The first of these articles (Abstract 2–12) describes the results of a randomized trial of immune-enhancing vs. standard enteral nutritional support, and the second study (Abstract 2–13) attempts to define the optimal protein requirements needed during the first 2 weeks of a critical illness. Taken together, these articles indicate that patients should receive about 1.2 to 1.5g of protein/kg per day and that the use of an immune-enhancing enteral formula will reduce ventilator days and the length of the ICU stay, although it does not improve survival. Additionally, based on an experimental study in endotoxin-challenged dogs, it appears that enteral feeding reverses sepsis-induced splanchnic ischemic and thus enteral feeding may exert beneficial effects on both the liver and the intestine during septic episodes (Abstract 2–14).

As in years past, I have included an article (Abstract 2–16) documenting that the right ventricular end-diastolic volume Swan Ganz catheter (RVEDVI) provides more accurate information than conventional catheters in a number of clinical situations. This year's study focuses on patients with respiratory failure. Another article of importance (Abstract 2–18) deals with the strategy of treating stored blood with a chemical (in this case phosphoenolpyruvate) so that the ability of the previously stored blood to release oxygen at the tissue levels is improved after the blood is transfused. This approach has significant clinical potential because oxygen release from stored blood is impaired.

Assessment of quality of life is an important variable in deciding whether to admit a patient to the ICU; it is also a factor in decision making once the patient is the ICU. Since many ICU patients cannot provide quality-of-life information, family members assume this responsibility. Based on a study (Abstract 2–19) of the reliability of next-of-kin decision making, it appears family members are good but not perfect proxies when it comes to estimating the patient's wishes related to quality-of-life issues. Another well-recognized quality-of-life issue is the use of adequate doses of narcotics and sedatives to achieve comfort and pain control. However, what is not recognized is the relatively high frequency of withdrawal symptoms that develop in these patients as narcotics and sedatives are withdrawn. Thus, the last article in this chapter (Abstract 2–20) deals with this important topic.

Edwin A. Deitch, M.D.

Has the Mortality of Septic Shock Changed With Time?

Friedman G, Silva E, Vincent J-L (Free Univ of Brussels, Belgium)

Crit Care Med 26:2078-2086, 1998 2–1

Purpose.—As survival of critically ill patients increases, so does the incidence of septic shock. It is unclear, however, whether advances in monitoring and therapy have improved mortality rates. A 40-year literature review was conducted to evaluate changes in the mortality rate of septic shock over time.

Methods and Findings.—The investigators analyzed 131 studies of mortality from septic shock published from 1958 to 1997. The studies included a total of 10,694 patients. The mean age of 57 years did not significantly change over time. The mortality rate was 50% overall, with a significant trend to reduced mortality with time. The mortality rate was 52% for patients with bacteremia as an entry criterion, compared with 49% for those without definite bacteremia. During the period studied, the number of chest-related infections increased while the number of gram-negative infections decreased. From 1958 to 1979, gram-positive and all other organisms accounted for just 10% of all cases of sepsis, including mixed infections. From 1980 to 1997, these organisms accounted for 31% of all infections.

Conclusions.—Published reports suggest that mortality from septic shock has decreased over the past 4 decades. The ability to draw conclusions is limited by the heterogeneous nature of the studies analyzed and the absence of severity scores in most cases. Other changes in the epidemiology of septic shock are documented as well, including an increased prevalence of gram-positive sepsis and of chest-related sepsis. These factors may serve to limit improvements in survival.

▶ In light of the numerous advancements in the care of the critically ill and the development of new therapies over the last 2 decades, it appears wise to take stock of how we are doing. When the therapeutic outcome "stats" of treating septic shock are critically evaluated, it appears that we are not doing all that well. Mortality has been minimally reduced. This sobering message is important and highlights that we have a long way yet to go in the treatment of patients with septic shock.

E.A. Deitch, M.D.

Gender Differences in Human Sepsis

Schröder J, Kahlke V, Staubach K-H, et al (Univ of Kiel, Germany; Univ of Lübeck, Germany; Ctr of Research, Borstel, Germany, et al)

Arch Surg 133:1200-1205, 1998 2–2

Introduction.—The prognosis of sepsis has changed little in recent years. Why some patients recover uneventfully while others progress to multiple-organ dysfunction and death is not known. Animal studies have found hormonal and immunologic differences between the sexes, associated with increased susceptibility to sepsis among males. Sex differences in human sepsis patients—including the influence of sex hormones and proinflammatory and anti-inflammatory mediators—were prospectively assessed.

Methods.—Fifty-two ICU patients with surgical sepsis were included in the study. Thirty-three patients were men and 19 were women (mean age, 53 and 55 years, respectively). The 2 groups were similar in cause and severity of sepsis. The mean Acute Physiology and Chronic Health Evaluation II score was 18.5 for men and 17.3 for women; multiple-organ dysfunction score was 10.8 and 9.9, respectively. At intervals from day 1 to day 14 after the diagnosis of sepsis, the patients underwent measurement of tumor necrosis factor-α, interleukin (IL)-6 bioactivity, IL-10 level (by enzyme-linked immunosorbent assay), total testosterone level, and 17β-estradiol (by radioimmunoassay). Clinical course and survival were compared between the sexes, along with hormone and cytokine levels.

Findings.—The outcomes of sepsis were significantly better for women than for men, despite the lack of any difference in multiple organ dysfunction score over time. Seventy percent of men died in the hospital, compared with 26% of women. For men, tumor necrosis factor-α bioactivity increased continuously after diagnosis; the difference between men and women became significant on day 10. There was no sex difference in IL-6 bioactivity. From days 1 to 10, women had higher IL-10 levels than men; the difference was significant on days 3 and 5. The men had subnormal total testosterone levels. At diagnosis, both sexes had elevated estradiol levels, with women having higher levels than men.

Conclusions.—Consistent with the results of animal studies, sepsis appears to have a better prognosis in women than in men. The survival advantage of women may be related to their higher levels of anti-inflammatory mediators, such as IL-10. The relative proportions of proinflammatory and anti-inflammatory mediators may be an important therapeutic target.

▶ Questions related to why some people die while others live after sustaining similar insults have led investigators to look at genetic and, most recently, gender-related variables. This prospective study documenting that females survive sepsis better than males validates recent animal experimental studies and previously published retrospective clinical studies. Although the mechanisms accounting for why females have enhanced survival remain cloudy, the observation is very important, especially in light of animal studies indicating that testosterone antagonists are beneficial in models of peritonitis. I personally find this topic fascinating and believe that further studies investigating the underlying mechanisms of this phenomenon will provide insights that will pay tremendous clinical dividends.

E.A. Deitch, M.D.

Reversal of Late Septic Shock With Supraphysiologic Doses of Hydrocortisone

Bollaert P-E, Charpentier C, Levy B, et al (Centre Hospitalier Universitaire, Nancy, France)

Crit Care Med 26:645-650, 1998 2–3

Objective.—Even with aggressive treatment, septic shock in the ICU carries a mortality of greater than 50%. There is evidence that low-dose corticosteroids can lead to rapid hemodynamic improvement for patients with late septic shock receiving catecholamine treatment. The effects of late hydrocortisone therapy in this group of patients were assessed in a randomized trial.

Methods.—Forty-one patients with septic shock who required more than 48 hours of catecholamine therapy were entered into the trial. They were randomized to receive 100 mg of IV hydrocortisone 3 times daily for 5 days or placebo. The effects of hydrocortisone on reversal of shock—defined as stabilization of systolic arterial pressure about 90 mm Hg for 24 hours or longer without catecholamine or fluid infusion—were assessed. The hemodynamic and survival effects were analyzed as well.

Results.—Shock was reversed within 7 days in 68% of the hydrocortisone group vs. 21% of the placebo group. There were no significant differences in hemodynamics, as assessed by serial invasive measurements during a 5-day period. The patients receiving hydrocortisone treatment showed significantly greater reversal of shock at 28 days' follow-up (Fig 2). At this time, mortality was 32% with hydrocortisone vs. 63% with placebo, and survival was significantly more likely for patients having reversal of shock within 7 days after the start of corticosteroid treatment. The results of a short corticotropin test were not significantly associated with outcome. The 2 groups were similar in their rates of gastrointestinal bleeding and secondary infection.

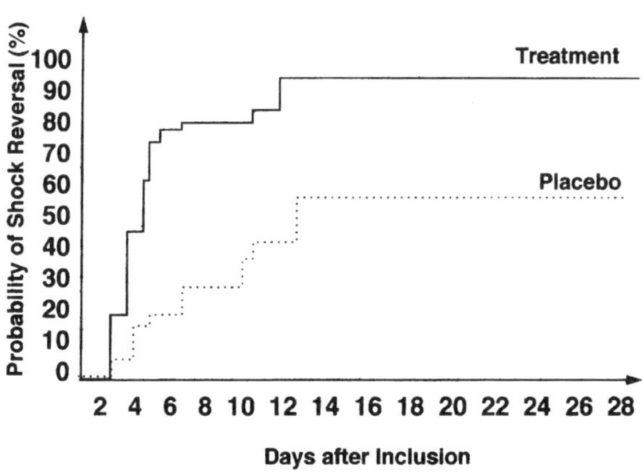

FIGURE 2.—Kaplan-Meier estimates of 28-day reversal of shock. (Courtesy of Bollaert P-E, Charpentier C, Levy B, et al: Reversal of late septic shock with supraphysiologic doses of hydrocortisone. *Crit Care Med* 26:645-650, 1998.)

Conclusions.—For patients in the ICU with pressor-dependent septic shock, moderate doses of hydrocortisone can increase the rate of shock reversal and, perhaps, survival. The benefits of hydrocortisone treatment may be more related to interactions between catecholamine treatment and adrenergic receptor regulation than to any specific effect on the course of sepsis. More research is needed to define the mechanism of this benefit, the optimal treatment period, and the true effect on survival.

▶ Steroids for the treatment of septic shock, or déjà vu all over again again. Perhaps not. This study is different in several important ways from previous multicenter studies that indicated steroid administration does not improve outcome in patients with septic shock. These differences in study design and patient enrollment seem to explain why this study showed steroids are beneficial, in contrast to previous studies and even conventional wisdom.

Bollaert et al., in this blinded prospective randomized trial, enrolled only patients in septic shock who were on pressor agents for 48 hours or longer, in contrast to previous studies that enrolled patients much earlier after the onset of shock. Secondly, the patients were treated for a much longer period with full-dose steroids (a minimum of 5 days) than patients in previous studies (2 days). Lastly, the steroids were not just stopped in the current study, but were tapered over 6 days. Thus, the patients enrolled in this study had refractory septic shock and were treated for prolonged periods, using resolution of shock as an end point.

Considering the study design, recent information on the biology of sepsis, and the effects of sepsis on steroids and of steroids on inflammatory factors, I am inclined to believe the results of this study. I am also becoming convinced that there is a clinically relevant difference between the early use of a short course of steroids (in previous studies) and the later use of a more prolonged course of steroids. Thus, I will be using this steroid strategy in my patients with refractory septic shock who fit the criteria outlined in this article. For those of you who desire a more in-depth review of the biology and rationale behind this late streoid approach, I recommend the editorial by Meduri et al.[1]

E.A. Deitch, M.D.

Reference

1. Meduri GU, Kanangat S: Glucocorticoid treatment of sepsis and acute respiratory distress syndrome: Time for a critical reappraisal. *Crit Care Med* 26:630-633, 1998.

Effect of Prolonged Methylprednisolone Therapy in Unresolving Acute Respiratory Distress Syndrome: A Randomized Controlled Trial

Meduri GU, Headley AS, Golden E, et al (Univ of Tennessee, Memphis, Baptist Mem Hosp, Memphis, Tenn; Veterans Affairs Med Ctr, Memphis, Tenn)

JAMA 280:159-165, 1998 2–4

Background.—To date, no pharmacologic therapy has been effective in modifying the clinical course of acute respiratory distress syndrome (ARDS). The mortality rate remains higher than 50%. The value of prolonged methylprednisolone treatment in patients with unresolving ARDS was studied.

Methods.—Twenty-four patients with severe ARDS were enrolled in the randomized, double-blind, placebo-controlled trial. In all patients, the lung injury score (LIS) had failed to improve by the seventh day of respiratory failure. Sixteen patients were given methylprednisolone at an initial daily dose of 2 mg/kg. The remaining 8 patients were given placebo. Treatment duration was 32 days. Four patients with LISs that did not improve by at least 1 point after 10 days of treatment were crossed over (blindly) to the alternative group.

Findings.—By treatment day 10, methylprednisolone recipients had reduced LISs, an improved ratio of PaO_2 to FIO_2, reduced multiple-organ dysfunction syndrome (MODS) scores, and successful extubation compared with placebo recipients. The ICU mortality rate was 0 in the methylprednisolone group and 62% in the placebo group. Hospital-associated mortality rates were 12% and 62%, respectively. The 2 groups had similar rates of infection per day of treatment. Pneumonia was commonly detected in the absence of fever.

Conclusions.—Prolonged methylprednisolone therapy in patients with unresolving ARDS improves LIS and MODS scores. Mortality is also significantly reduced. Timing of methylprednisolone administration affected treatment response. Few clinically important complications were associated with methylprednisolone.

► As stated by the authors, no pharmacologic therapeutic protocol has reduced the mortality rate of ARDS, including numerous *short-course* trials of high-dose methylprednisolone. Why are these authors' results different? The major reason, according to the authors, is that they have used a *prolonged* 32-day methylprednisolone regimen, where the patients receive 2 mg/kg/day for the first 2 weeks, which is tapered down over the next 18 days.

Although the number of patients studied is relatively small, the results are provocative and fit with an enlarging body of experimental information indicating that when a short course of steroids is stopped in models of acute lung injury, their protective effect is rapidly lost. Thus, the authors' finding that prolonged steroid therapy is beneficial fits the experimental data. Why might this be so? One potential answer lies with the fact that ARDS progresses from an early inflammatory disease to one in which progressive collagen deposition and alveolar fibrosis occur. The prolonged use of steroids appears to limit or prevent the fibrosing alveolitis typically observed in patients with prolonged ARDS. My impression, from a handful of patients treated with steroids for intractable ARDS, is that this regimen is likely to have significant clinical benefit. But, prolonged steroid therapy is not for every patient with ARDS. If used, it should be limited to the patient population described by the authors. That is, patients who have not responded to 7 to 10 days of conventional therapy and who do not have evidence of uncontrolled infection. I hope that this promising therapy will be tested and verified in further studies. Until then, when your back is against the wall and the patient fits the clinical description of the patients in this study, it might be reasonable to give steroids a try.

E.A. Deitch, M.D.

Effects of Inhaled Nitric Oxide in Patients With Acute Respiratory Distress Syndrome: Results of a Randomized Phase II Trial

Dellinger RP, and the Inhaled Nitric Oxide in ARDS Study Group (Univ of Missouri, Columbia; Baylor College of Medicine, Houston; St John's Mercy Med Ctr, St Louis)

Crit Care Med 26:15-23, 1998 2–5

Background.—Because of its short half-life and its potency as a mediator of smooth muscle relaxation, nitric oxide (NO) given by inhalation would be expected to produce vasodilation in well-aerated areas of the lung without systemic hemodynamic side effects. This vasodilatory effect in pulmonary vessels would be expected to increase blood flow to well-ventilated areas of the lung while shunting blood away from poorly ventilated areas. A randomized trial assessed the safety and physiologic effects of inhaled NO in patients with acute respiratory distress syndrome (ARDS), including the effects of various doses on clinical outcome parameters.

Methods.—The 14-month study included 177 patients with ARDS, as defined by the American-European Consensus Conference, at 30 U.S. hospitals. Within 72 hours of disease onset, all patients were randomized in double-blind fashion to receive inhaled NO, 1.25, 5.0, 20.0, 40.0, or 80.0 ppm, or nitrogen gas as a placebo. The effects of NO on PaO_2, mean pulmonary arterial pressure, mechanical ventilation parameters, and oxygenation index were assessed. The clinical effects of the various doses of NO, including mortality, number of days surviving without mechanical ventilation, and number of days surviving after meeting defined oxygenation criteria for extubation, were analyzed. A 20% or greater increase in PaO_2 was the study definition of an acute response to treatment.

Results.—Sixty percent of patients treated with inhaled NO had an acute response to treatment, regardless of the concentration given. An acute response was also noted in 24% of the placebo group. The NO and placebo groups were similar in terms of mortality and number of days alive and off mechanical ventilation or after meeting criteria for extubation.

Conclusions.—Inhaled NO is well tolerated by patients with ARDS. It has a clear effect on oxygenation in these patients, although a similar effect is noted in a substantial minority of patients receiving placebo. Larger trials are recommended to see whether the acute physiologic improvements noted in this study will translate into improved clinical outcomes.

► Is the answer "yes" or "no?" Does inhaled NO improve clinical outcome in patients with ARDS? According to the results of this study, to me the answer is a clear "no," although the authors' comments would lead one to believe the opposite. Why is it that the authors' data and clinical spin are not in synchrony? The answer is simple: The authors are advocates of NO and their intrinsic bias leads them to look at the glass as half-full rather than half-empty. This article illustrates the importance of looking at the data and not just at the authors' interpretation of their data. In the field of sepsis research, post hoc identification of subgroups that benefit from therapy has been common. Examples include antiendotoxin antibodies, cytokine antagonists, anticytokine antibodies, and even steroids. We all know how the story ended for these putative magic bullets. It seems to me that inhaled NO is fast joining the pantheon of failed therapeutic agents.

E.A. Deitch, M.D.

Inhaled Prostaglandin E_1 for Treatment of Acute Lung Injury in Severe Multiple Organ Failure

Meyer J, Theilmeier G, Van Aken H, et al (Westfälische Wilhelms-Universität, Münster, Germany)

Anesth Analg 86:753-758, 1998 2–6

Introduction.—Patients with acute lung injury have hypoxemia resulting from a mismatch between pulmonary ventilation and perfusion. The vasodilator prostaglandin E_1 (PGE_1) has a high pulmonary clearance; administered IV, it may be of value in the treatment of acute lung injury. Nitric oxide and prostacyclin inhalation can improve oxygenation through specific dilation of the pulmonary vasculature in ventilated areas of the lung. This study evaluated the results of PGE_1 inhalation therapy in patients with acute lung injury.

Methods.—The study included 15 patients meeting criteria for acute lung injury, i.e., partial pressure of arterial oxygen (PaO_2)/fraction of inspired oxygen (FIO_2) of less than 160 mm Hg. In addition to standard therapy in the ICU, all patients received PGE_1, delivered continuously via pneumatic nebulizer. The patients had a mean Acute Physiology and Chronic Health Evaluation System II score of 33 and a Multiple Organ Failure score of 10.

Results.—The patients underwent PGE_1 inhalation for a mean of 103 hours over 1 to 7 days. The mean dose was 41 µg/hr. During PGE_1

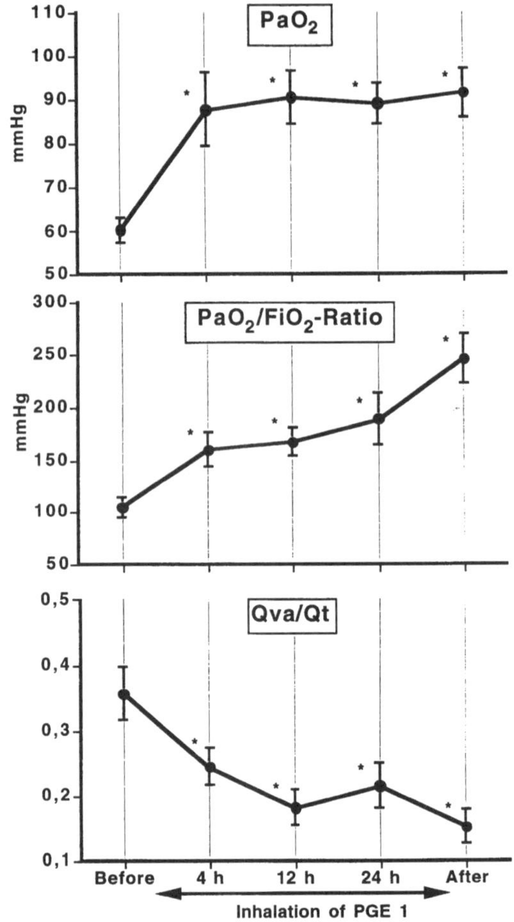

FIGURE 2.—Partial pressure of arterial oxygen (*Pa_{O_2}*), inspiratory oxygen fraction (*Fi_{O_2}*), and venous admixture (*Qva/Qt*) measured before and after prostaglandin E_1 (*PGE_1*) inhalation. *Asterisk* indicates *P* less than 0.05 vs. before PGE_1 inhalation (*n* = 15). (Courtesy of Meyer J, Theilmeier G, Van Aken H, et al: Inhaled prostaglandin E_1 for treatment of acute lung injury in severe multiple organ failure. *Anesth Analg* 86:753-758, 1998.)

inhalation, pulmonary function parameters improved significantly. The ratio of Pa_{O_2}/Fi_{O_2} increased from 105 to 160 mm Hg at 4 hours and 189 mm Hg at 24 hours (Fig 2). Mean pulmonary artery and central venous pressures decreased, but not significantly. There were no changes in mean arterial pressure, pulmonary capillary wedge pressure, cardiac output, or heart rate. Forty percent of the patients died in the ICU.

Conclusion.—Inhaled PGE_1 can improve oxygenation in patients with acute lung injury. It causes no systemic hemodynamic impairments or other adverse effects. A controlled trial is needed to see whether this form of therapy can increase survival.

► The strategy of using localized aerosolized delivery of a therapeutic agent directly into the lungs of patients with acute respiratory distress syndrome to obtain a beneficial pulmonary response, while avoiding potentially adverse systemic drug effects, has been successful with the use of nitric oxide. In this phase I study, the authors have used this strategy, with some success, to test the beneficial effects of the vasodilator PGE_1. The physiologic principle behind the use of inhaled PGE_1 is that limiting delivery of the drug to alveoli that are ventilated will selectively dilate only the pulmonary vasculature that is being ventilated, thereby improving ventilation/perfusion mismatches. Because PGE_1 administered IV would vasodilate essentially the entire pulmonary vasculature, IV PGE_1 would not be as effective in improving oxygenation as inhaled PGE_1.

Although this clinical trial did not assess mortality, it was encouraging that the PaO_2/FIO_2 ratio was improved within hours of the administration of PGE_1 and that this improvement was not lost over time. Another potential advantage of using nebulized PGE_1 is that no specialized equipment is needed. One just puts the drug in the nebulizer and waits for a response.

E.A. Deitch, M.D.

Aerosolized Antibiotics in Mechanically Ventilated Patients: Delivery and Response

Palmer LB, Smaldone GC, Simon SR, et al (State Univ of New York, Stony Brook)

Crit Care Med 26:31-39, 1998 2–7

Introduction.—Topical airway therapy with aerosols is an appealing approach to the treatment of nosocomial pneumonia in mechanically ventilated patients. However, there have been no reports of aerosolized antibiotic treatment directed to the lower airway in mechanically ventilated patients. A human model of gram-negative colonization in mechanically ventilated patients was used in a study of the delivery of aerosolized antibiotics to the lower respiratory tract, as well as the possible clinical responses to these antibiotics.

Methods.—The prospective serial study included 6 ventilator-dependent but medically stable patients with chronic respiratory failure. Each patient was colonized with gram-negative organisms and had a tracheostomy. The colonizing bacilli produced purulent secretions that could be serially sampled. Each patient received a total of nine 14- to 21-day courses of nebulized antibiotic therapy, consisting of gentamicin (80 mg) or amikacin (400 mg) every 8 hours. Each patient served as his or her own control. Radiolabeled aerosols and sputum antibiotic concentrations were used to measure antibiotic doses to the lung. Indicators of response to treatment included changes in the volume of respiratory secretions, culture results, and changes in inflammatory cells and inflammatory mediators in the respiratory secretions.

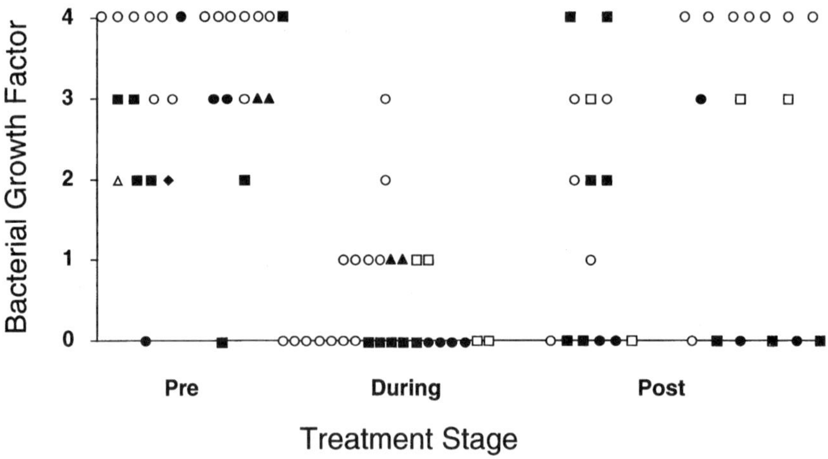

FIGURE 3.—Bacterial growth from tracheal aspirate cultures obtained during the 9 trials of aerosolized antibiotics. Cultures were obtained weekly 2 to 3 weeks before, during, and 2 to 3 weeks after delivery of aerosolized antibiotics. *Open circles*, *Pseudomonas aeruginosa*; *solid circles*, *Proteus mirabilis*; *solid squares*, *Serratia marcescens*; *solid triangles*, *Acinetobacter calcoaceticus*; *open squares*, *Providencia stuartii*; *open triangles*, *Enterobacter aerogenes*; *solid diamond*, *Klebsiella pneumoniae*. The quantity of growth is assessed on a graded scale of 0 to 4. (Courtesy of Palmer LB, Smaldone GC, Simon SR, et al: Aerosolized antibiotics in mechanically ventilated patients: Delivery and response. *Crit Care Med* 26:31-39, 1998.)

Results.—During treatment, the patients inhaled a mean of 35% of the drug initially placed in the nebulizer. In most cases, serum concentrations of antibiotic were unmeasurable. However, the volume of respiratory secretions was reduced significantly with antibiotic treatment. Serial culture studies showed elimination of the colonizing pathogens, including *Pseudomonas* spp., *Serratia marcescens*, and *Enterobacter aerogenes* in most treatment trials (Fig 3). Treatment reduced airway inflammatory mediators, in a way that was significantly related to the volume of respiratory secretions.

Conclusions.—The effective delivery of nebulized antibiotics to mechanically ventilated patients is demonstrated. The findings suggest that aerosolized antibiotic treatment can significantly reduce respiratory secretions and measures of airway inflammation. Further study is needed to determine the efficacy of nebulized aminoglycosides in the treatment of critically ill patients.

▶ The direct delivery of antibiotics to the colonized/infected surfaces of the lung makes a lot of sense. Therefore, this pilot study demonstrating that aerosolized antibiotics can be efficiently delivered to the lung in mechanically ventilated patients was chosen. The basic idea of delivering antibiotics directly into the airways is clinically attractive, since this is where the bacteria are present at highest concentrations. Furthermore, by delivering the antibiotics directly into the lungs, it should be possible to use lower antibiotic doses, thereby potentially reducing the risk of antibiotic-related toxicity. Unfortunately, the downside of this therapy is the potential emergence of antibiotic-resistant organisms. Although this method of antibiotic delivery is not ready for routine clinical use, over the last several years I have personally used aerosolized colistin in the treatment of pneumonia and pneumonitis in patients colonized with multiantibiotic gram-negative bacteria, with reasonably good results. I hope that this novel approach to delivering antibiotics will pan out in future studies.

E.A. Deitch, M.D.

A Comparison of Two Antimicrobial-impregnated Central Venous Catheters

Darouiche RO, for the Catheter Study Group (Baylor College of Medicine and Veterans Affairs Med Ctr, Houston; et al)

N Engl J Med 340:1-8, 1999 2–8

Introduction.—Previous studies have shown that rates of central venous catheter colonization and catheter-related bloodstream infection can be significantly reduced through the use of catheters impregnated with minocycline and rifampin or with chlorhexidine and silver sulfadiazine. However, no studies have directly compared the benefits of the 2 types of catheter. Minocycline/rifampin and chlorhexidine/silver sulfadiazine catheters were compared for their ability to prevent catheter colonization and catheter-related bloodstream infection.

Methods.—The prospective, multicenter trial included adult patients considered at high risk of catheter-related infection who were likely to require a central venous catheter for 3 days or longer. The patients were randomized to receive polyurethane, triple-lumen catheters impregnated with minocycline/rifampin on the luminal and external surfaces or with chlorhexidine/silver sulfadiazine on the external surface only. Catheter tips and subcutaneous segments were cultured by both the roll-plate and sonication methods after removal, with peripheral blood cultures performed as indicated. The analysis included a total of 738 catheters with evaluable culture results.

Results.—The 2 catheter groups were similar in their clinical characteristics and infection risk factors. The catheter colonization rate was 8.3% for minocycline/rifampin–impregnated catheters, compared with 22.8% for chlorhexidine/silver sulfadiazine–impregnated catheters. Catheters impregnated with minocycline and rifampin were also associated with a lower rate of catheter-related bloodstream infection (0.3% vs. 3.4%).

Conclusions.—This randomized trial suggests that anti-infective catheters impregnated with minocycline and rifampin carry a lower risk of colonization and infection than those impregnated with chlorhexidine and silver sulfadiazine. The authors emphasize that antimicrobial-impregnated catheters must complement, rather than replace, adequate aseptic technique.

▶ Central venous catheter–related bacteremia and infection are all too frequent and life-threatening complications in ICU patients in spite of meticulous regimens of catheter care. Consequently, a number of strategies have been tested to reduce this risk. One such strategy is the development of antibiotic-impregnated central venous catheters. The results of this prospective randomized double-blinded study clearly document that minocycline/rifampin–treated catheters have a low colonization and infection rate. In fact, the rate of infection with these catheters is 10- to 40-fold less than that observed with untreated or silver sulfadiazine–treated catheters. When one considers that more than 3 million central venous catheters are placed each year in the United States and about 50,000 patients die of catheter-related infections, the potential clinical benefits of this antibiotic-treated catheter is very significant. Although the minocycline/rifampin–treated catheters are more expensive than untreated catheters, the reduced need to change them as well as the lower infection rate associated with their use makes them a good buy.

E.A. Deitch, M.D.

Practice Parameters for Evaluating New Fever in Critically Ill Adult Patients

O'Grady NP, Barie PS, Bartlett J, et al (NIH, Bethesda, Md; New York Hosp; Johns Hopkins Hosp, Baltimore, Md; et al)

Crit Care Med 26:392-408, 1998 2–9

Background.—A new elevation of temperature in a critically ill patient sometimes leads to a routine set of orders. The orders call for various tests, often including repeated blood tests, that can be time consuming, expensive, and uncomfortable for the patient. Information is needed on how to investigate these fevers in a prudent and cost-effective fashion. Practice parameters for the evaluation of new fevers in ICU patients were developed by a task force of the Society of Critical Care Medicine and the Infectious Disease Society of America.

Methods.—The task force included 13 experts in various disciplines, including critical care medicine, infectious disease, and surgery. The members analyzed the published literature on the topic and classified it according to research design and scientific value. In forming consensus recommendations for clinical practice, the task force considered both the scientific evidence and the experts' opinions. After debate over draft documents, the nominal group process was used to reach a consensus.

Results.—The task force made specific recommendations related to initial fever evaluation, including how body temperature should be measured and the definition of fever for diagnostic purposes, performance of blood cultures, relationship between fever and intravascular catheters, stool evaluation, urinary tract infections, sinusitis, postoperative fever, wound infections, CNS infections, and noninfectious causes of fever. Given the many different causes of fever, both infectious and noninfectious, the task force concluded that the development of new fever in an ICU patient should trigger a careful clinical assessment, rather than an automatic battery of laboratory and radiologic tests. The specific recommendations reflect a cost-conscious approach to culture and radiologic studies, depending on the clinical findings. The recommendations provide for a directed approach to ascertaining the presence of infection so as to avoid additional tests and to consider the treatment options.

Discussion.—The task force's recommendations for the evaluation of new fever in critically ill patients are presented. The recommendations are based on the strength of scientific evidence and the opinions of experts from relevant specialties. The recommendations are intended to provide a starting point for the development of effective and cost-conscious approaches to the management of patient populations seen by intensivists and consultant physicians.

▶ Over the last few years, articles focusing on evidence-based practice patterns have begun to appear. The goal of many of these articles is to address focused areas of controversy or confusion. The current article, which addresses practice patterns for evaluating new fever in ICU patients, is the product of a task force commissioned by the Society of Critical Care Medicine and the Infectious Disease Society of America. It outlines approaches to 6 important and common questions that arise in the care of the ICU patient, including (a) what temperature should elicit laboratory and diagnostic tests, (b) when blood cultures should be obtained, and (c) when IV catheters should be cultured or removed. Because of the nature of the article, it does not lend itself well to summarization or commentary. In spite of this, it was chosen because of the large amount of clinically relevant material that it contains. Nonetheless, my message to you is clear: Read the paper and use it.

E.A. Deitch, M.D.

Unplanned Extubation: Risk Factors of Development and Predictive Criteria for Reintubation

Chevron V, Ménard J-F, Richard J-C, et al (Charles-Nicolle Hosp, Rouen, France)

Crit Care Med 26:1049-1053, 1998 2–10

Background.—Unplanned extubation is a frequent and serious complication of endotracheal intubation. Risk factors for unplanned extubation were investigated, along with the contribution of nursing workload and factors predictive of the need for reintubation.

Findings.—In a 10-month prospective study, unplanned extubation occurred in 40 of 281 intubated and ventilated patients (14%). Thirty-three percent of case patients with unplanned extubation were intubated orally, compared with 15% of controls. Among sedated patients, those with unplanned extubation were more likely to be agitated (60% vs. 19%). Nursing workload was no higher on days with unplanned extubations. Overall, reintubation was necessary in 37% of unplanned extubations. The most important predictive factor for reintubation was a Glasgow Coma Score of less than 11, followed by accidental unplanned extubation and a PaO_2/FIO_2 ratio of less than 200 mm Hg.

Conclusions.—Oral intubation and insufficient sedation place patients at increased risk of unplanned extubation. This complication does not appear to be related to nursing workload, at least on the unit studied. A Glasgow Coma Score of less than 11 is the most important predictive factor of the need for reintubation.

▶ Although about 10% or more of extubations in the ICU are unplanned, surprisingly little information is available identifing the high-risk patient or the circumstances potentially predisposing to this complication. When the potential and actual complications associated with unplanned extubation are considered, this lack of information takes on larger proportions. Thus, the value of this prospective clinical study that evaluated 18 separate variables is apparent. The authors found that 87% of the unplanned extubations were done by the patients, and patient-mediated extubation was associated with oral intubation and patient agitation (translated as inadequate sedation). These results are not surprising to anyone taking care of ICU patients. An agitated, inadequately sedated patient with an uncomfortable endotracheal tube in his throat will attempt to pull it out. In fact, similar risk factors were observed in a second study on unplanned extubations published this year.[1] It makes sense to be sure that agitated patients are adequately sedated, and whenever possible to use nasotracheal rather than orotracheal tubes.

In general, about 60% of patients with unplanned extubations require reintubation. Thus, the second portion of this study provides useful information in predicting which patients who extubate themselves or are accidentally extubated will require reintubation. In this series, patients with either a Glasgow Coma Score of less than 11 or a PaO_2/FIO_2 ratio of less than 200 mm Hg required reintubation.

The take-home message of this study is that particular attention should be paid to orally intubated patients and that agitated patients must receive adequate sedation to control their agitation.

E.A. Deitch, M.D.

Reference

1. Boulain T: Unplanned extubations in the adult intensive care unit: A prospective multicenter study. *Am J Respir Crit Care Med* 157:1131-1137, 1998.

Radial Artery Pressure Monitoring Underestimates Central Arterial Pressure During Vasopressor Therapy in Critically Ill Surgical Patients

Dorman T, Breslow MJ, Lipsett PA, et al (Johns Hopkins Univ, Baltimore, Md)

Crit Care Med 26:1646-1649, 1998 2–11

Introduction.—Direct intra-arterial pressure monitoring is needed for patients with septic shock who are receiving vasopressors. The radial artery is the most common monitoring site; however, radial artery pressure is not necessarily the same as central arterial pressure. Clinical observations suggest that higher arterial pressures are recorded from femoral artery catheters than from radial artery catheters. These measurements were compared in a prospective, observational study of critically ill patients with presumed sepsis.

Methods.—Fourteen patients in a surgical ICU who had a presumed diagnosis of septic shock and were receiving high-dose norepinephrine at a rate of greater than 5 µg/min were included in the study. In keeping with standard practice for hypotensive patients with presumed septic shock, all patients underwent intravascular volume repletion followed by vasopressors, adjusted to achieve a mean arterial pressure of 60 mm Hg or greater. The patients underwent simultaneous intra-arterial measurements of radial and femoral artery blood pressures.

Results.—Comparison of these peripheral and central pressures, respectively, found that the femoral site gave significantly higher systolic (143 vs. 86 mm Hg) and mean arterial pressure (81 vs. 66 mm Hg) values. In response to the higher measured mean arterial pressure values, the norepinephrine infusion rate was immediately reduced in 79% of patients. This dose reduction did not cause any change in cardiac output or pulmonary artery occlusion pressure. Simultaneous radial and femoral artery pressure recordings continued after norepinephrine was discontinued in 2 patients. The results showed no difference in mean arterial pressure measurements.

Conclusions.—In septic, hypotensive patients receiving high-dose vasopressors, radial artery pressure monitoring underestimates central arterial pressure. The resulting excessive vasopressor administration may be avoided by monitoring pressure in the femoral artery instead. Reduced use of vasopressors may improve blood flow to the organs, thus limiting the morbidity attributable to vasopressor therapy.

▶ This simple, practical, and clinically relevant study is based on the physiologic principle that pressures in peripheral arteries, such as the radial artery, can differ significantly from pressures in central arteries, such as the femoral artery. Their observation that radial artery hypotension may occur in the absence of central arterial hypotension is of major clinical importance in septic patients, since radial arterial hypotension may result in the inappropriate use of vasopressors. The take-home message is very clear: in case of doubt, measure the blood pressure in the femoral artery. Perhaps, just as in other aspects of life, when choosing a blood vessel for pressure monitoring in the septic patient on pressor support, bigger is better.

E.A. Deitch, M.D.

A Prospective, Randomized, Double-blind, Controlled Clinical Trial of Enteral Immunonutrition in the Critically Ill

Atkinson S, for the Guy's Hospital Intensive Care Group (Guy's Hosp, London)

Crit Care Med 26:1164-1172, 1998 2–12

Introduction.—It is agreed that the enteral route of nutrition is best for critically ill patients. However, there is continued debate over the advantages of the various enteral nutrition formulas. Impact is a recently introduced enteral immunonutrition (IMN) formula, supplemented with arginine, purine nucleotides, and ω-3 fatty acids, that was developed to enhance immune function in patients at risk of sepsis. The effects of enteral IMN on hospital mortality and length of stay were assessed in critically ill patients.

Methods.—The randomized, controlled trial included a heterogeneous group of 390 critically ill patients. Within 48 hours after ICU admission, the patients were assigned in double-blind fashion to receive the IMN formula Impact or an isocaloric, isonitrogenous formula. All patients were included in an intention-to-treat analysis. Of 369 patients who actually received some enteral nutrition, 101 were classified as having successful "early enteral nutrition." The effects of assigned formula on specified ICU and hospital outcomes were assessed.

Results.—The intention-to-treat analysis found no difference in hospital mortality rate between the 2 groups: 48% in the Impact group vs. 44% in the control formula group. Subgroup analyses also found no significant mortality differences. Acute Physiology and Chronic Health Evaluation II scores were significantly higher in the IMN group: 20.1 vs. 18.7 on intention-to-treat analysis and 20.1 vs. 18.5 among patients who actually received formula. Among patients with successful early enteral nutrition, median duration of mechanical ventilation was 6.0 days with IMN vs. 10.5 days with control formula. Median length of hospital stay was also significantly reduced for the IMN group: 15.5 vs. 20.0 days.

Conclusions.—Providing enteral IMN to critically ill patients does not reduce mortality. However, among patients in whom early enteral nutrition is successfully initiated, IMN is associated with significantly reduced morbidity in the form of reduced duration of mechanical ventilation and reduced hospital stay. Cost-benefit analyses should be performed to determine whether widespread adoption of IMN is warranted in the general ICU setting.

▶ This article brings to 13 the number of controlled, double-blind, randomized trials of enteral immunonutrition. Most of these studies have been carried out in burn, trauma, or ICU patients. Just as in this study, essentially all of these studies showed that feeding patients an immune-enhancing enteral diet reduced morbidity and shortened hospital stay, although in only 1 study was survival improved. Thus, it is clear that feeding high-risk patients an immune-enhancing rather than a "standard" enteral formula is worthwhile. Because a variety of different immune-enhancing formulas were used in these studies and all seemed to work equally well, the brand of diet does not appear to be critical.

So in response to the question of what's for dinner, in high-risk ICU patients, the answer is an immune-enhancing enteral formula.

E.A. Deitch, M.D.

Optimal Protein Requirements During the First 2 Weeks After the Onset of Critical Illness

Ishibashi N, Plank LD, Sando K, et al (Auckland Hosp, New Zealand)

Crit Care Med 26:1529-1535, 1998 2–13

Purpose.—With optimal nutritional support, it is possible to reduce the loss of body protein in critically ill patients. However, it can be very difficult to determine the optimal protein requirement for an individual. Protein requirements are commonly prescribed on the basis of body weight (i.e., protein intake of 1.4 to 1.5 g/kg/day); however, overhydration often increases body weight significantly. This retrospective study sought to assess the optimal protein requirements for critically ill patients with sepsis or trauma during the first 2 weeks after ICU admission.

Methods.—Twenty-three critically ill patients had complete, 10-day records of daily protein and energy intake, body composition, and resting energy expenditure. Eighteen patients were trauma victims, and 5 had sepsis. Changes in total-body protein over the 10-day study, which began as soon as the patients were in a hemodynamically stable condition, were assessed by in vivo neutron activation analysis. Based on their average daily protein intake, the patients were divided into 3 groups. To adjust for overhydration and variable body fat, protein intake was indexed to normally hydrated (corrected) fat-free mass (FFMc), with average protein intakes of 1.1, 1.5, and 1.9 g/kg/FFMc/day of protein.

Results.—The patients lost an average of 1.2 kg of total-body protein over the 10-day study, with the loss being significantly increased for patients at the lowest level of protein intake. This protein loss was reduced by 50% when the patients' protein intake was increased from 1.1 to 1.5 g/kg/FFMc/day. However, no further change in protein loss was achieved when protein intake was increased to 1.9 g/kg/FFMc/day. Expressed in body weight as measured at the beginning of the study, the optimal protein intake of 1.5 g/kg/FFMc/day was equivalent to 1.0 g/kg/day.

Conclusions.—Recommended protein intakes for critically ill patients may be excessive if based on the patient's body weight soon after the onset of critical illness. Overhydration can have a significant impact on apparent protein requirement, and may vary considerably early in the course of critical illness. Information about the patient's pre-illness body weight should be obtained and a protein intake of 1.2 g/kg/day should be prescribed accordingly. If premorbid information is not available, a prescription of 1.0 g of protein/kg/day will come close to the patient's optimal protein requirement.

▶ The nutritional care pendulum continues to swing. In the late 1970s and early 1980s, the war cry was that we were underfeeding our sick patients. "If a little is good, more is better" was soon applied to our protein and caloric nutritional goals. Within a decade, as the consequences of overfeeding became apparent, we changed to believing that we were feeding our patients too much. The net result is that, even as we approach the 21st century, nutritional support of the ICU patient is still based more on opinion than on data. Although this controversy exists, most would agree that enteral alimentation is superior to parenteral and that the key is to meet the patient's increased protein needs. But exactly, how much protein should be given is still uncertain, largely because of the technical difficulties of performing the complex physiologic studies required to answer this question.

The technically elegant but retrospective study described in this article indicates that administering more than 1.2 to 1.5 g/kg of protein is unnecessary. Although my bias would lean toward the higher side of this number (numerous studies document that ICU patients receive an average of only about 80% of the nutritional support ordered), the data are valuable, because they provide a much-needed target.

E.A. Deitch, M.D.

Influence of Enteral Nutrition-Induced Splanchnic Hyperemia on the Septic Origin of Splanchnic Ischemia

Kazamias P, Kotzampassi K, Koufogiannis D, et al (Univ of Thessaloníki. Greece)

World J Surg 22:6-11, 1998 2–14

Background.—In most ICUs, splanchnic ischemia of septic origin—and the resulting multiple-organ dysfunction—has become a leading cause of death among critically ill surgical patients. Enteral nutrition clearly induces postprandial hyperemia in ICU patients, but the possible effects of this phenomenon on splanchnic ischemia caused by sepsis are unknown. A study was performed in dogs with splanchnic ischemia to determine whether postprandial splanchnic hyperemia has hemodynamic benefits in the abdominal organs.

Methods.—Mongrel dogs were administered *Escherichia coli* endotoxin through the portal vein. They then received enteral nutrition via a jejunostomy or placebo. Before, during, and after endotoxin infusion and during and after feedings, the 2 groups were compared for systemic hemodynamic variables; blood flow in the portal vein, hepatic artery, and

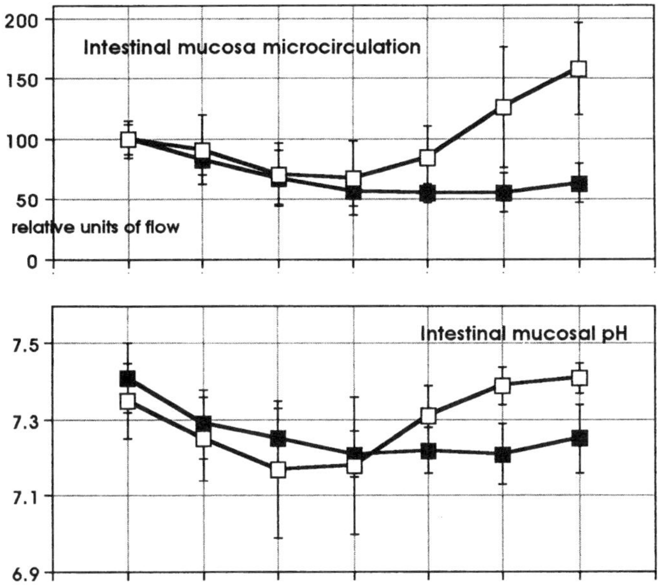

FIGURE 1.—Splanchnic hemodynamic alterations during the early phase after *Escherichia coli* lipopolysaccharide (LPS) infusion-induced sepsis in enteral nutrition (*open squares*) and placebo-fed (*closed squares*) animals. *T1-T7* represent study periods; *T1*: baseline; *T2*, termination of 30-minute LPS infusion; *T3*, *T4*, 30 and 60 minutes later; *T5*, termination of 30-minute feeding; *T6*, *T7*, 30 and 60 minutes later. (Courtesy of Kazamias P, Kotzampassi K, Koufogiannis D, et al: Influence of enteral nutrition-induced splanchnic hyperemia on the septic origin of splanchnic ischemia. *World J Surg* 22:6-11, copyright 1998, Springer-Verlag.)

superior mesenteric artery; microcirculation in the liver and intestine; hepatic tissue PO_2; intestinal pH; and hepatic energy change.

Results.—After endotoxin administration, all splanchnic hemodynamic measures declined significantly. In response to enteral feeding, all of these measurements increased significantly, compared with placebo administration (Fig 1).

Conclusion.—In this animal model, enteral nutrition appears to reverse endotoxin-induced splanchnic ischemia. Thus, splanchnic hyperemia after enteral nutrition may prevent enteral and hepatic dysfunction. The clinical relevance of the improvement in splanchnic hemodynamics remains to be determined.

► It is well known that after eating a meal, intestinal blood flow increases, and it has been speculated that at least part of the beneficial effects of enteral nutrition on the gut mucosa is related to this increase in splanchnic blood flow. Based on this knowledge, the authors tested the hypothesis that enteral feeding will help reverse the decrease in splanchnic perfusion that occurs during sepsis. They observed that enteral feeding improved blood flow to the gut and liver in septic dogs, as well as reversing intestinal mucosal acidosis, and restored the energy levels of the liver. These observations are important both conceptually and therapeutically. Conceptually, the observations provide new information on a potential mechanism by which enteral feeding improves organ function. Therapeutically, they support the importance of enteral feeding in patients with sepsis, including those with splanchnic ischemia.

E.A. Deitch, M.D.

Gastric Intramucosal Acidosis in Mechanically Ventilated Patients: Role of Mucosal Blood Flow

Elizalde JI, Hernández C, Llach J, et al (Universitat de Barcelona)
Crit Care Med 26:827-832, 1998 2–15

Introduction.—Gastric intramucosal pH (pHi) appears to be a useful indicator of outcome in critically ill patients. However, there is limited evidence to support the suggestion that impaired gastric mucosal blood flow is the cause of gastric intramucosal acidosis. Endoscopic techniques for estimating gastric blood perfusion are now available. These techniques were used to study the relationship between gastric mucosal acidosis and decreased gastric mucosal blood flow in patients receiving mechanical ventilation.

Methods.—The prospective study included 17 patients in stable hemodynamic condition receiving mechanical ventilation. In each patient, pHi was measured by tonometry. Two different endoscopic techniques for measuring gastric mucosal blood flow were performed as well: laser Doppler flowmetry and reflectance spectrophotometry. The flow measurements were compared in patients with intramucosal acidosis, defined as a pHi of 7.32 or less, and in those with normal pHi values.

Results.—Gastric intramucosal acidosis was present in 6 patients; the mean pHi was 7.24. The remaining 11 patients had normal pHi values (mean value, 7.44). The general characteristics and hemodynamic condition of the 2 groups were similar. According to laser Doppler flowmetry, gastric mucosal blood flow was reduced in the patients with intramucosal acidosis compared with patients with normal values (i.e., 1.4 vs. 2.1 V). On reflectance spectrophotometry, the patients with low pHi values also had a significantly lower hemoglobin content index than patients with normal values (61 vs. 81 arbitrary units). There was no significant difference in the oxygen saturation index, however.

Conclusions.—This study supports the link between gastric mucosal hypoperfusion and intramucosal acidosis in patients receiving mechanical ventilation. The findings suggest that measurement of gastric pHi could be a useful means of assessing the adequacy of gastrointestinal tract perfusion in critically ill patients. Gastrointestinal ischemia leading to intramucosal acidosis could result in bacterial translocation, which has been implicated in the development of multiple-organ failure.

► Why choose an article on gastric tonometry? This technique has been around for over a decade and, based on the literally hundreds of published articles dealing with this technique, several concepts have been established. For example, multiple clinical trials (but not all) have documented that the monitoring of gastric mucosal pH is a better predictor of outcome than measurements of global oxygen delivery in ICU and trauma patients. So, why choose this article showing that mucosal acidosis, as measured by gastric tonometry, reflects inadequate gastric mucosal blood flow? The answer is that, although gastric tonometry has been proposed as the only technique that directly reflects end-organ oxygen delivery, this assumption is not fully established. There are some conflicting experimental data and recent conflicting indirect human data that cast doubt on the concept that the development of mucosal acidosis reflects inadequate oxygen delivery to the gut. Thus, the value of this human study is that it is the first study to directly correlate decreased gastric mucosal microcirculatory blood flow and gastric mucosal acidosis.

Knowing that mucosal acidosis does indicate inadequate end-organ (gastric) blood flow will be important in setting up clinical trials directed at testing new therapies, as well as in clinical monitoring of established methods of improving oxygen delivery.

E.A. Deitch, M.D.

Right Ventricular End-Diastolic Volume Index as a Predictor of Preload Status in Patients on Positive End-Expiratory Pressure

Cheatham ML, Nelson LD, Chang MC, et al (Orlando Regional Med Ctr, Fla; Wake Forest Univ, Winston-Salem, NC)

Crit Care Med 26:1801-1806, 1998 2–16

Purpose.—For critically ill patients receiving intrinsic or extrinsic positive end-expiratory pressure (PEEP), it is essential to have acute information on preload status. In patients with acute respiratory failure, PEEP can increase right ventricular afterload and decrease ventricular preload, the result of increases in intrathoracic pressure. New thermodilution pulmonary artery catheters permit bedside assessment of right ventricular function through measurement of right ventricular ejection fraction and calculation of right ventricular end-diastolic volume index (RVEDVI). RVEDVI and pulmonary artery occlusion pressure (PAOP) were compared for accuracy as indicators of preload status in patients receiving PEEP for acute respiratory failure.

Methods.—Sixty-four patients with acute respiratory failure who were admitted to a surgical ICU were included in a prospective cohort study. All of the patients were receiving PEEP, titrated to target values of 0.92 or greater for arterial oxygen saturation, less than 0.5 for fractional concentration of oxygen in inspired gas, and 0.2 or less for intrapulmonary shunt. Both RVEDVI and PAOP were monitored in all patients, and compared for their ability to predict preload-recruitable increases in cardiac index (CI) at various levels of PEEP.

Results.—A total of 250 sets of hemodynamic measurements were obtained at PEEP values ranging from 5 to 50 cm H_2O. RVEDVI showed a better correlation with CI than PAOP did, regardless of PEEP value. The correlation between CI and PAOP became inverse at PEEP levels of 15 cm H_2O or greater, whereas the correlation between CI and RVEDVI always remained positive.

Conclusions.—In patients with acute respiratory failure receiving PEEP values of up to 50 cm H_2O, RVEDVI is a better predictor of CI than PAOP is. Particularly at higher PEEP levels, RVEDVI provides a better indicator of volume depletion and preload-recruitable increases in CI. Interpretation of PAOP values is difficult at PEEP values of 15 cm H_2O or greater. The use of arbitrary maximum PAOP values to limit volume resuscitation in patients receiving PEEP may lead to inadequate resuscitation in patients with acute respiratory failure.

▶ Over the last 5 years, several articles have appeared suggesting that RVEDVI measurements are more accurate than pulmonary artery pressure measurements in correctly identifying patients in whom the provision of additional volume will increase cardiac output. This prospective clinical trial adds further support to the notion that critically ill patients, especially those with acute respiratory distress syndrome who are receiving moderate to high levels of PEEP, are better served with the use of the new generation of thermodilution pulmonary artery catheters that allow direct measurements of right ventricular function. Simply stated, the results of this study indicate that in patients receiving PEEP, pulmonary capillary wedge pressures are not accurate in predicting those patients in whom volume administration will increase cardiac output. In contrast, RVEDVIs do. To quote the authors, "RVEDVI is a clinically useful indicator of intravascular preload status and accurately predicts preload recruitable increases in cardiac index." So when trying to determine whether ventilated patients receiving PEEP would benefit from more volume, think RVEDVI.

E.A. Deitch, M.D.

Decomplexification in Critical Illness and Injury: Relationship Between Heart Rate Variability, Severity of Illness, and Outcome

Goldstein B, Fiser DH, Kelly MM, et al (Univ of Rochester, NY; Arkansas Children's Hosp, Little Rock; Children's Natl Med Ctr, Washington, DC)

Crit Care Med 26:352-357, 1998 2–17

Purpose.—The activity of physiologic systems is nonlinear and dynamic, meaning that the systems change over time and respond to stimuli in nonlinear fashion. Signal variability is a characteristic of physiologically healthy systems, whereas aging or diseased systems show loss of variability, termed *decomplexification*. This study measured heart rate power spectra, as a measure of heart rate dynamics, to assess the presence of decomplexification of heart rate dynamics in children with critical illness or injury.

Methods.—The study included 135 consecutive patients admitted to a pediatric ICU. Heart rate power spectra were measured and correlated with various measures of severity of illness and outcome, including the Pediatric Risk of Mortality (PRISM) score, the Pediatric Cerebral Performance Category (PCPC), and the Pediatric Overall Performance Category (POPC).

Findings.—Minimum low-frequency and high-frequency heart rate power were significantly and negatively correlated with maximum PRISM score. r^2 values were 0.293 for log low-frequency heart rate power vs. PRISM and 0.243 for log high-frequency heart rate power vs. PRISM. Negative correlations were also noted with POPC or PCPC: $r^2 = 0.429$ for log low-frequency heart rate power and $r^2 = 0.271$ for log high-frequency heart rate power. Maximum heart rate power was not correlated with any of the scores.

Conclusion.—The findings confirm an inverse relationship between heart rate power spectra and severity of illness and outcome among pediatric ICU patients. Decomplexification of physiologic dynamics occurs in these patients. Heart rate power spectral analysis could be a useful tool for rapid physiologic assessment. Its value in assessing severity of illness and physiologic derangement and in predicting patient outcomes warrants further study.

▶ It has been recognized for over 30 years that the heart rate varies in response to autonomic and other normal physiologic responses in healthy individuals. However, only recently has loss of heart rate variability been studied as a sign of physiologic failure. This article showing that loss of heart rate variability correlates with prognosis in pediatric ICU patients is consistent with recent adult data. Although the current techniques for measuring heart rate variability are complex and tricky, if other investigators continue to find this noninvasive method clinically helpful, I anticipate that the technology will be made user-friendly enough to become part of the intensivist's armamentarium in the not-too-distant future. So, for the present, keep your eyes open.

E.A. Deitch, M.D.

Transfusion of Phosphoenolpyruvate-treated Blood Increases Oxygen Consumption in Acute Hemorrhage

Cornum RL, Martin RR, Bandy WC, et al (Brooke Army Med Ctr, Fort Sam Houston, Tex)

Am J Surg 175:469-471, 1998 2–18

Introduction.—The hemoglobin oxygen affinity (HOA) of blood is reduced by incubation with the high-energy glycolytic intermediate phosphoenolpyruvate (PEP). Previous studies have been unable to determine whether transfusion of blood with reduced HOA increases oxygen consumption. A study was performed in a canine model of acute anemia to determine the effects of PEP-treated blood on oxygen consumption.

Methods.—Anesthetized, splenectomized, instrumented dogs were subjected to isovolemic hemodilution to achieve a hematocrit of 10%. After 1 hour at this level, the animals received transfusion with PEP-treated blood or conventionally stored blood to reach a hematocrit level of 18%. Oxygen consumption during the period of anemia and after transfusion was assessed by measuring cardiac output, co-oximetry, and hemoglobin P_{50}.

Results.—During the hemodilution period, both groups showed doubling of hemodilution. Dogs receiving PEP-treated blood showed an oxygen consumption of 8.31 cc/kg/mm, compared with 3.73 cc/kg/mm in those receiving conventional stored blood. The 2 groups were similar in terms of arterial or venous PO_2 and pH. Posttransfusion measurements of hemoglobin P_{50} showed increased HOA values in the group treated with PEP-treated blood: 47 vs. 21.

Conclusions.—In this canine model of anemic hypoxia, transfusing blood with reduced HOA led to increased oxygen consumption. Treating blood with PEP can increase oxygen consumption at a similar hematocrit level. More study is needed to find ways to decrease the HOA of red blood cells in vivo.

▶ In patients requiring massive blood transfusions or in patients who are receiving blood transfusions to improve oxygen delivery, the transfusion of stored blood has one major disadvantage. Specifically, stored blood is less effective at binding oxygen than fresh blood because the red blood cell enzyme 2,3-DPG, which increases the affinity of blood for oxygen, is lost during the storage period. This decrease in the oxygen-carrying capacity of stored blood is likely to be bad, since it limits oxygen delivery to the tissues, especially in patients whose oxygen delivery is supply-dependent. This experimental study indicates that a practical solution to this problem is possible, since the authors found that by treating stored red blood cells with PEP, it was possible to both increase the affinity of stored blood for oxygen as well as improve oxygen delivery. The translation of simple strategies, such as this, to our patients is likely to be beneficial.

E.A. Deitch, M.D.

Reliability of the Next of Kins' Estimates of Critically Ill Patients' Quality of Life

Rogers J, Ridley S, Chrispin P, et al (Norfolk and Norwich Hosp, England)
Anaesthesia 52:1137-1143, 1997 2–19

Objective.—Quality of life is a key consideration in making decisions about whether a patient should be admitted to the ICU. However, the assessment of quality of life in an obtunded patient is an important problem in ICU practice. Few studies have examined the use of proxy respondents to provide information on health status in the ICU setting. This study analyzed family members' assessments of quality of life of critically ill patients, including the level of agreement between the assessments of patients and their next of kin.

Methods.—The Short Form 36 (SF-36), a validated assessment of quality of life, was administered to 99 adult ICU patients and their next of kin, both at ICU discharge and 6 months later. The relatives' assessments were analyzed for reliability, validity, and agreement with the patients' responses.

Results.—The next of kin's responses to the SF-36 met the study standards for reliability and validity. However, reliability was significantly lower in the mental health dimension, which addresses the patient's mood and anxiety level. The discharge scores of patients and relatives differed significantly in the 6 dimensions of the SF-36. However, the 2 sets of responses showed fair agreement, which improved between the discharge and 6-month follow-up assessments. Agreement was greatest for dimensions related to physical health.

Conclusions.—The next of kin of critically ill patients appear to give a good proximal assessment of the patient's functional quality of life. However, these assessments are limited in terms of qualitative aspects, particularly the mental health dimension. This information may help in understanding the biases in relatives' responses if quality-of-life assessments are considered in making management decisions.

▶ Assessment of quality of life is an important variable in deciding whether to admit a patient to the ICU as well as a factor in decision making after the patient is admitted to the ICU. Since many patients admitted to the ICU cannot provide quality-of-life information, family members frequently assume this responsibility. How accurate family members are in this role as proxy respondents has not been well studied. Hence, the value of this focused clinical trial demonstrating that families, while not perfect predictors, are in general reasonably accurate.

E.A. Deitch, M.D.

Acute Withdrawal Syndrome Related to the Administration of Analgesic and Sedative Medications in Adult Intensive Care Unit Patients

Cammarano WB, Pittet J-F, Weitz S, et al (Univ of California, San Francisco)
Crit Care Med 26:676-684, 1998 2–20

Background.—Critically ill patients receiving mechanical ventilation often are given high doses of opioids, benzodiazepines, or other drugs for a prolonged period. Rapid weaning in preparation for transfer from the ICU to the hospital ward can sometimes lead to acute withdrawal syndromes, complications of which may increase morbidity and thus hospital costs. The frequency of and risk factors for acute withdrawal syndrome were

TABLE 2.—Signs and Symptoms of Opioid and/or Benzodiazepine Withdrawal

Symptoms	Signs
Drug craving	Sweating
Restlessness, irritability	Tachycardia*
Increased sensitivity to pain	Vomiting
Nausea	Diarrhea
Cramps	Hypertension†
Muscle aches	Fever‡
Dysphoria	Seizure
Insomnia	Tachypnea§
Anxiety	
Myoclonus	
Delirium	

*Heart rate greater than 100 beats/min or increase of greater than 10 beats/min from baseline.

†Systolic blood pressure greater than 140 mm Hg or diastolic blood pressure greater than 90 mm Hg or an increase in either by 10 mm Hg above baseline.

‡Temperature greater than 38°C.

§Respiratory rate greater than 20 breaths/min or an increase by greater than 4 breaths/min over baseline.

(Modified from Himmelsbach C: *J Pharmacol Exp Ther* 67:239-249, 1939, and from George C, Robertson D: *Medical Toxicology* 2:367-382, 1987. Courtesy of Cammarano WB, Pittet J-F, Weitz S, et al: Acute withdrawal syndrome related to the administration of analgesic and sedative medications in adult intensive care unit patients. *Crit Care Med* 26(4):676-684, 1998.)

determined retrospectively in mechanically ventilated ICU patients receiving analgesic and sedative drugs.

Methods.—A total of 28 adult patients who spent more than 7 days in a trauma/surgical ICU, where they received mechanical ventilation, were studied. The patients' use of opioids and benzodiazepines was assessed by converting the respective doses to fentanyl and lorazepam units on the basis of potency and availability. Each patient was evaluated for acute withdrawal syndrome, based on the presence of more than 2 of a list of specified symptoms (Table 2).

Results.—The frequency of acute withdrawal syndrome possibly related to analgesic or sedative drugs was 32%. Compared with patients without withdrawal, those with acute withdrawal syndrome had higher mean daily and peak doses of fentanyl equivalents and higher mean daily doses of lorazepam equivalents. The withdrawal group was also more likely to receive neuromuscular blocking agents or propofol for longer than 1 day and had a longer duration of mechanical ventilation, benzodiazepine therapy, and propofol therapy. Withdrawal syndrome was significantly related to the presence of acute respiratory distress syndrome.

Conclusions.—Acute withdrawal syndrome is a common complication of drug weaning in mechanically ventilated patients who spend a prolonged period in the ICU. Risk is elevated for patients receiving large doses of sedative and analgesic drugs. Such large doses are commonly used in patients with adult respiratory distress syndrome, which places them at high risk of acute withdrawal syndrome.

▶ I found the premise and results of this pilot study on the development of opioid and benzodiazepine withdrawal syndrome both surprising and important. It was surprising that almost one third of the surgical ICU patients who received mechanical ventilation for more than 7 days had evidence of an acute withdrawal syndrome. This observation is important because the signs of opioid or benzodiazepine withdrawal, such as tachycardia, tachypnea, fever, agitation, restlessness, and diarrhea, might not be correctly diagnosed as being caused by a decrease in opioids or benzodiazepine administration. Failure to consider the possibility of a drug withdrawal syndrome would essentially preclude the ability to make a correct diagnosis and thus prevent proper therapy. Although this is a retrospective pilot study, the take-home message is important. We must consider the possibility that ventilated patients receiving high doses of sedatives, opioids, and neuromuscular blocking agents for long periods are at increased risk of having withdrawal symptoms as these agents are reduced.

E.A. Deitch, M.D.

3 Burns

Introduction

All physicians have learned from personal experience that chronic sleep deprivation can be devastating. So too can it be after burn injury. Based on a study of 237 burn patients (Abstract 3–1), it appears that sleep deprivation occurring during the hospitalization period can have long-term psychological and physiologic deleterious effects that last well after the patient is discharged. As reflected in several articles in this year's selections, improving the functional outcome of patients with major burns requires acute as well as postdischarge attention to sleeping patterns, nutrition, and exercise programs. This focus on continuance of aggressive supportive therapy after hospital discharge clearly takes on increasing importance as hospitalization periods shorten and the burden for recovery shifts from the inpatient to the outpatient arena. A further reflection of the new economics of medical care is the re-evaluation of indications for hospital admission in patients with low-voltage electrical injuries. Based on two clinical studies (Abstracts 3–4 and 3–5), one in children and one in adults, it appears that the vast majority of patients with low-voltage electrical injuries can be sent home after a brief period of observation in the emergency room. That is, admission for observation is not indicated if the ECG tracing upon arrival in the emergency room is normal, since the fear that these patients may go on to have occult life-threatening cardiac arrhythmias develop is unfounded.

As in years past, infection and smoke inhalation injury remain the most common causes of death in patients with large burns. To control bacterial contamination of the burn wound and fight infection, the patient must be able to mobilize functional neutrophils from the bone marrow. Yet, the ability to carry out this important process may become impaired after a burn injury. Why many burn patients are unable to optimally mobilize neutrophils from the bone marrow is unclear, but based on an elegant experimental study, the answer appears to be related to the inability of the bone marrow to respond to physiologic signals to produce and release neutrophils. Additional experimental studies indicate that the impaired production and release of neutrophils from the bone marrow is an important factor in infectious mortality, since drugs aimed at reversing this myeloid block improve survival in a rodent model of burn wound infection. These studies (Abstracts 3–6 and 3–7) on neutrophil physiology and function after thermal injury take advantage of recent advances in cellular and molecular biology. So, what you might say is, "These are animal studies and as clinicians we treat patients." OK. The next article chosen (Abstract 3–8) is one where basic science studies in animals has led to improved clinical care. In this study, the authors have shown that the mortality in pediatric burn patients with inhalation injury was reduced from 19% to 4% by the use of aerosolized heparin and acetylcysteine. This therapy was based on a decade of basic science studies in sheep and other animal models, thereby highlighting the ultimate clinical importance of advances made using animal models to better understand the pathophysiology of a disease process.

Basic science studies utilizing animal models have also provided insight into why so many burn patients develop altered levels of consciousness, delirium, or hallucinations. At least part of the answer appears to be that major burn injuries may be associated with reduced cerebral perfusion and the subsequent development of cerebral edema.

The last three abstracts in this year's selections (Abstracts 3–10 to 3–12) deal with the burn wound. The first of these highlights the role of an excessive immune response in the pathophysiology of hypertrophic burn scars, and the last two abstracts deal with practical aspects of burn wound care.

Edwin A. Deitch, M.D.

The 1998 Clinical Research Award: Sleep Disturbance After Burn Injury: A Frequent Yet Understudied Complication

Lawrence JW, Fauerbach J, Eudell E, et al (Johns Hopkins Univ, Baltimore, Md)

J Burn Care Rehabil 19:480-486, 1998 3–1

Background.—Sleep disturbance has been reported in various populations of surgical patients, but it is generally regarded as a relatively minor problem in burn patients. However, the few available data suggest that sleep disturbance is a common and often persistent problem in this population. The frequency and chronicity of sleep disturbance were evaluated in adult survivors of burn injuries.

Methods.—The study included 237 patients (average age, 42 years) who were hospitalized for burn treatment. Average total body surface area burned was 12%, with an average full-thickness burn component of 3%. In the hospital, all patients completed instruments measuring posttraumatic stress disorder, depression, anxiety, and quality of life; the posttraumatic stress and depression measures included items on sleep disturbance. Follow-up assessments were performed at 1 week after discharge in 149 patients and 2 months after discharge in 91 patients.

Results.—Sleep disturbance was reported while in the hospital and 1 week after discharge by approximately 50% of patients, and 2 months after discharge by 40% (Table 3). At all assessments, sleep disturbance was more strongly associated with emotional distress than with pain or extent

TABLE 3.—Percentage of Burn Survivors Endorsing Positive Symptoms on Davidson Trauma Scale During Hospitalization and 1 Week and 2 Months After Discharge

Question	Content	During Hospitalization	1 Week After Discharge	2 Months After Discharge
1	Painful thoughts of event	37	37	30
2	Distressing dreams of event	18	19	16
3	Felt like the event was reoccurring	12	13	13
4	Upset by reminders of event	26	24	27
5	Avoid thoughts or feelings about the event	20	22	21
6	Avoid situations or actions which remind you of the event	23	20	18
7	Unable to recall important parts of the event	15	13	16
8	Difficulty enjoying things	15	17	23
9	Felt distant/cut off from people	13	12	16
10	Unable to have sad or loving feelings/ felt numb	4	5	10
11	Hard to imagine living a fullfilling life	7	8	11
12	Difficulty falling or staying asleep	49	46	41
13	Irritability or outburst of anger	26	31	40
14	Difficulty concentrating	17	17	19
15	Felt on edge, been easily distracted, had to stay on guard	17	15	23
16	Jumpy or easily startled	19	16	23
17	Physically upset by reminders of the event	9	12	11

(Courtesy of Lawrence JW, Fauerbach J, Eudell E, et al: Sleep disturbance after burn injury: A frequent yet understudied complication. *J Burn Care Rehabil* 19:480-486, 1998.)

of burn. Sleep disturbance had a significant negative impact on quality of life.

Conclusions.—Sleep disturbance is a common, important, and often persistent complication of burn injuries. Improved sleep could have a number of beneficial effects during burn rehabilitation. Studies of prevention and treatment of sleep disturbance in burn patients are needed. The authors' clinic has had success with cognitive-behavioral therapy and treatment of intrusive posttraumatic symptoms.

▶ For burn survivors, Shakespeare may have put it best: "To sleep, perchance to dream. Aye, that is the rub." This important article emphasizes that even months after hospital discharge, burn patients may still be experiencing difficulty with sleep. In providing optimal burn care, it is important for treating physicians to recognize that sleep disorders may persist long after the patient has left the hospital. Frequently, just acknowledging that these problems exist gives comfort to both the patient and the family. The value of reassurance and sleeping pills should not be underestimated.

E.A. Deitch, M.D.

Increased Protein Intake During the Recovery Phase After Severe Burns Increases Body Weight Gain and Muscle Function

Demling RH, DeSanti L (Brigham and Women's Hosp Burn Ctr and Braintree Rehabilitation Hosp, Boston)

J Burn Care Rehabil 19:161-168, 1998 3–2

Objective.—In patients with severe burns, a catabolic or stress response can lead to rapid loss of lean body mass, particularly from skeletal muscle. Even with aggressive dietary and exercise interventions, the problems persist. Most lost lean body mass is restored in the recovery period; however, few data exist about the effects of protein intake and other nutrients on the rate of restoration of body weight. The impact of protein intake on weight gain and muscle function during the recovery phase in patients with severe burns was assessed.

Methods.—The study included 15 patients with severe, deep burns covering 30% to 50% of total body surface area. The patients were studied for 3 weeks in a rehabilitation facility after resolution of the acute phase. All patients received a high-calorie, high-protein diet. In addition, 1 group received a standard nutritional supplement to keep caloric intake at 30 to 35 kcal/kg/day and protein intake at 1.3 to 1.5 g/kg/day. Another group received a protein hydrolysate to provide a protein intake of 1.7 to 2.0 g/kg/day. Nutritional profiles and weight gain were compared between groups. In addition, muscle strength was measured using a physical therapy index of 0 to 10, with 10 denoting the most progress, based on completion of physical therapy sessions and fatigue level.

Results.—During the 3-week study period, average weight gain was 1.0 to 1.5 lb/week for patients receiving the standard diet vs. 2.5 to 3.0 lb/week for those receiving the high-protein diet. Weight gain during the 3 weeks was 3 or 4 lb in the standard group vs. 8.5 lb in the high-protein group. Both groups had significant improvement in strength and endurance, although the final physical therapy index was higher in the high-protein group: 7 vs. 4.

Conclusions.—In patients with severe burns, addition of a protein hydrolysate to increase protein intake leads to faster restoration of body weight and muscle function. Increasing protein intake to about 2 g/kg/day—about twice the recommended daily allowance—doubles weight gain in the recovery phase. The results strongly suggest that this weight gain is lean body mass. The role of increased protein quantity vs. the type of protein remains to be determined.

▶ The key point of this prospective clinical trial of patients with major burn injuries is that aggressive nutritional support should not end when the patient leaves the hospital. Although the nutritional support of hospitalized burn patients has been extensively studied during the last 25 years, and advances from these studies have resulted in major improvements in burn care, little is known about the optimal nutritional support for the burn patient after hospital discharge. Yet this is an important area for study, because recovery of lean body mass, body composition, and muscular strength occurs during the recovery phase, much of which may occur after hospital discharge. Because it is known that it takes 5 to 10 times as long to replace muscle mass during the recovery phase as it took to lose it during the acute catabolic phase of burn injury, prolonged nutritional support after hospital discharge is likely to be of major clinical importance. Therein lies the value of this clinical study documenting that weight gain and recovery of muscular strength is increased by the administration of high levels of dietary protein supplements. Because this phenomenon is likely to be operative in trauma or ICU patients as well as burn patients, I suggest that all clinicians who treat severely catabolic patients read this article and apply it to their practices.

E.A. Deitch, M.D.

Muscle Strength in Individuals With Healed Burns

St-Pierre DMM, Choinière M, Forget R, et al (McGill Univ, Québec; Hôtel Dieu Hosp of Montreal; Univ of Montreal)

Arch Phys Med Rehabil 79:155-161, 1998 3–3

Introduction.—The aim of burn rehabilitation is to restore the patient to his or her preburn level of functioning. Muscle weakness may be a persistent problem in burn survivors; however, there are few data on how muscle size and strength recover after a major burn. Skeletal muscle proteins may be particularly vulnerable to postburn hypermetabolism. The long-term effects of burns on muscle strength, including the impact of initial burn severity, were evaluated.

Methods.—The cross-sectional study included 36 burn survivors (mean age, 36 years). All had second- and third-degree burns over a mean 35.5% of total body surface area (TBSA). All patients were studied more than 1 year after discharge, with a mean follow-up of 37 months. The patients underwent measurements of maximal torque, work, and power developed by the elbow and knee flexors and extensors. The findings were compared with those of 30 unburned controls, matched for age, sex, body mass index, and physical activity level.

Results.—Torque, work, and power developed by the quadriceps muscles were significantly reduced among patients with burns of greater than 30% TBSA. Reductions of 15% to 20.5%, depending on the test velocity, were observed. Severely burned patients also had reduced muscle power at the elbow, with reductions of approximately 19% in flexion and extension at the faster velocities. However, patients with burns of less than 30% TBSA did not differ significantly from controls.

Conclusions.—There are long-term reductions in muscle strength in patients with severe burns of more than 30% TBSA. This muscle weakness may be the result of insufficient rehabilitation or limited muscle plasticity.

Further studies are needed to determine the cause of this lasting postburn muscle weakness.

▶ Limited range of motion, poor dexterity, loss of mobility, intolerance of prolonged standing or walking, and decreased muscle strength and endurance are frequently reported by burn patients as preventing them from engaging in the full range of leisure activities or returning to work. Yet little information is available on the time course of muscle recovery after thermal injury. Because patients and employers may have different ideas of when a patient should return to work, as well as different expectations of job performance once the patient re-enters the workforce, information on muscle strength recovery is critical. This article describes a long-term study documenting that muscle strength may be severely impaired even a full year after a major burn injury. So the next time a patient says he does not have the stamina or strength to do his job, instead of telling him to "suck it up," we might initiate a focused exercise/program to help him regain lost muscular strength.

E.A. Deitch, M.D.

Pediatric Electrical Burns: Management Strategies

Zubair M, Besner GE (Ohio State Univ, Columbus; Children's Hosp, Columbus, Ohio)

Burns 23:413-420, 1997 3–4

Objective.—Most electrical injuries occurring in the home involve children. Low-voltage electrical injuries—those involving sources less than 1,000 V—occur more frequently in younger children. Few studies have addressed the topic of electrical burns in children. Toward the development of safe and cost-effective approaches to pediatric burn injuries, a 25-year experience with such patients was reviewed.

Patients and Findings.—The experience included 127 children; their mean age was 5 years. There were more than twice as many boys as girls. There were 48 oral injuries, the result of biting an electrical cord; 33 outlet injuries, caused by putting an object into an electrical socket; 25 low-voltage household injuries, caused by indoor contact with a low-voltage wire or appliance; 18 outdoor high-voltage wire injuries; and 3 lightning strikes. Eighty-three percent of the injuries were low-voltage injuries (Table 3). Most patients with low-voltage electrical injuries did not require hospitalization. In contrast, high-voltage injuries were severe enough to warrant hospitalization in almost every case.

Conclusions.—Children with low-voltage electrical injuries do not generally require hospitalization. If these children remain asymptomatic after 4 hours of observation, they may safely be treated on an outpatient basis. This approach will reduce medical costs, in addition to the other benefits of avoiding hospitalization. Most low-voltage electrical injuries to young children are easily preventable.

TABLE 3.—Age Distribution Related to Voltage

Age	n	Voltage 100 V	10 000 V	>100 000 V
0-3	73	73	—	—
3.1-6	16	16	—	—
6.1-9	15	9	6	—
9.1-12	10	4	4	2
12.1-15	12	3	8	1
15.1-18	1	1	—	—
TOTALS	127	106	18	3

(Courtesy of Zubair M, Besner GE: Pediatric electrical burns: Management strategies. *Burns* 23:413-420. Copyright 1997, with permission from Elsevier Science Ltd, The Boulevard, Langford Lane, Kidlington OX5 16B, UK)

▶ This article was chosen for one reason and one reason only. It highlights the fact that most children with low-voltage injuries do not require hospital admission.

Although we are taught to worry about the development of respiratory arrest, cardiac arrhythmias, and myoglobin-induced renal failure after an electrical injury, these complications are uncommon after a low-voltage injury. Arrhythmias or respiratory arrest, when they do occur, generally occur at the scene or very shortly after the electrical injury. Thus, a child (or adult) with a low-voltage electrical injury who does not have an arrhythmia at the scene or upon arrival to the hospital, and does not have an arrhythmia develop within a few hours, is not likely to develop one. Therefore, admission for cardiac monitoring is not indicated, and the child should be allowed to go home.

E.A. Deitch, M.D.

Electrical Injury and the Frequency of Cardiac Complications

Arrowsmith J, Usgaocar RP, Dickson WA (Morriston Hosp, Swansea, UK)

Burns 23:576-578, 1997 3–5

Purpose.—Cardiac abnormalities caused by electrical injury are most often apparent at the time of the injury. However, they can also develop later, and 24-hour cardiac monitoring has been recommended for patients with electrical injuries. A 5-year experience with cardiac complications of electrical injuries was analyzed, with focus on the timing of the complications after the injury.

Methods.—The analysis included 145 patients with electrical injuries: 128 with low-voltage injuries and 17 with high-voltage injuries (greater than 1,000 V). A 12-lead ECG recorded within 72 hours after injury was available for 104 patients. Seventy-three of these patients underwent cardiac monitoring for at least 24 hours after injury.

Findings.—Four patients had ECG abnormalities, all noted on the initial ECG. Three of these patients had only occasional ectopic beats, which resolved during the 24-hour observation period. The remaining patient, who suffered a high-voltage injury, had atrial fibrillation, which was successfully treated with IV digoxin. Patients who lost consciousness at the time of the injury and those with high-voltage injuries were more likely to have cardiac complications.

Conclusions.—This analysis finds a 3% rate of cardiac abnormalities among patients with electrical injuries. For patients who did not lose consciousness at the time of injury and who have a normal admission ECG, cardiac complications are unlikely to develop later. These patients need not be admitted to the hospital for the sole purpose of cardiac monitoring.

▶ As highlighted in this article, overtreatment of electrical injuries is common. This overtreatment takes 2 common forms. First is the unnecessary admission and cardiac monitoring of patients with low-voltage contact-type electrical injuries. The second is the search for myoglobin in patients with small or superficial electrical injuries. The message of this article is clear and accurate: The majority of patients with low-voltage electrical injuries do not require hospital admission. In the absence of loss of consciousness or the presence of a documented dysrhythmia in the field or in the emergency room, the patient should be sent home.

E.A. Deitch, M.D.

Mechanisms of Neutropenia Involving Myeloid Maturation Arrest in Burn Sepsis

Shoup M, Weisenberger JM, Wang JL, et al (Loyola Univ, Maywood, Ill)

Ann Surg 228:112-122, 1998 3–6

Purpose.—Sepsis is a major cause of morbidity and death in trauma patients. To avoid sepsis, patients must be able to mobilize functional neutrophils from the bone marrow into the circulation. Burn patients with sepsis have impairments of bone marrow granulopoiesis leading to neutropenia, even though their circulating levels of granulocyte colony-stimulating factor (G-CSF) are normal. This study examined the mechanisms of decreased bone marrow neutrophil production in sepsis.

Methods.—B6D2F1/J mice were randomized into 3 groups. Two groups were subjected to burn trauma, one of which also received topical inoculation with *Pseudomonas aeruginosa* (1,000 colony-forming units); the third group served as a control. After 3 days, the animals' peripheral blood absolute neutrophil count and G-CSF levels were measured. Neutrophil differentiation patterns in bone marrow aspirates were assessed by Gr-1 antigen expression; G-CSF receptor status was measured as well. Histologic studies of the liver, lung, spleen, and burn site were performed.

Results.—Mice with burn sepsis had a reduced absolute neutrophil count but elevated levels of G-CSF in plasma (Table 1). The neutrophil differentiation pattern showed a shift toward immature mitotic myeloid cells. The burn sepsis group also had significantly reduced G-CSF receptor

TABLE 1.—Comparison of the Total White Blood Cell Count, Absolute Neutrophil Count, and Serum Granulocyte Colony-Stimulating Factor in Control, Burn, and Burn-Infected Mice

	Control	Burn	Burn Infection
WBC (per μl)	7085 ± 1387	8340 ± 896	3620 ± 638*
ANC (per μl)	2555 ± 433	2942 ± 557	764 ± 207*
Serum G-CSF (pmol/ml)	0.033 ± 0.006	0.119 ± 0.016	0.998 ± 0.193*

Note: Data represent mean ± standard deviation.
$*P < 0.01$ vs. control and burn-alone mice (N = 6).
Abbreviations: WBC, white blood cell count; *ANC,* absolute neutrophil count; *G-CSF,* granulocyte colony-stimulating factor.
(Courtesy of Shoup M, Weisenberger JM, Wang JL, et al: Mechanisms of neutropenia involving myeloid maturation arrest in burn sepsis. *Ann Surg* 228:112-122, 1998.)

messenger RNA levels in bone marrow, as well as reduced G-CSF–stimulated proliferation. Neutrophil infiltration into tissues was insignificant on histologic examination.

Conclusion.—In burn patients with sepsis, neutropenia and arrested myeloid maturation may be observed despite the presence of elevated G-CSF levels. The abnormal bone marrow findings are correlated with reduced expression of G-CSF receptor in the marrow. The results might help to explain the mechanism of neutropenia in sepsis.

► Have you ever wondered why some patients with sepsis get neutropenia? I have. Is it because the neutrophils are being used up in fighting the infection faster than they can be made? Probably not. This study helps explain this phenomenon of infection-induced neutropenia by showing that there is a maturation arrest of granulocytes in the bone marrow, which is associated with downregulation of G-CSF receptor expression. What this means is that even though the signal is given to increase production of neutrophils (i.e., increased blood G-CSF levels), the neutrophil precursors in the bone marrow have a decreased ability to respond. It is too early to say whether these observations will be translated into clinical therapy, but one must understand what is broken before it can be fixed.

E.A. Deitch, M.D.

Cyclooxygenase-2 Inhibitor NS-398 Improves Survival and Restores Leukocyte Counts in Burn Infection

Shoup M, He L-K, Liu H, et al (Loyola Univ, Maywood, Ill)

J Trauma: Injury Infect Crit Care 45:215-221, 1998 3–7

Background.—Cyclooxygenase (COX) plays a central role in the production of prostaglandin E_2 (PGE_2) from arachidonic acid. Production of PGE_2 may be increased when sepsis develops after trauma, particularly after burns. There is evidence that PGE_2 may play a role in the development of leukopenia during sepsis and, therefore, that COX inhibitors may

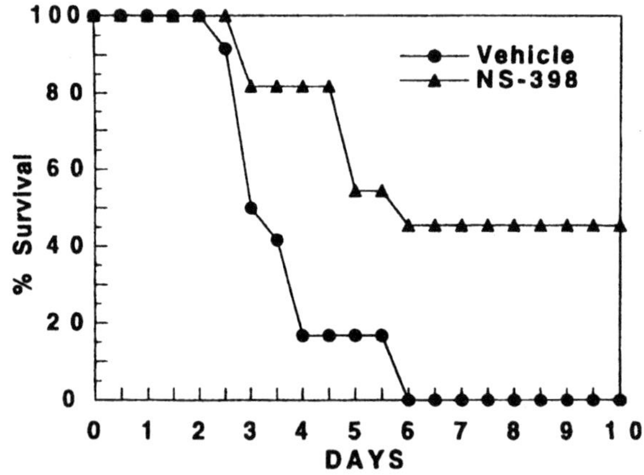

FIGURE 6.—Effect of NS-398 on survival in burn-infected mice. Burn-infected mice were separated into a placebo group and a test group. The animals in the placebo group received the vehicle, and those in the test group received NS-398 (10 mg/kg) intraperitoneally twice daily for 3 days, starting 4 to 6 hours after burn infection. n = 22. (Courtesy of Shoup M, He L-K, Liu H, et al: Cyclooxygenase-2 inhibitor NS-398 improves survival and restores leukocyte counts in burn infection. *J Trauma: Injury Infect Crit Care* 45:215-221, 1998.)

be of therapeutic value. Using a mouse study of burn sepsis, this study evaluated the treatment benefits of the COX-2 inhibitor NS-398.

Methods.—In the study model, mice were subjected to a 15% dorsal scald burn, followed by infectious challenge with topical *Pseudomonas aeruginosa*, 1,000 colony-forming units. The active-treatment group received NS-398, 10 mg/kg, 4 to 6 hours after infectious challenge and then twice daily for 3 days. The control group received placebo at these times. Fourteen-day survival was compared between groups, along with the 3-day white blood cell (WBC) count and absolute neutrophil count (ANC).

Results.—The significant increase in macrophage PGE_2 production was completely avoided in animals receiving NS-398. Mice receiving this COX-2 inhibitor also showed increased WBC counts (mean, 7,866 vs. 4,288/mm^3) and increased ANCs (3,663 vs. 1,068/mm^3). NS-398 also reduced macrophage depression of hematopoietic proliferation. Forty-six percent of mice receiving NS-398 survived, whereas none of those receiving placebo did (Fig 6).

Conclusions.—In this animal model of burn infection, treatment with the selective COX-2 inhibitor NS-398 inhibited macrophage PGE_2 production, preserved the ANC, and improved survival. The findings suggest a potential role for NS-398 in the treatment of neutropenic patients with sepsis. The mechanism of increased survival may involve protective effects of WBC production, particularly neutrophils.

▶ The therapeutic strategy shown to improve survival in this murine burn-plus-infection model takes advantage of recent advances in cellular and molecular biology. This article was chosen for that reason and to illustrate how basic science advances are leading to the development of potential therapeutic agents. To illustrate: It appears clear that PGE_2 plays a role in burn- and trauma-induced immunosuppression and thus may predispose to infection. Although nonsteroidal anti-inflammatory drugs (NSAIDs) can inhibit PGE_2 production, they are associated with potentially significant side effects, including gastric and renal toxicity. These side effects have limited the use of NSAIDs in clinical sepsis trials. Recent recognition that basal levels of PGE_2 are under the control of the enzyme COX-1, while inflammatory and injury-induced increases in PGE_2 are due to the activity of the COX-2 enzyme, allows one to inhibit the increased production of PGE_2 by selectively inhibiting COX-2 with selective drugs. Since these agents do not inhibit COX-1, side effects due to the total inhibition of PGE_2 are prevented. Strategies such as those used in this study have significant clinical potential and are likely to become more common in the future. Thus, it is important for clinicians to become familiar with this clinical approach.

E.A. Deitch, M.D.

Reduction in Mortality in Pediatric Patients With Inhalation Injury With Aerosolized Heparin/*N*-acetylcysteine Therapy

Desai MH, Mlcak R, Richardson J, et al (Univ of Texas, Galveston; Shriners Burns Inst, Galveston, Tex)

J Burn Care Rehabil 19:210-212, 1998 3–8

Purpose.—Smoke inhalation injury is a major cause of death after burns. These injuries are associated with fibrin cast deposition in the airways, as well as progressive carbon dioxide retention resulting from a ball-valve effect. Conventional treatment for these injuries focuses on reducing arterial carbon dioxide, maintaining airway patency, and ensuring adequate oxygenation. Based on promising results in animal studies, a combination of aerosolized heparin and acetylcysteine was evaluated for the treatment of smoke inhalation injury in children.

Methods.—Ninety consecutive children with burns and inhalation injury treated during a 10-year period were studied. In each case, inhalation injury was confirmed by bronchoscopy and was severe enough to require ventilatory support. Forty-seven children treated in the latter part of the experience were treated with aerosolized heparin and acetylcysteine. Every 4 hours for the first 7 days post burn, these patients received aerosolized heparin, 5,000 U, and aerosolized acetylcysteine 20% solution, 3 mL. The results were compared with those of 43 children treated in the initial part of the experience, who received conventional therapy. In both groups, the children remained intubated until they could maintain a PaO_2/FIO_2 ratio of greater than 400 on their own.

Results.—Six percent of the children receiving aerosolized heparin/acetylcysteine required reintubation for progressive respiratory failure, compared with 28% of those receiving conventional therapy. The rate of atelectasis was 43% vs. 70%, respectively. Mortality was 4% in the heparin/acetylcysteine group vs. 19% in the control group (Table 2).

TABLE 2.—Results (n = 90)

Characteristics	Control Group (n = 43) Mean	±	SD	Treatment Group (n = 47) Mean	±	SD
Ventilator (hrs)	187		79	81		93
Reintubation rate	12/43		28%	3/47		6%*
Mortality	8/43		19%	2/47		4%*
Atelectasis	30/43		69%	20/47		42%*

*$P < 0.05$.

(Courtesy of Desai MH, Mlcak R, Richardson J, et al: Reduction in mortality in pediatric patients with inhalation injury with aerosolized heparin/N-acetylcysteine therapy. *J Burn Care Rehabil* 19:210-212, 1998.)

Conclusions.—Aerosolized heparin/acetylcysteine therapy appears to improve outcomes for burned children with inhalation injury. Compared with conventional therapy, this new regimen reduces mortality, atelectasis, and the need for reintubation because of progressive pulmonary failure. This treatment effectively addresses the pathophysiologic mechanics of inhalation injury by reducing free radical ions and inhibiting fibrin cast formation.

► This clinical study indicating that survival in pediatric burn patients with inhalation injury can be improved by the use of aerosolized heparin and acetylcysteine, reinforces the concept that basic science studies in animals can lead to improved clinical care. During the last decade, these authors have intensively investigated the pathophysiology of inhalation injury and tried a myriad of potential agents in their animal models of smoke inhalation injury. The results of these experimental studies implicated oxygen radical formation and fibrin plugging as 2 key factors leading to respiratory failure after smoke inhalation. Consequently, they used a clinical therapeutic regimen that addresses the pathophysiology of inhalation injury. The only weakness of the study is that it was retrospective and used historical controls. Nonetheless, the clinical results are impressive and based on these results, I know that I will be using an aerosolized cocktail of heparin and acetylcysteine in my patients.

E.A. Deitch, M.D.

Effect of Cutaneous Burn Injury and Resuscitation on the Cerebral Circulation in an Ovine Model

Shin C, Kinsky MP, Thomas JA, et al (Univ of Texas, Galveston; Yonsei Univ, Seoul, Korea)

Burns 24:39-45, 1998 3–9

Background.—Altered consciousness, delirium, hallucinations, or seizures can occur in adults or children with major or minor burns. However, the cerebral hemodynamic effects underlying this burn-induced encephalopathy remain unclear. A study was performed in sheep to examine the effects of a major burn and resuscitation on the cerebral circulation.

Methods.—A 70% total body surface scald injury was induced in 8 anesthetized sheep. The animals received 30 minutes of resuscitation with Ringer's lactate, titrated to restore and maintain baseline oxygen delivery values. This protocol was designed to mimic current burn resuscitation practices. Assessments of intracranial pressure, cerebral perfusion pressure, brain water content, and brain blood flow were obtained with vascular catheters, a urinary catheter, and a Richmond bolt.

Results.—During resuscitation, the animals showed normal blood pressure, cardiac output, and urine output. Intracranial pressure increased gradually from 10.6 to 17.0 mm Hg, and cerebral perfusion pressure fell from 86.4 to 64.1 mm Hg. Early in the course of resuscitation, the animals' cerebrovascular resistance decreased to levels associated with maintenance of brain blood flow and oxygen delivery at baseline levels or greater. Six hours after injury, the sheep had an inappropriate increase in cerebrovascular resistance at a time of reduced cerebral perfusion pressure. This led to reductions to one half of baseline values in brain blood flow.

Conclusions.—This ovine model shows reduced cerebral perfusion pressure immediately after major cutaneous burn, and again after 6 hours of resuscitation. Though blood flow to the brain is maintained by cerebral autoregulation in the early phase after injury, blood flow fails after the development of brain edema and elevated intracranial pressure. More study is needed to establish the clinical significance of these findings, and to investigate resuscitation regimens that reduce postburn cerebral edema and maintain normal hemodynamics.

► It is clear that a number of burn patients develop encephalopathy even though they have no evidence of head injuries. It is also clear that a number of burn patients manifest subtle and rarely overt personality changes or changes in mental abilities that generally improve over time. Why these CNS changes occur, however, is far from clear. It has been widely assumed, but not proved, that the acute changes in mental status represent a type of metabolic encephalopathy, whereas the later personality changes represent a type of posttrauma stress disorder. The elegant basic physiologic study described in this article indicates that decreased cerebral blood flow may be contributing to the postburn CNS syndromes. Based on these experimental observations, burn injury, by decreasing cerebral blood flow and thus oxygen delivery, could lead to a type of hypoxic encephalopathy. If these results are verified in clinical studies, they would provide an explanation to the perplexing etiology of postburn changes in CNS function. Furthermore, by providing a physiologic explanation for burn-induced changes in mental status, this article opens the way for therapeutic approaches directed at preserving cerebral blood flow.

E.A. Deitch, M.D.

Interrelationship Between Immunocompetent and Structural Cells in Post-burn Scars

Stella M, Castagnoli C, Trombotto C, et al (CTO, Via Zuretti, Torino, Italy; Piedmont Found of Studies and Research in Burns; Ctr for Immunogenetics and Experimental Oncology, CNR, Turin, Italy)

Eur J Plast Surg 21:8-13, 1998 3–10

Introduction.—The development of hypertrophic scarring may involve various immunologic factors. Hypertrophic scars show a pattern of progressive change, with a variable active phase followed by a period of remission. The factors responsible for this pattern are uncertain, as are the prospects for manipulating these factors for therapeutic benefit. A series of morphological studies were performed to gain insight into the pathophysiology of hypertrophic scarring after burns.

Findings.—In the active phase, hypertrophic scars were characterized by abundant lymphocytic infiltrates. Seventy percent of these infiltrates were activated T cells, compared with just 30% activated T cells in normotrophic scars. The activated T cells produced various cytokines, producing anomalous expression of activation markers in the keratinocytes and fibroblasts of hypertrophic tissue. Markers observed included HLA-DR, intercellular adhesion molecule-1, CD36, and interleukin-2R. Of the various cytokines analyzed, interferon-γ (IFN-γ) was the only one to show a change during the remission phase of hypertrophic scarring (Fig 3). Lym-

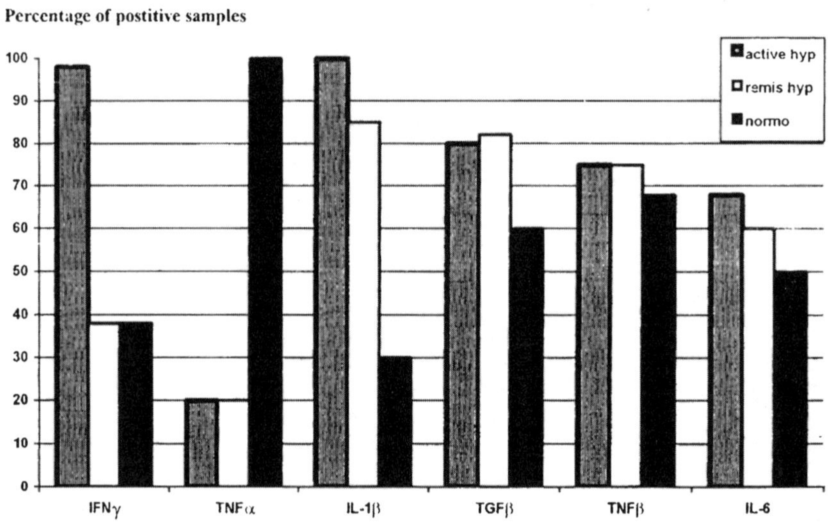

FIGURE 3.—Percentage of positive samples of active (n = 25), remission hypertrophic scars (n = 15), and normotrophic scars (n = 10) for the presence of different cytokines using immunoperoxidase technique and specific monoclonal antibodies. (Courtesy of Stella M, Castagnoli C, Trombotto C, et al: Interrelationship between immunocompetent and structural cells in post-burn scars. *Eur J Plast Surg* 21:8-13. Copyright 1998, Springer-Verlag.)

phocytes in the active phase showed high levels of IFN-γ expression, compared with those in the remission phase and control specimens.

Conclusions.—Hypertrophic scars show a highly complex pattern of interactions between cells, various mediators, and the cytokine network. Thus, many different pathways may be involved in the pathogenesis of these abnormal scars. The new findings suggest that IFN-γ and its receptor play a functional role in amplifying and terminating the hypertrophic state in postburn scars.

▶ Burn scars that become hypertrophic go through a series of phases. The first phase occurs shortly after the burn heals, where the wound is hypopigmented and erythematous, but flat. During the next few weeks to months, the burn becomes more elevated, red, thick, and painful. Finally, during the subsequent months to years, the burn matures, becomes softer, and to some extent, flattens out. However, all too often the net result is not cosmetically and at times functionally acceptable. Why does this process occur? Unfortunately, the answer is not known, although one hypothesis is that the burn wound becomes hypertrophic because of an uncontrolled local immunologic response. This was the hypothesis that this study was testing.

The authors' findings that active hypertrophic burn wounds have an increased number of activated lymphocytes and a different cytokine pattern than normal skin or even burn wounds in remission, support the notion that immunologic factors are involved in this process. Because IFN-γ is elevated when hypertrophic scars are active, and normal when these scars are in remission, it appears that this cytokine may be causally involved in this process. If so, it may be possible to modulate the extent of postburn hypertrophic scar formation by decreasing IFN-γ levels. This is a potentially exciting observation, because hypertrophic scar formation is one of the major unsolved problems in burn care.

E.A. Deitch, M.D.

Local Anesthetics Improve Dermal Perfusion After Burn Injury

Jönsson A, Brofeldt BT, Nellgård P, et al (Göteborg Univ, Sweden; Univ of California, Davis, Sacramento)

J Burn Care Rehabil 19:50-56, 1998 3–11

Background.—Studies have shown that amide local anesthetics inhibit the release of various inflammatory mediators involved in the pathophysiology of burns. They have also been shown to reduce activity in various inflammatory conditions. At certain concentrations, local anesthetics can also increase skin perfusion.

Methods.—The effect of topical and systemic administration of amide local anesthetics on dermal perfusion after deep partial-thickness skin burn injury was assessed with laser Doppler flowmetry. Burn injury was induced in the abdominal skin of anesthetized rats. In the first set of experiments, study rats were treated with a topical lidocaine-prilocaine cream (EMLA) (5%) for 6 hours beginning 5 minutes after the burn injury was induced. Control rats were treated with a placebo cream. In the second set of experiments, study rats were treated with IV lidocaine (2 mg/kg), then continuous IV lidocaine at a rate of 50, 100, or 150 μg/kg/min for 6 hours beginning 5 minutes after burn injury. Control rats were treated with saline solution.

Results.—In the first set of experiments, control animals had significantly reduced skin perfusion within an hour of burn injury, with further reduction occurring in the next 5 hours. Study animals treated with the lidocaine-prilocaine cream had significantly increased skin perfusion in the first 30 minutes after the burn injury as compared with before the burn injury. This was followed by a decrease in perfusion to levels lower than before the burn injury but significantly higher than levels in control animals in the first hour after burn injury. In study animals, skin perfusion slowly recovered to preburn levels by the end of the experiment. In the second set of experiments, animals treated with lidocaine had significantly improved skin perfusion in a dose-response fashion as compared with control animals. Maximum improvement in dermal perfusion was induced by IV lidocaine at a rate of 150 μg/kg/min as compared with burned control animals treated with saline solution.

Discussion.—The results in this rat model show that topical or systemic administration of local anesthetics can prevent progressive dermal ischemia after deep partial-thickness burn injury. This may result from direct action on the vasculature or indirectly through inhibition of various mediators of the inflammatory process.

► After a burn occurs, there is a progressive decrease in burn wound blood flow, resulting in progressive dermal ischemia and deepening of the burn. In cases of moderate partial-thickness burns, this progressive dermal ischemia may result in the conversion of a burn that might heal without significant scarring to one that heals with a hypertrophic scar. In deeper partial-thickness burns, progressive dermal ischemia may ultimately result in a full-thickness injury. Consequently, a lot of energy has been invested in studies designed to clarify the biology of postburn progressive dermal ischemia and to test potentially protective agents. The idea that administering a local anesthetic to the burn wound can reduce the degree of subsequent dermal ischemia is fascinating. For those who are interested in potential mechanisms, local anesthetics might improve dermal blood flow in 3 basic ways: (1) by inhibiting the release of vasospastic substances from sensory nerves; (2) by inhibiting neutrophil recruitment into the burn wound and limiting the release of toxic substances from neutrophils that do reach the burn wound; and (3) by decreasing the production of vasoactive and immunoinflammatory prostaglandins and leukotrienes.

Wouldn't it be nice if it was possible to reduce the depth of a burn wound by the administration of a substance that also decreases pain? Although dose considerations make it unlikely that lidocaine can be used for this purpose clinically, hopefully other agents will be found that can be used clinically.

E.A. Deitch, M.D.

The Unna 'Sleeve': An Effective Postoperative Dressing for Pediatric Arm Burns

Nakamura DY, Gibran NS, Mann R, et al (Univ of Washington, Seattle)
J Burn Care Rehabil 19:349-351, 1998 3–12

Objective.—With time-consuming, labor-intensive, and painful dressing changes, postoperative management of sheet grafts in children poses difficult problems. A plan was developed that would protect the grafts after surgery while eliminating the need for daily wound care. Based on good results with Unna boots after leg grafts, they evaluated the use of Unna "sleeves" for the postoperative care of children with skin grafts of the arms.

Methods.—The technique was evaluated in 11 children with a total of 13 arm burns. The burns were managed with excision and sheet grafting, with a total grafted area of 1% to 5% of total body surface area. The grafts were secured with Steri-Strips or sutures and covered with a layer of greasy gauze. This was followed by an Unna paste dressing, consisting of 3 to 5 layers of Unna paste applied in a spiral fashion. The Unna sleeve was covered with an elastic bandage and was left in place for an average of 6 days. Eight arms had a second Unna sleeve applied, to be removed about 1 week later.

Results.—The Unna sleeve avoided the need for additional graft wound care in all 13 extremities. The graft take rate was 100%, with no reconstructive surgery required. Avoiding graft dressing changes obviated the need for extended hospitalization, saved staff time, and reduced expenses for dressing supplies. Patient anxiety appeared to be reduced as well.

Conclusions.—This Unna sleeve technique provides an effective postoperative dressing for pediatric arm burns. It provides gentle, uniform pressure while protecting the grafts against mechanical shearing. The authors have extended this technique for use in their adult patients and outpatients as well.

▶ This practical article was chosen to illustrate a relatively pain-free method of treating patients who have had skin grafts. Not only does it decrease patient pain and postoperative work, but it allows patients to avoid hospitalizations. These authors have previously described this technique for lower extremity skin grafts. Try it. It works.

E.A. Deitch, M.D.

4 Trauma

Introduction

All of us are familiar with aphorisms like "men are from Mars and women are from Venus," but did you know that females appear to be more resistant to trauma-induced immune suppression and sepsis than men? They are, as shown by articles included in this chapter as well as in the chapter on Critical Care. The reason for this increased susceptibility to trauma-induced immune dysfunction is testosterone. Thus, it appears that too much testosterone can not only predispose one to trauma but can also adversely affect the immune response.

A whole range of important studies evaluating the accuracy and clinical value of new generations of CT scanners in trauma patients have been published this past year. Several have been selected, including the multi-institutional study by Livingston (Abstract 4–2) showing that patients with blunt abdominal trauma and a negative abdominal CT and no other reasons for hospital admission can be safely sent home from the emergency department. This study was chosen because it dispels the myth that patients with blunt abdominal trauma should be routinely admitted and observed in the hospital for 24 to 48 hours. Two articles chosen (Abstracts 4–3 and 4–4) demonstrate that the new spiral CT scans are extremely accurate in helping identify which patients with abnormal chest radiographs have aortic injuries. In fact, the sensitivity of spiral CT scans is so good that only patients with suspicious spiral CT scans require aortography. CT scanning has even been shown to be accurate enough to be used as a diagnostic modality for the triage of hemodynamically stable patients with gunshot wounds of the abdomen and flank. Although not clinically mature, as shown by the article by Bowersox (Abstract 4–6), advances in imaging have improved to the point that remote telemetry is being tested for battlefield use.

Few would disagree that optimal care is based on the combination of good clinical judgment, technical expertise, and a thorough understanding of the host's response to injury. However, the best clinical approach to certain injuries remains controversial. One such controversy concerns the operative management of patients with penetrating rectal injuries. Consequently, included in this year's selections is a prospective randomized clinical trial (Abstract 4–7) indicating that presacral drainage of rectal injuries is not mandatory. Another area of controversy has been the exact role of angiography in patients with penetrating extremity injuries and no hard signs of vascular injury. Based on the study by Dennis et al. (Abstract 4–8) and the recent literature, this controversy appears to be resolved. That is, in the absence of hard signs of vascular injury on physical examination, angiography is not required, because less than 2% of patients will have a significant vascular injury. In treating patients with solid organ abdominal injuries, as reflected in the evolution of the management of splenic injuries, support for the "less is more" approach continues to expand. In fact, over the last decade, there has been a progressive shift from operative to nonoperative management of a number of traumatic injuries. Thus, it was a pleasure to include a prospective randomized clinical trial (Abstract 4–10) documenting that an early thorascopic operative approach to patients with retained hemothoraces improves outcome and is superior to the repeated placement of chest tubes.

A series of articles dealing with the lung, either directly or indirectly, were chosen because pulmonary problems continue to have a major influence on morbidity and mortality. The first of these articles (Abstract 4–11) demonstrates that early tracheostomy is clearly beneficial and is an effective strategy for decreasing ventilator and ICU days. Because the diagnosis of pneumonia is especially difficult in intubated trauma patients, a prospective study by Croce et al. (Abstract 4–12) was chosen which provides critical information supporting the use of bronchoalveolar lavage (BAL) as an accurate method of diagnosing pneumonia. The next two abstracts (Abstracts 4–13 and 4–14) deal with the pathogenesis of trauma-induced lung injury and methods of prevention. The first study is an experimental study investigating the relationship between gut injury and distant organ (lung) injury. The results of this study suggest that gut barrier failure after hemorrhagic shock leads to lung injury via the release of gut-derived toxic factors into the intestinal lymphatics rather than the portal blood. Since intestinal lymph enters the blood stream through the thoracic duct, the lung is the first organ exposed to these toxic intestinally derived factors. The importance of this basic science paper is that it provides insight into the controversy of the role of the gut in the pathogenesis of acute respiratory distress syndrome. Indirect support for this concept of gut-driven distant organ failure comes from a clinical study in trauma patients showing that therapy directed at improving gastric mucosal pH reduces the incidence of multiple organ failure.

Lastly, several miscellaneous articles of interest were chosen that deal with a wide range of issues, including the topics of missed injuries, the potentially deleterious effects of early fracture fixture in patients with head injuries, methods of providing temporary coverage for patients with an open abdomen, and the first randomized trial of human polymerized hemoglobin as a blood substitute in patients with trauma.

Edwin A. Deitch, M.D.

Testosterone and/or Low Estradiol: Normally Required but Harmful Immunologically for Males After Trauma-Hemorrhage

Angele MK, Ayala A, Monfils BA, et al (Brown Univ, Providence, RI; Rhode Island Hosp, Providence)

J Trauma: Injury Infect Crit Care 44:78-85, 1998 4–1

Introduction.—There is clinical and epidemiologic evidence to suggest sex differences in susceptibility to and morbidity from sepsis. Severe hemorrhage leads to marked depression of immune function in males but not in females. This effect is prevented by prehemorrhage androgen depletion in male mice. This study sought to determine whether testosterone is responsible for the depressed immune response to trauma-hemorrhage in males.

Methods.—Experiments were performed in female C3H/HeN mice. The animals underwent 20 days of treatment with 5α-dihydrotestosterone (DHT) or vehicle. They were then subjected to either sham operation or laparotomy and hemorrhagic shock to a blood pressure of 35 mm Hg for 90 minutes. Both groups received adequate fluid resuscitation. Two groups of untreated male mice were studied as well; one group underwent hemorrhagic shock followed by resuscitation, and the other had sham operations only.

Results.—The DHT-treated female mice showed a rise in DHT level and a drop in estradiol level to levels similar to those observed in untreated male animals. Hemorrhage led to no depression of macrophage function in vehicle-treated females. This was not the case in DHT-treated females, which showed significantly reduced splenic and peritoneal macrophage IL-1 and IL-6 production. These effects were similar to those observed in macrophages from bled male mice.

Conclusions.—The immune depression in response to trauma-hemorrhage in male mice appears to result from high levels of testosterone, low levels of estradiol, or both. The findings suggest the possibility of hormonal treatments (i.e., testosterone-receptor blocking agents such as flutamide or estradiol) to prevent immune depression in male trauma patients.

▶ As reviewed in this study, multiple clinical and epidemiologic studies of patients with sepsis documented that males have higher morbidity and mortality rates than females and that this difference is not due to differences in severity of the septic state. Although interesting, this phenomenon was largely ignored until recently, when this group began a series of studies testing the hypothesis that males are more susceptible than females to injury-induced immune suppression. This article is of value because it provides further information that sex hormones can influence outcome. Perhaps, as suggested by the authors, hormonal therapy will ultimately be used clinically in males to reduce the risk of infection. The idea is intriguing.

E.A. Deitch, M.D.

Admission or Observation Is Not Necessary After a Negative Abdominal Computed Tomographic Scan in Patients With Suspected Blunt Abdominal Trauma: Results of a Prospective, Multi-institutional Trial

Livingston DH, Lavery RF, Passannante MR, et al (Case Western Reserve Univ, Cleveland, Ohio; Univ of Tennessee, Memphis; Univ of New Mexico, Albuquerque)

J Trauma: Injury Infect Crit Care 44:273-282, 1998 4–2

Objective.—Patients with blunt abdominal trauma who do not require emergent surgery are generally hospitalized for 24 to 48 hours of observation, despite the absence of serious demonstrable injuries and the performance of diagnostic studies that exclude intra-abdominal injury. This study prospectively evaluated the ability of abdominal CT to identify patients with minimal blunt abdominal trauma who do not require observation.

Methods.—The 22-month study included 2,299 consecutive patients with blunt abdominal trauma seen at 4 level I trauma centers. All patients underwent physical examination in the emergency department, followed by abdominal CT. The patients were admitted for observation, with outcomes measured at 20 hours.

Results.—Sixty-one percent of the patients had abdominal tenderness or bruising. However, only 22% had a positive CT scan (i.e., showing visceral injury or intraperitoneal fluid). The initial abdominal CT scan had a negative predictive value of 99.63%, based on the subsequent need for celiotomy among all patients who fully completed the study protocol.

Conclusions.—Contrary to usual practice, hospital observation is not required for all patients with blunt abdominal trauma. If an abdominal CT scan is negative, there is no benefit from hospitalization and observation. The physical examination finding of abdominal tenderness does not predict the presence of abdominal injury.

▶ This prospective multi-institutional study was selected because it successfully challenges the common but scientifically unfounded clinical practice of the routine admission of patients with blunt abdominal trauma for observation. On the basis of this study, no longer is it necessary to admit patients with blunt abdominal trauma if the CT scan is negative. That you can send these patients home is the take-home message of this excellent clinical study of more than 3,000 patients sustaining blunt abdominal trauma. The cost savings and the savings in terms of workload are tremendous.

E.A. Deitch, M.D.

Use of Spiral Computed Tomography for the Assessment of Blunt Trauma Patients With Potential Aortic Injury

Mirvis SE, Shanmuganathan K, Buell J, et al (Univ of Maryland, Baltimore)

J Trauma: Injury Infect Crit Care 45:922-930, 1998 4–3

Objective.—There is ongoing debate regarding the accuracy of thoracic CT in evaluation of patients with possible traumatic aortic injury (TAI). Because it offers fewer artifacts and better image quality, fast-spiral CT might be useful for the detection of TAIs. The use of contrast-enhanced spinal thoracic CT (CEST-CT) for the detection of TAI in patients with blunt thoracic trauma was studied.

Methods.—The investigators saw 7,286 patients with acute blunt trauma over a 2-year period. CEST-CT was performed on 1,014 patients (14% of the total) who had abnormal mediastinal contours on their admission chest radiographs or for whom technically acceptable chest radiographs were not obtained. The scans were evaluated for the presence and location of mediastinal hemorrhage, as well as pseudoaneurysm and other direct signs of aortic injury. The CEST-CT findings were compared with those of aortography or surgery, if performed, or with the patient's discharge status.

Results.—Mediastinal hemorrhage was seen on 10.7% of the CEST-CT scans. Of this group, 20.3% also had direct CT evidence of aortic injury. Thus, 2.2% of all 1,014 patients had direct evidence of aortic injury on CEST-CT. In each case, the injury was found in the proximal descending thoracic aorta. CEST-CT had a sensitivity of 100%, based on clinical follow-up. Specificity was 99.7%, positive predictive value 89%, negative predictive value 100%, and accuracy 99.7%.

Conclusions.—Spiral CT is a highly accurate imaging technique for the detection of TAI in patients with blunt trauma. It is useful in the detection and localization of blood within the mediastinum, as well as direct evidence of aortic injury. This technique offers a specific new approach to selecting blunt trauma patients for thoracic angiography.

▶ Advances in imaging technology allow us to better see what is inside the black box. This article showing the utility of spiral CT in the diagnosis of blunt aortic injuries illustrates that the newest generations of spiral-CT scanners are not only faster but also provide more accurate images. Based on the accepted difficulty in diagnosing an aortic injury on clinical or radiographic evidence, aortography has evolved into the diagnostic gold standard in patients with suspected aortic injuries. However, aortography has several disadvantages. It is invasive, requires the presence of an invasive radiologist and keeping the patient in the angiography suite for prolonged periods of time, and is frequently not feasible in the unstable patient with multiple injuries. Spiral CT has none of these limitations and is likely to replace aortography in all but the rare patient. At my institution, with the use of spiral

CT, aortography has gone from the diagnostic test of choice to a confirmatory test.

E.A. Deitch, M.D.

Prospective Study of Blunt Aortic Injury: Helical CT Is Diagnostic and Antihypertensive Therapy Reduces Rupture

Fabian TC, Davis KA, Gavant ML, et al (Univ of Tennessee, Memphis)
Ann Surg 227:666-677, 1998 4–4

Introduction.—If aortic rupture occurs in patients with blunt aortic injury (BAI), the result can be immediate death. Conventional chest CT is not effective in recognizing BAI, but helical CT—which offers faster scanning and better resolution—may be useful for this purpose. There is evidence to suggest that antihypertensive medication may help to prevent aortic rupture. Helical CT of the thorax (HCTT) was evaluated for use in the diagnosis of BAI. In addition, β-blockers—with or without nitroprusside—were evaluated for efficacy in the prevention of aortic rupture in BAI.

Methods.—The 4-year prospective study included 494 patients with significant blunt torso trauma. All underwent HCTT. In the first year of the study, aortography was performed in patients whose HCTT scan suggested mediastinal abnormalities. In the latter 3 years, aortography was performed only in patients whose HCTT findings suggest BAI, excluding those with mediastinal hematomas without direct evidence of aortic injury.

When aortic injury was suspected, a protocol of IV β-blockers was started, with nitroprusside added if needed to achieve a satisfactory blood pressure. This treatment was evaluated for its ability to prevent rupture before aortic repair, or to permit delayed aortic repair in patients with significant associated injuries.

TABLE 5.—Results of Helical CT of the Thorax (*HCTT*) and Aortography for the Diagnosis of Blunt Aortic Injury in 494 Study Patients

	HCTT		Aortography
True positive	71		56
True negative	353		201
False positive	70		2
Indeterminate		65	
"Aortic injury"		5	
False negative	0		5
Sensitivity	100%		92%
Specificity	83%		99%
Accuracy	86%		97%
Positive predictive value	50%		97%
Negative predictive value	100%		97%

HCTT = helical computed tomography of the thorax.

(Courtesy of Fabian TC, Davis KA, Gavant ML, et al: Prospective study of blunt aortic injury: Helical CT is diagnostic and antihypertensive therapy reduces rupture. *Ann Surg* 227:666-677, 1998.)

Results.—Seventy-one patients (14%) had BAI diagnosed. Helical CT of the thorax had a sensitivity of 100%, specificity of 83%, accuracy of 86%, positive predictive value of 50%, and negative predictive value of 100%. Values for aortography were 92% sensitivity, 99% specificity, 97% accuracy, 97% positive predictive value, and 97% negative predictive value (Table 5). There were no cases of spontaneous aortic rupture.

Conclusions.—Patients with blunt torso trauma who have no direct evidence of BAI on HCTT scanning do not need to undergo aortography. If the results of HCTT are indeterminate, aortography can be done. The use of HCTT for early diagnosis, coupled with antihypertensive treatment for patients with suspected aortic injury, minimizes the risk of aortic rupture and allows aortic repair to be delayed in patients with significant associated injuries.

► A common problem in patients with blunt trauma is determining whether they have an aortic injury. Because of the insensitivities of chest x-rays and conventional CTs, most trauma centers use aortograms as their major diagnostic test of choice, although some use transesophageal echocardiograms. While accurate, aortography is invasive, can be very time-consuming, and requires moving the patient to the angiography suite. Thus, if a screening test could be found that either obviated the need for routine aortography or reduced the number of patients in whom aortography was required, that would be good. The value of this prospective clinical trial is that helical CT may be such a test, especially because no aortic injuries were missed when findings on helical CT were negative. Furthermore, performing a helical CT of the thorax is quick and, in a patient undergoing an abdominal examination, adds less than a minute of extra time. Thus, if other clinical trials confirm these results, it is likely that helical scanning of the aorta will replace aortography as the initial screening test. However, because of the relatively high number of indeterminate tests with helical scanning, it is unlikely to totally replace aortography.

E.A. Deitch, M.D.

The Role of Computed Tomography in Selective Management of Gunshot Wounds to the Abdomen and Flank

Ginzburg E, Carrillo EH, Kopelman T, et al (Univ of Miami, Fla)

J Trauma: Injury Infect Crit Care 45:1005-1009, 1998 4–5

Background.—Although acceptance of the change in practice has been slow, surgery is no longer regarded as mandatory for all patients with penetrating abdominal trauma. With dynamic helical CT, it is possible to accurately assess projectile trajectory and the presence of intra-abdominal injuries. This retrospective study evaluated the accuracy of CT in the selective management of patients with gunshot wounds to the abdomen and flank.

Methods and Findings.—The review included 83 patients undergoing initial CT evaluation for gunshot wounds of the flank or abdomen. The CT scan showed no signs of peritoneal penetration in 53 patients, whereas another 15 had evidence of either peritoneal penetration or hepatic injury. There were no false negative CT results among these patients. The CT evidence of peritoneal penetration was questionable in 15 patients; 11 underwent endoscopy, and 3 had laparoscopy. The remaining patient was initially observed but eventually required surgery for a missed colonic injury. When equivocal CT findings were followed by cavitary endoscopy, sensitivity, specificity, positive and negative predictive value, and overall accuracy were all 100%.

Conclusions.—For properly selected, hemodynamically stable patients with gunshot wounds to the abdomen, initial screening with CT can determine the presence or absence of intraperitoneal penetration. If there is no peritoneal penetration, or if nonbleeding liver injuries are found, nonoperative management is safe. If peritoneal penetration is questionable, cavitary endoscopy should be performed. These preliminary results await confirmation in randomized, prospective trials.

▶ As the resolution of newer generations of CT scanners has improved, so has the ability to accurately determine the trajectory of penetrating missiles and the presence of intra-abdominal injuries. As shown in this clinical study, with today's availability of helical CT scanners, it now appears possible to identify a subgroup of patients with gunshot wounds to the abdomen and flank who can be safely managed nonoperatively. Candidates for this protocol of nonoperative management include patients with low-risk gunshot wounds (i.e., hemodynamically stable patients with tangential injuries and no peritoneal signs) and a screening dynamic, triple-contast helical CT scan that does not show evidence of intra-abdominal injury.

Although these patients represent only a modest-sized subgroup of patients with gunshot wounds to the abdomen or flank, avoiding an unnecessary laparotomy is well worthwhile from both the patient's and the hospital's perspective. The patient avoids the pain and potential complications of a laparotomy, and the hospital saves money. Thus, in view of several studies such as this one and my own good experiences with the use of helical CT scans to avoid surgery in low-risk patients with gunshot wounds, I believe that the traditional surgical aphorism that "gunshot wounds of the abdomen mandate abdominal exploration" no longer holds true. It is possible to avoid surgery in these low-risk patients with the use of CT scanning.

E.A. Deitch, M.D.

Use of an Intuitive Telemanipulator System for Remote Trauma Surgery: An Experimental Study

Bowersox JC, Cordts PR, LaPorta AJ (Stanford Univ, Calif; Tripler Regional Med Ctr, Honolulu, Hawaii; Evans Army Community Hosp, Colorado Springs, Colo)

J Am Coll Surg 186:615-621, 1998 4–6

Background.—Ninety percent of battlefield deaths occur before the casualty reaches definitive care, a figure consistent with the high fatality rate associated with penetrating truncal injuries. The U.S. Department of

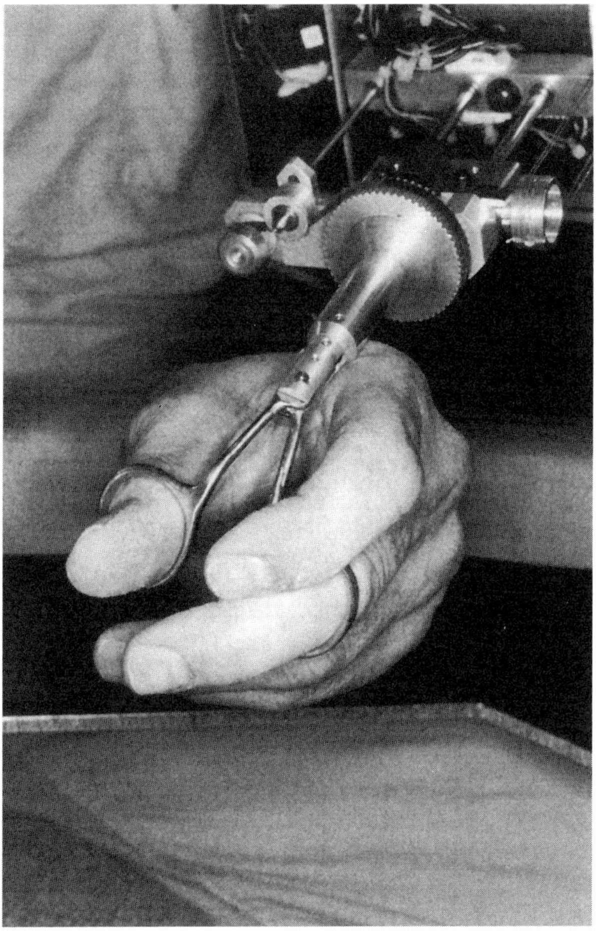

FIGURE 2.—Standard surgical instrument handle attached to a robotic manipulator arm at the surgeon's console. Hand motions are transmitted precisely to instrument tips on identical manipulator arms at the remote patient unit. (Courtesy of Bowersox JC, Cordts PR, LaPorta AJ: Use of an intuitive telemanipulator system for remote trauma surgery: An experimental study. *J Am Coll Surg* 186:615-621, 1998. By permission of the American College of Surgeons.)

Defense is interested in developing a robotic surgical telemanipulator system that surgeons could use to operate on patients at distant locations. A prototype telesurgical system is described.

Methods and Results.—The 4-degrees-of-freedom telemanipulator system included visual, auditory, and haptic devices that allowed the surgeon to see, hear, and feel the operative field. Instrument handles were connected to robotic manipulator arms at the surgeon's workstation (Fig 2). The surgeon's movements were transmitted to instrument tips attached to the telemanipulator arm at the remote patient site. The workstation and remote unit were connected by coaxial cables, with the potential of being separated by more than 200 meters. Using this system, surgeons performed surgical procedures on anesthetized swine at remote sites. Gastrotomy closures were successfully performed remotely, although it took nearly 3 times longer than normal. Other attempted procedures, including cholecystectomies, control of hemorrhage from liver lacerations, and enterotomy closures, were successfully performed. With force feedback and stereoscopic video, the surgeons found that the telesurgery system offered intuitive performance. However, procedures could be successfully carried out even without these sensory cues.

Conclusions.—This study demonstrates a prototype surgical telemanipulator for use in performing remote surgical procedures. This system permits intuitive telesurgery and complex manipulations, although with greatly prolonged operative times. This technology is unlikely to find practical application in trauma management anytime soon; however, surgical telemanipulator systems are already under development for use in minimally invasive therapy and educational applications.

▶ Will courses in computer games and video simulators become required topics in the education of medical students and residents? Maybe. This article was chosen to illustrate what the future may hold for surgeons. Although this system is not practical for providing operative trauma care in the field, it does hold promise as an educational tool and as a method for expanding laparoscopic surgery. Because several companies are working on similar types of systems for use in civilian operating rooms, it may not be too far-fetched to think that systems such as this may be on the horizon. If so, surgeons may need to spend more time playing video games with their children, a task that has distinct secondary gains.

E.A. Deitch, M.D.

The Role of Presacral Drainage in the Management of Penetrating Rectal Injuries

Gonzalez RP, Falimirski ME, Holevar MR (Christ Hosp and Med Ctr, Oak Lawn, Illinois; Univ of Illinois, Chicago)

J Trauma: Injury Infect Crit Care 45:656-661, 1998 4–7

Introduction.—The principles of management of penetrating rectal injuries, concentrating on diverting colostomy and presacral drainage, are based on experience with combat injuries. However, some authors have questioned whether low-velocity injuries in civilian practice might be managed differently. The effect of presacral drainage on infectious complications in patients with penetrating rectal injuries was evaluated in a randomized, prospective trial.

Methods.—Forty-eight patients with penetrating rectal injuries were included in the 45-month study. *Penetrating rectal injuries* are defined as large-bowel injuries occurring distal to the peritoneal reflection. Soon after the rectal injury was detected, the patients were randomized to undergo presacral drainage or no drainage. Ninety-two percent of the injuries were detected using proctoscopy. The study included all patients with rectal injuries; there were no exclusion criteria. Fecal diversion was performed in all patients. Presacral drainage was carried out using closed Jackson-Pratt drainage. The effects of this intervention on the rate of infectious complications was assessed.

Results.—All patients received gunshot wounds. Average age was 26 years for patients assigned to presacral drainage vs. 22 years for those assigned to the nondrainage group. Penetrating Abdominal Trauma Index score was 34.3 for the nondrainage group and 32.4 for the drainage group. There was no significant difference in the incidence of septic complication. Two patients in the drainage group developed abscesses, which were successfully managed using CT-guided drainage. One patient in the nondrainage group developed a rectocutaneous fistula, which resolved after an associated missile fragment was removed.

Conclusions.—This randomized trial found no difference in the infectious complication rate for patients with penetrating rectal injuries managed with or without presacral drainage. Given the mechanisms and severity of civilian injuries of this type, a re-evaluation of their management is warranted. Presacral drainage is an invasive procedure that may be unnecessary.

► Without question, lessons learned during wartime have greatly benefitted civilian trauma victims. However, not all the wartime surgical principles learned in the treatment of high-velocity gunshot injuries are required for the low-velocity gunshot injuries seen in civilian practice. An example in case is the treatment of rectal gunshot injuries. As stressed by the authors, the surgical management of rectal gunshot injuries that emerged after the Vietnam war was based on the following five principles: (1) diversion of the fecal stream via colostomy, (2) débridement and closure of the rectal injury when possible, (3) distal rectal irrigation, (4) presacral drainage, and (5) perioperative antibiotics. While essentially all trauma surgeons agree with diversion of the fecal stream and perioperative antibiotics, the other three principles are more controversial and patient related. For example, most surgeons would débride and repair the rectal injury if it was easy, but many would not perform an extensive dissection to accomplish this goal. The need for distal rectal irrigation and prophylactic presacral drainage is much more controversial. Thus, the value of this prospective, randomized clinical trial showing that presacral drainage does not confer any clinical benefits and rectal irrigation is not necessary. Based on the results of this study, it appears that one can safely omit both of these barbaric customs in most patients; I know I will.

E.A. Deitch, M.D.

Validation of Nonoperative Management of Occult Vascular Injuries and Accuracy of Physical Examination Alone in Penetrating Extremity Trauma: 5- to 10-Year Follow-up

Dennis JW, Frykberg ER, Veldenz HC, et al (Univ of Florida, Jacksonville)

J Trauma: Injury Infect Crit Care 44:243-252, 1998 4–8

Background.—A number of different approaches are used in the management of clinically occult vascular penetrating extremity trauma (PET). Arteriographically detected occult injuries are generally minimal and are easily managed nonoperatively. However, there is continued concern about managing PET solely on the basis of physical examination findings. This long-term follow-up study examined the use of physical examination alone to determine treatment for PET, including the safety and efficacy of nonoperative management for clinically occult arterial injuries.

Methods.—The study compared 2 groups of patients with PET. Group 1, treated from 1986 to 1989, included 43 patients with a total of 44 clinically occult penetrating injuries to the arteries of the extremities, demonstrated by arteriography. However, all patients were free of hard signs of vascular injury and were treated nonoperatively. Group 2, managed from 1989 to 1991, comprised 287 patients with a total of 309 clinically occult arterial injuries. These patients underwent physical examination only. Patient outcomes were evaluated at a mean follow-up of 5 and 9 years, respectively, including physical and ultrasonographic examination if possible.

Results.—The arteriographically identified injuries in group 1 consisted of 21 intimal flaps or irregularities, 19 arterial narrowings, 2 pseudoaneurysms, and 1 arteriovenous fistula. Clinical deterioration required surgery within 1 month in 9% of the patients; good results were achieved in all of them. Follow-up of 18 patients revealed that all were free of symptoms, with normal physical examination results, although ultrasonography revealed mild narrowing in 1 case. Another 6 patients were not examined but had no symptoms of vascular insufficiency and had sought no treatment for vascular problems. In group 2, only 1% of the patients underwent delayed surgery within the first week after PET. Follow-up information was available for 78 patients, none of whom had any vascular symptoms or had sought care for vascular problems.

Conclusions.—The long-term results of a policy of physical examination only in the initial management of PET, with nonoperative management of clinically occult arterial injury, are presented. This policy is safe and effective and may be regarded as a proven standard of care. In everyday trauma center practice, it will reduce costs, conserve personnel and resources, and increase the efficiency of treating associated injuries.

► The goal of this study was to provide long-term follow-up information on the efficacy of physical examination in the diagnosis of vascular injuries as well as the role of nonoperative management of nonocclusive vascular injuries. The main weakness of this study is the relatively low follow-up rates. But, as any one who treats patients with penetrating trauma knows, these patients frequently do not return for follow-up and are difficult or impossible to track down. Nonetheless, the authors make a compelling argument that no more than physical examination is required to determine treatment in patients with penetrating extremity trauma. Their findings, as well as the literature, document that the incidence of vascular injuries in patients without hard physical signs of vascular trauma is only 10% to 15%. Furthermore, only about 10% of patients with occult vascular injuries require surgical repair of their injuries. That is, the false negative or missed injury rate of physical examination is only about 1% to 2% in the absence of hard physical signs (i.e., active hemorrhage, absent distal pulses, large pulsatile or expanding hematoma, distal ischemia, or a bruit or thrill over the wound). Said another way, physical examination is 98% to 99% accurate in excluding a clinically significant injury. In view of the results of this study and the aggregate information in the literature, I agree with the authors that physical examination is a sensitive and accurate way to screen patients with penetrating extremity trauma for vascular injuries and that, in the absence of hard signs on physical examination, no further diagnostic tests are required.

E.A. Deitch, M.D.

Changing Patterns in the Management of Splenic Trauma: The Impact of Nonoperative Management

Pachter HL, Guth AA, Hofstetter SR, et al (New York Univ; Bellevue Hosp Ctr, New York)

Ann Surg 227:708-719, 1998 4–9

Background.—In patients with splenic trauma, either blunt or penetrating, the injured organ is preserved whenever possible. In an 11-year series including 193 patients with splenic injuries, the authors noted that most patients were managed by splenorrhaphy or splenectomy, with only 13%

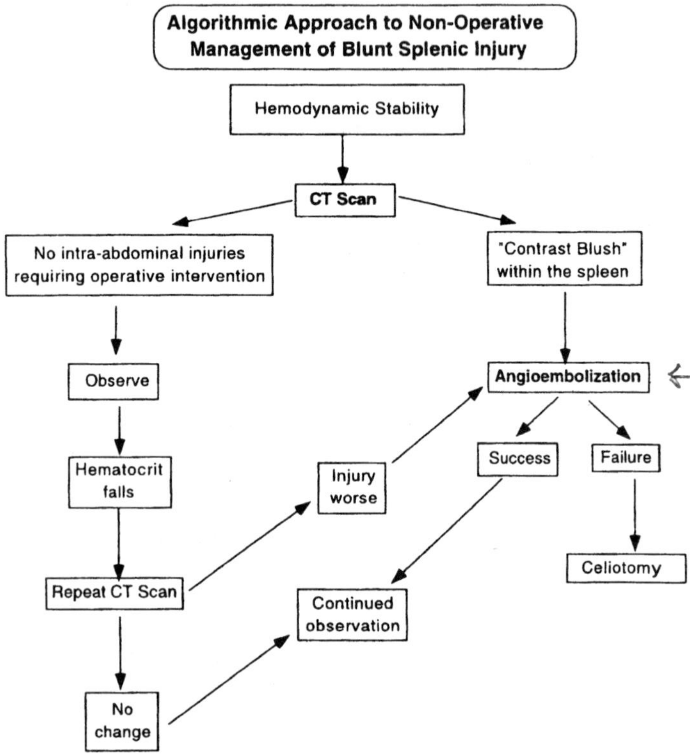

FIGURE 2.—Algorithmic approach to nonoperative management of blunt splenic injury. (Courtesy of Pachter HL, Guth AA, Hofstetter SR, et al: Changing patterns in the management of splenic trauma: The impact of nonoperative management. *Ann Surg* 227:708-719, 1998.)

managed nonoperatively. Changes in the management of splenic injury in the 6 years since that report were presented.

Patients.—From 1990 to 1996, 190 consecutive patients with splenic injuries were treated. One hundred forty-seven had blunt injuries, 18 had gunshot wounds, and 25 had stab wounds. To be managed nonoperatively, the patients had to be in stable hemodynamic condition and have no evidence of shattered spleen or other abnormal findings detected on CT scan requiring celiotomy. Nonoperative management was used in 96% of patients with blunt injuries, including 15 with preexisting splenic pathology related to other diseases. Twenty-four percent of the patients with stab wounds, all of whom had isolated splenic injuries, were managed nonoperatively as well.

Splenectomy was performed in 29% of patients and splenorrhaphy in 17%. Patients in the nonoperative management group had a mean transfusion requirement of only 0.8 units, with 85% receiving no transfusions at all. The failure rate of nonoperative therapy was 2%; these patients subsequently underwent splenectomy. Another patient eventually required splenectomy after undergoing partial splenic resection. None of the patients in the nonoperative group had missed enteric injuries.

Conclusions.—Most splenic injuries are now managed nonoperatively. About two thirds of blunt splenic injuries can be managed nonoperatively, as can selected isolated stab wounds (Fig 2). This approach is associated with minimal transfusions, low morbidity and mortality, and a 98% success rate.

▶ This article and its associated algorithms clearly illustrate that the management of most *hemodynamically stable* patients with splenic trauma (especially blunt) has evolved from splenectomy to splenorrhaphy to nonoperative therapy. The road to the nonoperative management of splenic trauma has been a long one, with many detours to be sure that patient care was not compromised. At first, only patients with less severe (grade I and II) injuries were managed nonoperatively. Now the grade of injury is a less important factor than hemodynamic stability, with nonoperative management frequently being successful even in patients with very severe injuries. If one plans on using a nonoperative approach, it is important to remember that certain radiographic signs predict failure, the most important of which is the presence of a "contrast blush" on CAT scan. Because extravasation of contrast material in the injured spleen, resulting in a hyperdense contrast blush, is an indicator of ongoing active hemorrhage, the presence of this radiographic sign is a warning that nonoperative management may fail. As a surgeon, it is emotionally difficult to be enthusiastic as the therapy for an established operative condition shifts to the nonoperative realm. However, when it comes to splenic trauma in the hemodynamically stable patient without other indications for surgery, we are there.

E.A. Deitch, M.D.

Early Evacuation of Traumatic Retained Hemothoraces Using Thoracoscopy: A Prospective, Randomized Trial

Meyer DM, Jessen ME, Wait MA, et al (Univ of Texas, Dallas)

Ann Thorac Surg 64:1396-1401, 1997 4–10

Objective.—Unless the blood is adequately evacuated from the pleural space in patients with thoracic trauma, there is a risk of extended hospitalization and complications such as empyema and fibrothorax. Techniques for avoiding these complications have included placement of additional thoracostomy tubes or early thoracotomy. This randomized study evaluated the use of video-assisted thoracoscopy (VATS) to manage retained hemothorax after chest trauma.

Methods.—The 4-year study included 39 patients with retained hemothoraces after thoracic trauma. Twenty-four patients (group 1) were assigned to undergo a second tube thoracostomy as their initial management, whereas 15 (group 2) were assigned to VATS. Group 1 patients in whom second-tube thoracostomy failed were then randomized to VATS or thoracotomy. The treatments were compared for duration of thoracostomy tube drainage, length of hospital stay, and hospital costs.

Results.—The mean duration of tube drainage was 4.5 days in group 1 vs. 2.5 days in group 2. The mean postprocedure hospital stays were 7.2 and 3.6 days, respectively, and the total hospital stays were 8.1 and 5.4 days, respectively. The mean hospital costs were $13,300 in group 1 vs. $7,700 in group 2. None of the patients died, and none of the patients assigned to VATS required conversion to open thoracotomy. The initial second-tube thoracostomy failed in 10 of 24 patients assigned to group 1. Five patients each went on to VATS or thoracotomy, with no difference in outcome.

Conclusion.—For patients with chest trauma with retained hemothorax, additional chest tube drainage commonly fails, leading to the need for additional treatment. Performing early VATS in this situation can decrease the duration of tube drainage, shorten hospital stay, and cut hospital costs. The authors propose early VATS as a more efficient and economical strategy for the management of retained hemothorax.

▶ Over the last decade, there has been a progressive shift from operative to nonoperative management of a number of traumatic injuries. It is, thus, a pleasure to highlight an article showing that an early operative approach to patients with retained hemothoraces improves outcome. In essence, this prospective clinical trial comparing the placement of additional chest tubes vs. early treatment with VATS in patients with retained hemothoraces indicates that VATS-based treatment is clinically and economically superior. Why might this be so? One reason is that with VATS, pleural blood clots can be completely removed at surgery, whereas with chest tube drainage, the blood must liquify before it can be evacuated. Additional potential advantages of VATS in patients with hemothoraces is that this approach facilitates the identification of areas of ongoing bleeding and aids in the optimal positioning of chest tubes.

A few points about VATS treatment of hemothoraces are worth stressing. First, early use of VATS (the first 2-5 days postinjury) is more effective than later institution of this therapy (7-21 days postinjury), because clot removal is easier at this time. Secondly, the early use of VATS to completely remove retained blood from the pleural cavity will almost certainly reduce the risk of empyema development and the incidence of fibrothorax.

E.A. Deitch, M.D.

Reduced Use of Resources by Early Tracheostomy in Ventilator-Dependent Patients With Blunt Trauma

Armstrong PA, McCarthy MC, Peoples JB (Wright State Univ, Dayton, Ohio)

Surgery 124:763-767, 1998 4–11

Objective.—There is ongoing debate about when to perform tracheostomy for ventilator-dependent patients with blunt trauma. Traditionally, the procedure is done 10 to 14 days after intubation in patients who have not been weaned from mechanical ventilation. Some investigators have proposed early tracheostomy to reduce total days of mechanical ventilation and the incidence of nosocomial pneumonia, but this approach has never been critically assessed. A retrospective study of early tracheostomy for ventilator-dependent blunt trauma patients is presented.

Patients.—The experience included 157 victims of blunt trauma who underwent tracheostomy over 5.5 years. Tracheostomy was performed within 6 days after admission in 62 patients, the early tracheostomy (ET) group; it was done at 7 days or later in 95 patients, the late tracheostomy (LT) group. Decisions about timing of tracheostomy were based on severity of chest injury, presence of adult respiratory distress syndrome, and severe head injury with a Glasgow Coma Scale score of 6 or less. Later in the experience, there was a trend toward early tracheostomy for patients expected to remain on mechanical ventilation for several weeks.

Outcomes.—The ET and LT groups were similar in sex distribution, injury severity scores, probability of survival scores, and mortality. Patients in the ET group remained in the ICU for a mean of 15 days, compared with 29 days for patients in the LT group. Mean hospital stay was 33 and 68 days, respectively. Charges for room and ventilator care only were estimated at less than $37,000 per patient in the ET group, in contrast to nearly $74,000 in the LT group.

Conclusions.—For ventilator-dependent patients with blunt abdominal trauma, early tracheostomy reduces the length of ICU and hospital stay, and the attendant costs. These advantages are achieved with no increase in morbidity and mortality. Other advantages of ET include avoiding further intubation injury, ensuring airway stability, and improving patient comfort.

► This study indicates that blunt trauma patients having an early tracheostomy, defined as one performed in the first 6 days postinjury, had shorter ICU and hospital stays than patients having their tracheostomies performed after 7 days. This shortening of hospital stay saved money and had no clinically apparent down side.

Skeptics of early tracheostomy would argue that the study was retrospective and therefore biased. They might also say that at least some patients in the early tracheostomy group would likely have been weaned within 10 to 14 days and thus would have avoided a tracheostomy altogether. Since I believe in early tracheostomies, I would answer these skeptics by saying that the authors performed their early tracheostomies in patients who they believed would require prolonged intubation, and they reserved late tracheostomies for patients who they thought had a greater likelihood of being successfully weaned. Thus, in my opinion, the bias would favor the group getting late, not early, tracheostomies.

The results of this study that early tracheostomy shortens ICU stay are not new and have been reported by many other groups. In addition, early tracheostomy has a number of additional benefits, not the least of which is that it is more comfortable for the patient, avoids the risk of unplanned self-extubation, and improves pulmonary toilet. For these reasons, early tracheostomy should be considered in high-risk patients, such as those with Injury severity scores greater than 30, multitrauma patients with severe head injuries, and patients with severe acute respiratory distress syndrome. In these patients, early tracheostomy is best performed within the first 3 or 4 days postinjury.

E.A. Deitch, M.D.

Utility of Gram's Stain and Efficacy of Quantitative Cultures for Posttraumatic Pneumonia: A Prospective Study

Croce MA, Fabian TC, Waddle-Smith L, et al (Univ of Tennessee, Memphis)
Ann Surg 227:743-755, 1998 4–12

Introduction.—Posttraumatic nosocomial pneumonia can be difficult to diagnose, particularly after multiple trauma. It has been suggested that bronchoalveolar lavage (BAL) with quantitative culture may help to differentiate between pneumonia and systemic inflammatory response and that Gram staining of the lavage fluid may serve as a useful guide to empiric antibiotic therapy. BAL with quantitative culture and Gram stain were evaluated for use in the diagnosis of posttraumatic pneumonia.

Methods.—The 2-year prospective study included 232 mechanically ventilated trauma patients with clinical signs of pneumonia. The patients underwent a total of 443 bronchoscopies with BAL, including Gram staining and quantitative culture of the BAL fluid. Antibiotic therapy was continued at a culture threshold of 10^5 CFU/mL or higher. If the culture results were below this threshold, antibiotic therapy was stopped and systemic inflammatory response syndrome was diagnosed. For cultures showing pneumonia, the causative organisms were compared with the results of Gram staining.

Results.—Thirty-nine percent of the patients had a diagnosis of pneumonia. The number of BALs performed had no effect on the overall incidence of pneumonia. Bronchoalveolar lavage had a false negative rate of only 7% (Table 4). Eighty percent of the patients with gram-positive pneumonia were correctly identified by Gram stain; however, only 40% of

TABLE 4.—Diagnostic Accuracy of Quantitative Cultures, Clinical Criteria, and Gram's Stain

	BAL	Clinical	Gram's Stain
Sensitivity (%)	89	100	57
Specificity (%)	100	14	60
Accuracy (%)	96	47	60
Positive predictive value (%)	100	43	47
Negative predictive value (%)	93	100	69

Abbreviation: BAL, bronchoalveolar lavage.
(Courtesy of Croce MA, Fabian TC, Waddle-Smith L, et al: Utility of Gram's stain and efficacy of quantitative cultures for posttraumatic pneumonia: A prospective study. *Ann Surg* 227:743-755, 1998.)

the patients with gram-negative pneumonia were correctly identified. The results of Gram staining suggested gram-negative organisms in 52% of the patients with gram-positive pneumonia, as well as in 77% of those with gram-negative disease. During the first week of intensive care, BAL was most likely to identify *Haemophilus influenzae* and gram-positive organisms. Thereafter, *Acetinobacter* and *Pseudomonas* organisms were more frequently identified.

Conclusions.—This study demonstrates the effectiveness of bronchoscopy with BAL to diagnose pneumonia in mechanically ventilated trauma patients. The causative organisms change with duration of ICU stay, suggesting the need for adjustments in empiric antibiotic therapy over time. Gram staining of BAL fluid does not correlate well with the results of quantitative culture and, therefore, should not be used to guide antibiotic therapy until culture results become available.

▶ The diagnosis of pneumonia in trauma patients, especially those with pulmonary contusions or acute respiratory distress syndrome, is very difficult. This difficulty is compounded by the fact that fever, leukocytosis, and abnormal chest x-ray findings are relatively common in the trauma patient population. For that reason, a number of diagnostic procedures have been developed to aid in establishing the diagnosis of pneumonia. BAL is one such technique that appears to work. Thus, the findings of this large prospective trial highlighting the accuracy of BAL are not surprising. However, what is both surprising and important is the failure of Gram staining of the BAL to aid in determining empiric antibiotic therapy. That is, the Gram stain was incorrect in predicting whether the pneumonia was caused by gram-positive or gram-negative bacteria in 40% of the patients. Thus, the Gram stain should *not* be used for antibiotic selection. On the other hand, the authors found that the time after injury that the pneumonia developed was very helpful in predicting the causative organisms. In early pneumonias, defined as occurring in the first postinjury week, gram-positive bacteria and *H. influenzae* accounted for 85% of the pneumonias, whereas in pneumonias developing later, gram-negative organisms were the culprits in 85% of the patients. Overall, this is an excellent article that should be read by all, since it contains so much useful information and is likely to become a landmark clinical study.

E.A. Deitch, M.D.

Gut-derived Mesenteric Lymph but Not Portal Blood Increases Endothelial Cell Permeability and Promotes Lung Injury After Hemorrhagic Shock

Magnotti LJ, Upperman JS, Xu D-Z, et al (Univ of Medicine and Dentistry of New Jersey, Newark)

Ann Surg 228:518-527, 1998 4–13

Purpose.—Experimental studies suggest an association between shock and gut injury, demonstrating that gut-induced sepsis leads to distant organ failure. However, clinical studies showing no detectable bacteremia or endotoxemia in the portal blood of trauma victims question these associations. It is possible that gut-associated sepsis may be mediated by factors traveling in the mesenteric lymph to the lung and systemic circulation, rather than through the portal circulation. The hypothesis that endothelial cell permeability and lung injury will be affected by mesenteric lymph generated after hemorrhagic shock was tested in an in vitro study using endothelial cell monolayers and a rat model of hemorrhagic shock.

Methods.—In the in vitro study, human umbilical vein endothelial cell monolayers were exposed to media, sham-shock portal vein plasma, postshock portal vein plasma, sham-shock lymph, or postshock lymph. The movement of a rhodamine (10K) probe across the monolayer was used to measure monolayer permeability. In the in vivo study, Sprague-Dawley rats underwent sham or actual hemorrhagic shock, and animals in both groups underwent division of the mesenteric lymphatics before or after shock. Postshock lung injury was measured by assessments of lung permeability, pulmonary myeloperoxidase levels, alveolar apoptosis, and bronchoalveolar fluid protein content.

Results.—In vitro, the permeability of endothelial cell monolayers increased in response to postshock lymph, but not to medium, postshock plasma, or sham shock lymph or plasma. In vivo, induction of hemorrhagic shock led to increased lung permeability to Evans blue dye, increased alveolar apoptosis, and reduced pulmonary myeloperoxidase levels. All of these changes were avoided when the mesenteric lymphatics were divided before shock was induced. The changes were lessened, but not prevented, when the mesenteric lymphatics were divided at the end of shock but before reperfusion.

Conclusions.—The relationship between gut barrier failure after hemorrhagic shock and distant organ injury may occur through gut-derived inflammatory factors traveling through the gut lymphatics, rather than through the portal circulation. Endothelial cell permeability is increased by exposure to postshock mesenteric lymph in vitro; interruption of mesenteric lymph flow avoids shock-induced lung injury in vivo. The next step is to identify the causative factor present in postshock lymph.

▶ This basic science article was chosen because it provides insight into the controversy over the role of the gut in the pathogenesis of sepsis, acute respiratory distress syndrome, and multiple organ failure. Since the emergence of the concept of bacterial translocation in the mid-1980s, the role of the gut as the hidden source of bacteria and toxic products that initiate, fuel, or perpetuate the septic response has been hotly debated. In spite of a large amount of clinical and experimental evidence implicating the gut in the pathogenesis of multiple organ failure, failure to find bacteria or endotoxin in the portal vein of trauma patients led many to question whether shock or injury-induced gut injury did, in fact, contribute to the septic response in the critically ill or injured. The current study goes a long way toward resolving this controversy by showing that gut-derived inflammatory products are reaching the lung and systemic circulation via the gut lymphatic rather than through the portal circulation. In fact, since intestinal lymph enters the blood stream through the thoracic duct, making the lung the first organ to be exposed to toxic intestinally-derived factors, the results of this study may help explain the unique susceptibility of the lung to fail in high risk patients.

E.A. Deitch, M.D.

The Impact of Antioxidant and Splanchnic-Directed Therapy on Persistent Uncorrected Gastric Mucosal pH in the Critically Injured Trauma Patient

Barquist E, Kirton O, Windsor J, et al (Univ of Rochester, NY; Univ of Miami, Fla; Univ of Connecticut, Hartford)

J Trauma: Injury Infect Crit Care 44:355-360, 1998 4–14

Purpose.—Among ICU patients, an abnormal gastric intramucosal pH (pH_i), as measured by gastric tonometry, is associated with poor outcomes. These patients are at increased risk of multiple organ dysfunction syndrome (MODS), even with supranormal oxygen delivery. A new splanchnic therapy resuscitation protocol and its effects on persistent uncorrected pH_i in critically injured trauma patients are assessed.

Methods.—The prospective clinical trial included patients with persistent uncorrected pH_i at 24 hours. Seven were historic control subjects, managed before institution of the new splanchnic/antioxidant protocol. This protocol included the xanthine oxidase inhibitor folate, 10 mg IV; the hydroxyl radical scavenger mannitol, 25-g IV bolus followed by continuous infusion at 4 g/hr; and low-dose isoproterenol. Splanchnic-sparing inotropic and vasodilator agents were given to optimize systemic cardiac output at a pH_i of less than 7.25.

Results.—The use of splanchnic therapy significantly reduced organ system failures. Mean number of organ system failures was 1.9 in the control group vs. 0.9 in the splanchnic therapy group. As a result, duration of ICU stay decreased from 35 to 18 days. Hospital stay decreased from 51 to 29 days.

Conclusions.—A new antioxidant/splanchnic therapy protocol for ICU patients with persistent intramucosal acidosis was evaluated that includes use of gastric tonometry to guide resuscitation, administration of "splanchnic-sparing" β-adrenergic agents rather than α-adrenergic agents, and antioxidant therapy. This approach may reduce organ system dysfunction and failure, thus decreasing ICU stay, costs, and mortality. A randomized, prospective trial of antioxidant/splanchnic therapy is required to confirm the efficacy of this type of therapy in the critically ill trauma patient.

► Although this was a small clinical study and used historic controls, it does carry an important message. That is, therapy directed at improving tissue perfusion, as reflected by the gastric mucosal pH, is more effective in preventing organ failure than therapy directed at improving global criteria of oxygen delivery in high-risk trauma patients. The therapeutic manuevers used were are follows: (1) folate and mannitol were administered as antioxidant therapy; (2) splanchnic blood flow preserving β-adrenergic agents (isoproterenol and dobutamine) rather than splanchnic vasoconstricting α-adrenergic agents (epinephrine and dopamine) were used as inotropes; and (3) vasodilators, such as nitroglycerin, nitroprusside, or prostaglandin E_1, were used as necessary to maintain the gastric mucosal pH at 7.25 or higher.

Without a doubt, their splanchnic-directed therapeutic approach is complicated, and the number of patients studied is small; however, the results are encouraging. Although it may be too early to jump on this bandwagon, it is not too early to be optimistic.

E.A. Deitch, M.D.

Prospective Evaluation of Early Missed Injuries and the Role of Tertiary Trauma Survey

Janjua KJ, Sugrue M, Deane SA (Liverpool Hosp, Australia)
J Trauma: Injury Infect Crit Care 44:1000-1007, 1998 4–15

Purpose.—In trauma management, there is a risk of missed injuries and delayed treatment. Even with established approaches to the primary and secondary trauma survey, there is a chance of missed injuries. Thus, the tertiary trauma survey—a standardized clinical reassessment performed within 24 hours after admission—has been proposed to further reduce the rate of missed injuries. The role of the tertiary trauma survey was evaluated as part of a prospective study of missed injuries in the trauma center.

Methods.—The study included all 206 trauma patients admitted to 1 trauma center over a 5-month period. The tertiary trauma survey—including a repetition of the primary and secondary survey, but also a review of radiographs, blood tests, and other diagnostic studies—was performed within 24 hours in all cases. The incidence and clinical significance of

TABLE 6.—Clinically Significant Missed Injuries

Clinically Significant Missed Injuries	Number of Injuries
Type	
Fractures	30
External soft tissues	8
Internal soft tissues and organs	12
Nerve injuries	9
Outcome of injuries	
Pain	18
Delay in treatment	26
Complications	12 (deaths = 2)
Residual disability	10
Type of treatment	
Operative	12
Nonoperative	33
No treatment	1

(Courtesy of Janjua KJ, Sugrue M, Deane SA: Prospective evaluation of early missed injuries and the role of tertiary trauma survey. *J Trauma: Injury Infect Crit Care* 44(6):1000-1007, 1998.)

missed injuries was assessed. Factors contributing to missed diagnoses were analyzed, and benefits of the tertiary trauma survey were evaluated.

Results.—Sixty-five percent of patients had missed injuries. The total number of missed injuries was 309, accounting for 39% of all injuries observed. Fifty-six percent of early missed injuries were detected by the tertiary trauma survey. Its use resulted in detection of 90% of clinically significant missed injuries within 24 hours. Thirty patients (14.5%) had clinically significant missed injuries, which led to complications in 11 patients and death in 2, both related to missed C1-C2 fracture (Table 6). A total of 224 errors were made, contributing to missed diagnoses, 55% were clinical, 37% were radiologic, 6% were patient related, and 2% were technical. Patients with multiple injuries and traffic accident victims were more likely to have missed injuries.

Conclusion.—Many trauma patients have missed injuries, even after primary and secondary trauma survey. These assessments cannot be regarded as definitive; a tertiary trauma survey is needed to reduce the rate of missed diagnoses, thus minimizing harmful effects on patient outcome. The study identifies factors responsible for missed diagnoses; the authors are conducting further studies to evaluate the effects of remedial measures.

▶ This prospective study on missed injuries in trauma patients provides important food for thought. All of us are rightly proud of our clinical abilities, although we occasionally miss injuries. Yet rarely do we prospectively or critically assess how well we are really doing. The value of this study is that it provides a reality check for us all. By instituting a rigorous policy of tertiary review of all trauma patients within 24 hours of admission, the authors found a high rate of missed injuries. Although only a fraction of these injuries were clinically significant, clinically significant missed injuries were found in 14.5% of their patients.

Because of the importance of the methods used in this tertiary survey, 2 elements bear repeating. First, the tertiary survey is carried out within 24 hours and is especially valuable when the patient is regaining consciousness and physical activity. Secondly, the tertiary trauma survey is more than a repeat physical examination. It includes a review of all radiographs and tests obtained. In summary, this article verifies the importance of clinical compulsiveness.

E.A. Deitch, M.D.

Timing Fracture Repair in Patients With Severe Brain Injury (Glasgow Coma Scale Score <9)

Townsend RN, Lheureau T, Protetch J, et al (Allegheny Gen Hosp, Pittsburgh, Pa; Kaplan Hosp, Rehovot, Israel)

J Trauma: Injury Infect Crit Care 44:977-982, 1998 4–16

Introduction.—Many patients with blunt trauma have multiple life-threatening injuries, and the timing of their treatment is a key consider-

TABLE 3.—Influence of Timing of Operation on Hypotension

Time to OR Hours	(n)	OR SBP < 90 mm Hg* Mean Hours to OR	Percent With Hypotension	CPP < 70 mm Hg* (Mean CPP ± 0^2 Within Group)	
0.0-2.00	(22)	1.6	68.2	58.8 ± 11.2	83.3%
2.01-12.00	(24)	4.3	37.5	61.0 ± 17.1	61.5%
12.01-24.00	(3)	16.6	33.3	62.4 ± 7.5	100.0%
24.01-244.00	(12)	17.4	8.3	60.3 ± 13.3	80.0%

*P = 0.007.

Abbreviations: OR, operating room; *SBP*, systolic blood pressure.

(Courtesy of Townsend RN, Lheureau T, Protech J, et al: Timing fracture repair in patients with severe brain injury (Glasgow Coma Scale Score <9). *J Trauma: Injury Infect Crit Care* 44:977-982, 1998.)

ation. Timing is an especially important consideration for patients with severe head injury and femoral fracture. In this situation, femoral fracture should be repaired only after potential causes of secondary brain injury have been addressed, such as intraoperative hypotension or large fluid shifts. The effects of timing of fracture repair in patients with severe brain injury was analyzed in a retrospective study.

Methods.—A hospital trauma registry was used to identify 61 patients with moderate to severe head injury (Glasgow Coma Scale score of 8 or less). The time-to-surgery was within 2 hours in 22 patients, 2 to 12 hours in 24 patients, 12 to 24 hours in 3 patients, and 24 to 244 hours in 12 patients (Table 3). The effects of surgical timing on complications, including hypotension, and patient outcomes were analyzed.

Results.—The longer the time-to-surgery, the less was the risk of intraoperative hypotensive events. Risk of such events was 8 times higher for patients operated on within 2 hours than for those operated on after 24 hours. Including all patients operated on within 24 hours, the risk of hypotension was twice as high as in patients operated later. Of 31 patients undergoing intracranial pressure monitoring, 74% had cerebral perfusion pressure of less than 70 mm Hg. This risk persisted beyond 24 hours.

Conclusions.—For patients with severe head injury and femoral fracture, orthopedic surgery is best deferred until risks are minimized by adequate resuscitation. Patients undergoing earlier fracture repair are at increased risk of secondary brain injury. Delaying surgery for 24 hours may help to prevent hypoxia, hypotension, and low cerebral perfusion pressure.

► The combination of a closed head injury and a long-bone fracture is relatively common in patients sustaining motor vehicle accidents. Thus, the question of the optimal timing of operative fracture fixation in this group of patients arises not infrequently. This article documents that intraoperative hypotensive episodes are more common when fracture fixation is done before rather than 24 hours after the injury. Because hypotensive episodes can significantly increase mortality and worsen long-term neurologic outcome by causing secondary brain injury, the avoidance of hypotensive episodes in patients with severe head injuries is of critical importance. Thus on the basis of this study and studies showing similar results, it is now clear that fracture fixation in the subgroup of patients with significant closed head injuries should be delayed. The question that is difficult to answer is exactly how long this delay should be. The easy answer is, "until resuscitation is fully complete." However, it is well known that patients may still be in a compensated state of shock even with a normal blood pressure. Thus, I use resolution of lactate and normalization of base excess to establish that the patient is fully resuscitated. The usefulness of lactate and base excess as optimal end points of resuscitation has been recently reviewed[1] and I recommend this thoughtful article to you.

E.A. Deitch, M.D.

Reference

1. Porter JM, Ivatury RR: In search of the optimal end points of resuscitation in trauma patients: A review. *J Trauma* 44:908-914, 1998.

Covering the "Open Abdomen": A Better Technique

Sherck J, Seiver A, Shatney C, et al (Stanford Univ, Calif; Santa Clara Valley Med Ctr, San Jose, Calif)

Am Surg 64:854-857, 1998 4–17

Introduction.—Several conditions occurring in critically ill patients are managed using the "open abdomen" technique. These conditions—such as severe abdominal trauma, abdominal compartment syndrome, abdominal wall necrotizing fasciitis, and necrotizing pancreatitis—may make it impossible to close the fascia after laparotomy. Though a number of different techniques for temporary coverage of the exposed viscera have been proposed, all have significant disadvantages. This study reports a new, temporary, sutureless coverage technique for the open abdomen.

Technique.—Once the decision to leave the abdominal fascia open has been made, any available omentum is placed over the viscera. A clear plastic or silicone sheet then covers the omentum, extending beneath the parietal peritoneum and fascia. Sump tubes are placed over this layer, exiting through separate skin incisions. Adhesive fluid is applied to the skin around the wound, and a layer of iodophore-impregnated adhesive plastic drape seals in the abdominal contents. A second drape is then placed over the abdomen, with no sutures and no additional dressings (Fig 2). The covering is not moved until it is necessary to access the abdominal cavity again. When possible, after the pathologic condition has resolved, the fascia is closed, followed by delayed-primary or secondary closure of the skin incision.

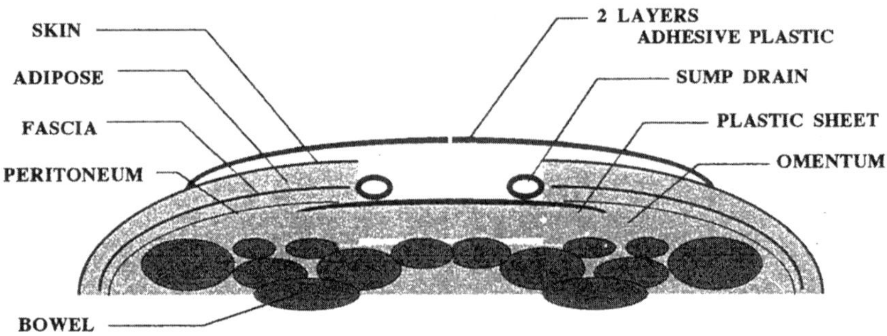

FIGURE 2.—Cross-sectional diagram of sutureless closure technique. (Courtesy of Sherck J, Seiver A, Shatney C, et al: Covering the "open abdomen": A better technique. *Am Surg* 64:854-857, 1998.)

Outcomes.—This technique of temporary abdominal coverage was used in 50 patients, age range 3 to 89 years. Twenty-seven patients had severe abdominal trauma, with an average injury severity score of 27. The most common specific indications were removal of packs placed for hemorrhage, "second-look" to determine bowel viability, and need for multiple débridements. None of the patients experienced wound infection, fasciitis, or bowel obstruction. There were 32 survivors; none of the 18 deaths was related to the abdominal coverage technique. In most cases, simple closure of the abdominal fascia was performed within 72 hours of the original operation.

Conclusions.—This technique provides a simple and readily available approach to temporary coverage of the open abdomen. It protects the abdominal organs, simplifies nursing care, and allows safe, delayed closure of the abdomen. The technique has important advantages over previous approaches.

▶ As the use of damage-control laparotomies has become more prevalent in the care of severely injured patients, a number of "how I do it" techniques for temporary closure of the abdomen have been reported. This article is such a paper. I chose it because the technique described seems both simple and effective.

E.A. Deitch, M.D.

The First Randomized Trial of Human Polymerized Hemoglobin as a Blood Substitute in Acute Trauma and Emergent Surgery

Gould SA, Moore EE, Hoyt DB, et al (Univ of Illinois, Chicago; Univ of Colorado, Denver; Univ of California, San Diego)

J Am Coll Surg 187:113-122, 1998 4–18

Objective.—Human polymerized hemoglobin (PolyHeme) has been developed as a blood substitute. It is a universally compatible, immediately available, disease-free, oxygen-carrying resuscitative fluid that has shown good safety characteristics in preliminary studies. A prospective, randomized trial of PolyHeme in the management of acute blood loss was reported.

Methods.—The phase II trial included 44 trauma patients with an average Injury Severity Score of 21. For resuscitation, the patients were randomized to receive allogeneic red blood cells (RBCs) or PolyHeme, up to 6 U. The 2 treatments were compared for safety and therapeutic benefit.

Results.—PolyHeme caused no serious or unexpected adverse events. The mean PolyHeme infusion was 4.4 U, producing a plasma hemoglobin (Hb) of 3.9, or 40% of total circulating Hb. The 2 groups were similar in total Hb before the start of treatment: 10.4 g/dL in the control group vs. 9.4 g/dL in the experimental group. Red blood cell Hb decreased to 5.8 g/dL in the experimental group, compared with a level of 10.6 g/dL in the control group, with no difference in total Hb. In the first day, the control group received a mean of 10.4 U of allogeneic red blood cells, compared with 6.8 U in the experimental group. Values through day 3 were 11.3 and 7.8 U, respectively.

Conclusion.—PolyHeme appears to be a safe and clinically useful blood substitute in patients with acute blood loss. Although use of PolyHeme is associated with a reduction in RBC Hb, it preserves total Hb and reduces the requirement for allogeneic blood. Phase III trials are underway to establish the clinical role of PolyHeme in the management of acute blood loss.

▶ This article on the use of what appears to be a nontoxic and safe polymerized hemoglobin blood substitute is likely to be a landmark study. The take-home message of this prospective, randomized clinical trial is that human polymerized hemoglobin was as effective as blood transfusions in patients experiencing acute blood loss. There are many advantages of having a safe and effective blood substitute for the treatment of acute blood loss. These include immediate availability, compatibility with all blood types, and freedom from the risks of transfusion reactions or the transmission of blood-borne diseases such as hepatitis and AIDS. An additional potential benefit of this blood substitute is its biologically inert nature. This is important in the light of recent studies indicating that blood can alter various components of the host's immune system and potentiate infection, and it can contribute to the development of a proinflammatory septic state. Thus, if further studies validate the safety and effectiveness of this human polymerized hemoglobin blood substitute, it could revolutionize the field of transfusion medicine.

E.A. Deitch, M.D.

5 Infection

Introduction

Several subjects about surgical infection are featured in the 1999 YEAR BOOK OF SURGERY. The first two articles deal with surgical wound infections. The study by Manian and Meyer (Abstract 5–1) investigated infection rates in elective surgery patients whose hospital admissions occurred on the same day as their operations and compared them with patients who were already hospitalized or who had emergency procedures. Except for one small group of neurosurgical patients, there was no difference in surgical site infection rates in the two groups. Zoutman and colleagues (Abstract 5–2) studied the cost of surgical wound infections at a Canadian tertiary care center. Like other studies, they found that wound infection contributed markedly to prolonged hospitalization and to the cost of hospitalization.

A study by Merad et al. (Abstract 5–3) investigated prophylactic drainage of colon resection anastomoses. This is an old subject that has been discussed for some time: is the rate of infections higher if anastomoses are drained? The authors found that drainage does not decrease the rate or severity of anastomotic leaks; furthermore, as others have found, drainage can potentially be harmful.

Two articles discussing abdominal abscesses are presented. The first article by Yeh and colleagues (Abstract 5–4) studied a series of hepatic abscesses in patients with malignant disease. Abscesses must, of course, be differentiated from hepatic metastases. The authors found that the mortality rate of hepatic abscess was substantially higher in those patients who have had hepatic, pancreatic, or biliary malignancies compared with patients with tumors of other origins. The second paper, by Röthlin and colleagues (Abstract 5–5), discussed the size of catheters required for percutaneous drainage of abdominal abscesses. They compared 7-F and 14-F drains. They found that small catheters were as effective as larger catheters in treating the abscesses. Many surgeons, of course, would regard even the 14-F catheter as a small catheter.

Infected necrotizing pancreatitis continues to be a challenge to surgeons, and it continues to have a high mortality rate. Formerly, these patients were always operated on and usually required removal of necrotic, infected pancreas and the thickened crankcase oil-like material in these abscesses. A study by Freeny et al. (Abstract 5–6) proposed percutaneous catheter drainage in these patients. They demonstrated that it is safe and effective in most patients. The mortality rate was low (12%). Obviously, patient selection is extremely important. The decision about who will or will not be best treated by percutaneous drainage is the most important decision. Another paper on infected necrotizing pancreatitis by Gentile and others (Abstract 5–7) discussed the use of polyglycolic acid mesh, especially for those patients with abdominal abscesses. The use of mesh allows repeat access to the retroperitoneum so that explorations and subsequent débridement can be conducted in the intensive care unit.

Schuler and colleagues (Abstract 5–8) discussed the use of CT scans in patients with appendicitis whose clinical symptoms were insufficient for surgery. They found the abdominal CT scan to be helpful in almost 58% of the patients studied. This paper is interesting because it does a cost analysis and permits the reader to develop a strategy based on cost and negative exploration rate.

Two papers deal with peritonitis. The first paper by Navez et al. (Abstract 5–9) discussed laparoscopic management of acute peritonitis, a procedure that many surgeons might consider inappropriate because of their inability to thoroughly explore the abdomen. Nevertheless, the authors achieved a high diagnostic accuracy (84.8%). Caution is warranted, however, because of the inability to accurately explore the abdomen in many patients and the increased operating time added by laparoscopy. The benefits of laparoscopic management were avoiding laparotomy in 6.5% of the patients and altering the incision site in 8.7%.

A fascinating subject, tertiary peritonitis, has been discussed by Nathens and others (Abstract 5–10). Tertiary peritonitis is persistent or recurrent intra-abdominal infection after adequate therapy for primary or secondary peritonitis. These can be among the most challenging patients to treat because of the difficulty in managing the primary source of infection as well as the lingering and persistent infection.

Muñoz and colleagues (Abstract 5–11) discussed postsurgical mediastinitis. This infection can be the most challenging and the mortality rate is high. The article is a good review of this complication.

Clostridium difficile has been discussed by Kent and others (Abstract 5–12). This bacterium infected 5.6% of patients in a tertiary care hospital. It can cause substantial morbidity in surgical patients. As previously demonstrated, patients who received antibiotics were more likely to have this infection develop than those who did not. The increased use of antibiotics with a broader spectrum will predictably increase the infection rate with *Clostridium difficile* in the future.

Finally, two uncommon infections have been discussed. The first is an article by Athié and colleagues (Abstract 5–13) that discussed management of ileal perforation caused by *Salmonella typhi.* This article is from Mexico where the authors see a large number of patients with ileal perforations. Because of the large number of individuals from Mexico in the United States, these infections may also be seen in this country. The last article by Passaro and others (Abstract 5–14) discussed wound botulism associated with black tar heroin among drug users. This type of infection might also be seen by surgeons, especially in the western United States, where this form of heroin is widely used.

Richard J. Howard, M.D., Ph.D.

Surgical-Site Infection Rates in Patients Who Undergo Elective Surgery on the Same Day as Their Hospital Admission

Manian FA, Meyer L (St John's Mercy Med Ctr, St Louis)
Infect Control Hosp Epidemiol 19:17-22, 1998 5–1

Objective.—Whether patients undergoing elective surgical procedures on their admission day have a higher rate of surgical site infections (SSI) than patients hospitalized before surgery is unknown. SSI rates for these 2 groups of patients were compared and reasons for higher-than-expected SSI rates in neurosurgical patients undergoing elective surgery on the day of admission were explored in a 900-bed, tertiary-care community hospital performing >10,000 surgeries on patients requiring postoperative hospital stays.

Methods.—SSI rates were compiled on patients having surgery between 1990 and 1994 and for all neurosurgical patients from July 1994 to May 1995. Surgical site infections and wound class were described according to the Centers for Disease Control and Prevention proposed criteria. Climatological data were collected.

Results.—Between 1990 and 1994, there were 18,794 group I patients and 29,670 group II patients. Overall SSI rates increased significantly from 0.9% in 1990 to 1.7% in 1994 (relative risk (RR), 1.8) (Figure). Whereas the SSI rate was significantly different for the 2 groups in 1990, rates were similar by 1994. Among the 511 neurosurgery patients, the SSI rate for

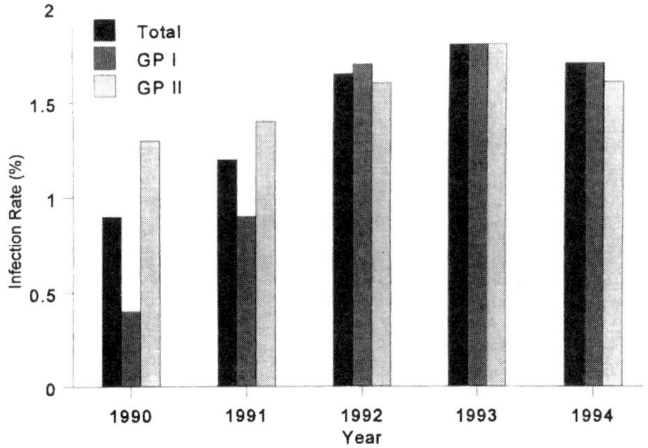

FIGURE.—Surgical-site infection rate by year among patients requiring postoperative hospitalization. Group I: patients undergoing elective surgery on the same day as their hospital admission. Group II: patients already hospitalized or undergoing surgery on non-elective basis. (Courtesy of Manian FA, Meyer L: Surgical-site infection rates in patients who undergo elective surgery on the same day as their hospital admission. *Infect Control Hosp Epidemiol* 19:17-22, 1998.)

neurosurgical group I patients in 1994 was significantly higher than for neurosurgical group II patients (3.4% vs. 0.4%). Rates for group I and II patients in other surgical services were similar. During warm months, observed SSI rates were higher than expected (4.7% vs. 1.4%). Group I patients were significantly less likely to have an ASA score 3 or higher, a risk index of 1 or higher, and a craniotomy, and were significantly more likely to have a clean surgical wound class and spinal surgery. Group I patients undergoing spinal surgery had observed rates significantly higher than expected rates during warm months (2.8% vs. 1.1%)(RR, 2.6).

Conclusion.—Overall SSI rates for group I and II patients are similar. For neurosurgical patients, those having surgery on admission day have a higher SSI rate than patients hospitalized before surgery.

▶ This study examined surgical-site infections in patients who had elective surgery on the same day as their hospital admission (group 1) and in patients who were already hospitalized for 1 or more days before surgery or who had emergency surgery on the same day as their hospitalization (group 2). Surgical-site infection rates increased during the study periods from 1990 to 1994. While group 1 patients had more surgical-site infections in 1990, there was no difference from 1992 to 1994. Only in the subset of patients who had neurosurgical procedures was the wound infection rate higher in patients having elective surgery (group 1) than in group 2 patients. This study demonstrates some of the difficulties of studying wound infections. It is difficult to study all the parameters that may impact wound infections, and it may be difficult to explain the findings. For instance, it is too bad the authors did not divide groups according to the common stratification system of wounds (clean, clean-contaminated, contaminated, and dirty) or other stratifications schemes that take into account the number of discharge diagnoses or comorbid conditions. Even with the large number of operative procedures followed in this study, the number of surgical-site infections was small. Therefore, subdividing patients further would have resulted in groups too small for an appropriate statistical analysis. It would have been interesting, however, to determine whether the wound class in patients having elective outpatient surgery was different from those who had emergency operations or operations as inpatients. It is logical to believe group 1 patients had more clean operations than group 2 patients and some differences may have been seen if the patients could have been stratified along these lines. The tendency toward early discharge of patients who may be in either group 1 or group 2 means that reliable surgical-site infection data will become more difficult to obtain than it has been in the past.

R.J. Howard, M.D., Ph.D.

Total and Attributable Costs of Surgical-Wound Infections at a Canadian Tertiary-Care Center

Zoutman D, McDonald S, Vethanayagan D (Queen's Univ, Kingston, Ontario, Canada)

Infect Control Hosp Epidemiol 19:254-259, 1998 5–2

Objective.—Surgical wound infections involve high costs to the hospital, the patient, and society. Infection-control programs can reduce the rate of these infections, but they require a substantial investment. One factor in determining the costs of surgical wound infection is the proportion of hospital care specifically dedicated to the surgical wound. The Appropriateness Evaluation Protocol (AEP) was used to assess the total and attributable costs of surgical wound infections.

Methods.—The study was conducted at a Canadian university referral center that performed more than 5,500 surgical procedures of all types in 1991. The analysis included all clean or clean-contaminated procedures performed by all surgical services during that year. Inpatients with wound infections were identified, and their charts were reviewed according to the AEP, a validated instrument for assessing appropriateness of care. All hospital costs associated with treatment during the wound-infection period—including inpatient days and outpatient and emergency visits—were accounted for. Costs were expressed in 1991 Canadian dollars.

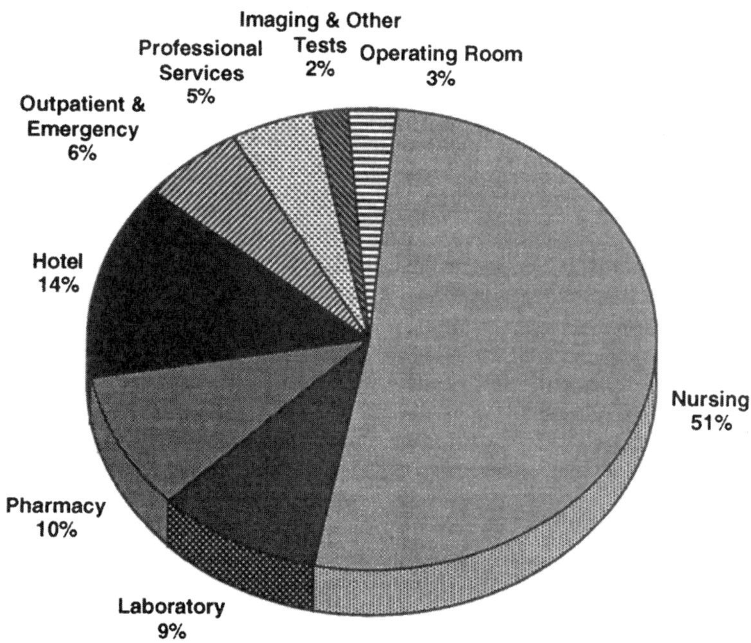

FIGURE.—Distribution of gross inpatient and outpatient costs of surgical wound infections. (Courtesy of Zoutman D, McDonald S, Vethanayagan D: Total and attributable costs of surgical-wound infections at a Canadian tertiary-care center. *Infect Control Hosp Epidemiol* 19:254-259, 1998.)

Results.—A total of 108 wound infections occurred, a rate of nearly 2%. These infections led to 28 repeat surgical procedures in 22 patients, and 9 patients with wound infections died. The infections led to 1,116 inpatient days, at a cost of nearly $395,000. In addition, there were 55 emergency visits and 42 clinic visits, at a cost of more than $27,000. According to the AEP, 833 inpatient days could be directly attributed to the surgical wound infections, an average of more than 10 days per case. Inpatient costs attributable to these infections totaled more than $320,000, approximately $4,000 per infection. Nursing care accounted for the majority of the additional costs (Figure). Eighty-four percent of drug costs were for antibiotics to treat the infections.

Conclusions.—This study documents the high hospital costs attributable to surgical wound infections. The results suggest an average 10-day increase in length of stay for each surgical wound infection. The AEP is a valid and practical tool for determining the increased length of stay attributable to such infections. Using this information, hospitals can assess the economic impact of infection-control programs to prevent surgical wound infections.

▶ By any measure, postoperative complications are expensive. Aside from the very real and human cost in terms of pain, suffering, and time away from family and work, the financial cost of all postoperative complications is high. This study investigates the cost of wound infections; these were measured in 1991 Canadian dollars, so appropriate inflationary and rate-of-exchange adjustments would have to be taken into consideration. The authors tried to be complete in their cost-accounting techniques. Many costs that may not have been included in previous studies, such as hotel costs for patients' additional stay near a hospital or a physician's office and outpatient costs as well, are included here.

R.J. Howard, M.D., Ph.D.

Prophylactic Abdominal Drainage After Elective Colonic Resection and Suprapromontory Anastomosis: A Multicenter Study Controlled by Randomization

Merad F, Yahchouchi E, Hay J-M, et al (Hôpital Louis Mourier, Colombes, France; Centre Hospitalier Intercommunal, Poissy, France; Hôpital Hauterive, Paris; et al)

Arch Surg 133:309-314, 1998 5–3

Objective.—There is debate over the use of abdominal drainage after colon surgery to prevent postoperative infection. None of the few controlled trials of this issue have found any significant difference between patients who underwent such drainage and those who did not. However, all of these studies have been small, with a high risk of β error. A multicenter trial was performed to assess the value of prophylactic abdominal drainage after colonic resection.

Methods.—The study included 319 patients who underwent elective colonic resection followed by immediate anastomosis of the suprapromontory colon. There were 184 women and 135 men (mean age 67 years) in the study. Each was being operated on for treatment of carcinoma, benign tumors, or colitis at any point between the ascending and sigmoid colons. The patients were randomized to receive abdominal drainage with suction or nonsuction drains or no abdominal drainage. During surgery, the anastomoses were tested for airtightness and were repaired if necessary. Diatrizoate sodium enemas were used to detect subclinical leakage. The groups were compared for postoperative complications possibly affected by drainage, including deep complications that can be detected early with drainage, complications potentially enhanced by drainage, and complications directly caused by drainage.

Results.—The final analysis included 317 patients, after exclusion of 2 protocol violations. The 2 groups were comparable, although the nondrainage group included more patients with ascites. Seventy-one anastomoses were repaired after airtightness testing revealed leakage. The rate of postoperative complications possibly influenced by drainage was 8% overall, with no significant difference between the drainage and nondrainage groups. One case of intestinal fistula was directly attributed to drainage. Complication rates were similar with suction and nonsuction drains.

Conclusions.—Prophylactic abdominal drainage after colonic resection does not reduce either the risk or the severity of postoperative complications. Nor is there any significant difference between suction and nonsuction drainage. Abdominal drainage can occasionally cause, rather than prevent, complications.

► Some surgeons always drain colonic anastomoses. Many others never do. Still other surgeons drain them for only a short time (24-48 hours). In this combined study of a large number of patients in France, no difference was found in the rate or the severity of anatomic leakage in drained and undrained anastomoses. However, 8% of the patients had postoperative complications that were possibly influenced by drainage. The authors point out that this is the fifth, but largest, controlled trial that failed to demonstrate any difference in anatomic leakage between drained and undrained anastomoses. Whether this study will affect the practice of surgeons is unclear. At best, drains themselves may cause some problems and seem to add little to serious problems such as anastomotic leaks.

R.J. Howard, M.D., Ph.D.

Pyogenic Liver Abscesses in Patients With Malignant Disease: A Report of 52 Cases Treated at a Single Institution

Yeh T-S, Jan Y-Y, Jeng L-B, et al (Chang Gung Med College, Taipei, Taiwan)

Arch Surg 133:242-245, 1998 5–4

Objective.—Cancer patients with pyogenic liver abscess have a poor prognosis. The clinical course of pyogenic liver abscess in patients with different types of cancer were investigated, and outcomes in abscesses caused by hepatopancreatobiliary malignant disease and other malignant disease were compared.

Methods.—Of 52 patients, aged 9 to 77 years, with pyogenic liver abscesses and malignant disease, 32 (group 1, 15 women) had cancers originating from the hepatic parenchyma, biliary system, and pancreas, and 20 (group 2, 8 women) had cancers originating from other sites. The prognosis of the liver abscess, age, causes, management, and outcome in the 2 groups were compared.

Results.—Thirteen (41%) group 1 patients and 16 (80%) group 2 patients had anticancer treatments. Significantly more group 1 than group 2 patients had jaundice (91% vs. 30%), leukocytosis, hypoalbuminemia, hyperbilirubinemia, and strongly inverted albumin-globulin ratio, and significantly more group 2 patients than group 1 patients had nausea and vomiting (52% vs. 34%). More group 1 (34%) than group 2 patients (10%) had abscesses communicating with the intrahepatic biliary tree. Group 1 patients had more polymicrobial pus cultures than group 2 patients (50% vs. 25%). Group 1 pus and blood cultures contained predominantly *Klebsiella pneumoniae* and *Escherichia coli* whereas group 2 pus and blood cultures contained a more diverse group of organisms. Hospital mortality rates were 28% for group 1 and 10% for group 2. Hospital mortality for patients with liver abscesses and cancer was significantly worse than for patients with liver abscesses and no cancer (21% vs. 11%). Within 6 months, 23 group 1 patients had died of uncontrolled sepsis or progressive cancer, whereas 17 group 2 patients were still alive after 1 year.

Conclusion.—Patients with pyogenic liver abscess and hepatobiliary disease have a worse prognosis than patients with pyogenic liver disease and no hepatobiliary malignant disease.

► This substantial series of hepatic abscess occurring in patients with cancer originates from Taiwan. The patients were divided into two groups, those with tumors originating in liver biliary system or pancreas and those with metastatic disease from distant sites. The mortality rate differed significantly with the former group having a mortality rate of 72% and the latter only 15%. Most patients died of uncontrolled sepsis or progressive cancer within 6 months of diagnoses. The mortality rate of pyogenic liver abscess in patients with underlying malignant disease is almost twice as high as that in patients with cancer. Even if the abscess can be successfully drained, the underlying cancer may prevent satisfactory healing of the abscess cavity.

Patients in the first group were treated mainly by surgery. Those with metastatic cancer were treated mainly by percutaneous drainage. The authors believed percutaneous drainage could be tried initially in both groups, but it is not clear why patients with metastatic disease were treated mainly by percutaneous drainage and those with tumor originating in the liver, biliary, or pancreatic glands required laparotomy. This study demonstrates the difficulties of treating pyogenic liver abscesses and high mortality rate in patients with malignant disease.

R.J. Howard, M.D., Ph.D.

Percutaneous Drainage of Abdominal Abscesses: Are Large-bore Catheters Necessary?

Röthlin MA, Schöb O, Klotz H, et al (Zürich Univ, Switzerland)

Eur J Surg 164:419-424, 1998 5–5

Objective.—Although large-bore drains are usually used for abdominal abscesses in open surgery, thin catheters are easier to insert for percutaneous drainage. Results of percutaneous treatment of patients was analyzed retrospectively.

Methods.—Between January 1990 and December 1995, 64 consecutive patients with abdominal abscesses were treated by percutaneous drainage using a 25-cm long pigtail catheter with internal and external diameters of 1.5 and 2.33 mm (n = 40) or a 30-cm long sump drain with internal and external diameters of 3.0 and 4.66 mm (n = 24). Success rates were compared.

Results.—Percutaneous drainage was successful in 34 (85%) patients and large-bore drainage was successful in 20 (83%) patients. There were recurrences in 3 percutaneous drainage patients and 1 large-bore drainage patient, all of whom required surgery. Duration of drainage averaged 7.9 days in the percutaneous drainage group and 11 days in the large-bore drainage group. There were 6 failures in the percutaneous drainage group, 4 as a result of pancreatic abscess, and 4 in the large-bore drainage group, 1 as a result of pancreatic abscess. There was 1 complication in the percutaneous drainage group and 2 in the large-bore drainage group.

Conclusion.—Percutaneous drainage is as effective as large-bore drainage in patients with abdominal abscesses.

► Surgeons are frequently dissatisfied with percutaneous drainage of abscesses in part because radiologists sometimes put in catheters that surgeons believe are too small. Surgeons may be concerned that a small catheter may not successfully drain thickened abscess contents. Failed percutaneous drainage may require open drainage and placement of a large catheter. This study from Switzerland compares results of patients drained with small (7F) pigtail catheters to those drained by large (14F) catheters. The success rates of drainage were the same in both groups. (Some surgeons would still suggest that even a 14F catheter is small by their standards.) Many of the drainage failures were in patients who had pancreatic abscess.

R.J. Howard, M.D., Ph.D.

Percutaneous CT-Guided Catheter Drainage of Infected Acute Necrotizing Pancreatitis: Techniques and Results

Freeny PC, Hauptmann E, Althaus SJ, et al (Univ of Washington, Seattle; Virginia Mason Med Ctr, Seattle)

AJR 170:969-975, 1998 5–6

Objective.—Acute pancreatitis, complicated by parenchymal necrosis, frequently results in multiorgan failure and death. Whereas surgery is the preferred treatment, it results in high mortality rates. Results of a series of patients with infected acute necrotizing pancreatitis treated initially with only computed tomography (CT)-guided percutaneous catheter drainage are presented.

Methods.—Between 1991 and 1995, 34 patients (8 women), aged 31 to 71, were treated with percutaneous drainage for uncontrolled sepsis. Parenchymal necrosis was documented using contrast-enhanced CT.

Results.—The extent of necrosis was less than 30% in 10 patients, 30% to 50% in 10, and more than 50% in 14. The mean CT severity index was 8.2. Sixteen patients were cured, 8 required elective surgery, 9 required surgery to control sepsis or hemorrhage, and 4 (12%) died of multisystem organ failure after necrosectomy. Fourteen patients had central gland necrosis and 12 had body-tail necrosis. Duration of drainage time averaged 89 days. Eight patients had complications, including 3 with respiratory and renal failure and shock, 1 with shock and bleeding, 3 with respiratory failure, and 1 with renal failure.

Conclusion.—Percutaneous catheter drainage of infected acute necrotizing pancreatitis cured 47% of patients and controlled sepsis in 74%.

▶ This article describes the use of polyglycolic acid mesh for treating abdominal abscess associated with necrotizing pancreatitis. The authors suggest CT-guided catheter drainage can provide results comparable to open drainage. Thirty-four of 123 patients who underwent percutaneous catheter drainage between 1991 and 1995 had pancreatic necrosis. The mortality rate was only 12%, which is as low as possible for this group of very seriously ill patients. The authors do not indicate how many patients required open drainage, were treated by open drainage during this same period, or what might have led to open drainage. Important in this treatment was maintenance of catheter patency by irrigation once every 8 hours. Catheters were exchanged multiple times (an average of 4 times per patient), which does not reflect upon this procedure. Certainly patients with open drainage usually require multiple operative procedures. Sixteen of the 34 patients were cured by catheter drainage alone and 18 required surgery. The site of necrosis was an important predictor of cure rate, because only 4 of 14 patients with central gland necrosis were cured by percutaneous catheter drainage whereas 60% of patients with body-tail necrosis were cured by percutaneous drainage alone. These latter patients were more likely to have complications and be seriously ill. An important point is that no patient seemed to have been compromised by an initial trial of catheter drainage. CT-guided percutaneous drainage was used exclusively in patients with infected necrotizing pancreatitis as distinct with patients with infected fluid collections, pseudocysts, or abscess. For these patients, initial catheterization drainage certainly seems worth trying, especially because delayed operative drainage did not seem to adversely affect the patients who eventually required surgery.

R.J. Howard, M.D., Ph.D.

The Utility of Polyglycolic Acid Mesh for Abdominal Access in Patients With Necrotizing Pancreatitis

Gentile AT, Feliciano PD, Mullins RJ, et al (Oregon Health Sciences Univ, Portland)

J Am Coll Surg 186:313-318, 1998 5–7

Objective.—Despite operative management, patients with necrotizing pancreatitis have mortality rates from 11% to 40%. Experience with the use of polyglycolic mesh for patients with delayed presentation of necrotizing pancreatitis and patient outcomes are retrospectively reviewed.

Methods.—Between 1985 and 1994, debridement and drainage were performed on 40 patients (12 women), aged 30 to 81, with histologically confirmed necrotizing pancreatitis. Eleven of 18 patients requiring multiple debridements were closed with absorbable polyglycolic acid (Dexon) mesh (Fig 1). Four of 11 patients, who underwent distal pancreatectomy and required additional procedures, were closed with mesh. Outcomes were compared for patients with a single debridement, patients with multiple debridements, and patients closed with mesh.

Results.—The primary causes of necrotizing pancreatitis were alcohol (30%), gallstone (28%), hyperlipidemia (12%), and iatrogenic injury (10%). Patients with infected pancreatic necrosis had higher mortality rates than those without infection. The average hospital stay was 35 days. Prolonged mechanical ventilation was necessary for 42% of patients. In-hospital mortality was 30% with multiple organ failure as the primary cause in 9 of 12 deaths. Sepsis was present in 11 of 12 patients who died. The number of operations was not correlated with mortality. The infection rate was 60%. Eleven (45%) of 24 infected patients died. Six patients had postoperative enterocutaneous fistulas. Postoperative intestinal fistulas were more common in patients closed with mesh. The presence of mesh facilitated multiple access procedures (Fig 2).

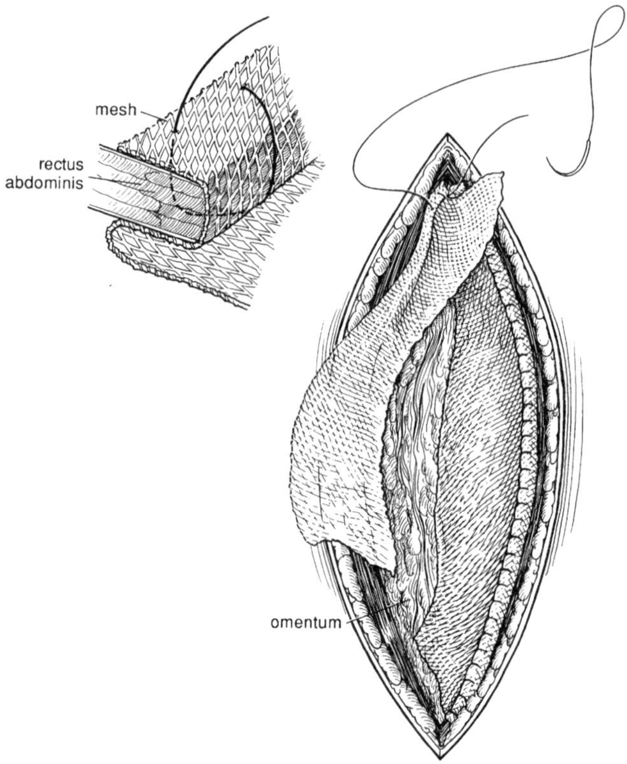

FIGURE 1.—Abdominal-wall reapproximation using an elliptical piece of polyglycolic acid (Dexon) mesh. The mesh is sewn circumferentially to the abdominal muscular fascia using a mattress suture of O-Dexon (**inset**). (Courtesy of Gentile AT, Feliciano PD, Mullins RJ, et al: The utility of polyglycolic acid mesh for abdominal access in patients with necrotizing pancreatitis. *J Am Coll Surg* 186:313-318, 1998. By permission of the American College of Surgeons.)

Conclusion.—Use of polyglycolic mesh facilitated multiple access procedures in patients with necrotizing pancreatitis. Patients closed with mesh had higher rates of fistula formation.

▶ In recent years the mortality rate of necrotizing pancreatitis has decreased somewhat, although it still remains extremely high. When combined with infection, the mortality rate of necrotizing pancreatitis is even higher. Infected necrotizing pancreatitis is certainly one of the most serious intraabdominal conditions. Because of the poor outcome of these patients, surgeons have been seeking innovative ways to treat the most serious infections, including leaving the abdomen open to allow further drainage, close needle aspiration to look for infection, nonoperative treatment in the absence of signs of infection, and even percutaneous catheter drainage. Despite all these treatment variations, the mortality remains high. The use of polyglycolic acid mesh allows repeat access to the retroperitoneum so repeated expirations and subsequent débridements can occur without difficulty. While this technique facilitated repeat débridement, the hospital mor-

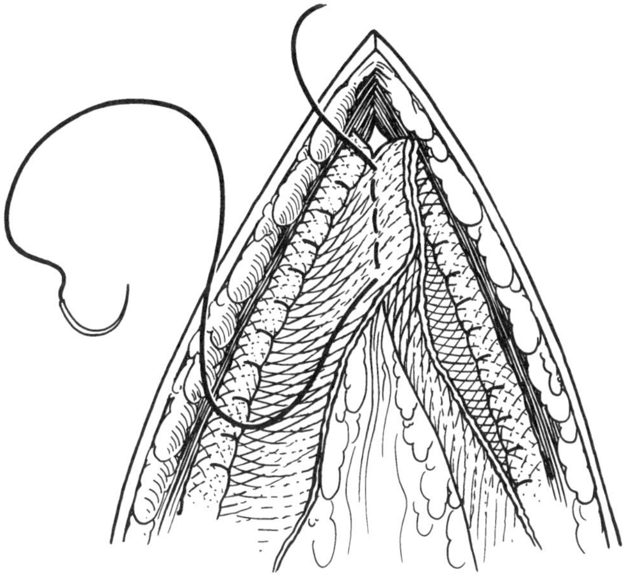

FIGURE 2.—Repeat access into the abdominal cavity is through a midline cleft in the mesh (Ref. 19). (Courtesy of Gentile AT, Feliciano PD, Mullins RJ, et al: The utility of polyglycolic acid mesh for abdominal access in patients with necrotizing pancreatitis. *J Am Coll Surg* 186:313-318, 1998. By permission of the American College of Surgeons.)

tality rate remained high. Repeat débridement is essential for infected pancreatic necrosis until the surgeon is convinced the necrotic tissue has been adequately removed, all infection has been adequately drained, and signs of healing begin to occur.

R.J. Howard, M.D., Ph.D.

Is There a Role for Abdominal Computed Tomographic Scans in Appendicitis?

Schuler JG, Shortsleeve MJ, Goldenson RS, et al (Mount Auburn Hosp, Cambridge, Mass)

Arch Surg 133:373-377, 1998 5–8

Objective.—The rate of negative appendectomy is as high as 30%, and up to 40% in women. The accuracy of abdominal computed tomographic scanning (ACTS) for the diagnosis of suspected appendicitis was retrospectively analyzed.

Methods.—Between November 1, 1995 and December 31, 1996, ACTS was performed on 97 patients (group 2) (38 male), aged 15 to 88 years, with suspected appendicitis. Patients were given 950 mL of water or juice containing 50 mL of iothalamate meglumine for 2 hours before the scan. Patients exhibiting contrast in the cecum were infused with 150 mL of iothalamate meglumine or 150 mL of iopamidol at a rate of 2 mL/sec and rescanned. Results were compared with those of 52 patients (group 1) (27 male), aged 17 to 68, who underwent appendectomy on the basis of clinical findings and history. All appendectomy specimens were evaluated pathologically.

Results.—In group 1, 41 patients had appendicitis for a negative appendectomy rate of 21%. With the exception of 1 patient requiring sigmoid resection for diverticulitis, 10 patients could have been treated nonsurgically. In group 2, 49 patients had appendicitis and 1 had endometriosis of the appendix. Three normal appendices were removed in 52 procedures for a negative appendectomy rate of 5.8%. ACTS was positive in 49 patients, false positive in 1 patient with cecal diverticulitis, and false negative in 1 patient. ACTS had a sensitivity, positive predictive value, negative predictive value, and accuracy of 98%, 92%, 98%, and 96%, respectively. ACTS correctly diagnosed the absence of appendicitis of 43 patients. ACTS definitively diagnosed appendicitis in 30 of 50 patients and definitely ruled out appendicitis in 10 patients.

Conclusion.—ACTS was of definite benefit to 57.7% of patients, but it was difficult to know ahead of time which patients were likely to benefit. ACTS can lower the negative appendectomy rate in the hands of an experienced radiologist.

▶ Acute appendicitis is usually an easy clinical diagnosis in the majority of patients, but it can be an extremely difficult diagnosis to make. Unfortunately many patients do not read the textbooks of surgery about how acute appendicitis is supposed to present clinically. Many articles demonstrate the advantages of radiologic testing, such as ultrasound, barium enema, nuclear medicine scanning, and now CT scanning to assist the clinician in diagnosing acute appendicitis. This study demonstrates CT scanning also can help diagnose patients with "equivocal" appendicitis. Of 149 patients, 97 were thought to have an equivocal diagnosis of appendicitis. The other 52 had immediate appendectomy. This number of patients with "equivocal" appendicitis is greater than I am personally used to encountering. It may represent a difference in the patient population. The authors clearly demonstrate that a CT scanning can help increase the diagnostic accuracy of the clinician in patients with equivocal clinical presentations. They also demonstrate that with Medicare payment (which is low for CT scanning) it would save hospitals money to CT scan every patient as long as his or her negative appendectomy rate is 13% to 15% or more, because the CT scan would allow the clinician to achieve a 7% appendectomy rate, which would result in cost savings.

I see a problem with using a CT scan or other radiologic modalities for diagnosing every patient who comes into the emergency room with acute abdominal pain. Physicians may rely more on x-ray studies than on history and physical examinations leading to excessive testing and costs.

While this study did demonstrate a higher than expected incidence of "equivocal" acute appendicitis, nevertheless, it did show radiologic testing can be helpful in a select group of patients. Clearly, the radiologist must be skilled in evaluating radiographic studies. We found this true in the initial use of ultrasonography in diagnosing equivocal acute appendicitis. Until the radiologists became familiar with the use of this test, they had a very high false-positive rate. A similar finding may also occur with CT scanning unless the radiologist is familiar with the radiographic signs of acute appendicitis.

R.J. Howard, M.D., Ph.D.

Laparoscopic Management of Acute Peritonitis

Navez B, Tassetti V, Scohy JJ, et al (Hôpital Saint-Joseph, Gilly (Charleroi), Belgium; Hôpital Civil, Strasbourg, France)

Br J Surg 85:32-36, 1998 5–9

Purpose.—Peritonitis was previously regarded as a contraindication to laparoscopy. The reason for this contraindication was fear of malignant hypercapnia or toxic shock syndrome. An experience with laparoscopy for the management of peritonitis is reviewed.

Patients.—The retrospective study included 231 patients who underwent laparoscopy during episodes of acute peritonitis. The patients (121 females and 110 males; mean age, 54 years) were treated at 2 centers over a 5-year period. Diagnoses included appendicular peritonitis in 91 patients, perforated gastroduodenal ulcers in 69, colonic perforations in 35, and other diagnoses in 36. Peritonitis was generalized in 54% of the patients.

Outcomes.—The postoperative mortality rate was 4%. In 85% of the patients, laparoscopy identified the exact cause of peritonitis. In 25%, laparoscopy led to a change in the preoperative diagnosis. It avoided unnecessary laparotomy in 6.5% of the patients and led to modification of the incision site in 9%. Conversion to laparotomy was necessary in 15% of the patients overall: 25% of those with appendicular peritonitis, 16% of those with gastroduodenal perforation, and 83% of those with colonic perforation (Table 2). There were no cases of malignant hyperthermia but 2 cases of postoperative septic shock; both patients survived.

TABLE 2.—Causes of Peritonitis, Diagnostic and Therapeutic Results

Aetiology of Peritonitis	Total	Correct Laparoscopic Diagnosis	Conversions	Complications	Mean Hospital Stay (Days)
Appendicitis	91	91	23 (25)	8 (9)	8
Perforated ulcer	69	63	11 (16)	9 (13)	13
Perforation of the colon	35	10	29 (83)	9 (26)	18
Pelvic inflammatory disease	14	14	0	0	6
Small bowel perforation	7	6	4	4	15
Biliary peritonitis	6	5	2	2	10
Postoperative peritonitis	5	5	0	0	7
Primary peritonitis	1	0	0	0	12
Acute pancreatitis	1	1	0	0	12
Urinary peritonitis	1	1	0	0	6

(Courtesy of Navez V, Tassetti V, Scohy JJ, et al: Laparoscopic management of acute peritonitis. *Br J Surg* 85:32-36, 1998. Blackwell Science Ltd.)

Conclusions.—The experience suggests that laparoscopy can be safely carried out in patients with peritonitis. Laparoscopy can confirm the preoperative diagnosis and clarify treatment planning, sometimes avoiding the need for laparotomy. It is particularly useful in patients with appendicular or gastroduodenal perforation. Patients with colonic perforation are more likely to require laparotomy, but even they may be managed laparoscopically with increasing surgical experience.

► Laparoscopy has now come to treatment of patients with peritonitis, something that previously was thought not to be appropriate because of the risk of hypercapnia and dissemination of infection. These authors, however, were successful in treating most patients with peritonitis, which was usually due to a perforated appendix or perforated ulcer. They were less successful with perforations of the colon. In patients with colonic perforations in whom treatment was successful, they either drained abscesses or performed laparoscope-assisted colostomy. The authors acknowledged that laparoscopic treatment for postoperative peritonitis is a new concept that should be used with caution. Of special concern is that, with intense inflammation, it may be difficult to explore all parts of the abdomen without injuring the intestine. There may be a real danger of missing abscesses between loops of intestine, below the diaphragm, or in the pelvis. Many patients with peritonitis are elderly and extremely ill. Laparoscopy may add undue amounts of time to the operative procedure. The procedure may still have to be converted to an open operation. Nonetheless, this report is promising because it shows that most patients with peritonitis (although not patients with colonic perforations) can be successfully treated laparoscopically.

R.J. Howard, M.D., Ph.D.

Tertiary Peritonitis: Clinical Features of a Complex Nosocomial Infection

Nathens AB, Rotstein OD, Marshall JC (Univ of Toronto; Toronto Gen Hosp)
World J Surg 22:158-163, 1998 5–10

Background.—Tertiary peritonitis exists when intra-abdominal infections persist or recur after appropriate therapy for primary or secondary peritonitis fails. The mortality rate associated with this condition is high, and therapy is typically ineffective. Reviewed are the clinical course and microbiological findings of critically ill patients in whom tertiary peritonitis developed.

Methods.—During 5 years, 59 patients who had undergone laparotomies for intra-abdominal infections before or during their ICU admissions and had secondary bacterial peritonitis were studied. All patients had been in the ICU at least 24 hours, and all received appropriate therapy for their infections. Tertiary peritonitis was defined as a persistent or recurrent intra-abdominal infection identified at least 48 hours after treatment for secondary peritonitis. Microbiological findings, clinical courses, and outcomes were compared between those patients who had tertiary peritonitis and those who did not.

Findings.—Of the 59 patients with secondary peritonitis, 44 (74%) also had tertiary peritonitis. The 2 groups did not differ significantly in age, diagnosis at admission, premorbid health status, or Acute Physiology and Chronic Health Evaluation II score at admission. However, patients with tertiary peritonitis stayed in the ICU significantly longer (21.8 ± 14.9 vs. 8.5 ± 7.9 days), and they had significantly greater organ dysfunction (organ dysfunction scores of 13.3 ± 5.1 vs. 7.7 ± 3.3). At the first treatment, the microbiological findings were similar in patients with secondary and tertiary peritonitis. In patients with secondary peritonitis, the most common isolates were *Escherichia coli*, *Enterococcus*, and *Bacteroides fragilis*. In patients with tertiary peritonitis, however, the microbiological findings shifted during the ICU stay to a predominance of *Enterococcus*, *Candida* species, and *Staphylococcus epidermidis*. Both groups received a similar number of antibiotics, but the course for patients with tertiary peritonitis was not altered by appropriate antimicrobial therapy. Almost twice as many patients with tertiary peritonitis died (28 of 64, or 64% vs. 5 of 15, or 33%), and most of these deaths (25 of 28, or 89%) occurred in the ICU. Those who died of tertiary peritonitis underwent significantly fewer percutaneous drainage procedures than did survivors (0.3 ± 0.6 vs. 1.2 ± 0.88) but significantly more open drainage procedures (3.9 ± 3.4 vs. 2.8 ± 1.5). Laparotomies revealed the infectious foci to be disperse.

Conclusions.—Neither antimicrobial therapy or surgical treatment could halt the development of tertiary peritonitis. The altered microbial environment in these patients consisted of relatively nonpathogenic organisms, which may reflect advancing immune dysfunction, a translocation of infecting species from the gastrointestinal tract, or both. Furthermore, the worse organ function scores in patients with tertiary peritonitis indicates a deterioration of organ function in this condition.

► Nathens and colleagues try to make sense of an extremely difficult subject, tertiary or recurrent peritonitis. One reason for the difficulty, no doubt, is that these patients are not that frequently seen in ICUs; the authors saw only 44 patients with tertiary peritonitis admitted to the surgical ICU of a major hospital during a 5-year period. These patients can differ markedly from one to the other in terms of age, cause of peritonitis, other medical illnesses, and the severity of both the secondary and the tertiary peritonitis. Yet tertiary peritonitis is a problem that every large hospital must face. These patients have an extremely high mortality rate—63.6% in this series. In addition, 44 of 59 patients with intra-abdominal infections admitted to the surgical ICU had tertiary peritonitis, which is a figure that seems to be high. The main difference between patients with secondary vs. tertiary peritonitis is the microbiological findings. The most common organisms cultured from patients with secondary peritonitis were common anterotic pathogens such as *E. coli* and *B. fragilis* and *Enterococcus*. On the other hand, those with tertiary peritonitis had organisms with low intrinsic virulence such as *Enterococcus*, *Candida* and *S. epidermidis*. It is not yet known what the best way to treat these patients is. Some have advocated scheduled reoperation on these patients, whereas others propose reoperation only for clinical indications. From the authors series, there was no difference between survival and mortality rates based on the operative plan.

The authors do suggest that tertiary peritonitis may be a manifestation of end-stage organ dysfunction caused by sepsis. Furthermore, they suggest that it is plausible that patients are dying with infection rather than of infection. This might lead the reader to conclude that what is really needed is treatment of the organ dysfunction and that treating the intra-abdominal infection is less important. If this interpretation is correct, it does seem to fly in the face of current surgical teaching.

R.J. Howard, M.D., Ph.D.

Postsurgical Mediastinitis: A Case-Control Study

Muñoz P, Menasalvas A, Bernaldo de Quirós JCL, et al (Hosp Gen Universitario "Gregorio Marañón, Madrid)
Clin Infect Dis 25:1060-1064, 1997 5–11

Objective.—Postsurgical mediastinitis (PSM), although rare, carries a high morbidity and mortality rate. Results of a 9-year case-control study to identify risk factors and poor prognostic factors for patients with PSM are discussed.

Methods.—Between 1985 and 1993, 81 (2.2%) of 3,711 patients who underwent sternotomy were diagnosed with PSM in a 2,000-bed general university hospital in Madrid, Spain. Charts of 73 PSM patients and 73 controls who had undergone median sternotomy but did not become

TABLE 2.—Comparison of Postsurgical Risk Factors for Cases With Postsurgical Mediastinitis and for Controls

Variable	Cases (n = 73)	Controls (n = 73)	P value	RR
Fever within first 3 days after surgery	39 (53.4)	12 (16.4)	<.001	
Mean ICU stay in d (range)	13 (3-55)	8 (1-111)	.03	
Reoperation*	29 (39)	6 (8.2)	<.001	9.2
Vasoactive drugs*	30 (41)	14 (19.1)	.002	3.5
Pacemaker	12 (16.4)	4 (5.4)	.02	
Mean duration of mechanical ventilation in d (range)	6 (1-40)	2 (1-30)	<.001	
Mean duration of treatment with central line in d (range)	8 (1-45)	3 (1-25)	<.001	
Fever after third postoperative day*	56 (76)	0	<.0001	406

NOTE: Data are number (%) of patients unless otherwise indicated.
Abbreviation: ICU, intensive care unit.
*Independent risk factors for postsurgical mediastinitis in the multivariate analysis.

infected after surgery were reviewed for risk factors that existed before onset of mediastinitis.

Results.—Significant preoperative risk factors included emergency surgery (27.3% of cases vs. 13.3% of controls) and New York Heart Association (NYHA) functional class IV (46.5% of cases vs. 21.9% of controls). Significant surgical risk factors included heart transplantation and coronary artery bypass graft (Table 2). There were 13 (17.8%) deaths among PSM patients, 10 directly attributable to PSM vs. 2 (2.7%) deaths among controls ($P<0.01$). According to multivariate analysis bacteremia (relative risk, 21.5), use of an intraaortic balloon (relative risk, 14.9), older age (RR, 1.14/year), and extended mechanical ventilation (RR, 1.1/day) were independent risk factors for mortality.

Conclusion.—Older patients, patients who required extended mechanical ventilation and an intraaortic balloon pump, and patients who had bacteremia were at higher risk for PSM.

▶ Postsurgical mediastinitis is a rare problem following sternotomy. It is important because it is difficult to treat, and the mortality rate is high among individuals who develop this complication. All patients received cefazolin prophylaxis. The study would have been more interesting if the authors had commented on whether infected patients received prophylaxis antibiotics at the appropriate time in relation to their operations. The factors associated with developing mediastinitis have been found in postoperative infections of other sites; that is, emergency surgery, operations on immunocompromised hosts (in this case, heart transplantation), reoperations, and presence of fever. This is a good review of this dreaded complication of median sternotomy.

R.J. Howard, M.D., Ph.D.

The Impact of *Clostridium difficile* on a Surgical Service: A Prospective Study of 374 Patients

Kent KC, Rubin MS, Wrobleski L, et al (Beth Israel Deaconess Med Ctr, Boston; Harvard Med School, Boston)

Ann Surg 227:296-301, 1998 5–12

Introduction.—*Clostridium difficile* colitis (CDC) is a common nosocomial infection that causes discomfort, inconvenience, and sometimes severe illness in patients admitted with unrelated medical or surgical conditions. The incidence, risk factors, and clinical course of CDC were assessed in patients admitted exclusively to a surgical service.

Methods.—During a 5-month period, 374 patients admitted to general, vascular, thoracic, and urologic surgical services were prospectively followed for the development of CDC. Patients admitted for treatment of CDC were excluded. Rectal cultures were taken from each patient before 9 days or within 24 hours of admission, then at 2-day intervals thereafter. Patients were considered to have symptomatic CDC if they had more than

3 bowel movements within 24 hours and a positive cytotoxin assay or culture.

Results.—CDC developed in 21 of 374 patients (5.6%). Risk factors independently predisposing patients to development of CDC included admission from a skilled care facility, use of the antibiotic cefoxitin, and an operative procedure for bowel obstruction. Other factors associated with CDC were colectomy, treatment with any antibiotic, nasogastric tube suction, advanced age, and previous antibiotic treatment. Abdominal pain and fever occurred frequently in patients with CDC. All patients had prolonged hospitalization as a result of CDC; 1 patient required urgent colectomy.

Conclusion.—Patients undergoing surgery frequently experience CDC, especially those undergoing intestinal surgery. The course of CDC was not severe in most patients and the infection responded well to oral metronidazole or vancomycin. Patients with CDC can experience significant morbidity, as evidenced by the 1 patient who required urgent laparotomy. A variety of factors may predispose patients to development of CDC. They should be treated aggressively, especially if there is associated intestinal stasis.

▶ Constipation and diarrhea are relatively common after surgical procedures. Several years ago, *Clostridium difficile*, an enterotoxigenic anaerobic bacterium, was identified as the cause of diarrhea in hospitalized patients. This cause is frequently thought of only after a patient may have had diarrhea for several days. Thus, the patient may become ill (and occasionally die) from CDC, and the hospitalization may be prolonged.

This study from the Beth Israel Deaconess Medical Center in Boston found that CDC was relatively common (5.6%) among patients admitted to the surgical services. As might be expected, most of these infections occurred in patients having general surgery. Also, as previously demonstrated, patients receiving antibiotics (especially cefoxitin) were more likely to have this infection than those who did not receive antibiotics.

Antibiotics may eliminate the natural host flora, allowing *C. difficile* to overgrow and cause disease. Although they do not specifically state it, the authors suggest that cefoxitin was used only for surgical prophylaxis in many of these patients. Thus, they suggest that even a brief course of antibiotics may predispose patients to CDC. Many hospitals have substituted cefotetan for cefoxitin in patients requiring prophylaxis for intestinal surgery. Thus, there is a possibility that this antibiotic might also predispose to CDC. This paper points out that CDC is relatively common in postoperative patients and that anyone with persistent diarrhea should be examined for the presence of this infection.

R.J. Howard, M.D., Ph.D.

Twenty-five Years of Experience in the Surgical Treatment of Perforation of the Ileum Caused by *Salmonella typhi* at the General Hospital of Mexico City, Mexico

Athié CG, Guízar CB, Alcántara AV, et al (Natl Autonomous Univ of México)

Surgery 123:632-636, 1998 5–13

Purpose.—Typhoid fever remains an important worldwide health problem. Intestinal perforation may occur as a result of delayed hypersensitivity to salmonellae; the resulting peritonitis is fatal unless the patient receives prompt and adequate treatment. There is ongoing debate over the most appropriate type of surgery for these intestinal perforations. A 25-year experience with the surgical management of intestinal perforations caused by *Salmonella typhi* is reported.

Methods.—From 1970 through 1994, 352 patients with ileal perforation caused by *S. typhi* were treated at a Mexico City hospital. In addition to antibiotic therapy, all patients underwent surgery. Two hundred thirty-six patients in group A, treated from 1970 through 1984, were managed with conventional resection and anastomosis or primary closure. One hundred sixteen patients in group B, treated during and after 1985, were managed with directed intestinal resection of 10 cm on either side of the perforation based on anatomopathologic studies with serial sections.

Results.—The 352 patients accounted for 2.24% of all patients undergoing surgery for nontraumatic acute abdominal conditions. In each patient, the perforation was found in the antimesenteric border. Patients in group A had high rates of anastomotic dehiscence, intestinal fistula, and new perforations. Morbidity was 33.47% in this group, and mortality was 7.20%. In group B, morbidity was reduced to 1.72%; both complications were anastomotic dehiscences. Mortality was also 1.72%.

Conclusions.—This large experience with surgical management of ileal perforation caused by *S. typhi* strongly supports the use of directed intestinal resection. In this procedure, 10 cm is resected on each side of the distal and proximal perforation. Ileostomy should be reserved for patients at high risk because of conditions in the peritoneum and intestinal loops. Even in patients with a single perforation, primary closure should be avoided because of intestinal wall alterations in the area surrounding the perforation.

► The authors sum up a long experience in the management of ileal perforations due to *Salmonella typhi*. They have seen a total of 352 cases. Mortality of patients who had either primary closure or a conventional resection clearly differs from mortality of patients treated on the basis of anatomic and histologic study of the involved ileum at the time of operation. Because of severe complications in the immediate postoperative period following either primary closure or conventional resection, the authors performed a directed intestinal resection of 10 cm on either side of the last distal and proximal perforation of all patients (group B) in 1985. This change in policy resulted in a much lower mortality. The mortality rate also was far below that of previous literature reports. Because of the rate of migration from other countries, it may not be unusual for surgeons to confront patients having ileal perforation because of this organism. Surgery should be cognizant of the latest treatment.

R.J. Howard, M.D., Ph.D.

Wound Botulism Associated With Black Tar Heroin Among Injecting Drug Users

Passaro DJ, Werner SB, McGee J, et al (Stanford Univ, Calif; Ctrs for Disease Control and Prevention, Atlanta, Ga)

JAMA 279:859-863, 1998 5–14

Objective.—Injectable drug users (IDUs) are at increased risk of wound botulism (WB), a potentially lethal infection. Because all forms of botulism are reportable in California, a case-control study was conducted in California to compare IDUs with WB to other heroin users to identify risk factors associated with the disease.

Methods.—Cases of all IDUs (n = 26, 15 female; median age, 41.5 years) confirmed with WB between January 1, 1994 and March 1, 1996 were compared with cases of control IDUs (n = 110) without WB, enrolled in methadone programs, with respect to factors associated with development of WB.

Results.—Fourteen WB patients were non-Hispanic white, 11 were Hispanic, and none were HIV-positive. Black tar heroin (BTH) was injected by 96% of WB patients (27 g/mo) and 97% of controls (31 g/mo). WB patients injected significantly higher quantities of heroin subcutaneously or intramuscularly than controls (22.3 vs. 6.3 g), were significantly more likely to inject drugs this way than controls (92% vs. 44%), and used these routes of administration more times every month than controls (67 vs. 24). There was a dose-response relationship between the amount of heroin injected subcutaneously or intramuscularly and risk of WB (χ^2=26.5). Cleaning the skin, cleaning syringes, and exchanging needles did not protect against WB. According to multivariate analysis, injecting BTH subcutaneously or intramuscularly was associated with development of WB.

Conclusion.—Injecting BTH subcutaneously or intramuscularly was significantly associated with development of WB.

▶ The transmission of viral diseases by injecting drug users is well known. Many cases of human immunodeficiency virus, hepatitis B virus, and hepatitis C virus have been transmitted in this way. This study describes 26 patients who transmitted botulism by use of black tar heroin. Most of the patients had subcutaneous or intramuscular injections. Surgeons may be called to treat cutaneous or muscular abscess from injection of illicit substances. They may be unfamiliar with signs and symptoms of botulism that can be transmitted by this fashion.

R.J. Howard, M.D., Ph.D.

6 Transplantation

Introduction

Transplantation continues to make strides in improving outcomes and is being extended to individuals previously denied this therapy. The past year has seen an individual in France undergo a hand transplant, and in January a patient in Louisville, Ky, underwent hand transplantation. The improved results and extension to individuals who previously were not thought to be candidates led to a marked growth in the waiting list of the United Network for Organ Sharing (UNOS). The first article by Lin and colleagues (Abstract 6–1) discusses the center-specific graft survival rates between 1988 and 1994. While these data are somewhat old, they do provide a basis for comparison between centers. These data are also available to patients on the internet so they can compare transplant center results.

The increased waiting times for transplantation and increased numbers of patients on the waiting list has fueled a controversy in the United States on the allocation of organs. Much of 1998 was spent debating various liver allocation schemes. The secretary of Health and Human Services proposed a national waiting list so that organs would go to the sickest patients first. Many individuals actively opposed this plan, which now has been deferred for a year. While the discussion has quieted temporarily, the debate will no doubt again become heated later in 1999. It may be that changes in the allocation system will also affect other organs. The net effect may be that some smaller centers may find it difficult to perform transplants in their patients. I believe that no matter what allocation system one adopts, the same number of transplants will be done. Organ availability is the rate-limiting step to transplantation. Any allocation system will merely choose where they are done and who gets transplanted.

With the growing organ shortage an ever-increasing attempt is being made to use organs previously not considered suitable for transplantation. Nghiem and others (Abstract 6–2) discuss their experience using en bloc infant kidneys and demonstrate that outcomes are reasonable enough to use them in most patients. Whiting and colleagues (Abstract 6–3) discuss the economic cost of expanded criteria donors, and they note that using these donors is more expensive than using regular donors.

The three-year results of the randomized multiple center study of mycophenolate mofetil is discussed by Mathew et al. (Abstract 6–4). They find that even in three years there was no significant difference among the groups in terms of graft outcome, even though there was less rejection in the early period after transplantation.

Another way of increasing the number of usable organs is to divide livers and use both pieces for transplantation (split liver transplantation). An article by Rela and others (Abstract 6–5) demonstrates that there is a minimal price to pay in technical complications for splitting livers and, therefore, this is a viable way to increase the donor supply. Two other articles dealing with liver transplantation discuss late graft loss up to 10 years after liver transplantation and the effect of lamivudine on recurrent hepatitis B following liver transplantation (Abstracts 6–6 and 6–7).

Sollinger and colleagues (Abstract 6–8) discuss their experience with 500 pancreas–kidney transplants at the University of Wisconsin. This article is a good summary of the outcomes of pancreas–kidney transplantation from this leading transplant institution. The hope was that pancreas transplantation would slow or reverse the secondary complications of diabetes. An article by Fioretto and colleagues (Abstract 6–9) from the University of Minnesota, another pioneering institution in pancreas transplantation, demonstrates that the lesions of diabetic nephropathy can be reversed after pancreas transplantation.

Abu-Elmagd and colleagues (Abstract 6–10) from the University of Pittsburgh demonstrate that results with intestinal transplantation have improved. Many problems remain, but the pioneering investigators from this institution have demonstrated that persistence and hard work can overcome many of the formidable barriers to intestinal transplantation.

Finally, Zaidi et al. (Abstract 6–11) demonstrate increased survival in a pig-to-primate renal xenotransplantation model using genetically modified donor animals.

Richard J. Howard, M.D., Ph.D.

Center-Specific Graft and Patient Survival Rates: 1997 United Network for Organ Sharing (UNOS) Report

Lin H-M, Kauffman M, McBride MA, et al (United Network for Organ Sharing, Richmond, Va; Milton S. Hershey Med Ctr, Hershey, Pa; Univ of Alabama, Birmingham; et al)

JAMA 280:1153-1160, 1998 6–1

Introduction.—As required by the Transplant Amendment Act of 1990, the United Network for Organ Sharing (UNOS) reports center-specific survival rates for all solid organ transplants performed in the United States. On the basis of previous reports, UNOS has developed objective criteria for use in identifying programs with lower than expected survival rates. The short-term and long-term results of U.S. organ transplant procedures—both nationally and for individual transplant programs—are reported.

Methods.—The analysis included a total of 97,587 kidney, liver, pancreas, heart, lung, and heart-lung transplants performed in 92,966 patients from 1988 to 1994. The procedures were performed by 742 different transplant programs. Donor and recipient factors affecting graft and patient survival were determined by multivariate regression analysis. Survival rates were considered in 2 eras (1988-1992 and 1992-1994) to compare center-specific performance with expected performance, adjusted for risk. The survival data were also used to identify transplant programs with survival rates that were better or worse than expected.

Results.—One-year follow-up data were available for more than 98% of the transplants, and conditional 3-year follow-up data were available for more than 91%. Transplants performed in era 2 were associated with significantly better graft and patient survival than those performed in era 1. The exception was heart transplants, for which patient and graft survival rates were unchanged. The 1-year graft survival rate after cadaver organ transplantation was 81.5% for heart transplants, 81.0% for kidney transplants, 73.5% for pancreas transplants, 70.4% for lung transplants, 69.9% for liver transplants, and 61.9% for heart-lung transplants. Values for 3-year conditional graft survival were 9.13% for pancreas transplants, 90.1% for heart transplants, 89.7% for kidney transplants, 89.0% for liver transplants, 80.1% for heart-lung transplants, and 74.7% for lung transplants. At 76% (for liver transplants) to 98% (for heart-lung transplants) of programs, actual 1-year graft survival was equal to or better than expected survival, adjusted for risk. Centers with significantly lower than expected survival rates usually performed fewer than the national average number of transplants per year.

Conclusions.—UNOS data show improving graft and patient survival rates after solid organ transplantation. Conditional 3-year graft survival exceeds 90% for most organs; most of the risk occurs in the first year after transplantation. For most transplant programs, survival figures are at least as good as expected. The differences between centers are most significant in the first year posttransplant, with little effect on long-term survival.

► The increase in graft survival rates over the past 15 to 20 years has been quite amazing. The improvement has been due to the work of a tremendous number of physicians and investigators, resulting in better surgical technique, development of new immunosuppressive drugs, and better ability to treat and prevent problems that occur after transplantation. This report from the UNOS gives national data between January 1988 and April 1994. These data provide comparison data that individual centers can use for comparing their own data. Unfortunately, the data are old. In some areas the field has already moved beyond what is presented here and survival rates are even better than the most recent period of May 1992 to 1994.

R.J. Howard, M.D., Ph.D.

En Bloc Transplantation of Infant Kidneys: Ten-Year Experience

Nghiem DD, Schlosser JD, Hsia S, et al (Allegheny Univ, Pittsburgh, Pa)
J Am Coll Surg 186:402-407, 1998 6–2

Objective.—Long-term results of en bloc infant kidney transplantation are few and controversial. Ten-year results of such en bloc transplants from Allegheny General Hospital in Pittsburgh are presented.

Methods.—Of the 794 renal transplants performed between February 1987 and September 1997, 78 adult recipients followed up for at least 6 months received cadaveric en bloc infant kidneys. Donors' and recipients' ages, weight, creatinine level, HLA antigen matching, panel reactive antibodies, cold ischemia time, surgical complications, original disease, and long-term graft function and survival were analyzed.

Results.—Glomerulonephritis was the most common cause of end-stage renal disease, followed by diabetes, glomerulosclerosis, polycystic kidney disease, and membranoproliferative glomerulonephritis. The mean age, weight, and serum creatinine level of donors were 31.2 months, 10.9 kg, and 0.3 mg/dL. The average age and weight of recipients were 36.3 years and 71.5 kg. Cold ischemia time averaged 23.4 hours; kidneys were mismatched for 2.6 HLA-A, B, and DR antigens; and the average follow-up was 43 months. Thrombosis occurred in 5 kidneys (6.4%), ureteral leaks in 2 (2.6%), and short-term dialysis in 5 (6.4%). Deaths were caused by infection (n = 2), heart attack and stroke (n = 6), and hepatoma (n = 1). All patients had functioning grafts at the time of death. Seven patients

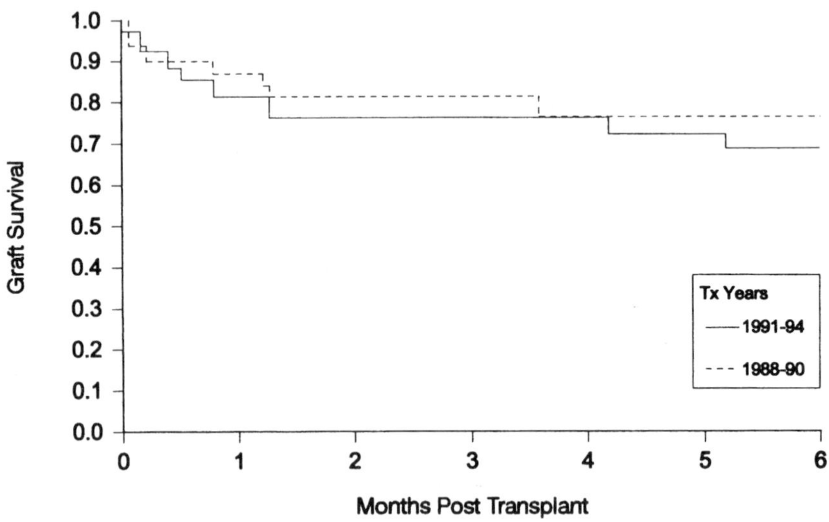

FIGURE 2.—En bloc graft survival for early and late transplant years. Early graft loss in both eras resulted from venous thrombosis and from rejection. The significantly higher graft loss in the recent series was probably related to the selection of high-risk kidneys requiring extensive venous and arterial reconstructions. *Abbreviation: Tx*, transplant. (Courtesy of Nghiem DD, Schlosser JD, Hsia S, et al: En bloc transplantation of infant kidneys: Ten-year experience. *J Am Coll Surg* 186:402-407, 1998. By permission of the American College of Surgeons.)

with renal stenosis were successfully treated with dilation. Six grafts were rejected, including 1 because of noncompliance. Massive proteinuria developed in 3 patients with recurrent disease. Graft survival at 43 months was 79%. Creatinine levels at 1, 3, 9, and 10 years were 1.2, 1.0, 0.8, and 0.8 mg/dL, respectively. There was a significant difference in serum creatinine levels between single, en bloc, adult, and living-related kidneys, with en bloc kidneys having the lowest levels. Graft survival in the en bloc and single-kidney groups was similar (Fig 2). However, there was a significantly higher graft failure rate in the en bloc group than in the single-kidney group during the first few months as a result of thrombosis and rejection (20.4% vs. 8.5%, respectively).

Conclusion.—Long-term function in successfully transplanted en bloc infant kidneys is excellent.

► A growing disparity between patients waiting for cadaveric organ transplants and the number of organs available has led transplant surgeons to extend the acceptable criteria for potential donors. Articles dealing with this were reviewed in the 1998 YEAR BOOK OF SURGERY.[1] The current article by Nghiem and colleagues discusses the experience of 78 adult recipients of cadaveric en bloc infant kidney transplants performed at Allegheny General Hospital. Five en bloc kidneys thrombosed (6.4%). This number is higher than seen with adult kidneys. There were also 2 ureteral fistulas, which were repaired successfully. The average creatinine levels were low and the creatinine clearances were in the normal range, suggesting that en bloc infant kidneys have sufficient renal mass and can hypertrophy to accommodate the large body size of the adult and result in normal renal function. The authors do note that the technique of recovery of organs from infant donors is critical, since pedicular dissection can result in devascularization of the ureter or division of small renal arteries. The combination of these problems resulted in the discarding of 30 pairs of infant kidneys during a 10-year period.

R.J. Howard, M.D., Ph.D.

Reference

1. 1998 YEAR BOOK OF SURGERY, pp 132-141.

Economic Costs of Expanded Criteria Donors in Renal Transplantation

Whiting JF, Golconda M, Smith R, et al (Univ of Cincinnati, Ohio; Health Alliance of Greater Cincinnati, Ohio)

Transplantation 65:204-207, 1998 6–3

Objective.—There is an effort to use "expanded criteria" donors (ECDs) to alleviate the shortage of kidneys despite the increased morbidity. The costs associated with the use of ECDs in kidney transplantation at the Health Alliance of Greater Cincinnati were identified retrospectively.

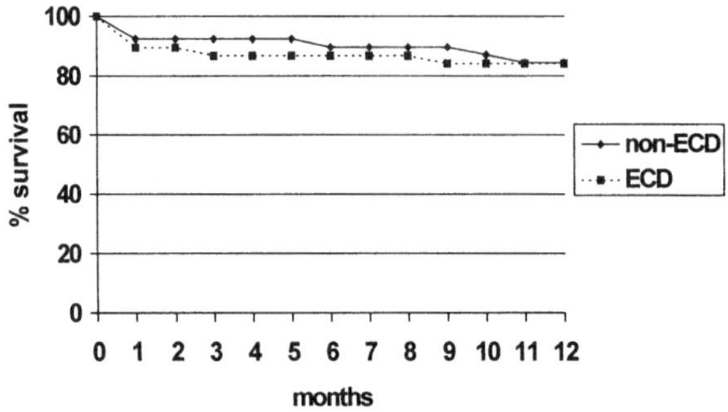

FIGURE 1.—Graft survival of recipients of kidneys from expanded criteria donors (*ECDs*) and non-ECDs. (Courtesy of Whiting JF, Golconda M, Smith R, et al: Economic costs of expanded criteria donors in renal transplantation. *Transplantation* 65:204-207, 1998.)

Methods.—Of 78 patients having renal transplants in 1995, 38 received ECD kidneys. Total hospital costs were calculated for each patient for the initial transplantation.

Results.—Graft and patient survival at 1 year were similar for ECD and non-ECD kidneys (Fig 1). Patients receiving ECD kidneys had a significantly longer cold ischemic time, required more hemodialysis, had a longer hospital stay, and had a higher serum creatinine level at 1 year after transplantation. Patients receiving ECD kidneys had a nonsignificantly higher incidence of rejection, received more antilymphocyte induction therapy, and had a higher number of readmissions. Patients receiving ECD kidneys had total average and median costs that were $12,190 and $10,911 higher, respectively, than recipients of non-ECD kidneys. For patients receiving ECD kidneys, costs were $15,311 higher for patients older than 60 years or for retransplant patients than when ECDs were transplanted into lower-risk patients, and $20,680 more than for low-risk patients receiving non-ECD kidneys. Length of stay and use of antilymphocyte therapy were significantly correlated to costs according to linear regression analysis.

Conclusions.—Transplantation using ECD kidneys is significantly more costly than transplantation using non-ECD kidneys. Additional studies need to investigate the long-term cost-effectiveness associated with the use of ECD kidneys.

▶ As more and more patients are placed on organ waiting lists, the disparity between the number of organs available and the number of patients needing organ transplants increases. This organ shortage has led transplant surgeons to expand their definition of an acceptable organ. These "expanded criteria" donors are being used more frequently in renal and other transplants.

Last year in YEAR BOOK OF SURGERY, we reviewed 2 papers dealing with ECDs and organs that had been turned down by all other transplant centers (the kidneys that nobody wanted). These papers found that graft survival was as good as that achieved with organs from donors that were considered to be "conventional."

The number of articles dealing with this issue has expanded this year. In the January 27, 1998 issue of *Transplantation*, 3 studies were published dealing with ECDs. The first study, by Whiting et al. from Cincinnati (summarized above), found that graft survival was identical in patients receiving conventional organs or organs from ECDs. Transplants using organs from ECDs, however, were associated with significantly increased costs. The increased costs resulted from an increased length of stay and from the increased number of patients requiring dialysis after transplantation. These differences led to increased pharmacy charges and increased room and board charges. The second study, by Lee et al.[1] from Stanford, used kidneys that nobody wanted. They found that even after a year, graft survival was similar in patients receiving organs from conventional donors and patients receiving organs from donors that no one wanted. On the other hand, the third study, by Kumar et al.[2] from the University of Pennsylvania, found that kidneys from older donors had inferior graft survival compared with organs from younger donors. This issue deserves continuing examination.

R.J. Howard, M.D., Ph.D.

References

1. Lee CM, Scandling JD, Pavlakis M, et al: Review of the kidneys that nobody wanted. Determinants of optimal outcome. *Transplantation* 65:213-219, 1998.
2. Kumar MSA, Panigrahi D, Dezii CM, et al: Long-term function and survival of elderly donor kidneys transplanted into young adults. *Transplantation* 65:282-285. 1998.

A Blinded, Long-term, Randomized Multicenter Study of Mycophenolate Mofetil in Cadaveric Renal Transplantation

Mathew TH, for the Tricontinental Mycophenolate Mofetil Renal Transplantation Study Group (Queen Elizabeth Hosp, Woodville, South Australia)
Transplantation 65:1450-1454, 1998 6–4

Objective.—The effect of the new immunosuppressant drug mycophenolate mofetil (MMF) on acute renal allograft rejection was investigated in a prospective, randomized, double-blind clinical trial at 21 transplant centers in Australia, Europe, and Canada.

Methods.—A total of 503 patients receiving their first (n = 443) or second (n = 60) renal transplants were randomly allocated to receive 100 to 150 mg of azathioprine (AZA) (n = 166), 2 g of MMF (n = 173), or 3 g of MMF (n= 164) daily for 3 years. Patients also received cyclosporine and prednisone. Graft and patient survival, graft function, and safety were assessed.

Results.—Of the 503 patients, 83 patients receiving AZA, 85 receiving MMF 2 g, and 83 receiving MMF 3 g completed the study. In addition to those who completed the protocol at 1 year, some patients failed to complete the study because of adverse events (27 AZA, 31 MMF 2 g, and 34 MMF 3 g); unsatisfactory therapeutic response (11 AZA, 10 MMF 2 g,

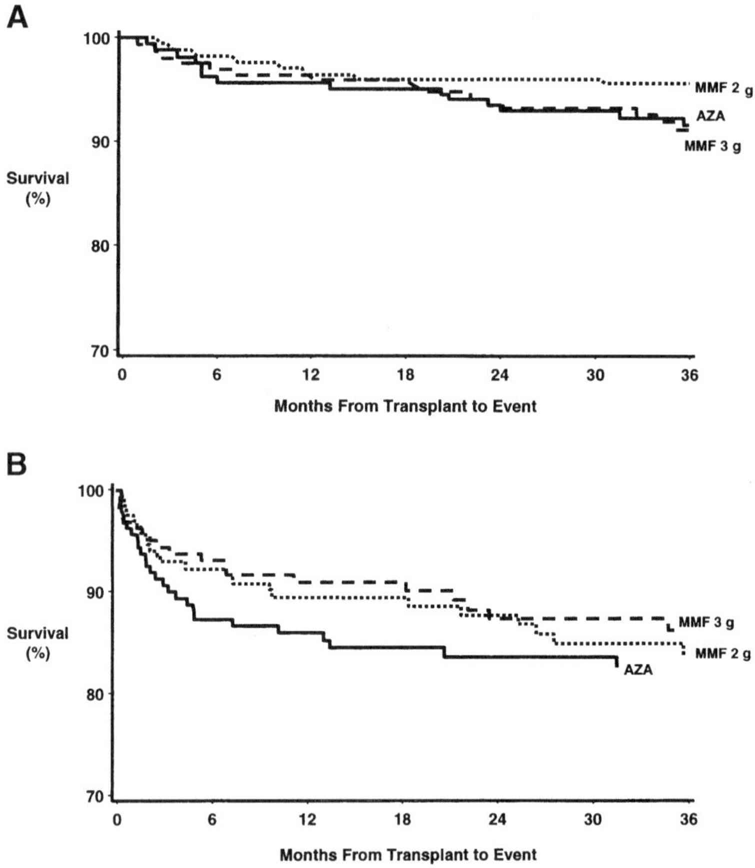

FIGURE 1.—Analysis of graft and patient survival (ie, patients alive with functioning graft). **A**, intent-to-treat analyses were performed with on-study plus posttermination data; therefore, all patients who received at least 1 dose of study drug are included. **B**, on-study (+90 days) analyses were performed with data in all patients up to the time they were terminated from the study plus 90 days after termination. (Courtesy of Mathew TH, for the Tricontinental Mycophenolate Mofetil Renal Transplantation Study Group: A blinded, long-term, randomized multicenter study of mycophenolate mofetil in cadaveric renal transplantation. *Transplantation* 65:1450-1454, 1998.)

and 3 MMF 3 g); noncompliance (9 AZA, 8 MMF 2 g, and 11 MMF 3 g); death (6 AZA, 3 MMF 2 g, and 5 MMF 3 g); and other causes (7 AZA, 10 MMF 2 g, and 10 MMF 3 g). At 6 months, the graft rejection rate was 19.7% in the MMF 2 g group, 15.9% in the MMF 3 g group, and 35.5% in the AZA group. The treatment failure rate at 6 months was significantly lower for MMF 2 g and MMF 3 g (38.2% and 34.8%) than for AZA (50%). At 3 years patient and graft survival was nonsignificantly better with MMF 2 and MMF 3 than with AZA (Fig 1). Intent-to-treat and on-study survival rates at 3 years were 81.9% and 84.0% for MMF 2 g, 84.8% and 86.4% for MMF 3 g, and 80.2% and 82.7% for AZA, respectively. Rejection rates at 3 years in the intent-to-treat group was

9.9% in the AZA group, 5.8% in the MMF 2 g group, and 3.0% in the MMF 3 g group. The respective mortality rates were 8.6%, 4.7%, and 9.1%. Renal function was similar in all 3 groups. MMF-treated patients had a higher incidence of gastrointestinal, hematologic, infection, and malignant events.

Conclusion.—Whereas MMF significantly reduced rejection episodes within the first 6 months, it did not improve survival at 3 years.

▶ This combined report of the Tricontinental Mycophenolate Mofetil Renal Transplant Study Group combines large-scale clinical trials conducted in North America, Europe, and Australia. These studies previously showed that the incidence of acute renal allograft rejection in the first 6 months after transplantation was decreased compared with that in placebo- or azathioprine-treated patients. This late (3-year) analysis is a further follow-up of the patients in the original trial. One might expect that decreased graft rejection in the first 6 months after transplantation would translate into better long-term graft survival. Since early acute rejection is the primary factor associated with chronic rejection, one might also expect a lower incidence of chronic rejection in these patients, although that was not one of the end points studied. Although graft and patient survival showed a trend toward advantage for MMF (that is, only patients alive with functioning grafts), the differences did not reach statistical significance (see Fig 1). Additional analysis, however, did show that patients who experienced biopsy-proven acute rejection during the first 6 months after transplantation were 4 times more likely to lose their grafts at 3 years than patients who experienced no early rejection. These patients were not subdivided according to immunosuppression treatment. In the 3-g MMF group, there were fewer graft losses due to rejection (3.0%) than in the 2-g MMF (5.8%) or the azathioprine-treated group (9.9%) at 3 years. Thus, there is some suggestion that prevention of early rejection can affect late graft loss due to rejection. Nevertheless, it is disappointing that this new immunosuppressive agent, which costs significantly more than azathioprine, is not associated with better graft outcomes at 3 years than the standard azathioprine treatment. (These authors use proteinuria and renal dysfunction as markers of chronic rejection.) There was no difference between the two groups in these parameters. Part of the reason that these authors were unable to show a statistically significant advantage for MMF treatment is the small size of their groups. To show a statistical difference for a survival advantage of 4% to 5%, the authors would have needed approximately 1,800 patients per treatment group, something that is just too expensive and too difficult to carry out for virtually all pharmaceutical companies.

R.J. Howard, M.D., Ph.D.

Split Liver Transplantation: King's College Hospital Experience

Rela M, Vougas V, Muiesan P, et al (King's College Hosp, London)
Ann Surg 227:282-288, 1998 6–5

Objective.—Whereas a split liver transplant (SpLT) can increase the number of grafts available for recipients, early results reveal technical complications and a selection of poor-risk patients. Experience with 41 SpLTs at 1 center are reported.

Methods.—Of 201 liver transplants performed on children between October 1989 and October 1996, 122 (61%) were SpLTs. Donor age ranged from 8 to 47 years. Patients were followed up for a median of 12 months.

Results.—Patient and graft survival was 90% and 88%. Three of the 4 patients who died received a left lateral segment, and 2 received the first 2 SpLTs performed. The remaining 2 deaths were the result of disseminated lymphoma (n = 1) and chest sepsis (n = 1). Patient and graft survival in recipients of right lobe segments were 95% and 95%. Patient and graft survival in recipients of left lateral segments were 86% and 82%, respectively. Other complications included a superficial wound dehiscence, a late hepatic artery thrombosis, and a segment IV infarction in 1 patient each, bleeding in 2 children, and peritonitis secondary to multiple small-bowel perforations in 2 children with biliary atresia. There were 6 biliary complications.

Conclusion.—Split liver transplantation, although a demanding surgical procedure, is a satisfactory procedure for adults and children with liver failure. Results are equally successful for recipients of right and left lobes. Good patient selection and good organ selection are very important.

► Split liver transplantation is a method that allows young children to receive transplants of the left lobe from an adult donor without the necessity of discarding the right lobe of the liver (reduced-size transplantation). If the hilar structures are carefully divided in the SpLT technique, the right lobe can be transplanted into an adult, thus getting 2 transplants from 1 donor. Some are reluctant to do this in light of the possibility of increased technical complications in the adult recipients because of the smaller structure. The authors present their experience with 41 SpLT recipients. In fact, 2 patient deaths involved the first 2 splits that were associated with technical complications. The authors demonstrate that, by using a careful technique, they can achieve excellent patient and graft survival in adults and children alike. The technique of splitting the liver is critical and requires attention to detail to make sure that the liver can be split in the first place and that the hilar structures are not compromised.

R.J. Howard, M.D., Ph.D.

Ten Years of Liver Transplantation: An Evolving Understanding of Late Graft Loss

Abbasoglu O, Levy MF, Brkic BB, et al (Baylor Univ, Dallas, Tex)
Transplantation 64:1801-1807, 1997 6–6

Objective.—Despite progress in long-term outcome of orthotopic liver transplantation (OLT), late graft loss is still a concern. The long-term outcome and the causes of late graft loss in OLT recipients was analyzed, prospectively.

Methods.—Between April 1985 and August 1995, 1,174 consecutive OLT were performed in 1,045 patients, aged 17 to 71. Patients were followed for a median of 48 months. Overall 5- and 10-year actuarial survival rates for patients were 68.4% and 55.9%. Overall actuarial survival rates for grafts were 60% and 48.3%.

Results.—A total of 884 patients survived their first year. There were 159 grafts lost after the first year, 132 because of death and 27 because of retransplantation in 25 patients. Patients who survived their first year had actuarial 5- and 10-year survival rates of 81.4% and 67.2% and actuarial graft survival rates of 80.1% and 64.9%. Grafts were functioning in 97 patients who died. Late graft loss was the result of recurrent disease (30.2%), cardiovascular diseases and stroke (17.7%), infections (15.1%), chronic rejection (9.4%), de novo malignancy (8.8%), biliary strictures (5.0%), acute pancreatitis (2.5%), and other (11.3%). Risk factors for late graft rejection included pretransplant diabetes, pretransplant heart disease, posttransplant renal failure, cytomegalovirus (CMV) infection, and ≥2 rejection episodes.

Conclusion.—OLT patients who live beyond the first year have excellent survival rates. The main causes of late graft loss are recurrent diseases, new malignancies, cardiovascular diseases, and stroke.

▶ During that past decade, the early and late graft survival in patients receiving liver transplants has increased substantially. Current results of liver transplantation are as good as those of kidney transplantation. Relatively few patients lose grafts from rejection both early and late compared to kidney transplant recipients. The vast majority of late graft loss is because of patient death from recurrent disease, cardiovascular disease, infections, or malignancy. Only a small number of patients (27 of 159) had a retransplant for liver failure after one year. Many of the deaths were from the effects of immunosuppressive drugs, such as infection, cardiovascular disease, malignancy, and from recurrent liver disease. With the continuing improvement of the results of liver transplantation, the reasons patients die will resemble more closely those of the general population.

R.J. Howard, M.D., Ph.D.

Efficacy of Lamivudine in Controlling Hepatitis B Virus Recurrence After Liver Transplantation

Nery JR, Weppler D, Rodriguez M, et al (Univ of Miami, Fla)
Transplantation 65:1615-1621, 1998 6–7

Objective.—Liver transplantation in patients with hepatitis B virus (HBV) is controversial because of the high risk of allograft reinfection. The effect of lamivudine, a potent HBV inhibitor, in a group of HBV-infected liver transplant recipients is reported.

Methods.—Forty (8 female) HBV-infected liver transplant recipients, aged 25 to 68 years, were treated with lamivudine (100 to 150 mg daily). Famciclovir (500 mg 3 times daily) was used as adjunct antiviral therapy in 12 patients. Patients were divided into 4 groups: group 1, rescue therapy (n = 8); group 2, elective conversion (n = 13); group 3, de novo HBV infection (n = 3); and group 4, primary treatment (n = 16). Posttransplant follow-up ranged from 8 to 64 months, and antiviral treatment follow-up ranged from 9 to 39 months.

Results.—Patient and graft survival at last follow-up was 97.5%. HBV recurred in 7 patients (17.5%). Among the 20 patients with viral replication before lamivudine treatment, the recurrence rate was 35%. There were 5 responders in group 1, 13 in group 2, 3 in group 3, and 12 in group 4. Recurrences were all mild. There were no side effects and no treatment interruptions. The estimated costs of treatment with lamivudine for the first and subsequent years were $1,401.86 and $1,343.20. The corresponding costs for famciclovir were $6,895.80 and $6,679.50. Comparable costs of hepatitis B immunoglobulin were $102,563.60 and $40,714.80.

Conclusion.—Treatment of HBV-infected liver transplant patients with lamivudine is safe, efficacious, and cost-effective.

► Concern for recurrent disease has led some liver transplant centers to not perform transplants in patients with liver failure due to active hepatitis B. Others have performed transplants in patients with nonreplicative hepatitis B who are chronically positive for HBsAg but whose HBV DNA is low. In this series of patients with chronic hepatitis B, 82.5% remained free of viral recurrence. We are not told the preoperative HBV DNA levels of the 7 patients in whom hepatitis B recurred. It would have been interesting to try to relate the risk of recurrence with preoperative DNA concentrations. It is interesting that viral replication disappeared in 19 of 20 patients after the beginning of lamivudine administration. Addition of lamivudine seems to be an important treatment in patients who receive transplants because of hepatitis B.

R.J. Howard, M.D., Ph.D.

Experience With 500 Simultaneous Pancreas–Kidney Transplants
Sollinger HW, Odorico JS, Knechtle SJ, et al (Univ of Wisconsin, Madison)
Ann Surg 228:284-296, 1998 6–8

Background.—With the availability of new immunosuppressants, the results of pancreatic transplantation have improved significantly. The past decade has seen a progressive increase in survival after simultaneous pancreas–kidney allografts (SPKs), 1-year survival now exceeds 80%. A large experience with SPKs was reviewed to assess the long-term outcomes of such transplants.

Methods.—A total of 500 SPKs were performed at the authors' center from 1985 to 1997. University of Wisconsin solution was used to preserve all pancreases. Seventy-eight percent of the procedures were performed with bladder drainage (BD); more recent patients were managed with enteric drainage (ED). Immunosuppressive regimens changed over time, with the most recent patients were managed with mycophenolate mofetil.

Results.—The 1-year patient survival rate was 96%, 5-year survival was 89%, and 10-year survival was 76% (Fig 2). Kidney function rates were 89%, 80%, and 67%; pancreatic function rates were 88%, 78%, and 67%, respectively. The overall pancreatic conversion rate was just 0.8%, whereas the primary nonfunction rate was 0.2%. Acute tubular necrosis occurred in 4% of the kidneys. Twenty-four percent of the procedures necessitated conversion from BD to ED, most often because of leakage (14% of the cases), urethritis with extravasation (7%), and chronic hematuria (3%). In no case did enteric conversion lead to graft loss, and graft survival was similar in the ED and BD groups. There were 45 cases of pancreas rejection, and 27 patients died with a functioning pancreas. After

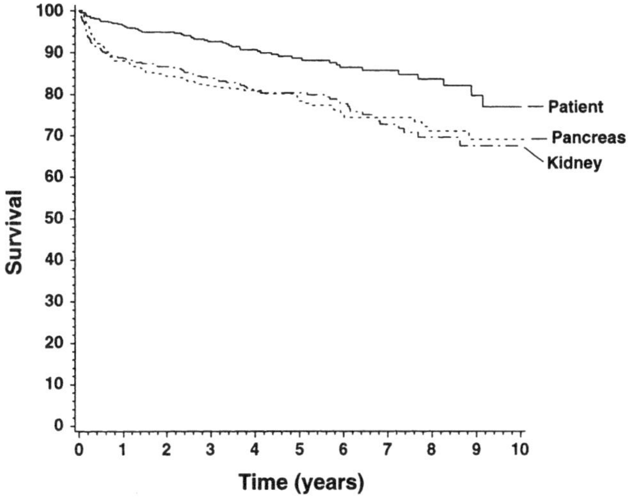

FIGURE 2.—Overall patient, pancreas graft, and kidney graft survival—500 consecutive simultaneous pancreas-kidney (SPK) transplants. (Courtesy of Sollinger HW, Odorico JS, Knechtle SJ, et al: Experience with 500 simultaneous pancreas–kidney transplants. *Ann Surg* 228:284-296, 1998.)

the introduction of mycophenolate mofetil, 1-year survival was 98%, the kidney function rate was 94%, and the pancreas function rate was 93%. This immunosuppressive regimen reduced the rate of steroid-resistant rejections from 48% to 15%.

Conclusions.—This is the largest series of SPKs ever reported, as well as the longest follow-up after pancreatic transplant with BD. Long-term survival is superior to that achieved with any other type of transplant, except for HLA-identical living-related donor transplants. Simultaneous pancreas–kidney transplantation is a very successful treatment for well-selected patients with diabetes and renal failure. The use of ED has reduced the rate of urinary tract infections, and advances in immunosuppressive therapy have greatly reduced the risk of rejection.

▶ The current success of pancreas transplantation is a result of the persistent efforts of a small number of surgeons, most notably those from the University of Wisconsin and the University of Minnesota, to improve the results of pancreas transplantation. Only a short time ago the results of pancreas transplantation were not good, with a 1-year graft survival rate far below 50%. These current data from the University of Wisconsin demonstrate that pancreatic graft survival is comparable to kidney graft survival. A main problem of pancreas transplantation has been dealing with the exocrine pancreatic drainage. Surgical technique has evolved from occluding the pancreatic duct to draining the pancreatic enzymes directly into the peritoneal cavity to bladder drainage and, more recently, directly to intestinal drainage. The transplant community can be thankful for the persistence of this small number of surgeons. Less clear are the long-term results of pancreas transplantation on the secondary complication, diabetes mellitus. Initially, the hope was that successful pancreas transplantation would stabilize or even reverse the retinopathy and neuropathy that developed in these patients. This benefit has not yet been demonstrated in patients. The patients who seem to benefit most from pancreas transplantation are those who have such brittle diabetes that they may vary between insulin shock and diabetic ketoacidosis within a short time. But merely being relieved of the obligation to take daily insulin is adequate justification for many patients to undergo pancreas transplantation.

R.J. Howard, M.D., Ph.D.

Reversal of Lesions of Diabetic Nephropathy After Pancreas Transplantation

Fioretto P, Steffes MW, Sutherland DER, et al (Univ of Padua, Italy; Univ of Minnesota, Minneapolis)

N Engl J Med 339:69-75, 1998 6–9

Background.—Previous research has shown that in patients with type 1 diabetes mellitus without uremia kidney transplantation, pancreatic transplantation did not ameliorate established lesions of diabetic nephropathy

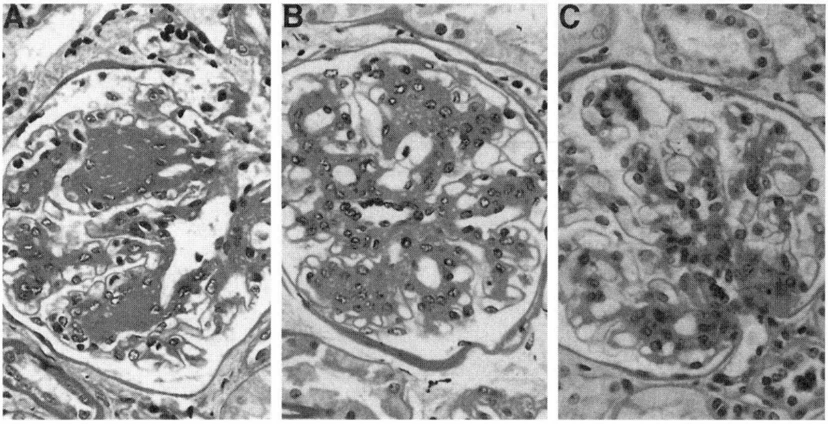

FIGURE 2.—Photomicrographs of renal biopsy specimens obtained before and after pancreas transplantation from a 33-year-old woman with type 1 diabetes of 17 years' duration at the time of transplantation (periodic acid–Schiff, ×120). **Panel A** shows a typical glomerulus from the baseline biopsy specimen, which is characterized by diffuse and nodular (Kimmelstiel-Wilson) diabetic glomerulopathy. Mesangial-matrix expansion and the palisading of mesangial nuclei around the nodular lesions are evident. In **Panel B**, a typical glomerulus 5 years after transplantation shows the persistence of the diffuse and nodular lesions. **Panel C** shows a typical glomerulus 10 years after transplantation, with marked resolution of diffuse and nodular mesangial lesions and more open glomerular capillary lumina. (Courtesy of Fioretto P, Steffes MW, Sutherland DER, et al: Reversal of lesions of diabetic nephropathy after pancreas transplantation. *N Engl J Med* 339:69-75. Copyright 1998, Massachusetts Medical Society. Reprinted by permission of *The New England Journal of Medicine*. All rights reserved.)

within 5 years. However, the effects of longer periods of normoglycemia have not been studied.

Methods.—Eight patients with type 1 diabetes, no uremia, and mild-to-advanced lesions of diabetic nephropathy at the time of pancreas transplantation were assessed. Kidney function was evaluated and renal biopsy performed before pancreas transplantation and at 5 and 10 years after transplantation. Biopsy samples were assessed morphometrically.

Findings.—After transplantation, all patients had persistently normal glycosylated hemoglobin values. Median urinary albumin excretion rate was 103 mg/day before transplantation and 30 mg/day and 20 mg/day at 5 and 10 years after surgery, respectively. The average creatinine clearance rate decreased from 108 mL/min/1.73 m^2 before surgery to 74 mL/min/1.73 m^2 at both 5 and 10 years after surgery. Glomerular and tubular basement membrane thickness was similar at baseline and at 5 years after surgery, but was reduced at 10 years. The mesangial fractional volume increased from baseline to 5 years postoperatively, then was decreased at 10 years, primarily because of a decline in mesangial matrix (Fig 2).

Conclusions.—Pancreas transplantation can reverse the lesions of diabetic nephropathy. However, more than 5 years of normoglycemia are required.

▶ The great hope of pancreas and islet cell transplantation originally was that establishing euglycemia would stabilize or even reverse secondary effects of diabetes mellitus, especially retinopathy, neuropathy, and nephropathy. While pancreas transplantation can clearly reestablish a normal response to glucose and eliminate the need for insulin, there has been little evidence that it has an effect on the secondary effects of long-standing diabetes. This paper is the first that demonstrates reversal of the lesions of diabetic nephrectomy in patients who have been rendered euglycemic by pancreas transplantation. Reversal of the lesions required at least 5 years of normal glycemia. Although this is only a small study of 13 patients, it nevertheless provides great hope for the future of pancreas and islet cell transplantation, because a clear benefit has been demonstrated. Merely establishing the euglycemia state is well worth the cost and problems associated with pancreas transplantation in many patients because of the disabling nature of their diabetes.

R.J. Howard, M.D., Ph.D.

Clinical Intestinal Transplantation: New Perspectives and Immunologic Considerations

Abu-Elmagd K, Reyes J, Todo S, et al (Univ of Pittsburgh, Pa)

J Am Coll Surg 186:512-527, 1998 6–10

Objective.—The requirement for chronic heavy immunosuppression, which too frequently results in lethal infection, has limited intestinal transplantation. Two changes in management strategy, avoidance of transplantation from cytomegalovirus (CMV)-positive donors to CMV-negative recipients and administration of perioperative adjunct donor bone marrow, were instituted to try to improve the outlook after intestinal transplantation.

Methods.—Between 1990 and 1997, 98 patients (48 females), aged 6 months to 58 years, received 104 cadaveric intestinal grafts, including 35 intestine only, 48 intestine plus liver, and 15 multivisceral grafts (Fig 1). Bone marrow augmentation was provided in 20 patients (18%). A group of 22 transplantation patients without bone marrow augmentation served as controls. Indications for transplantation included short-gut syndrome, dysmotility syndrome, intestinal neoplasm, and enterocyte dysfunction. Patients received tacrolimus and prednisone immunosuppression. They were followed up for an average of 24 months. The 47 survivors have been followed up for an average of 32 months. Patient and graft survival were determined, and risk factors for mortality, graft loss, and morbidity were analyzed.

Results.—Of the 47 survivors with intact grafts (2 after retransplantation), 15 have had their grafts for more than 5 years. Actuarial 1- and 5-year patient survival rates of 72% and 48% were similar for isolated and composite graft recipients, with most of the deaths occurring during the first 30 months. Patients younger than 2 years had the highest mortality rate (50%), resulting mainly from technical difficulties. The highest survival rate (68% at 5 years) occurred in the 2- to 17-year age group.

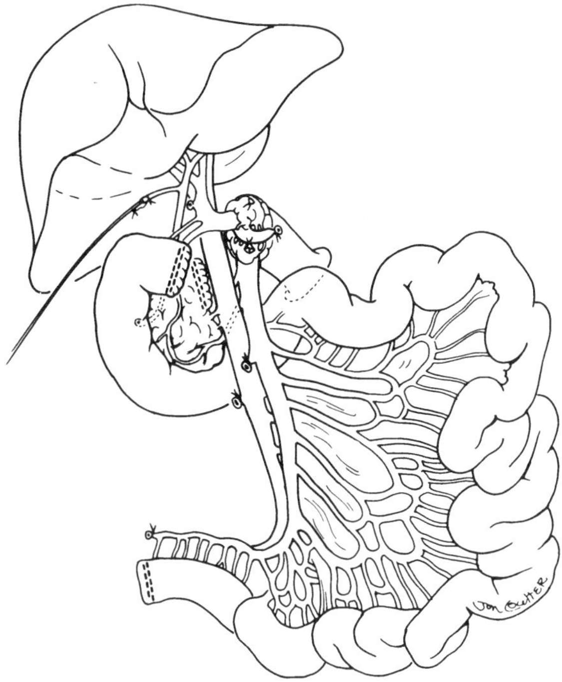

FIGURE 1.—Composite liver and intestinal graft with preservation of the duodenum in continuity with the graft jejunum and hepatic biliary system. Note transection of the pancreas to the right of the portal vein with preservation of the pancreatoduodenal arterial and venous arcade. The technique (used in four cases) reduces the time of the recipient operation and avoids the potential risks of biliary reconstruction. (Courtesy of Abu-Elmagd K, Reyes J, Todo S, et al: Clinical intestinal transplantation: New perspectives and immunologic considerations. *J Am Coll Surg* 186:512-527, 1998. Reprinted by permission of the American College of Surgeons.)

Patients receiving bone marrow augmentation had 6-month and 2-year actuarial survival rates of 89% and 72%, which were similar to rates in control patients of 77% and 57%. Estimated graft survival rates of 64% and 40% at 1 and 5 years were similar for both intestine-only and composite grafts. Grafts in patients receiving bone marrow augmentation had 6-month and 2-year survival rates of 75% and 61%, similar to the rates of 77% and 52% for control patients. Risk factors included high tacrolimus blood levels, steroid bolus therapy, use of antilymphoid therapy, length of operation, CMV disease, inclusion of a segment of colon with the graft, the number of intestinal rejection episodes, development of B-cell lymphoma, cold ischemia time, number of previous abdominal operations, and male donor to male recipient.

Conclusion.—The morbidity and mortality of these 3 intestinal transplantation techniques are too high for the techniques to become generally applicable.

▶ Clinical intestinal transplantation continues to be experimental and is performed only at selected centers. This article from the University of

Pittsburgh details 104 allografts performed in 98 consecutive patients since 1990. In 63 of the 104 patients, the intestine was transplanted as a composite, usually with the liver. This article details many aspects of this most interesting series, including a group of 20 patients who received unmodified adjunct donor bone marrow cells along with their transplants. Most significant is the finding that graft survival is substantially better than that shown in previous reports. In addition, 43 (91%) of 47 currently surviving patients are completely off parenteral nutrition. Continued improvement in immunosuppression, better treatment of rejection, and ability to deal with infections and graft vs. host disease have continued to result in better survival of intestinal transplants. Many problems remain before clinical intestinal transplantation will become widely applicable, but certain centers, such as the University of Pittsburgh, should continue to gain knowledge and work out the clinical problems associated with this organ.

R.J. Howard, M.D., Ph.D.

Life-supporting Pig-to-Primate Renal Xenotransplantation Using Genetically Modified Donors

Zaidi A, Schmoeckel M, Bhatti F, et al (Univ of Cambridge, England; Imutran Ltd, Cambridge, England; Papworth Hosp, Cambridge, England)

Transplantation 65:1584-1590, 1998 6–11

Introduction.—Pig-to-human transplants are discordant xenografts, resulting in hyperacute rejection caused by preformed antispecies antibody. Previous attempts to prolong the survival of these xenografts have focused on removal of the preformed antibodies, splenectomy to suppress antibody production, and potent immunosuppression. Another approach might be to make the transplanted organ less vulnerable to preformed antibodies. This experimental study used pigs genetically modified to express the human regulator of complement activity to extend the survival of porcine xenografts.

Methods.—The investigators developed a colony of pigs transgenic for human decay-accelerating factor. The transgenic protein showed a high level of function on both endothelium and tissue parenchyma, and appeared to modify the rejection process in preliminary studies. Seven kidneys from transgenic pigs were transplanted into cynomolgus monkey, from which both native kidneys were removed. As a control, 6 kidneys from nontransgenic pigs were transplanted. Both groups received immunosuppression with cyclosporine, steroids, and cyclophosphamide.

Results.—Median graft survival was twice as long in the transgenic group than in the control group: 13.0 vs. 6.5 days. The transgenic kidneys also provided better function than control kidneys (Fig 1). Hyperacute rejection occurred in none of 7 kidneys in the transgenic group vs. 1 of 6 in the control group. The 2 transgenic kidneys which survived the longest—27 and 35 days—showed no histologic evidence of rejection. In the

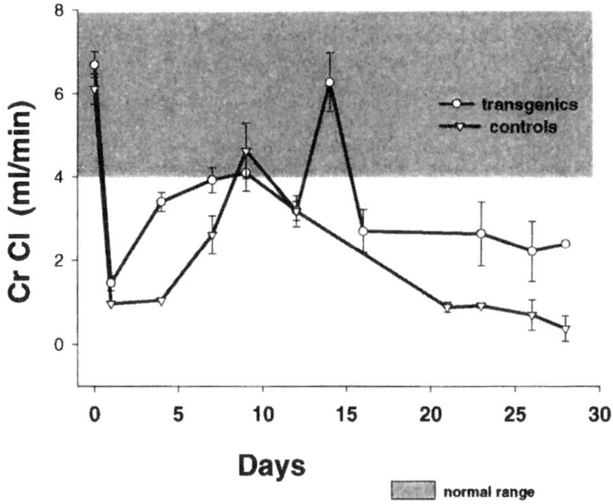

FIGURE 1.—Creatinine clearance after renal xenograft transplantation using transgenic or control organs. (Courtesy of Zaidi A, Schmoeckel M, Bhatti F, et al: Life-supporting pig-to-primate renal xenotransplantation using genetically modified donors. *Transplantation* 65:1584-1590, 1998.)

control group, all kidneys underwent antibody-mediated rejection, either hyperacute or acute vascular.

Conclusions.—In this pig-to-primate transplant model, xenograft kidneys from human decay-accelerating factor transgenic pigs show prolonged survival. The experience includes no episodes of hyperacute rejection of transgenic kidneys, which may also be protected against acute vascular rejection. The findings also demonstrate the basic physiologic compatibility between a pig and a non-human primate.

► Xenografts are the great hope of clinical transplantation, because there will be no limit on organ supply. Graft survival of unmodified xenotransplantation is usually measured in minutes or hours. The ability to genetically modify animals has allowed new approaches to xenograft transplantation. One approach seeks to replace pig transplantation antigens on the surface of cells with human transplantation antigens so that the human host will recognize the pig as human. This article describes a different approach, that of genetically modifying pigs to express the human regulator of complement activity, human decay-accelerating factor. With this modification graft, survival was increased from an average of 6.5 to 13 days. Although much improvement remains to be accomplished, such approaches may one day provide us with an unlimited supply of organs for transplantation. Many other issues also remain to be addressed. These include the possible transmission of zoonoses and whether the function of certain organs, such as the kidney or liver, of animals is similar enough to those of humans to permit normal metabolic function.

R.J. Howard, M.D., Ph.D.

7 Endocrine

Introduction

The first article by Denham and colleagues (Abstract 7–1) discusses cost-effectiveness for preoperative scanning of the parathyroid glands. In the authors' view, it is specific enough to allow unilateral exploration instead of bilateral exploration. The main benefit may be localization of glands, thus allowing minimally invasive surgery, a technique that is now gaining favor in the United States. It was popularized by Norman, who in the next article discusses his technique and results of minimally invasive parathyroidectomy (Abstract 7–2). Parathyroid adenomas may be removed through a small incision placed directly over the gland. Patients can also have the operation done on an outpatient basis or they can be discharged after an overnight stay.

Kerby et al. (Abstract 7–3) discusses operative treatment of tertiary hyperparathyroidism that occurs after kidney transplantation. From a very large renal transplantation program at the University of Alabama, the authors were able to find only 38 patients who required parathyroidectomy during the 29-year period. Thus, the problem is not very common.

Chen and others (Abstract 7–4) discuss parathyroidectomy in the elderly. Many surgeons may be reluctant to operate on elderly patients. The authors suggest that the results in elderly patients are no worse than those in young patients and that amelioration of symptoms can lead to a marked improvement in quality of life for these patients.

Treatment options for thyroid cancer are discussed in the first few papers. Kelemen et al. (Abstract 7–5) describes sentinel lymphadenectomy in patients with thyroid neoplasms. The technique adopted for melanoma and breast cancer patients is added to the evaluation of lymph node status in people with thyroid cancer as well. An article by Noguchi and colleagues (Abstract 7–6) maintains that modified radical neck dissection improves the prognosis in papillary thyroid cancer. These authors present the results of a very large series of over 2,800 patients. Sherman and colleagues (Abstract 7–7) also discuss the results of thyroid cancer treatment. This multicenter study benefits from large numbers of patients.

Total thyroidectomy for benign thyroid disease is described by Liu et al. (Abstract 7–8). While the disease may be cured and the risk of thyroid cancer eliminated in susceptible individuals, it commits the patient to a life of thyroid replacement therapy. The differences between acute suppurative thyroiditis and aggressive malignant thyroid tumors are discussed by Lin and colleagues (Abstract 7–9). These different thyroid diseases can nevertheless resemble each other clinically in certain circumstances.

A seldom-reported subject is thyroid reoperation. This subject is covered by Wilson et al. (Abstract 7–10) and reports a rather high (22%) complication rate among 32 patients. Because of adhesions and loss of normal tissue planes, it can be expected that thyroid reoperations are associated with a high rate of complications.

A comparison of laparoscopic and posterior open adrenalectomy is carried out by Thompson et al. (Abstract 7–11). While it is more expensive, laparoscopic adrenalectomy is clearly preferred by patients and will be the standard form of adrenalectomy where applicable.

Russell and colleagues (Abstract 7–12) discuss the preoperative management of pheochromocytoma. It is an uncommon problem in the United States (estimated 800 cases per year). With better understanding of the pathophysiology and better anesthesia, the mortality rate has decreased as have the wide fluctuations in blood pressure. Finally, the lethality of multiple endocrine neoplasia, type I (MEN-I) is discussed by Doherty and colleagues (Abstract 7–13) from Washington University. They have collected what is probably the largest number of patients with MEN-I syndrome and have the best database to study these patients to determine mortality rates and causes of death.

Richard J. Howard, M.D., Ph.D.

Cost-Effectiveness of Preoperative Sestamibi Scan for Primary Hyperparathyroidism Is Dependent Solely Upon the Surgeon's Choice of Operative Procedure

Denham DW, Norman J (Univ of South Florida, Tampa)

J Am Coll Surg 186:293-304, 1998 7–1

Introduction.—A 1991 NIH Consensus Panel concluded that preoperative localization of diseased parathyroid glands in patients with primary hyperparathyroidism is not a cost-effective procedure. However, surgeons and physicians have continued to publish reports showing excellent results of sestamibi scanning in patients with parathyroid disease. In some cases, parathyroid scanning may permit unilateral exploration using local anesthesia. A 10-year meta-analysis was conducted to assess the sensitivity and specificity of sestamibi scanning and its value in directing unilateral surgical exploration.

Methods.—The meta-analysis included 175 reports describing surgical approaches to the parathyroid gland. Of these, 24 studies included sensitivity and specificity data on the use of sestamibi scanning for localizing solitary adenomas. Subtraction images were used in 10 of these studies, and dual-phase sestamibi in 14. To evaluate the cost-effectiveness of scanning all patients with sporadic primary hyperparathyroidism, the investigators examined the costs associated with certain variables that could be reduced by using a limited procedure.

TABLE 1.—Meta-analysis of the Sensitivity and Specificity of Sestamibi Scans*

Author (Reference)	Scan	n	Sensitivity	Specificity
Bergenfelz et al (69)	S	39	86	97.5
Caixas et al (70)	D	70	97.8	100
Carter et al (71)	D	16	85	100
Casas et al (72)	S	22	88	100
Chapuis et al (20)	D	70	80	100
Chen et al (73)	D	55	93	93
Fjeld et al (74)	S	16	75	100
Hindie et al (75)	S	65	95	98
Khan et al (76)	S	14	87	100
Light et al (15)	D	15	87	100
Malhotra et al (77)	D	32	100	100
Martin et al (52)	D	50	82	98
Norman et al (22)	D	14	92.6	100
Norman and Chheda (28)	D	18	90	100
Norman†	D	50	93	100
O'Doherty (13)	S	49	97.5	100
Perez-Monte et al (78)	D	47	91	NA
Shaha et al (79)	D	19	89.5	100
Sofferman et al (23)	D	33	94	97
Taillefer et al (80)	D	23	90	95
Thompson et al (81)	S	20	NA	100
Thule et al (82)	S	13	93	100
Wei et al (83)	S	23	92	100
Wei et al (84)	S	11	100	100
Total		784	90.74	98.74

*A total of 784 patients from 24 studies with either subtraction (S) or dual (D) technique scans were included.
†Unpublished data.
Abbreviation: NA, not available.
(Courtesy of Denham DW, Norman J: Cost-effectiveness of preoperative sestamibi scan for primary hyperparathyroidism is dependent solely upon the surgeon's choice of operative procedure. *J Am Coll Surg* 186:293-304, 1998. Reprinted by permission of the American College of Surgeons.)

Results.—Sestamibi scanning had an average sensitivity of 91% and specificity of 99% (Table 1). Of the total 6,331 patients analyzed, 87% had solitary adenomas. Unilateral exploration was estimated to reduce costs by an average of $650. Given the sensitivity of sestamibi scanning, this savings could be achieved in up to 90% of patients with solitary adenomas. Since 87% of patients had solitary adenomas, 78% of all patients would appear to be candidates for unilateral exploration based on the results of sestamibi scanning. This compared favorably with the 51% rate at which a policy of scanning all patients becomes cost-effective.

Conclusions.—Based on a 10-year meta-analysis, sestamibi scanning appears sufficiently specific enough to permit unilateral dissection in patients with primary hyperparathyroidism. At the same time, sensitivity is high enough to be cost-effective. A policy of routine preoperative sestamibi scanning can be truly cost-effective only if the surgeon uses the information gained to plan a smaller, more directed operation, as appropriate.

▶ Every year an article is presented in YEAR BOOK of SURGERY discussing the preoperative localization of parathyroid adenomas. Every year, I swear this will be the last article that I present on this subject. Every year I am wrong. Perhaps, this is the definitive article. Attitudes on preoperative localization have gone from feeling that only preoperative localization studies are not needed to patients need only to localize an experienced surgeon to identify the parathyroid adenoma. Nevertheless, preoperative localization studies may help surgeons who do not routinely perform parathyroidectomy. Probably most parathyroids in this country are removed by such surgeons. Perhaps this is the "definitive" article on localization indicating that preoperative scanning is currently specific enough to allow unilateral exploration and whether the surgeon plans to do a unilateral or bilateral localization should determine whether preoperative radiographic localization is obtained. Preoperative localization is also required for surgeons who do minimally invasive operations with short (2.5-cm) incisions directly over the adenoma. (See the article by Norman, Abstract 7–2.)

R.J. Howard, M.D., Ph.D.

Minimally Invasive Parathyroidectomy for Primary Hyperparathyroidism: Decreasing Operative Time and Potential Complications While Improving Cosmetic Results

Norman J, Chheda H, Farrell C (Univ of South Florida, Tampa)

Am Surg 64:391-396, 1998 7–2

Objective.—The cause of primary hyperparathyroidism (HPTH) in most patients is a single adenoma. Because of poor localization studies, most patients with HPTH undergo complete bilateral neck exploration and examination of all 4 glands. Recent evidence has suggested that technetium-99m-sestamibi scintigraphy can accurately diagnose single adenomas. The efficacy and safety of unilateral neck exploration with minimal dissection for patients with a single primary HPTH on scintigraphy were examined prospectively.

Methods.—Sestamibi scans performed in 18 patients with evidence of primary HPTH indicated a single adenoma. These patients underwent minimal unilateral neck exploration. Incision length, operative time, and duration of hospital stay were compared with 25 patients with suspected HPTH who underwent bilateral neck exploration for a single adenoma.

Results.—Compared with patients having bilateral neck exploration, incision length was significantly shorter in patients undergoing minimal exploration (3.0 vs. 9.6 cm), operative time was significantly shorter (49 vs. 127 minutes), and hospital stay was significantly shorter (15.2 vs. 29.6 hours). The range for operative times was 90 to 210 minutes for the bilateral exploration group vs. 25 to 70 minutes for the unilateral exploration group. All patients having unilateral exploration had normal calcium within 24 hours after surgery. Bilateral exploration failed to locate the single adenoma in 1 patient who required reexploration. All explorations but 1 bilateral exploration were performed under local anesthesia. There were no complications.

Conclusion.—In patients with HPTH, minimal unilateral exploration for a single adenoma indicated by sestamibi scan is safe and effective, and significantly decreases operative time, length of incision, and hospital stay.

► In recent years surgeons have become minimalists. Instead of large incisions, surgeons now take pride in small incisions and certainly patients favor small incisions, which can accomplish safely the goals of large procedures. Laparoscopic techniques have made possible this tendency toward small incisions in abdominal surgery. This article demonstrates that with good, reliable, preoperative localization, single parathyroid adenomas can be safely removed through a small incision. This incision allows exposure of only a single parathyroid gland. The placement was made according to the results of a technetium-99m-sestamibi scan. With experience the surgeon was able to perform this procedure with local anesthesia and monitored anesthesia care. The small operation also allowed patients to be discharged early and to even have the procedure performed as outpatients. While ten patients did require slight extension of the initial two and one-half centimeter incision, it remained four centimeters or less in all patients. Generally, the deeper the adenoma the longer the incision that was required to reach it. Use of a small incision and unilateral expiration requires reliable, accurate preoperative localization. Several reports suggest that use of technetium-99m-sestamibi scans by skilled radiologists can achieve these results.

R.J. Howard, M.D., Ph.D.

Operative Treatment of Tertiary Hyperparathyroidism: A Single-Center Experience

Kerby JD, Rue LW, Blair H, et al (Univ of Alabama, Birmingham)

Ann Surg 227:878-886, 1998 7–3

Objective.—Whereas some patients with chronic renal failure who continue to have hyperparathyroidism (tertiary hyperparathyroidism) after successful transplantation, few require subtotal parathyroidectomy. A retrospective review of 38 patients who required operative reduction of the parathyroid glands for treatment of tertiary hyperparathyroidism (TH) is presented.

Methods.—Of 3,909 patients who received 4,344 renal transplants between May 1968 and July 1997, 38 required parathyroid surgery for TH. Graft survival and demographic characteristics in this group were compared with a control group (n = 899) matched for age, sex, race, and number of transplants and with the entire transplant population.

Results.—All patients were hypercalcemic. Twenty patients had no symptoms, and the remainder had an array of symptoms. The time between transplantation and parathyroidectomy averaged 997 days. Total parathyroidectomy with parathyroid autograft was performed in 26 of 34 patients, subtotal parathyroidectomy in 7, and a 2-gland resection in 1 patient with parathyroid adenoma. Two patients underwent reoperation

TABLE 7.—Histopathology

Patient Number	Cell Composition: Oxyphil	Chief	Water Clear	Vascular	Fat	Diagnosis	Total Weight (g)
3	7	81	0	5	7	Diffuse	1.92
4	7	80	0	3	10	Diffuse	NA
5	25	68	0	6	1	Nodular	10.35
7	36	58	0	4	2	Diffuse	0.67
8	0	95	0	4	1	Nodular	2.32
9	33	58	0	9	0	Diffuse	2.62
10	16	64	7	10	3	Nodular	1.6
11	25	68	0	7	0	Nodular	9.7
12	37	56	0	7	0	Diffuse	0.1
15	8	75	2	7	8	Nodular	2.59
16	28	62	0	6	4	Diffuse	1.71
17	7	87	0	4	2	Diffuse	NA
18	42	49	0	6	3	Diffuse	2.43
19	1	89	0	8	2	Adenoma	2.14
20	52	35	0	9	4	Nodular	4.38
21	4	73	3	3	17	Diffuse	0.48
22	16	73	1	9	1	Diffuse	1.75
23	15	75	0	10	0	Nodular	1.67
24	41	27	20	12	0	Nodular	6.04
25	15	66	0	5	14	Diffuse	2.25
26	3	91	1	4	1	Diffuse	0.95
27	14	71	0	4	11	Diffuse	1.77
29	56	29	0	15	0	Nodular	5.48
30	81	15	0	4	0	Diffuse	NA
32	29	53	0	18	0	Diffuse	NA
33	12	77	0	10	1	Diffuse	1.21
34	54	40	0	4	2	Diffuse	NA
35	13	74	1	8	4	Diffuse	1.82

(Courtesy of Kerby JD, Rue LW, Blair H, et al: Operative treatment of tertiary hyperparathyroidism: A single-center experience. *Ann Surg* 227:878-886, 1998.)

because of persistent disease. Complications in 36 procedures included 1 recurrent laryngeal nerve injury and 1 wound separation. Patients were hospitalized for an average of 5.42 days. At pathologic examination, parathyroid hyperplasia was diagnosed in 33 patients and benign adenoma in 1 (Table 7). At follow-up, 27 patients were still alive and 22 have good renal function. Five experienced chronic rejection, and 4 lost their grafts. Long-term graft survival rates were similar for the study group and the matched control group.

Conclusion.—Tertiary hyperparathyroidism can be treated successfully with operative reduction of the parathyroid gland.

► Correction of renal malfunction with kidney transplantation theoretically should correct secondary hyperparathyroidism, which occurs in many patients with renal failure. When secondary hyperparathyroidism is not corrected, even though the renal failure is corrected, it is designated tertiary hyperparathyroidism. The authors, from a very large renal transplant program, were able to find only 38 patients who required parathyroidectomy for tertiary hyperparathyroidism after transplantation over a 29-year period. Thus, the problem is not very common. Of the 38 patients, 24 had diffuse hyperplasia and 9 had nodular hyperplasia, diseases that are very widespread in patients with secondary hyperparathyroidism who are undergoing dialysis. This disease may have continued after transplantation. Only 1 of 38 patients had an adenoma. The patient with an adenoma may indeed have had primary hyperparathyroidism, since that disease probably occurs in patients with renal failure just as it occurs in those with normal renal function. If fact, it is surprising that more of their patients did not have adenomas inasmuch as primary hyperparathyroidism occurs in about one of 1,000 individuals. Serum calcium levels should be monitored after transplantation, since this may be the easiest method of detecting tertiary hyperparathyroidism.

R.J. Howard, M.D., Ph.D.

Parathyroidectomy in the Elderly: Do the Benefits Outweigh the Risks?
Chen H, Parkerson S, Udelsman R (Johns Hopkins Hosp, Baltimore, Md)
World J Surg 22:531-536, 1998 7–4

Introduction.—Advances in medical technology have produced a tenfold increase in the population of persons over age 65 years in the United States. Several reports indicate that age is no longer a contraindication to major surgical procedures, thanks to ongoing improvements in anesthesia and surgery. With increasing costs of health care and ballooning Medicare expenses, allocation of funds for the treatment of elderly patients has been questioned. The incidence of hyperparathyroidism (HPT) in the elderly is over 1.5%; parathyroidectomy is the treatment of choice in these patients. The outcomes of elderly patients with HPT were evaluated to determine the risks and benefits of this surgery.

Methods.—Data were prospectively gathered over the 5-year period from August 1990 to May 1996 on a consecutive series of 211 patients who underwent parathyroid exploration by 1 endocrine surgeon. Of these, 184 underwent exploration for primary hyperparathyroidism. Thirty-six patients (20%) in this cohort were over 70 years of age and were classified as elderly. Demographic and outcome data from elderly patients were

TABLE 4.—Patient Outcomes

Patients	No.	Cure Rate (%)	Morbidity (%)	Mortality (%)	LOS
Elderly	36	94.4	5.5*	0	2.1 ± 0.2
Young	148	98.0	1.4†	0	1.7 ± 0.1
p	NA	NS	NS	NS	NS

*Represents 2 patients who were rehospitalized for treatment of transient hypocalcemia and a deep venous thrombosis, respectively.

†Represents 1 previously explored patient who sustained a unilateral recurrent nerve injury and 1 patient with multiple endocrine neoplasia and a forearm parathyroid graft failure.

Abbreviations: LOS, length of stay in days (mean ± SEM); *NA*, not applicable; *NS*, not significant.

(Courtesy of Chen H, Parkerson S, Udelsman R: Parathyroidectomy in the elderly: Do the benefits outweigh the risks? *World J Surg* 22:531-536, copyright 1998, Springer-Verlag.)

compared with the same data on the 148 patients who were younger than age 70 years.

Results.—Elderly patients had significantly more symptoms of mental impairment, bone disease, and fatigue. Younger patients had a significantly higher rate of nephrolithiasis than their elderly counterparts. Elderly patients had significantly more advanced disease, with higher preoperative parathyroid hormone levels. The respective cure rates were similar in elderly and younger patients: (94.4% vs. 98%) as were morbidity (5.5% vs. 1.4%) and mortality (0% vs. 0%) (Table 4).

Conclusion.—Elderly patients were referred for surgery with more advanced disease than younger patients. Contrary to earlier series reporting high morbidity rates, significant mortality rates, and longer length of stay, elderly patients in this series who underwent parathyroidectomy experienced high cure rates, low morbidity, zero mortality, short length of stay, and high patient satisfaction. The benefits of surgery outweigh its risks in elderly patients with HPT. Elderly patients with HPT should be referred for surgical treatment at a lower threshold of disease.

▶ The authors' point out that HPT is more common in the elderly than in the general population. In the elderly, it may account for mental impairment (in the authors series, 42% of the patients who were older than 70 years had mental impairment) and 39% of this group had fatigue. As our population ages, expending medical resources on the elderly—who have a shortened life span compared with younger patients and, thus, will gain less benefit—may come under intense discussion because of limited resources.

Nevertheless, this article shows that the elderly have no higher rate of morbidity and mortality from parathyroidectomy than younger patients. This paper is consistent with a variety of other studies that have examined the results of operative procedures in the elderly and have found that many procedures can be done safely in this population. Therefore, it seems reasonable that most individuals should not be denied quality-of-life–enhancing procedures only because of their ages. Cure rates in the elderly were comparable to those of younger patients, and the elderly patients' own opinions were that their symptoms were significantly ameliorated by the procedure.

It seems to me that the main criterion for an operative procedure should not be absolute age but the physiologic ability to tolerate the operative procedure. Nevertheless, in the future, choices may have to be made if resources become even more limited than they are currently. Such was the case in some countries where "elderly" patients of more than 65 years were not considered candidates for beginning hemodialysis, a criterion that has disappeared in most western countries.

R.J. Howard, M.D., Ph.D.

Sentinel Lymphadenectomy in Thyroid Malignant Neoplasms
Kelemen PR, Van Herle AJ, Giuliano AE (Saint John's Health Ctr, Santa Monica, Calif; Univ of California, Los Angeles)
Arch Surg 133:288-292, 1998 7–5

Objective.—Among patients with well-differentiated thyroid cancer, the presence of lymph node metastases is associated with high recurrence rates. There is controversy as to the surgical management of occult lymph node metastases, with options including blind nodal sampling, "berry-picking" procedures, and modified radical neck dissection. Previous reports from the authors' center have described the use of sentinel lymph node dissection (SLND) for patients with melanoma and breast cancer. The results of intraoperative lymph node mapping and SLND in patients with suspected thyroid tumors were evaluated.

Methods.—The 2-year study included 17 patients referred for evaluation of a suspicious thyroid nodule with no palpable cervical adenopathy. The patients were 14 women and 3 men, median age 48 years. Intraoperative lymphatic mapping was performed by injecting the exposed thyroid lobe with 1.0% isosulfan blue dye, mean volume 0.5 mL. The dye quickly spread to the sentinel lymph node, which was excised. These nodes were analyzed for the presence of micrometastases using routine processes and keratin immunohistochemical studies.

Results.—In all but 1 patient, who had benign thyroid disease treated with lobectomy, total thyroidectomy was performed after SLND. Twelve of the 17 nodules proved to be thyroid cancers; the other 5 were follicular adenomas or colloid nodules. In 2 patients, the lymphatics mapped to the retrosternum, causing lymphatic mapping to be regarded as a failure. In most cases, the sentinel nodes were paratracheal; the exceptions were 2 female patients who also had stained jugular nodes. Positive sentinel nodes were found in association with 42% of tumor nodules. Five patients underwent central neck dissection. In 2 of these, the sentinel lymph node was the only metastatic node.

Conclusions.—This experience suggests that SLND is feasible for patients with thyroid cancer. Just as in patients with melanoma or breast cancer, SLND appears to detect nonpalpable nodal metastases. Further study is needed to establish the role of SLND in the clinical management of thyroid cancer.

▶ Sentinel lymph node biopsy has become popular for breast cancer and melanoma. These authors now apply these same techniques to find sentinel lymph nodes in patients with malignant thyroid neoplasms. Many surgeons currently do not biopsy lymph nodes in patients with malignant thyroid cancers or only biopsy obviously enlarged lymph nodes. Some surgeons biopsy whatever nodes they can find. These authors attempted to locate the sentinel node after injecting isosulfan blue dye into the thyroid tumor. Of 12 patients with thyroid cancer, five (42%) were associated with positive sentinel lymph nodes, indicating this technique can detect nonpalpable node metastases with the same ease as melanoma and breast cancer. The clinical significance, however, remains to be determined. This technique requires a certain amount of expertise. Because of the excellent survival of patients with differentiated thyroid cancer, the high positivity rate is surprising. Deciding what to do with this knowledge (that there may be positive nodes even if they are not detected) is unclear. Of the 12 patients with proven thyroid cancer, none had palpable cervical adenopathy preoperatively—just the situation where accurately detecting metastases nodes would be most valuable.

R.J. Howard, M.D., Ph.D.

Papillary Thyroid Carcinoma: Modified Radical Neck Dissection Improves Prognosis

Noguchi S, Murakami N, Yamashita H, et al (Oita Med Univ, Japan)
Arch Surg 133:276-280, 1998 7–6

Objective.—Whereas modified radical neck dissection for thyroid carcinoma reduces recurrence rate, its effect on survival has not been established. In a subgroup of patients with papillary thyroid carcinoma, modified radical neck dissection improved survival, even when these patients had advanced disease.

Methods.—A retrospective study of 2,966 patients treated curatively at Noguchi Thyroid Clinic and Hospital Foundation in Oita, Japan between 1946 and 1991 was performed. Cause-specific survival rates were determined, and risk factor analysis was performed.

Results.—Seventy-five patients (2.5%) had total thyroidectomy, 1,233 (41.6%) had subtotal thyroidectomy, 1,217 (41.0%) had lobectomy, and 441 (14.9%) had partial lobectomy. Modified radical neck surgery was performed in 2,139 patients (72.1%), partial node excision in 252 (8.5%), and no node excision in 575 (19.4%). Patients undergoing modified radical neck surgery had macroscopic metastases, invasive primary tumor, or cancer. Males had a significantly higher incidence of nodal metastases than females (92.1% vs. 85.5%, respectively). Patients with invasion or adhesion of the primary tumor had improved survival after modified radical neck dissection. Whereas survival rates of those undergoing and not undergoing modified radical neck dissection were similar, among patients with metastases those who underwent modified radical neck surgery had improved survival. In women over age 60, modified radical neck surgery significantly improved survival. Ten- and 20-year cause-specific survival rates for patients having and not having modified radical neck surgery were 92.4% and 73.2% vs. 80.3% and 56.7%, respectively. Of 97 patients with recurrent disease, 83 were successfully treated with a second surgical procedure and 1 survived with disease. The remaining 13 died of their disease. Female sex, older age, diameter of the tumor, extrathyroid invasion, and presence of metastatic disease were significant risk factors, according to multivariate analysis.

Conclusion.—Patients with thyroid cancer who have nodal metastases or invasive disease and women who are over age 60 can benefit from modified radical neck surgery.

► This study examined a very large number of patients (2,966) treated for thyroid cancer over a 45-year period. Of 2,859 patients with tumors of 1 cm or larger, 72% underwent modified radical neck dissection. Nineteen percent underwent no node dissection. The authors do not state why some patients were treated with lymph node dissection and some were not. With this large group of patients, they were able to demonstrate that modified radical neck dissection improved the cause-specific survival rate in patients who had extrathyroidal invasion. This finding seems logical, and in a further subset analysis of the patients the authors were able to demonstrate that patients in whom the primary tumor invades beyond the thyroid capsule and in women older than 60 modified radical neck dissection can lead to improved survival. The patients also differed in the operations that they had. The extent of resection of the thyroid gland could also have an effect on survival. This study from Japan noted a very high incidence of nodal metastases (92.1% in men and 85.5% in women). Studies from the United States generally are associated with a lower prevalence of nodal metastasis. This high prevalence of nodal metastases strongly suggests that modified radical neck dissection should be done in Japan. Whether this finding should be applied to the United States would require more investigation.

R.J. Howard, M.D., Ph.D.

Prospective Multicenter Study of Thyroid Carcinoma Treatment: Initial Analysis of Staging and Outcome

Sherman SI, Brierley JD, Sperling M, et al (Univ of Texas, Houston; The Princess Margaret Hosp, Toronto; Univ of Cincinnati, Ohio; et al)

Cancer 83:1012-1021, 1998 7–7

Introduction.—Thyroid carcinoma is a rare disease with a good prognosis, although up to 10% of patients with this diagnosis will die of the disease. For many years, a wide range of primary treatments have been used, with no consensus as to the optimal choice for various patient groups. The National Thyroid Cancer Treatment Cooperative Study (NTCTCS) Registry has created a new prognostic staging classification system for predicting outcome in patients with all types of thyroid carcinoma. An initial analysis of this system, including prospective validation and comparison with other staging classifications, is reported.

Methods.—A total of 1,607 patients from 14 institutions were prospectively entered into the registry between 1987 and 1995. Clinicopathologic staging was performed according to age at diagnosis, tumor histologic type, tumor size, intrathyroid multifocality, extraglandular invasion, metastases, and tumor differentiation. Stages I and II were considered low

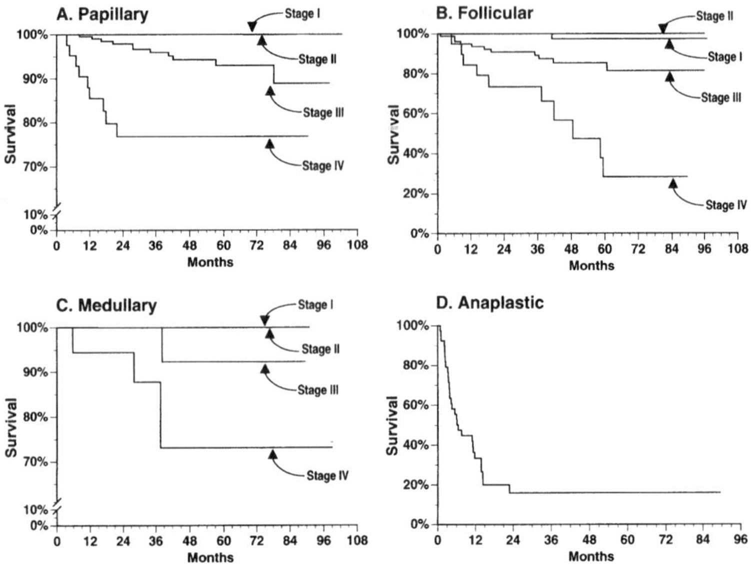

FIGURE 1.—Product-limit estimates of disease-specific survival after diagnosis of thyroid carcinoma, according to NTCTCS Registry stage assigned at entry. A, Papillary carcinoma. $P < 0.001$ for differences in survival among the four stages. B, Follicular carcinoma (including oxyphilic variant). $P < 0.001$. C, Medullary carcinoma. $P = 0.11$. D, Anaplastic carcinoma. (Courtesy of Sherman SI, Brierley JD, Sperling M, et al: Prospective multicenter study of thyroid carcinoma treatment: Initial analysis of staging and outcome. *Cancer* 83:1012-1021, 1998. Reprinted by permission of Wiley-Liss, Inc., a subsidiary of John Wiley & Sons, Inc.)

risk, and stages III and IV were considered high risk; all anaplastic carcinomas were considered stage IV.

Findings.—Forty-three percent of the patients were classified as having stage I disease, 24% stage II, 25% stage III, and 9% stage IV. Patients with follicular carcinomas were more likely to fall into the high-risk stages than those with papillary carcinoma. Major determinants of disease stage for patients with papillary carcinoma were patient age, tumor size, macroscopic extraglandular invasion, and metastases; for patients with follicular carcinoma, patient age, tumor size, extracervical metastases, and poor tumor differentiation were determinants of stage.

Follow-up data covering a median of 40 months were available for 1,562 patients. There were 78 deaths from thyroid carcinoma or treatment-related complications. Five-year disease-specific survival was 100% for patients with stage I or II disease and 92% for those with stage III disease, compared with 49% for those with stage IV disease (Fig 1). Likelihood of freedom from disease was 94% in stage I, 93% in stage II, 78% in stage III, and 25% in stage IV. Compared with other staging classifications, the NTCTCS Registry system offered high predictive values for disease-specific mortality and freedom from disease, regardless of tumor type.

Conclusions.—The NTCTCS Registry staging classification system is valid for the prediction of short-term prognosis in patients with thyroid carcinoma. More study is needed to validate its use in predicting long-term prognosis. This study underscores the prognostic significance of tumor size, extraglandular invasion, and other histologic features.

▶ Large multicenter studies have the advantage of being able to get large numbers of patients and the disadvantage of a lack of standard ways of treating or even diagnosing disease. As with any cancer operation, surgical skill is an important parameter. In this study, multiple surgeons were undoubtedly involved, which introduces further variation. Nevertheless, because there are so many patients and because the data are analyzed by stage and type of cancer (see Fig 1), surgeons can use this study to compare their own results with a large multicenter experience. In addition, they can provide information about the likely outlook for their particular stage and type of cancer.

R.J. Howard, M.D., Ph.D.

Total Thyroidectomy for Benign Thyroid Disease

Liu Q, Djuricin G, Prinz RA (Rush-Presbyterian-St Luke's Med Ctr, Chicago)
Surgery 123:2-7, 1998 7–8

Objective.—Whether total thyroidectomy is appropriate for benign disease is controversial. The safety and efficacy of total thyroidectomy for gross benign disease involving both lobes were evaluated in 106 consecutive patients.

Methods.—Between October 1982 and July 1995, thyroidectomy was performed in 106 patients (33 men), aged 16 to 82 years. Indications included radiated gland (n = 36), bilateral nodules (n = 35), suspicious biopsy findings (n = 18), and toxic goiter (n = 17). Serum calcium level and vocal cord function were assessed at baseline, at the first and second postoperative visits, and at 1- to 3-month intervals as necessary.

Results.—Total thyroidectomy was performed in 98 patients. Completion thyroidectomy was performed in 5 patients with recurrent benign nodular goiter (BNG) and in 3 patients with recurrent follicular adenoma. Two patients had unilateral recurrent laryngeal nerve (RLN) palsy before surgery. Pathologic examination revealed BNG in 49 patients, follicular adenoma in 26, hyperplasia in 19, and Hashimoto's thyroiditis in 12. Complications included postoperative hemorrhage in 2 patients (1.9%) and unilateral RLN palsy in 3 patients, which resolved in 2 patients at 3 and 4 months. Early in the postoperative period, 28 patients had subnormal total serum calcium levels, and 8 (8.5%) of these had hypocalcemia. At follow-up, no patient had permanent hypoparathyroidism.

Conclusion.—Total thyroidectomy can be performed safely and with a low complication rate in patients with nodular goiter, hyperthyroidism, and thyroiditis to prevent recurrence and eliminate malignant disease in patients with irradiated glands. Total thyroidectomy is safe and effective for patients with benign bilateral disease.

► Although total thyroidectomy for benign disease can achieve the authors' goal of avoiding reoperation for goiter and hyperthyroidism and eliminating any risk of malignant change in irradiated thyroid glands, problems associated with total thyroidectomy may well outweigh potential benefits. First of all, it commits the patient to lifelong thyroid replacement therapy. Furthermore, although there was no permanent hypoparathyroidism or recurrent nerve injury in the authors' series, the risk of these 2 dreaded complications does increase with total thyroidectomy compared with subtotal thyroidectomy. Whereas the risk of cancer in irradiated thyroid glands is higher than in glands that have not been irradiated, the incidence is still low. It can be reduced further by removing almost all of the thyroid gland but leaving a small margin of gland laterally. This would reduce the likelihood of recurrent nerve injury and of parathyroid injury and the need for thyroid replacement therapy while still achieving the authors' goal of reducing (albeit the precise amount is unknown) the risk of thyroid cancer. Although total thyroidectomy may be an acceptable procedure in expert hands, whether this should be routinely done by all surgeons is unclear.

R.J. Howard, M.D., Ph.D.

Acute Suppurative Thyroiditis and Aggressive Malignant Thyroid Tumors: Differences in Clinical Presentation

Lin K-D, Lin J-D, Huang M-J, et al (Chang Gung Mem Med Ctr, Taiwan, Republic of China)

J Surg Oncol 67:28-32, 1998 7–9

Purpose.—Acute suppurative thyroiditis (AST) is a very rare condition accompanied by high fever, leukocytosis, and acute swelling in the area of the thyroid. These are largely the same features associated with the early course of aggressive malignant thyroid tumors (AMTT), which must be recognized and treated promptly. The clinical and laboratory differences between AST and AMTT were analyzed.

Methods.—The retrospective study included 30 patients with clinical features similar to those of AST who were managed over a 13-year period. In each patient the eventual diagnosis was either AST, based on a positive thyroid pus culture or (if sterile) on prompt disappearance of thyroid lesions in response to antibiotics, or AMTT, based on histologic examination of thyroid biopsy material. The clinical and laboratory data were analyzed to determine the best approach to early diagnosis and appropriate treatment.

Results.—The diagnosis was AST in 25 patients and AMTT in 5. The AST group included 9 men and 16 women, and the AMTT group consisted of 1 man and 4 women. Significant differences included age, a mean of 35 years in the AST group vs. 64 years in the AMTT group; history of dysphonia, present in 28% of the AST group vs. 80% of the AMTT group; involvement of the right thyroid lobe, 8% vs. 60%; and lesion size, 3 cm vs. 6 cm. The presence of anemia was another distinguishing factor, with mean hemoglobin values of 12 g/dL in the AST group vs. 10 g/dL in the AMTT group. Pus cultures from thyroid aspirates were sterile in 16% of the AST group vs. 100% of the AMTT group. All of these factors gave reason to suspect cancer if the thyroid lesion did not resolve after antibiotic therapy. Sixty percent of the patients with AMTT died of this disease.

Conclusions.—This study identifies key clinical and laboratory differences between AST and AMTT, which should help to achieve timely diagnosis and treatment. The latter condition carries a poor prognosis, which might be improved with early, aggressive surgery. Prompt diagnosis and treatment also improve the chances of full recovery from AST.

► Highly aggressive malignant thyroid tumors and AST can have similar clinical presentations. Unfortunately, no clinical symptom or sign was helpful in clearly distinguishing between these two diagnoses. Even laboratory findings (white blood cell count and sedimentation rate) were similar. Only the presence of pus clearly differentiated suppurative thyroiditis from cancer, but even here 16% of the cultures were negative. Because AST may be rapidly fatal when proper diagnosis and treatment do not occur, it is important that physicians suspect this diagnosis. Because of the poor outlook for patients with AMTT, a presumptive diagnosis and treatment for suppurative thyroiditis can be advisable. Prompt needle aspiration, with or without the use of ultrasound or CT guidance, can lead to early diagnosis. Another helpful finding in the aspirate was the presence of neutrophils in patients with thyroid infection.

R.J. Howard, M.D., Ph.D.

Thyroid Reoperations: Indications and Risks

Wilson DB, Staren ED, Prinz RA (Rush Med College, Chicago)

Am Surg 64:674-679, 1998 7–10

Background.—There is ongoing controversy regarding the appropriate extent of primary thyroid surgery and the need for reoperation, whether for benign or malignant disease. Reoperation is technically difficult and carries an increased risk of complications. A large series of repeat thyroid operations was reviewed to define the indications for reoperation and the associated risk of complications.

Patients.—Over a 12-year period, one of the authors performed thyroidectomies in 362 consecutive patients. Of these, 32 underwent reoperation. The patients were 21 women and 11 men (average age, 55 years). Eight patients had 2 or more reoperations; in 28 patients, the primary operation was performed at another center. In 14 patients, reoperation was performed because of symptomatic recurrence of a multinodular goiter. In 5 patients, the indication for repeat surgery was a change in histologic diagnosis from benign adenoma to thyroid cancer. All other patients required additional treatment for cancer. Reoperation consisted of completion thyroidectomy in 31 patients. Of the remaining patients, 3 underwent unilateral or bilateral modified radical neck exploration. One patient underwent median sternotomy for removal of a substernal goiter, and 1 had subtotal thyroidectomy.

Outcomes.—The overall complication rate was 22%. Two patients had recurrent laryngeal nerve injury, which was permanent in 1 patient who had repeated operations for goiter. In one patient with preoperative unilateral vocal cord with paralysis, function returned after median sternotomy. In another case nerve injury from the original surgery was permanent. Postoperative hypocalcemia of less than 8 mg/dL was present in 3 patients but resolved within 1 to 6 months. One case of postoperative hemorrhage required tracheostomy for airway control. A case of seroma resolved within 2 months.

Conclusions.—This experience highlights the indications for repeat thyroid surgery for patients with benign and malignant disease. Careful preoperative evaluation is needed to identify those patients who stand to gain the most from reoperation. Although the risk of complications is acceptable, it is higher than with primary thyroidectomy. The best approach is to avoid the need for reoperation by performing definitive primary surgery.

▶ Because of the scarring and loss of normal tissue planes, reoperations in the neck for either thyroid or parathyroid disease can be challenging. The complication rate is higher with reoperations than with primary procedures. Indeed, complications occurred in 7 of 32 patients (22%) in the authors' series. Recurrent laryngeal nerve injury, perhaps the most severe complication, occurred in 2 patients; it was permanent in one. If cancer is diagnosed in thyroid specimens only after permanent section analysis, reoperation can be performed promptly before scarring occurs and with a lower risk. Early operation was done in only 4 patients in this series. It has been my experience that if thyroid reoperations are to be done, they should be done promptly (if that is feasible) because, unlike abdomen scarring, adhesions do not tend to "soften up" or "thin out" with time. Therefore, reoperations continue to be more hazardous and associated with more complications.

R.J. Howard, M.D., Ph.D.

Laparoscopic Versus Open Posterior Adrenalectomy: A Case-Control Study of 100 Patients

Thompson GB, Grant CS, van Heerden JA, et al (Mayo Found, Rochester, Minn)

Surgery 122:1132-1136, 1997 7–11

Objective.—Few large studies have compared laparoscopic adrenalectomy (LA) with conventional open anterior or posterior adrenalectomy.

TABLE 2.—Results*

	PA	LA	p Value
Operating room time (min)	127	167	0.0002
Blood transfusions (total group)	None	2 units	NS
Narcotic (morphine sulphate) equivalents	48	28	0.002
Ketorolac tromethamine (Toradol) doses	1.7	0.7	0.75
Antiemetic doses	5.7	3.1	0.50
Hospital stay (days)	5.7	3.1	0.0001
Early complications (%)	18	6	0.25
Late complications (%)	54	0	0.0001
Return to normal (weeks)	7	3.8	0.0001
Patient satisfaction (1-10)	7	9	0.0001
Adjusted hospital charges (median)	$6,000	$7,000	0.05

Abbreviation: NS, Not significant.
*Mean values unless otherwise specified.
(Courtesy of Thompson GB, Grant CS, van Heerden JA, et al: Laparoscopic versus open posterior adrenalectomy: A case-control study of 100 patients. *Surgery* 122:1132-1136, 1997.)

The benefits and disadvantages of LA and posterior adrenalectomy (PA) performed by the same surgical group were compared.

Methods.—Between 1992 and 1996, of the 61 LAs attempted in 57 patients, 54 were successful in 50 patients. Results were compared with those of 50 demographically matched PA controls. Data on operating room time, blood transfusions, analgesic/antiemetic requirements, hospital stay, early and late complications, return to normal daily activities, patient satisfaction, and adjusted median hospital charges were compared. Patients (82%) were followed up for an average of 25 months.

Results.—Seven LA patients (12%) required conversion to an open anterolateral procedure. The early LA and PA complication rates were 6% and 18%, respectively (Table 2). The advantages of LA over PA included analgesic requirements (28 vs. 48 narcotic equivalents), hospital stay (3.1 vs. 5.7 days), late complications (0 vs. 54%), return to normal activities (3.8 vs. 7 weeks), and patient satisfaction (9 vs. 1 on a 1-10 scale). Disadvantages included a significantly longer operating time (167 vs. 127 minutes) and slightly higher median hospital charges ($7,000 vs. $6,000).

Conclusion.—Laparoscopic adrenalectomy is a safe and effective procedure that is superior to PA with respect to patient satisfaction, length of hospital stay, return to normal activities, analgesic requirements, and late complications. Compared with PA, LA operating times and hospital stays are slightly longer.

▶ As most studies comparing laparoscopic and conventional surgery show, LA is more expensive than open adrenalectomy. It is also technically more demanding. Nevertheless, it can be done safely and effectively, and patient preference will drive the continuing application of minimally invasive surgical techniques for this and other surgical procedures in the future.

R.J. Howard, M.D., Ph.D.

The Preoperative Management of Phaeochromocytoma

Russell WJ, Metcalfe IR, Tonkin AL, et al (Univ of Adelaide, South Australia)
Anaesth Intensive Care 26:196-200, 1998 7–12

Background.—Patients with pheochromocytoma generally receive preoperative α-adrenergic receptor drugs. However, this practice has never been tested on a prospective clinical trial. During surgery, patients with pheochromocytoma may show large swings in blood pressure, the management of which has not been established. The authors reviewed the effectiveness of preoperative alpha-receptor blockade in terms of intraoperative stability in patients undergoing surgery for pheochromocytoma.

Methods.—The study included 14 consecutive patients undergoing surgery for pheochromocytoma at 1 hospital during a 13-year period. Each received preoperative α- and β-adrenoceptor blockade, tailored to produce the lowest preoperative blood pressure and the least variability in heart rate. Phenoxybenzamine was used in 12 patients, and labetalol and prazosin in 1 each. The needs for additional hypertensive treatment before tumor removal and for blood pressure support afterward were scored to create a simple blood pressure stability score: patients with higher scores had greater instability.

Results.—Blood pressure was more stable with phenoxybenzamine than with labetalol or prazosin. The duration of phenoxybenzamine treatment had no effect on operative stability. Continuing phenoxybenzamine treatment for longer than 10 days did not result in better perioperative blood pressure stability than treating for less than 1 week. Operative stability was unrelated to the patients' degree of postural hypotension after phenoxybenzamine treatment. However, patients with a higher intraoperative peak total catecholamine level had greater operative stability.

Conclusions.—In patients undergoing surgery for pheochromocytoma, 3 to 5 days of maximal phenoxybenzamine treatment before surgery appears to offer good blood pressure stability. Risk factor analysis suggests that patients with high catecholamine production have a higher rate of cardiovascular instability. Postural hypotension with treatment does not appear to be a good indicator of operative stability.

▶ Pheochromocytoma is an uncommon lesion (an estimated 800 cases per year in the United States). Operative removal was previously associated with wide swings in blood pressure and, occasionally, death. The mortality rate of operation for pheochromocytoma has become much lower as a better understanding of the pathophysiology of this tumor has been gained. Patients with pheochromocytoma require extensive preoperative preparation and careful intraoperative management to prevent the effects of hormone secreted by this tumor. Surgeons who operate on these lesions should know about preoperative and intraoperative preparation of these patients, well discussed in this article.

R.J. Howard, M.D., Ph.D.

Lethality of Multiple Endocrine Neoplasia Type I

Doherty GM, Olson JA, Frisella MM, et al (Washington Univ, St Louis)

World J Surg 22:581-587, 1998 7–13

Introduction.—The mutated gene in patients with multiple endocrine neoplasia type I (MEN-I) has been identified; DNA testing is about to be undertaken to identify carriers. The frequency of significant, life-threatening complications has not been determined. Most patients have progressive indolent disease that rarely causes death. There is a subgroup of patients with MEN-I who seem to die of malignant complications of the disease, frequently at an early age. A patient database was reviewed to determine the cause and age of death in MEN-I kindreds over age 18 years.

Methods.—The Washington University Department of Surgery Multiple Endocrine Neoplasia Program database contains 34 distinct MEN-I kindreds with 1,838 family members at genetic risk of having MEN-I. Records were reviewed retrospectively of all patients who died. Reliable data were available for 103 of 158 patients who died. Accident and suicide deaths were excluded. Survival curves were compared for patients who died from causes related to MEN-I, carriers who died from a nonendocrine cause, and unaffected kindred members. Ages of death were compared between affected and unaffected members of MEN-I kindreds.

Results.—Of 59 patients who were MEN-I affected (46% of cohort), 27 and 32, respectively, died of MEN-I–specific illness and non–MEN-I causes. Median MEN-I–specific deaths occurred at a significantly younger age (47 years) compared with patients with MEN-I who died of a nonendocrine cause and kindred members who did not die of MEN-I disease (60

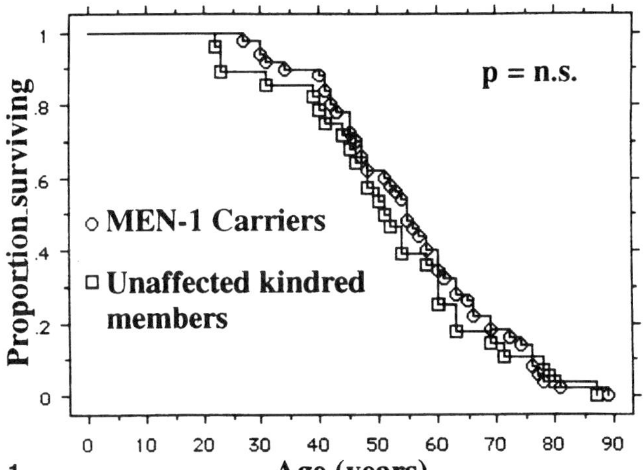

1

FIGURE 1.—Kaplan-Meier cumulative survival plot comparing the age at death of known multiple endocrine neoplasia I (MEN-I) carriers (*circles*) to apparently unaffected kindred members (*squares*). There is no statistical difference between the curves (Tarone-Ware test, $P = 0.45$). (Courtesy of Doherty GM, Olson JA, Frisella MM, et al: Lethality of multiple endocrine neoplasia type I. *World J Surg* 22:581-587, copyright 1998, Springer-Verlag.)

and 55 years, respectively). The median age of MEN-I–affected patients was 55 years; for unaffected kindred members, it was 51 years, a nonsignificant difference (Fig 1). Causes of death for patients with MEN-I–specific disease were as follows: 12 islet cell tumors, 6 ulcer disease, 3 hypercalcemia/uremia, 6 carcinoid tumors, and 9 nonendocrine malignancies.

Conclusion.—Forty-six percent of patients who were MEN-I carriers died of MEN-I–related causes at a median age of 47 years. Two thirds of MEN-I deaths (18/27) were caused by malignant endocrine tumors. There was a substantial subset of MEN-I carriers who died early, particularly of malignant endocrine neoplasms. Aggressive screening is needed in kindreds with MEN-I to identify and initiate treatment of malignancies.

▶ Surgeons at Washington University of St. Louis have collected what is, no doubt, the largest number of patients with MEN-I. They compared the survival rate among these patients and with that of unaffected family members. Surprisingly, there was no difference in mortality rate between MEN-I carriers and unaffected kindred members, something that many people would be surprised at because of the propensity of MEN-I–affected individuals for neoplastic disease. Finding that overall there was no difference in age at death between MEN-I carriers and unaffected kindred members is particularly surprising because 46% of MEN-I–affected patients died of causes related to MEN-I

R.J. Howard, M.D., Ph.D.

8 Nutrition and Metabolism

Introduction

In this year's section on nutrition and metabolism, we examine a melange of research-oriented and clinically oriented studies. Much of the basic research in the field in the past year has been an attempt to improve our understanding of the nutritional and metabolic derangements that occur after surgery, sepsis, and other surgically related catabolic disease states. Clinical studies have attempted to better define the indications for nutritional support. The best of these studies have focused on meaningful end points (e.g., reduction in hospital stay, decrease in cost, and improvement in outcome) rather than on biochemical markers, changes in body weight, or less objective indices. As our knowledge and insights grow, new and previously unappreciated components of the body's response to critical illness also become apparent. The complexity of the human body and its resilience continue to awe us.

Virtually any patient today can safely be given nutritional support, but the exact indications for the provision of exogenous nutrients require further definition. Given the nature of surgical diseases and the current health care environment, it becomes crucial for surgeons to be familiar with the administration of nutritional support for a variety of reasons:

- The kinds of diseases that surgeons treat and the surgical procedures required to treat them can cause marked abnormalities in organ metabolism and nutrient utilization
- Poor nutritional status can adversely affect the outcome of surgical patients
- Surgical patients have diseases and undergo treatments that often preclude the use of oral feedings
- Nutritional support can be expensive and is associated with complications that can be severe, necessitating knowledge of its indications and administration
- Managed care is affecting reimbursement for nutritional support services

- Specific nutrients, which have not historically been included in standard nutritional regimens, can support organ function and improve outcome

Although definitive indications for the use of nutritional support in many patients are unclear and efficacy in many circumstances is unclear, the provision of nutritional support should be based on one of three different rationales: (1) therapy to prevent death from malnutrition (e.g., patients with the short gut syndrome); (2) therapy to prevent starvation-induced complications (infectious complications, impaired wound healing); or (3) therapy to have a favorable impact on the natural history or treatment of a specific disease. This latter category is based on correcting existing nutritional deficiencies arising from a disease or treatment with the intent that outcome will improve. Rationale No. 2 is problematic because it is difficult to know exactly when a particular patient has become nutritionally "at-risk." Clearly, the timing of nutritional intervention will be affected by the patients' pre-existing nutritional status, the magnitude of their hypermetabolism, and the anticipated time before being able to resume normal oral intake. Thus, the use of nutritional support is often based on a subjective assessment made by the experienced surgeon.

Meta-analyses of existing studies allow for the following conclusions: (1) enteral nutrition is always preferable to the parenteral route and should be used if the gut is functional but only if indicated (small amounts of enteral nutrition can be beneficial even if simultaneous parenteral nutrition is required to meet calorie and nitrogen needs); (2) preoperative nutritional support should only be used if the patient has substantial weight loss (at least 15% of body weight); (3) patients sustaining major trauma should be aggressively nourished beginning in the immediate postinjury period, and using the enteral route if feasible; and (4) there is growing evidence that the use of specific nutrients (e.g., glutamine) in pharmacologic amounts can improve outcome in selected groups of patients.

Wiley W. Souba, M.D., Sc.D.

Basic and Clinical Research in Nutrition and Metabolism

Sequential Changes in the Metabolic Response in Severely Septic Patients During the First 23 Days After the Onset of Peritonitis

Plank LD, Connolly AB, Hill GL (Auckland Hosp, New Zealand)
Ann Surg 228:146-158, 1998 8–1

Introduction.—Patients with severe sepsis have a characteristic metabolic response in which hypermetabolism occurs, fat and protein are consumed, and body water and salt are conserved. This response has not been quantified in the context of modern surgical care. Patients with severe sepsis secondary to peritonitis were evaluated to quantify sequential changes in metabolic response.

Methods.—In a series of 12 patients with severe sepsis secondary to perforation of an abdominal viscus, energy expenditure and body composition were measured as soon as the patients were hemodynamically stable and at 5, 10, and 21 days. Sequential measurements of acute-phase proteins and cytokine responses were taken.

Results.—Resting energy expenditure increased to 49% above predicted levels throughout follow-up. Total energy expenditure was 1.25 times the average resting energy expenditure during the 10-day evaluation period. Body fat was oxidized when energy intake was not adequate to realize energy balance. During the first 2 days after onset of sepsis, there was a positive fluid balance of 12.51. After that, body water changes were closely parallel to changes in body weight and were usually the result of changes in extracellular water. During the 21-day evaluation period, patients lost a mean of 1.21 kg (13%) of total body protein. Sixty-seven percent of the protein loss came from skeletal muscle in the first 10 days; thereafter, loss was predominantly from viscera. Intracellular potassium levels were low but did not worsen after hemodynamic stability was reached. A reprioritization of hepatic protein synthesis that was obligatory and independent of changes in total body protein was observed. Cytokine responses revealed a complexity, redundancy, and overlap of mediators.

Conclusion.—Severe sepsis is related to hypermetabolism, lipolysis, proteolysis, and extracellular water gain. For the first time, these changes have been quantified and are more prolonged and greater than was previously believed. These changes are similar to those observed in major trauma; the changes in body water are greater in sepsis. Further investigation should evaluate how to prevent the massive loss of skeletal muscle and visceral protein in patients with severe sepsis.

Plasma Levels of High-Energy Compounds Compared With Severity of Illness in Critically Ill Patients in the Intensive Care Unit

Jabs CM, Sigurdsson GH, Neglen P (UAE Univ, Al Ain, Univ of Bern, Switzerland)

Surgery 124:65-72, 1998 8–2

Introduction.—Animal trials have shown that plasma metabolic changes reflect deterioration of the energy state of tissues. No trial has evaluated the plasma levels of high-energy molecules and their products in critically ill patients and compared these levels with patients' clinical condition. Plasma adenine and creatine energy pools were analyzed in 13 critically ill patients in an intensive care unit (ICU) and correlated with the clinical condition simultaneously evaluated by Acute Physiology and Chronic Health Evaluation (APACHE) II scoring. The prognostic value of metabolic disturbances was assessed.

Methods.—Patient age range was 18-70. Patients had either major trauma, severe septic shock, or cardiogenic shock and an APACHE II score of 16 or greater. The APACHE II scores were recorded daily, and patients

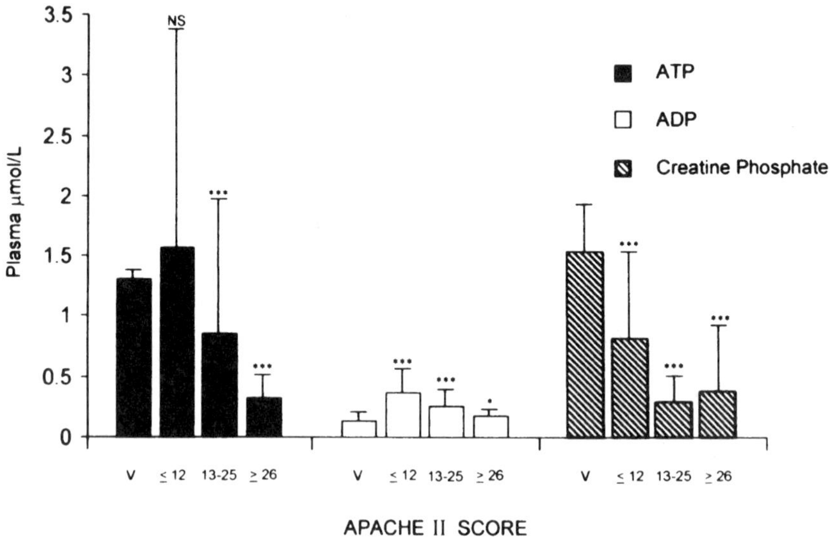

FIGURE 1.—Mean plasma concentrations (± SD) of ATP, ADP, and creatine phosphate in groups of patients with APACHE II scores of 12 or less, 13 to 25, and 26 or greater at time of sampling compared statistically with group of healthy volunteers. *Abbreviations*: *NS*, not significant. $^*P < 0.05$. $P < 0.001$. (Courtesy of Jabs CM, Sigurdsson GH, Neglen P: Plasma levels of high-energy compounds compared with severity of illness in critically ill patients in the intensive care unit. *Surgery* 124:65-72, 1998.)

underwent daily evaluations of adenosine triphosphate, adenosine diphosphate, adenosine, inosine, hypoxanthine, creatine phosphate, creatine, uric acid, and lactic acid. Fifteen healthy volunteers acted as controls.

Results.—All 4 patients with an APACHE II score of 12 or less at some time during their ICU stay survived. All 5 patients with an APACHE II score of 26 or higher died. The initial APACHE II score was a median of 21 (range, 16-25) in the 7 survivors and 24 (range, 7-28) in the 6 nonsurvivors. This difference was not significant. Final median APACHE II scores for survivors and nonsurvivors were 11 (range, 3-16) and 29 (range, 20-47), respectively. The difference was significant. The plasma metabolites were categorized according to patients' APACHE II score of the day. There was a positive relationship between severity of metabolic derangement and the APACHE II score (Fig 1). Higher APACHE II scores yielded depleted plasma contents of adenosine triphosphate and creatine phosphate and progressively increasing levels of creatine and uric acid. Critically ill patients had significantly increased levels of adenosine, inosine, hypoxanthine, and lactic acid.

Conclusion.—Specific patterns of altered plasma metabolism were observed were grouped patients according to APACHE II scores. Patients with higher scores had patterns of altered adenylate energy status that sometimes resulted in unfavorable clinical outcome. The initial APACHE II scores, early individual plasma levels of single high-energy compounds, and certain metabolic patterns were not of prognostic value. Deterioration of physiologic parameters was coexistent with specific metabolic changes.

▶ The article by Plank et al. (Abstract 8–1) is of critical importance for surgeons because it quantifies the loss of functional tissue in surgical patients with abdominal sepsis undergoing exploration. Over a 3-week period, patients lost about 13% of total body protein, despite the provision of adequate nutritional support. This points out the inability of exogenous protein to block the catabolic response; at best, we can hope to match the nitrogen losses. Contrary to common thought, body fat did not change; the exogenous substrates provided to these patients appear to be converted to fat rather than to protein. Simultaneously, there was a huge gain in water. Much of this water is located in and around the gastrointestinal tract, which may contribute to bowel dysfunction in critically ill patients. It would be interesting to know whether enteral nutrition is superior to parenteral nutrition in its ability to promote the accretion of lean body mass. Some studies would suggest that it is.

Cytokine levels in critically ill patients rise initially and then normalize by 7-10 days. However, the hypermetabolism can persist and, as shown by Jabs et al. (Abstract 8–2), may be associated with an abnormal plasma profile of certain metabolites relating to tissue energy charge. Unfortunately, the article did not include serial measurements of plasma high-energy metabolites to determine whether such measurements could be useful prognostically or therapeutically or whether they correlated with protein losses or nutritional intervention.

W.W. Souba, M.D., Sc.D.

Early Effects of Catecholamine Therapy on Mucosal Integrity, Intestinal Blood Flow, and Oxygen Metabolism in Porcine Endotoxin Shock

Sautner T, Wessely C, Riegler M, et al (Univ of Vienna)

Ann Surg 228:239-248, 1998 8–3

Introduction.—The intestine has recently received considerable attention in patients with sepsis and septic shock because it is a potential source of bacteria. Bacterial translocation in these conditions is well defined; yet little is known regarding the consequences of conventional treatment of septic shock with various catecholamines on intestinal integrity or permeability. The early effects of endotoxin (ET) shock with epinephrine, norepinephrine, or dopexamine on splanchnic circulation, oxygen metabolism, sigmoid mucosal pHi, bacterial translocation, and morphologic integrity of the ileal, colonic, and sigmoid mucosa were assessed.

Methods.—Twenty-three landrace pigs underwent ET shock that was induced by ET infusion over 30 minutes; they were observed for 4 hours. Animals were continuously infused with either 250 μg/kg ET (*Escherichia coli*) in saline solution or with saline solution alone and then monitored for 240 minutes. Animals were randomized into 1 of 4 groups: fluid resuscitation (FR) alone, FR plus epinephrine hydrochloride, FR plus norepinephrine, or FR plus dopexamine hydrochloride. They were observed for systemic and splanchnic blood flow and oxygen metabolism, sigmoid colon mucosal pHi, and bacterial translocation determined by culture of portal venous blood, mesenteric lymph nodes, liver, spleen, and lung specimens. Histologic sections of ileal, colonic, and sigmoid mucosa were examined morphometrically to determine effects of therapy.

Results.—Every catecholamine increased cardiac output and systemic oxygen delivery; intestinal blood flow and oxygen delivery were unchanged. Sigmoid mucosal pHi diminished in all pigs. The reduction was most noticeable in the epinephrine group. Pigs in this group had greater than 40% damage of the ileum and colon. Animals who received ET alone, norephinephrine, or dopexamine had only moderate lesions with signs of restitution. Bacterial translocation was not observed in any of the animals.

Conclusion.—Intestinal perfusion is not reflected in systemic hemodynamics and oxygen metabolism. No additional impairment of intestinal integrity was observed with administration of norephinephrine or dopexamine in ET shock. Epinephrine therapy was associated with a significant decrease in mucosal pHi and considerable early mucosal damage. Its use in patients with septic shock is hazardous.

Testosterone: The Crucial Hormone Responsible for Depressing Myocardial Function in Males After Trauma-Hemorrhage

Remmers DE, Cioffi WG, Bland KI, et al (Brown Univ, Providence, RI)

Ann Surg 227:790-799, 1998 8–4

Introduction.—Specific and nonspecific immune functions are depressed after trauma hemorrhage and may be responsible for increased susceptibility to sepsis after insult. Several reports indicate that susceptibility to and death from sepsis are higher in males than in females. Recent trials have reported that in vivo cardiac performance is markedly depressed in male animals after trauma hemorrhage and resuscitation. Testosterone levels were depleted in rats before trauma hemorrhage and resuscitation to determine whether testosterone levels in males had any effect on cardiac performance.

Methods.—Male Sprague-Dawley rats were castrated or sham-castrated (skin of scrotum only incised and closed with sutures) 14 days before trauma was induced under general anesthesia. Laparotomy was performed, animals were bled, and a mean arterial pressure of 40 mm Hg was maintained until 40% of the maximal shed volume was returned in the form of Ringer's lactate solution. Animals were resuscitated with 4 times the shed blood volume in the form of Ringer's lactate solution over 60 minutes. Heart performance was monitored with a left ventricular catheter connected to an in vivo heart performance analyzer. Indices of left ventricular performance were measured up to 4 hours after trauma, hemorrhagic shock, and resuscitation and included maximal rate of the pressure increase ($+dP/dt_{max}$) and decrease ($-dP/dt_{max}$).

Results.—Trauma hemorrhage and resuscitation reduced the in vivo heart performance in sham-castrated rats, as indicated by diminished values of $+dP/dt_{max}$ and $-dP/dt_{max}$. Precastrated rats had significantly higher values of $+dP/dt_{max}$ and $-dP/dt_{max}$, than sham-castrated rats after trauma hemorrhage and resuscitation.

Conclusion.—Testosterone antagonism in males could be effective in maintaining myocardial function after adverse circulatory conditions. This approach is neither practical nor advocated in male patients who experience trauma hemorrhage. Testosterone receptor blockade after trauma may be a novel and useful adjunct for maintaining normal myocardial performance in male patients.

Recombinant Human Growth Hormone Modulates Th1 and Th2 Cytokine Response in Burned Mice

Takagi K, Suzuki F, Barrow RE, et al (Shriners Burns Inst, Galveston, Tex; Univ of Texas, Galveston)

Ann Surg 228:106-111, 1998 8–5

Introduction.—Growth hormone (GH) is an anabolic agent used in patients with burns to improve wound healing and protein metabolism. The effect of GH on lymphocyte cytokine production in patients who are immunosuppressed has not been determined. Immunosuppressed mice were evaluated after burn to determine if the production of type I cytokines (INF-γ, IL-2) and type 2 cytokines (IL-4, IL-10) were altered in burned animals by GH therapy and whether distinctly different patterns of Th1-like or Th2-like responses could be observed.

Methods.—Burn injury was induced in BALB/c mice under general anesthesia by exposing a 3 × 4-cm area to the flame of a Fisher burner for 10 seconds. Fluid resuscitation was administered with 4 mL of normal saline intraperitoneally to each mouse. Animals were treated with either subcutaneous recombinant human GH (rhGH) or saline every other day. Animals were sacrificed at 1 or 11 days after burn and the spleen was harvested to evaluate the production of Th1 and Th2 cytokines from isolated splenic lymphocytes.

Results.—On both days 1 and 11 after burn, Th1 cytokine production by splenic lymphocytes from burned mice treated with GH was higher, than mice treated with saline. The production of Th1 cytokine was greater in burned mice than nonburned mice. Production of Th2 cytokines were diminished in burned animals.

Conclusion.—Burn trauma causes Th cells to differentiate toward the Th2 phenotype. This is modified by rhGH, which generates the Th1-dominant response. This alteration of the Th1/Th2 response induced by GH may be an important mechanism in protecting patients with burns or other injuries from opportunistic infections, which could become fatal complications.

▶ Embedded into the body's inventory of protective mechanisms is a complex set of well-regulated defense responses that are initiated within moments of injury or insult. These responses are involuntary, but they are essential for survival. They are designed to maintain body homeostasis at a time when key physiologic processes are threatened and are initiated by various components of the response to injury such as volume loss, tissue damage, fear, and pain. These responses are regulated by specific genes that encode the biosynthesis of key hormones, cytokines, and peptides—compounds that allow the body to respond to such insults with remarkable resilience. (Abstracts 8–3 to 8–5). From an evolutionary standpoint, these biologic responses are the result of a process that favors survival of the fittest in the struggle to survive and preserve the species. From a teleologic standpoint, they are designed to benefit the organism, enhance recovery, and assure a relatively speedy return to health.

Later factors that reinitiate or perpetuate these responses include invasive infection and starvation. The events are generally related to the severity of injury; that is, the greater the insult, the more pronounced the specific response. In some circumstances, the elaboration of stress mediators can be excessive. In other circumstances, the therapies that we use to treat patients (e.g., pressors, steroids) may have undesirable side effects. In either case, the net result is that the body's responses may become exaggerated to the point that they are detrimental. Therefore, strategies to block these maladaptive responses (e.g., receptor blockade) or combat the undesirable side-effects (e.g., treatment of catabolism with protein synthesis promoting agents) may be of value. This field of research will become of key importance in the next decade.

W.W. Souba, M.D., Sc.D.

Alteration of the Intestinal Intraepithelial Lymphocytes During Total Parenteral Nutrition

Kiristioglu I, Teitelbaum DH (Univ of Michigan, Ann Arbor; C.S. Mott Children's Hosp, Ann Arbor, Mich)

J Surg Res 79:91-96, 1998 8–6

Introduction.—Use of total parenteral nutrition (TPN) is associated with various major septic complications, including generalized sepsis, pneumonia, and catheter-associated infections. The source of sepsis may be the gastrointestinal tract. An animal model of TPN reported two thirds of rats had bacterial translocation (BT) develop. The mode by which this translocation occurs is not known. It may be related to the breakdown of intestinal epithelial barrier function. The effect of TPN administration on the phenotypic composition of intraepithelial lymphocytes (IEL) was assessed, along with alterations in the expression of cytokines in the IEL.

Methods.—Male C57BL/6 mice were randomized to receive either TPN with no oral feedings or intravenous saline and mouse chow. Mice were evaluated on day 7 for BT. Isolated IEL were stained for CD4, CD8, and CD44 and underwent flow cytometry. The mRNA was obtained from remaining IEL for cytokine expression. Reverse transcriptase polymerase chain reaction was done to identify TGF-β1 and INF-γ mRNA expression. The densities were standardized to expression of β-actin.

Results.—The rate of BT to mesenteric lymph nodes was 40% for the TPN group and 12.5% for controls. There was a significant reduction in CD4+, CD8−; CD4+, Cd8+ and the CD8+, CD44+ IEL subpopulations in animals fed TPN only. Compared to controls, the mRNA expression for INF-γ was increased by 53% and TGF-β1 mRNA expression was diminished by 75% in the IEL of mice fed TPN only.

Conclusion.—Administration of TPN only caused significant alterations in the phenotypic subpopulations of the IEL. There were also changes in the spontaneous expression of cytokine mRNA. These alterations in the IEL phenotype and function may be an important mechanism by which epithelial integrity is lost.

Gut Bacterial Translocation During Total Parenteral Nutrition in Experimental Rats and Its Countermeasure

Nakasaki H, Mitomi T, Tajima T, et al (Tokai Univ, Oiso, Japan)
Am J Surg 175:38-43, 1998 8–7

Introduction.—The use of total parenteral nutrition (TPN) during extended periods causes gross atrophy of the intestinal mucous membrane and a potential decrease in the local immune activity within the gastrointestinal tract. Bacterial translocation may occur under these conditions. Methods to prevent this from occurring are urgently needed. A TPN rat model was used to evaluate the action of proteoglycan (PSK), a biological response modifier, which seems to suppress bacterial translocation and maintain local immune activity within the gastrointestinal tract during TPN.

Methods.—Male specific pathogen-free Wistar rats were enrolled in 1 of 3 groups: free-feeding, received food and water ad libitum; TPN, standard TPN solution via a central catheter; and PSK, simultaneous TPN via the central catheter and oral PSK daily (1,000 mg/kg). At 2 weeks, rats were anesthetized and samples of bile and portal venous blood were collected to measure the amount of S-IgA. The small bowel was resected along its total length and the number of Peyer's patches were counted. Peyer's patches were analyzed histologically; frozen specimens were created for immunohistochemical examination. Specimens were examined for bacterial translocation.

Results.—Cultures of mesenteric lymph nodes taken after TPN only revealed a bacterial rate as high as 60%. Immunohistochemical analysis revealed a decrease in the number of plasma cells and a reduction in S-IgA production and secretion. A similar decrease in S-IgA within bile and portal venous blood was also seen. Continuous oral administration of PSK offered a protective effect against the degeneration of gut-associated lymphoid tissue (GALT). Constant levels of MHC-I, MHC-II, T helper cells, and interleukin-2 producing cells were observed supporting the protective role of PSK against degeneration of GALT, with a subsequent decrease in bacterial translocation.

Conclusion.—PSK can restore impaired local immunity in the intestinal tract to normal levels and suppress the bacterial translocation in patients undergoing TPN treatment.

Increased Intestinal Permeability and Altered Mucosal Immunity in Cholestatic Jaundice

Welsh FKS, Ramsden CW, MacLennan K, et al (St James' Univ, Leeds, England; Regional Blood Donor Ctr, Edinburgh, Scotland)

Ann Surg 227:205-212, 1998 8–8

Introduction.—Sepsis and its sequelae are the major causes of morbidity and mortality in patients with jaundice; this risk correlates with severity of jaundice. Few trials have evaluated gut barrier function in relevant clinical situations in humans. Gut barrier function was evaluated in patients with jaundice to determine if it was impaired and to determine the effects of any altered barrier function on intestinal morphology or gastrointestinal immune function. Intestinal permeability was assessed before and after internal biliary drainage.

Methods.—Twenty-seven patients with extrahepatic obstructive jaundice and 27 research subjects who were nonicteric underwent evaluation of intestinal permeability using the lactulose-mannitol test. Endoscopic biopsies of the second part of the duodenum underwent morphologic examination and were evaluated for the presence of mucosal immunologic activation. Systemic antiendotoxin core IgG antibodies, serum interleukin-6, and C-reactive protein were quantified to detect evidence of chronic exposure to endotoxin.

Results.—The median lactulose-mannitol ratio was significantly elevated in patients who were jaundiced. Upregulation of HLA-DR expression on enterocytes and gut-associated lymphoid tissue was indicative of immune activation. There was a significant rise in acute phase response and circulating antiendotoxin core antibodies in patients who were jaundiced. Intestinal permeability returned to normal levels after internal biliary drainage.

Conclusion.—A reversible impairment in gut barrier function was observed in patients with cholestatic jaundice. Increased intestinal permeability was correlated with local immune cell and enterocyte activation. The rise in intestinal permeability was restored toward normal by internal biliary drainage.

Medium-chain Compared With Long-chain Triacylglycerol Emulsions Enhance Macrophage Response and Increase Mucosal Mass in Parenterally Fed Rats

Hinton PS, Peterson CA, McCarthy DO, et al (Univ of Wisconsin, Madison)

Am J Clin Nutr 67:1265-1272, 1998 8–9

Introduction.—The absence of luminal nutrients during total parenteral nutrition (TPN) causes a loss of intestinal mass and impaired immune function that the type of parenteral lipid emulsion can regulate. Parenteral medium-chain triacylglycerol (MCT) emulsions may be of greater benefit than long-chain triacylglycerol (LCT) emulsion when used in TPN, because MCTs are cleared more rapidly from plasma than LCTs and are more rapidly and completely oxidized; this offers a readily available energy source. The effects of MCTs plus LCTs administered during TPN were evaluated in rats to determine if this approach would enhance macrophage responses and resist TPN-induced gut atrophy, compared to animals infused with LCTs alone.

Findings.—Male Sprague-Dawley rats underwent TPN that provided 16% or 48% of nonprotein energy from MCTs plus LCTs or LCTs alone or 100% of nonprotein energy from dextrose for 6 or 12 days. Body weight gain was similar among all groups. After 6 days, serum concentrations of β-hydroxybutyrate were greater with MCTs plus LCTs, compared to LCTs alone. After both 6 and 12 days, triacylglycerol concentrations in liver were higher with LCTs than with MCTs plus LCTs. After 6 days, MCTs plus LCTs increased by 50% the percentage and number of splenic macrophages, compared to LCTs alone, in accord with diminished triacylglycerol concentrations in spleen. Compared to LCTs alone, MCTs plus LCTs increased in vitro tumor necrosis factor-α secretion by splenic or circulating macrophages in response to lipopolysaccharide (2-fold after 6 days and 7-fold after 12 days). Jejunal mucosal mass was 30% greater after 6 days in rats fed MCTs plus LCTs, compared to those who received LCTs alone. Groups did not differ significantly in the incidence of bacterial translocation to the mesenteric lymph nodes.

Conclusion.—Inclusion of MCTs in parenteral lipid emulsions diminished jejunal mucosal atrophy and enhanced macrophage functions after 6 and 12 days of TPN, despite coinfusion with moderate amounts of LCTs.

▶ Under certain circumstances, the gut can be a source of sepsis and serve as the motor of the systemic inflammatory response syndrome. Normally, an intact brush border and intercellular tight junctions prevent the movement of toxins into the intestinal lymphatics and circulation. We can alter these conditions in critically ill patients. Maintaining a gut mucosal barrier that effectively excludes luminal bacteria and toxins requires an intact epithelium and normal mucosal immune mechanisms.

Microbial translocation is the process by which microorganisms migrate across the mucosal barrier and invade the host. Translocation can be promoted in the following three general ways:

- Altered permeability of the intestinal mucosa (caused by hemorrhagic shock, sepsis, distant injury, or administration of cell toxins)
- Decreased host defense (secondary to glucocorticoid administration, immunosuppression, or protein depletion)
- Increased bacteria in the intestine (caused by bacterial overgrowth, intestinal stasis, or the feeding of bacteria to experimental animals)

A number of retrospective and epidemiological studies have associated infection in specific patient populations with bacterial invasion from the gut. These studies have demonstrated an increase in mucosal permeability in normal volunteers receiving endotoxin and in infected burn patients. Because many of the factors that facilitate bacterial translocation occur simultaneously in surgical patients and their effects may be additive or cumulative, patients in an intensive care unit can be extremely vulnerable to the invasion of enteric bacteria or to the absorption of their toxins. The provision of luminal nutrition is an effective method of decreasing the incidence of gut-derived sepsis.

W.W. Souba, M.D., Sc.D.

Albumin Synthesis Rates Are Not Decreased in Hypoalbuminemic Cachectic Cancer Patients With an Ongoing Acute-Phase Protein Response

Fearon KCH, Falconer JS, Slater C, et al (Royal Infirmary, Edinburgh, Scotland; SURRC, East Kilbride, Glasgow, Scotland; Royal Infirmary, Glasgow, Scotland)
Ann Surg 227:249-254, 1998 8–10

Background.—Little is known about the factors affecting the changes in protein metabolism observed in cancer patients with cachexia. Recent reports have suggested an important role for the host proinflammatory cytokine network, including the initiation of an hepatic acute-phase protein response (APPR). An ongoing APPR may be reflected in increased levels of C-reactive protein and reduced levels of albumin, both observed in patients with advanced cancer. This study examined the presence of suppressed albumin synthesis among cachectic patients with evidence of an ongoing acute-phase response.

Methods.—A flooding-dose [$^2H_5$]-phenylalanine technique was used to assess albumin synthesis rates in 6 patients with pancreatic cancer who were losing weight and had an ongoing APPR, as indicated by a C-reactive protein level of greater than 10 mg/L. Levels of the proinflammatory cytokines tumor necrosis factor (TNF) and interleukin (IL)-6 were measured as well, together with soluble TNF receptors and serum cortisol and insulin. Six healthy controls were studied for comparison.

TABLE 2.—Plasma Volume and Albumin Synthetic Rate in Normal Subjects and Patients With Cancer

	Control Subjects (n = 6)	Cancer Patients (n = 6)	p
Plasma albumin (g/L)	42 (40-45)	32 (23-36)	<0.01
Plasma volume (mL)	3122 (2483-4326)	2623 (2449-2881)	NS
Intravascular albumin mass (g)	133 (105-177)	88 (56-93)	<0.01
Albumin secretion time (min)	28 (22-32)	25 (19-28)	NS
Albumin fractional synthetic rate (%/day)	10.3 (7.1-11.3)	13.9 (13.5-18.5)	<0.01
Albumin total synthetic rate (g/day)	11.7 (8.5-18.7)	12.7 (7.7-15.7)	NS

Note: Values are medians with range in parentheses.
Abbreviation: NS, not significant.
(Courtesy of Fearon KCH, Falconer JS, Slater C, et al: Albumin synthesis rates are not decreased in hypoalbuminemic cachectic cancer patients with an ongoing acute-phase protein response. *Ann Surg* 227:249-254, 1998.)

Results.—The median serum albumin value was 32 g/L in the cancer patients vs. 42 g/L in controls (Table 2). Serum C-reactive protein was 72 vs. less than 5 mg/L, respectively. Neither group had detectable TNF, although one of the soluble TNF receptor levels was increased in cancer patients. There were no significant differences in serum IL-6, insulin, or cortisol. The cancer patients had a lower intravascular albumin mass (88 vs. 133 g). However, they had a higher rate of intravascular albumin fractional synthesis (13.9% vs. 10.3% per day). There was no significant difference in the total rate of intravascular albumin synthesis: 12.7 g per day in the cancer patients vs. 11.7 g per day in the controls.

Conclusion.—The hypoalbuminemia observed in cachectic patients with pancreatic cancer and evidence of an ongoing APPR does not appear to result from a reduced rate of albumin synthesis. Further study of the factors affecting positive and negative acute-phase proteins in vivo may help in designing interventions to interrupt nutritional and metabolic decline in cancer patients.

Regulation of Albumin mRNA and Its Promoter-binding Nuclear Factors Under Different Perioperative Nutritional Methods in Hepatectomized Rats

Morimoto T, Tsujinaka T, Yano M, et al (Osaka Univ, Japan)
Am J Surg 175:221-226, 1998 8–11

Introduction.—Compared with parenteral nutrition (PN), enteral nutrition (EN) can reduce morbidity and mortality in critically ill patients. There is evidence that EN may modulate the production of proteins involved in regulating albumin synthesis. A study was performed in rats to examine the effects of PN and EN on regulation of perioperative albumin synthesis.

Methods and Results.—Rats received 7 days of artificial nutrition via PN or EN, followed by 70% hepatectomy. Seventy-two hours later, rats in the PN group had significantly lower levels of serum albumin and albumin

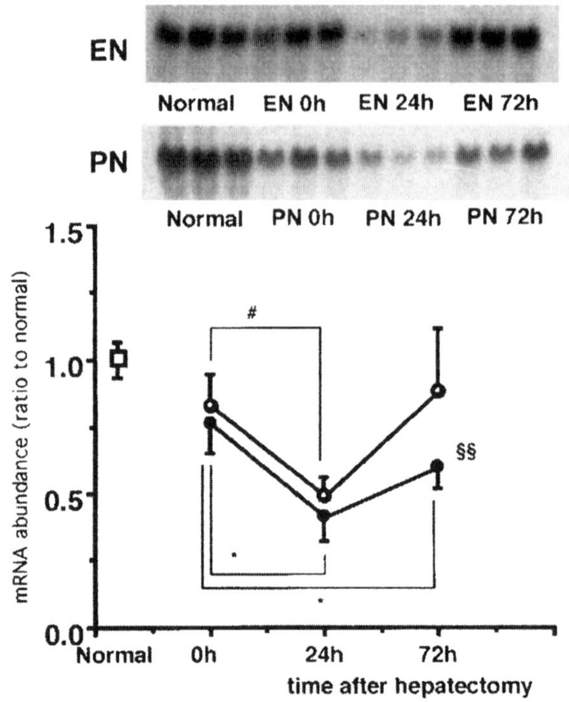

FIGURE 2.—Changes in the level of albumin messenger RNA (*mRNA*) before and after hepatectomy and effects of parenteral nutrition (*PN*) vs. enteral nutrition (*EN*). **Upper section**, Northern blotting of each of 3 representative samples obtained from normal, PN, and EN rats. **Lower section**, data indicate the relative intensity of densitometry defined as arbitrary densitometric units. Data are expressed as mean ± standard deviation of 5 rats in each group. *White squares* indicate normal rats; *black circles*, the PN group; *white circles*, the EN group; *0h*, 7 days after initiation of artificial nutrition and before hepatectomy; *24h*, 24 hours after hepatectomy; *72h*, 72 hours after hepatectomy; *Asterisk* indicates *P* less than 0.05 (vs. PN 0h, analysis of variance; *number symbol* indicates *P* less than 0.05 (vs. EN 0h, analysis of variance); *double section mark* indicates *P* less than 0.05 (PN vs. EN at the same time point, Student's *t* test). (Reprinted from the *American Journal of Surgery* courtesy of Morimoto T, Tsujinaka T, Yano M, et al: Regulation of albumin mRNA and its promoter-binding nuclear factors under different perioperative nutritional methods in hepatectomized rats. *Am J Surg* 175:221-226, copyright 1998, with permission from Excerpta Medica Inc.)

messenger RNA (mRNA) than those in the EN group (Fig 2). Before and after hepatectomy, animals in the EN group had significantly higher albumin promoter-binding nuclear factors: i.e., CCAAT/enhancer-binding protein α and D-site—binding protein.

Conclusion.—In this model, serum albumin is well maintained after hepatectomy in rats receiving perioperative EN, compared with those receiving PN. The mechanism of this effect is early recovery of albumin mRNA and its nuclear factor mRNA levels. The results suggest that perioperative EN for hepatectomy patients may be preferable to PN in terms of albumin synthesis.

▶ Most surgeons use serum albumin as a marker of malnutrition. Although it is not specific, it can be helpful. Fearon et al. (Abstract 8–10) show that the hypoalbuminemia that occurs in cancer patients is not caused by a decrease in hepatic biosynthesis, as we have assumed in the past. Rather, it is probably the result of an increase in albumin degradation (turnover) or intravascular volume expansion. These findings have implications from a nutritional standpoint. If albumin synthetic rates are maintained (or increased), should nutritional support be provided? What is the significance of a low serum albumin level in cancer patients? It is important to remember that although serum albumin values can be used to predict nutritional risk[1] and a low serum albumin concentration at the time of hospital admission can predict death and length of stay[2], hypoalbuminemia is not specific to poor nutritional status.[2,3]

W.W. Souba, M.D., Sc.D.

References

1. The Veterans Affairs Total Parenteral Nutrition Cooperative Study Group: Perioperative total parenteral nutrition in surgical patients. *N Engl J Med* 325:525-532, 1991.
2. Herrmann FR, Safran C, Levkoff SE, et al: Serum albumin level on admission as a predictor of death, length of stay, and readmission. *Arch Intern Med* 152:125-130, 1922.
3. Chandra RK: Nutrition, immunity, and infection: Present knowledge and future directions. *Lancet* 1: 688-691, 1983.

Adaptive Alterations in Cellular Metabolism With Malignant Transformation

Fischer CP, Bode BP, Souba WW (Harvard Med School, Boston)
Ann Surg 227:627-636, 1998 8–12

Introduction.—To go through malignant transformation, cells must exploit nutrients for energy, protein synthesis, and cell division. Cancer cells derive much of their energy from glucose and glutamine, the latter of which plays a key role in protein and DNA biosynthesis. The metabolic changes associated with malignant transformation were examined by comparing the utilization of glutamine and glucose in normal fibroblasts and fibrosarcoma cells.

Methods and Results.—Rat fibrosarcoma cells showed a sixfold increase in glutamine transport rates, compared with normal rat fibroblasts. Glutamine transport in normal fibroblasts was mediated by 2 systems: system ASC and system A. In contrast, only system ASC was operative in malignant fibrosarcoma cells, with a V_{max} 15 times higher than in fibroblasts. Fibrosarcoma cells showed reduced glutaminase activity and glutamine oxidation to carbon dioxide, even though transport was increased. Glutamine oxidation was 1.8-fold higher than glucose oxidation in fibroblasts, whereas glucose oxidation was 3.5-fold higher than glucose oxidation in fibrosarcomas. Glutamine transported by fibrosarcomas synthesized 3 times as much protein as that transported by normal fibroblasts. Fibrosarcoma cells grew faster than normal fibroblasts, even with their increased rates of glutamine utilization and glucose oxidation.

Conclusion.—This study links malignant transformation of cells to increased cellular glutamine transport. This alteration is mediated by a single high-affinity, high-capacity plasma membrane carrier protein. As glutamine oxidation falls in fibrosarcoma cells, glutamine is used for protein synthesis. At the same time, the malignant cell becomes a glucose oxidizer. It is the malignant phenotype per se, and not the increased rate of cell growth, that is responsible for the increased glutamine transport and glucose oxidation exhibited by fibrosarcoma cells.

▶ The changes the authors observed appear to be related to the malignant phenotype and not merely to an increase in cell growth rates. However, one piece of information not provided by this study concerns the changes in substrate metabolism that occurred in atypical cells or cells that were transformed but not tumorigenic—only normal and malignant cells, those at 2 ends of the spectrum, were examined. It would be interesting to define the specific molecular events that result in the changes in transport the authors described and the timing of their expression. As a normal cell undergoes the multistep transformation process, are there specific genetic events that lead to an increase in glutamine transport which are necessary for transformation to occur? Is an upregulation in transporter gene expression sufficient for the progression to the malignant phenotype to occur, or, more likely, only necessary? Are there differences in glutamine transport rates and transporter characteristics between well-differentiated and poorly differentiated tumors, between proliferating and nonproliferating tumor cells? These questions remain unanswered.

W.W. Souba, M.D., Sc.D.

Clinical Aspects of Nutritional Support

Prevalence and Causes of Undernutrition in Medical Outpatients

Wilson M-MG, Vaswani S, Liu D, et al (St Louis Univ; St Louis Veterans Affairs Med Ctr)

Am J Med 104:56-63, 1998 8–13

Background.—Although the prevalence of diagnosed undernutrition in community-dwelling elderly individuals is reportedly less than 5%, one fifth to one third of such individuals may have evidence of undernutrition, some of which may be considered subclinical. The prevalence, causes, and frequency of recognition and treatment of undernutrition in older and younger medical outpatients were studied.

Methods.—The charts of 1,017 adults were reviewed. Eighty-five patients met the study inclusion criteria and were followed up for 2 years. Patients' nutritional, cognitive, and affective status as well as nutritional attitudes were assessed.

Findings.—Undernutrition was present in 11% of older patients and in 7% of younger patients. The odds ratio for older vs. younger age was 1.65.

The primary cause of undernutrition, considered treatable in almost 90% of the patients, differed between age groups. Undernutrition was recognized in 43% of the older patients and in 12% of the younger patients, and appropriate treatment was begun in 14% and 5%, respectively. The older patients had higher scores on the EAT-26 oral control subscale than did younger patients, but their scores on the EAT-26 dieting subscale were similar.

Conclusions.—In both older and younger medical outpatients, undernutrition was relatively common. Although usually amenable to treatment, undernutrition was often undetected and undertreated. Older undernourished patients had higher oral control needs than younger patients.

Total Parenteral Nutrition in the Critically Ill Patient: A Meta-analysis

Heyland DK, MacDonald S, Keefe L, et al (Queen's Univ, Kingston, Ont, Canada; Kingston Gen Hosp, Ont, Canada)

JAMA 280:2013-2019, 1998 8–14

Introduction.—To prevent the complications associated with malnutrition, nutritional support has become a standard of care for hospitalized patients. Yet the effect of total parenteral nutrition (TPN) on morbidity and mortality remains uncertain, and evidence supporting its use is limited. An analysis of randomized trials examined the relationship between TPN and complication and mortality rates in critically ill patients.

Methods.—Data were obtained from a search of MEDLINE (including pre-MEDLINE) for studies from 1980 to April 1998. Eligible trials included adult surgical or critically ill patients, compared any form of TPN with standard care (oral diet plus IV fluids), and reported the outcome measures of complications, length of stay, and mortality. The studies were scored for methodologic quality.

Results.—Twenty-six randomized trials involving 2,211 patients met study criteria. When the findings of these trials were combined, there was no effect of TPN on mortality (relative risk, 1.03). Although patients who received TPN had a lower complication rate than those given standard care, the difference was not statistically significant. No differences in mortality were seen when trials that included only malnourished patients were compared with other trials. Trials with higher methods scores and trials published since 1989 showed no effect of TPN on mortality. The earlier studies and those with lower methods scores showed a significant treatment effect. Complication and mortality rates were significantly higher in studies limited to critically ill patients than in studies that included surgical patients.

Conclusion.—TPN may have some benefits, but the overall results of this meta-analysis show no reductions in mortality or major complication rates in surgical or critically ill patients when compared with standard care. Trial results are influenced by patient population, use of lipids, methodological quality, and year of publication.

Patterns and Problems of Adult Total Parenteral Nutrition Use in US Academic Medical Centers

Schloerb PR, Henning JF (Univ of Kansas, Kansas City)
Arch Surg 133:7-12, 1998 8–15

Introduction.—A recent meta-analysis concluded the use of total parenteral nutrition (TPN) benefits cases of severe malnourishment, but its routine use in unselected patients is not justified. One study has reported an increase in complications when patients undergoing major pancreatic resections were randomized to TPN. Two surveys of the University Health-Systems Consortium (UHC) sought to determine TPN formulas and amounts of TPN nutrients administered to 2 hypothetical abdominal trauma patients.

Methods.—The first questionnaire, sent by the UHC to pharmacy directors of all 74 members and 32 network partners, asked about the TPN formula used at each institution. In a second survey, respondents were asked to provide TPN prescriptions for 2 clinical examples: a 21-year-old previously healthy man (weight, 70 kg; height 6 feet) who sustained abdominal injury in a motor vehicle accident and had near normal vital signs after undergoing laparotomy with suture closure of ruptured duodenum and drainage of the pancreatic area; a 70-year-old previously healthy woman (weight 70 kg; height 5 feet) who sustained the same injury and operation. The young man was to receive 2,162 kcal and the older woman, 1,534 kcal.

Results.—In the first survey, TPN solutions with 20% concentrations or greater of dextrose were reported by 78% of the 72 respondents. Most institutions used 4% to 5% amino acids in TPN. Most replies to the second survey were from pharmacists; only 5.8% were from physicians. Although average values of amino acids and dextrose, fat emulsion, and infusion rates were in accord with common practice, TPN formulations varied widely. Dextrose use exceeded 15% with 80% of respondents and was 25% with 14% of respondents. At the rates of TPN administration reported, the man received a mean of 2,081 mL per day and the woman, 1,600 mL per day. Most institutions (65 of 86) used only 20% fat emulsion. The female patient received less amino acids than the male patient.

Conclusion.—There was a discrepancy between TPN values in the first and second surveys. The excessive amounts of glucose administered may explain previous adverse effects associated with TPN. Findings suggest using a standard TPN formula, with no more than 15% dextrose administered at a rate to provide no more than 4 mg/kg of glucose per minute.

► The observation that malnutrition is common in hospitalized patients was initially reported 25 years ago.[1,2] Today, the incidence remains high—unfortunately, many malnourished patients are untreated or undertreated even with the feasible use of nutrition support. On the other hand, many patients receive enteral or parenteral nutrition even though the rationale is invalid.

Virtually all patients can be fed intravenously or enterally because of the development of 2 important techniques: the infusion of hypertonic nutrient solutions by central venous catheterization and the intraluminal administration of specific enteral diets through a feeding tube. As Heyland et al. (Abstract 8–14) indicate, it is often difficult to identify the patient who is "at risk" for developing malnutrition-related complications. The identification of protein-calorie malnutrition has been based on objective measurements including weight loss, serum protein concentrations, anthropometric measurements, energy, and immunologic indices. Unfortunately, no single measurement is highly sensitive and specific in identifying malnutrition. Clinical assessment is as effective as objective measurements in categorizing a patient's nutritional status. It should be emphasized that the lack of evidence that nutritional support affects clinical outcome favorably in a particular circumstance does not necessarily condemn its use.

W.W. Souba, M.D., Sc.D.

References

1. Bistrian B, Blackburn B, Hallowell E, et al: Protein status of general surgical patients. *JAMA* 230: 858-860, 1974.
2. Bistrian B, Blackburn B, Vitale J, et al: Prevalence of malnutrition in general medical patients. *JAMA* 235: 1567-1570, 1976.

Effects of Glutamine Supplementation on Circulating Lymphocytes After Bone Marrow Transplantation: A Pilot Study

Ziegler TR, Bye RL, Persinger RL, et al (Emory Univ, Atlanta, Ga; Harvard Med School, Boston)

Am J Med Sci 315:4-10, 1998 8–16

Introduction.—The supplementation of enteral and parenteral nutrition (PN) solutions with the amino acid glutamine (Gln) has been extensively studied, for Gln is apparently a conditionally essential nutrient during catabolic stress. A pilot study evaluated the effects of Gln supplementation on circulating lymphocytes and lymphocyte subsets after allogeneic bone marrow transplantation (BMT).

Methods.—Data were obtained from a subset of 20 patients from the authors' previously reported double-blind, randomized trial in 45 patients on the benefits of Gln-PN after BMT. The subset of 20 patients included those who had flow cytometry studies performed within 14 days after hospital discharge. Patients had received either PN supplemented by LGln (Gln-PN) or standard Gln-free PN (Std-PN) after BMT. To evaluate lymphocyte recovery in the 20 patients, investigators obtained the total leukocyte count, total lymphocyte count, and percentage of lymphocytes at weekly intervals during PN therapy.

Results.—The 9 patients receiving Gln-PN were similar to the 11 control patients in age, sex, gender, body weight, primary diagnosis, initial leuko-

TABLE 4.—Weekly Leukocyte and Lymphocyte Counts (Cells/μL) and Percentage of Lymphocytes During Hospitalization

Week	Total Leukocytes*		Total Lymphocytes*		% Lymphocytes*†	
	Std-PN	Gln-PN	Std-PN	Gln-PN	Std-PN	Gln-PN
Week 2 (day 14)	714 ± 273	625 ± 144	149 ± 77	209 ± 38	22 ± 4	42 ± 6
Week 3 (day 21)	2887 ± 397	3488 ± 927	296 ± 48	406 ± 91	11 ± 3	16 ± 5
Week 4 (day 28)	7150 ± 1484	3733 ± 462	422 ± 107	595 ± 102	8 ± 2	16 ± 3

Data are reported as mean number of cells ± standard error.
*P <0.0001 effect of time by 2-factor analysis of variance.
†P = 0.0135 effect of glutamine by 2-factor analysis of variance.
Std-PN = standard parenteral nutrition; Gln-PN = glutamine-supplemental parenteral nutrition.
(Courtesy of Ziegler TR, Bye RL, Persinger RL, et al: Effects of glutamine supplementation on circulating lymphocytes after bone marrow transplantation: A pilot study. *Am J Med Sci* 315:4-10, 1998.)

cyte and lymphocyte counts, and diet protocols. The 2 groups had a similar percentage of patients in whom acute graft-vs.-host disease developed before flow cytometry analysis. Patients in the Gln-PN group had a higher percentage of blood lymphocytes during hospitalization. Flow cytometry showed those who received Gln-PN had an increased total lymphocyte count, greater numbers of total T lymphocytes, and higher CD4+ and CD8+ T-lymphocyte counts in peripheral blood compared with controls. The weekly total leukocyte and lymphocyte counts rose similarly in the 2 groups, as expected, during hospital weeks 2, 3, and 4 (Table 4). Clinical foci of infection were detected in 5 of 11 Std-PN patients but in none of the 9 Gln-PN patients.

Conclusion.—The administration of Gln-PN enhances circulating lymphocyte cell number in adult patients after BMT. No adverse effects of the amino acid were observed. Findings are consistent with previous studies suggesting an important role for Gln in lymphocyte metabolism.

Total Parenteral Nutrition With Glutamine Dipeptide After Major Abdominal Surgery: A Randomized, Double-blind, Controlled Study

Morlion BJ, Stehle P, Wachtler P, et al (Ruhr-Univ of Bochum, Germany; Univ of Bonn, Germany; Univ of Hohenheim, Germany)

Ann Surg 227:302-308, 1998 8–17

Introduction.—Commercially available amino acid solutions do not contain free glutamine (Gln), yet profound intracellular Gln depletion is a typical feature of hypercatabolic states. Recent studies suggest the parenteral provision of Gln benefits surgical patients and shortens hospital stay. A randomized study assessed the efficacy of Gln dipeptide-enriched total parenteral nutrition (TPN) on metabolic, immunologic, and clinical variables in patients undergoing elective abdominal surgery.

Methods.—Study participants were 28 patients with a mean age of 68. All received 5 days of TPN given continuously 24 hours with 0.24 g of nitrogen (isonitrogenous) and 122 kJ/kg daily (isoenergetic) via a central venous catheter. Controls received 1.5 g of amino acids $kg^{-1}day^{-1}$, and the

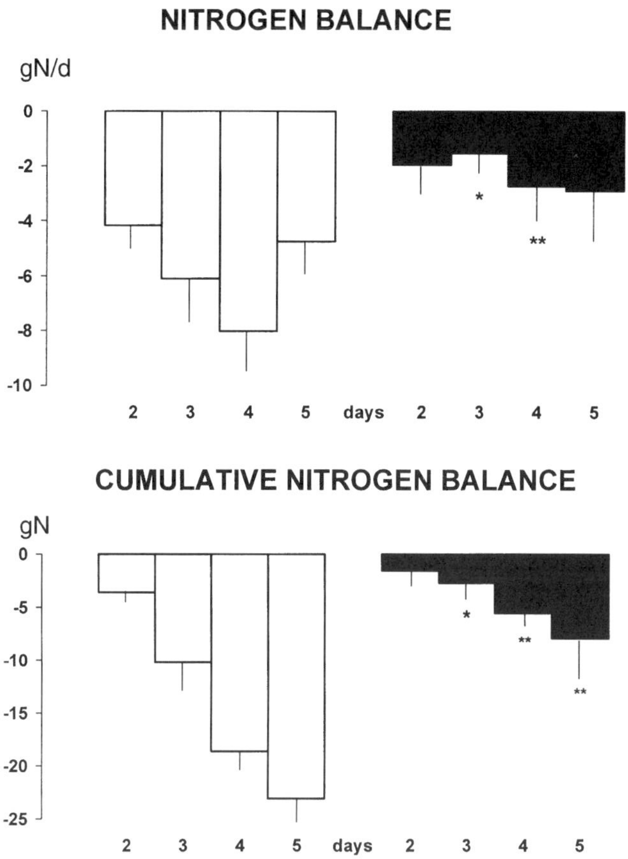

FIGURE 1.—Day-to-day and cumulative nitrogen balance in patients receiving TPN supplemented with L-alanyl-L-glutamine (black columns) or conventional TPN (open columns). Mean ± standard error of the mean, significant between groups; *$p < 0.05$, **$p < 0.01$. *Abbreviation: TPN,* total parenteral nutrition. (Courtesy of Morlion BJ, Stehle P, Wachtler P, et al: Total parenteral nutrition with glutamine dipeptide after major abdominal surgery: A randomized, double-blind, controlled study. *Ann Surg* 227:302-308, 1998.)

Gln group received 1.2 g of amino acids and 0.3 g of L-alanyl-L-glutamine (Ala-Gln) $kg^{-1}day^{-1}$. Urine was collected throughout the study, and venous heparin blood samples were obtained before surgery and on days 1, 3, and 6 after surgery.

Results.—Postoperative recovery was normal in all patients, and the 2 groups had similar plasma protein concentrations and routine clinical biochemical indices. Nitrogen balances on postoperative days 3 and 4 were significantly better in patients receiving Gln dipeptide (Fig 1). The dipeptide-supplemented group had improved nitrogen balances during 5 days, improved lymphocyte recovery on day 6, and improved generation of cysteinyl-leukotrienes from polymorphonuclear neutrophil granulocytes. In addition, the supplemented group had a postoperative hospital stay 6.2 days shorter than the control group.

Conclusion.—Recent clinical studies have shown patients needing nutritional support benefit from feedings enriched with Gln or Gln dipeptides. The outcome of this trial confirms the value of Gln dipeptide-containing TPN for patients experiencing catabolic stress.

Effects of Glutamine Supplements and Radiochemotherapy on Systemic Immune and Gut Barrier Function in Patients With Advanced Esophageal Cancer

Yoshida S, Matsui M, Shirouzu Y, et al (Kurume Univ; St Mary's Hosp)

Ann Surg 227:485-491, 1998 8–18

Introduction.—Patients with advanced esophageal cancer who are treated with neoadjuvant radiochemotherapy experience major side effects including decreases in lymphocyte count, impairment of lymphocyte function secondary to radiation exposure, and the toxicity of anticancer drugs. Experimental studies have found glutamine supplementation enhances immune function and reduces the toxicity of chemotherapy. A randomized study examined the effects of oral glutamine supplements on lymphocyte and gut barrier function in patients undergoing radiochemotherapy for advanced esophageal cancer.

Methods.—Thirteen patients took part in the study: 7 were randomized to glutamine and 6 to a control group. Patient characteristics were similar in the 2 groups, and nutritional status was equivalent. The mean total irradiation dose was 36.0 Gy in the control group and 36.2 in the glutamine group. Chemotherapy consisted of cisplatin and 5-fluorouracil, ad-

TABLE 4.—White Blood Cell, Lymphocyte, T Cell, B-Cell Counts, and Lymphocyte Blast Information

	Group	Pretreatment	Day 7	Day 14	Day 28
WBC	control	6112 ± 874	6798 ± 1541	4143 ± 441	2696 ± 485
($/mm^3$)	glutamine	6974 ± 582	5270 ± 537	4162 ± 446	2852 ± 278
Lymphocyte	control	1383 ± 69	567 ± 96	387 ± 64	420 ± 81
($/mm^3$)	glutamine	1740 ± 169	1007 ± 151*	633 ± 150	551 ± 121
T-cell	control	1117 ± 139	467 ± 80	330 ± 52	393 ± 112
($/mm^3$)	glutamine	1474 ± 172	854 ± 106*	556 ± 127	489 ± 106
B-cell	control	133 ± 32	45 ± 14	28 ± 7	16 ± 6
($/mm^3$)	glutamine	165 ± 43	86 ± 13*	34 ± 12	19 ± 3
PHA (dpm)	control	37424 ± 3305	19478 ± 2121	19284 ± 3848	26836 ± 6959
	glutamine	39012 ± 5638	33860 ± 1433†	30399 ± 2455*	31751 ± 1415
ConA (dpm)	control	31797 ± 3677	19177 ± 1897	16515 ± 2904	25324 ± 4304
	glutamine	35595 ± 3893	29473 ± 2302†	31372 ± 2523†	25810 ± 2167
Standard	control	161 ± 13	187 ± 30	221 ± 64	146 ± 69
(dpm)	glutamine	186 ± 38	165 ± 44	184 ± 31	126 ± 21

White blood cell, lymphocyte, T-cell, B-cell count, and lymphocyte blast formation.
Standard was defined as the baseline formation of lymphocyte blasts without stimulation of the lymphocytes.
*$p < 0.05$ vs. control.
†$p < 0.01$ vs. control.
WBC: white blood cell; *PHA*: phytohemagglutin; *Con A*: concanvalin A; *dpm*: disintegrations per minute.
(Courtesy of Yoshida S, Matsui M, Shirouzu Y, et al: Effects of glutamine supplements and radiochemotherapy on systemic immune and gut barrier function in patients with advanced esophageal cancer. *Ann Surg* 227:485-491, 1998.)

ministered by IV infusion and with similar total doses in the 2 patient groups. Glutamine was given orally (30 g/day) at the start of radiochemotherapy and continued for 28 days.

Results.—Glutamine levels in plasma were decreased in controls 7 days after the start of radiochemotherapy, but this decrease did not occur in glutamine-supplemented patients. The glutamine levels in controls recovered to levels of the glutamine group on day 14, and both groups had similar levels on days 21 and 28. Glutamine supplementation prevented the reduction in lymphocyte count seen in controls on day 7. The 2 groups had similar lymphocyte counts on days 14 and 28. Glutamine supplementation also led to greater T- and B-cell counts on day 7, maintained lymphocyte blast formation stimulated by phytohemagglutinin (Table 4), and reduced phenolsulfonphthalein in the urine on day 7.

Conclusion.—In these patients undergoing radiochemotherapy for advanced esophageal cancer, oral glutamine supplementation protected lymphocytes and attenuated gut permeability. The use of glutamine may improve outcome in these patients.

Randomised Trial of Glutamine-Enriched Enteral Nutrition on Infectious Morbidity in Patients With Multiple Trauma

Houdijk AP, Rijnsburger ER, Jansen J, et al (Free Univ Hosp, Amsterdam; Univ of Amsterdam; Ohio State Univ, Columbus)

Lancet 352:772-776, 1998 8–19

Background.—Glutamine deficiency is common in patients with multiple trauma, as are infections. Studies suggest a role for glutamine in preventing infection. Glutamine supplementation was provided by means of enteral feeding and infectious morbidity in patients with multiple trauma was evaluated.

Methods.—Patients with multiple trauma (Injury Severity Score 20 or higher) who were expected to survive 48 hours or longer were randomly assigned to receive either balanced, isonitrogenous, isocaloric enteral nutrition (3.5 g glutamine/100 g protein; n = 39) or glutamine-supplemented enteral nutrition (30.5 g glutamine/100 g protein; n = 41). Two patients in the control group and 6 in the treatment group were excluded because of death within 48 hours, transfer, HIV infection, or age of 65 or older. Feeding problems and death after 48 hours or more excluded more patients, so that ultimately the control group contained 31 patients who received enteral nutrition for more than 5 days, and the test group contained 29 patients who received enteral feedings for more than 5 days. Every 8 hours, each patients were assessed for the development of pneumonia, sepsis, bacteremia, and other infectious processes.

Findings.—Enteral nutrition was used for 11.9 days in the control group and for 12.8 days in the glutamine-enriched group. Median hospital stays did not differ significantly between the controls (27.4 days) and the glutamine-enriched group (32.0 days), nor did the days on mechanical ventilation (9.0 vs. 7.6 days). There were 2 deaths in each group; 3 patients (2 in the test group, 1 control) died of brain injury and 1 control patient died of pneumonia. Compared with the test group, the controls experienced significantly higher rates of pneumonia (14 of 31, or 45%, vs. 5 of 29, or 17%), bacteremia (13, or 42%, vs. 2, or 7%), and sepsis (8, or 26%, vs. 1, or 3%).

Conclusions.—In these patients with multiple trauma, those receiving enteral feeding with a glutamine-supplemented formula experienced significantly fewer episodes of pneumonia, bacteremia, and sepsis. The mechanism for this protective effect is not known. Whether glutamine-enriched enteral feedings have a significant effect on mortality in these patients remains to be elucidated.

Immunostimulating Effect of Oral Glutamine

Gismondo MR, Drago L, Fassina MC, et al (Univ of Milan, Italy; Bracco SpA, Milan, Italy)

Dig Dis Sci 43:1752-1754, 1998 8–20

Introduction.—L-Glutamine is one of the principal metabolic fuels for all rapidly dividing cells, such as immune system cells. The intestine is one of the main immune organs. Researchers examined the effect of glutamine on the intestinal lymphocytic population (CD3, CD4, CD8), and the seric production of interleukin 2 (IL-2).

Methods.—The 48 female athymic (nude) mice used in the study were divided into 2 groups: 24 (group A) were fed a standard diet and water supplemented with 4% glutamine for 10 days; the remaining 24 mice (group B) served as controls and received a standard diet and water

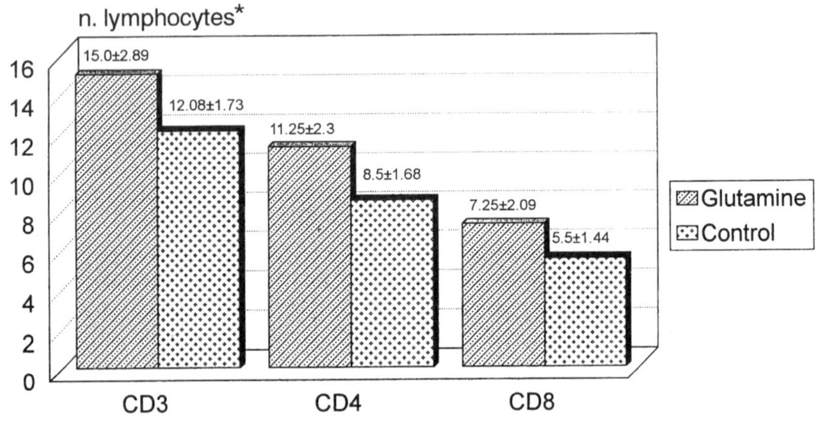

FIGURE 1.—Effect of glutamine on intestinal lymphocyte population in an immunosuppressed mouse model. (Courtesy of Gismondo MR, Drago L, Fassina MC, et al: Immunostimulating effect of oral glutamine. *Dig Dis Sci* 43:1752-1754, 1998. Plenum Publishing Corporation.)

without glutamine supplementation for 10 days. Sections of jejunum and ileum from 12 mice in each group were taken for lymphocyte counts in the mucosa and submucosa. The most representative sections from each animal were taken to count the number of intestinal lymphocytes in 20 different microscope fields. Twelve treated mice and 12 untreated mice were used to evaluate serum levels of IL-2.

Results.—The group treated with glutamine exhibited an increase of each class of intestinal T lymphocytes compared to the control group (Fig 1). The difference between groups A and B was statistically significant. Glutamine-treated animals also had a statistically significant increase in IL-2 serum concentrations compared to controls (mean, 604.24 vs. 104.86 pg/mL, respectively).

Conclusion.—Glutamine, the most abundant amino acid in the bloodstream, plays an important role as nitrogen carrier through the different tissues of the organism. Findings of this study suggest orally administered glutamine positively affects serum levels of IL-2 and the intestinal population of T cells, demonstrating the amino acid's role in the complex mechanisms of the immune system. The immunostimulating activity of oral glutamine could have clinical relevance in cases of trauma, surgery, and starvation.

► It is now clear that diet composition as well as delivery route play an important role in maintaining gut structure and function. In addition, the use of nutritional support in patients has given birth to a new clinical science—nutritional pharmacotherapy, defined as the use of nutrients that have more pharmacological effects than nutrient effects per se. Although several specific nutrients have been studied, glutamine has received the most attention. Historically, glutamine has been classified as a nonessential or nutritionally dispensable amino acid. Since this categorization implies that glutamine can be synthesized in adequate quantities from other amino acids and precursors, it has not been considered necessary to include glutamine in nutritional formulas. It has been eliminated from total parenteral nutrition solutions because of its relative instability and short shelf-life compared to other amino acids. With few exceptions, glutamine is in oral and enteral diets only

TABLE.—Most Important Clinical Trials Evaluating the Use of Supplemental Glutamine

Study Group/Diagnosis	Glutamine Dose/Route	Effects of Glutamine
Bone marrow transplant[1]	0.57 gm/kg/day IV	Improved nitrogen balance Decrease in clinical infections Reduction in hospital stay by 7 days
Patients with GI dysfunction[2]	0.23 gm/kg/day IV	Decrease in intestinal permeability Increase in villus height
Very low birth weight infants[3]	0.31 gm/kg/day enterally	Lower incidence of infection Shorter time to achieve full enteral feeds Reduced length of hospital stay
Intensive care patients[4]	25 gms/day IV	Improved survival at 6 months Cost savings for hospital
Short gut patients[5]	Glutamine + growth hormone + modified diet	Increased nutrient absorption by the gut Diminished the need for TPN

at the relatively low levels characteristic of its concentration in most animal and plant proteins (about 7% of total amino acids). Several studies (see Table), besides the ones reviewed (Abstracts 8–16 to 8–20) have demonstrated glutamine may be a conditionally essential amino acid during catabolic states.

W.W. Souba, M.D., Sc.D.

References

1. Ziegler TR, Young LS, Benfell KB, et al: Clinical and metabolic efficacy of glutamine-supplemented parenteral nutrition after bone marrow transplantation. *Ann Int Med* 116:821-828, 1992.
2. Van Der Hulst, RRWJ, Van Kreel, BK, Von Meyenfield MF, et al: Glutamine and the preservation of gut integrity. *Lancet* 341: 1363-1365, 1993.
3. Lacey JM, Crouch JB, Benfell K, et al: The effects of glutamine-supplemented parenteral nutrition in premature infants. *JPEN* 20:74-80, 1996.
4. Griffiths RD, Jones C, Palmer TE: Six-month outcome of critically ill patients given glutamine-supplemented parenteral nutrition. *Nutrition* 13: 295, 1997.
5. Byrne TA, Persinger RL, Young LS, et al: A new treatment for patients with short-bowel syndrome. Growth hormone, glutamine, and a modified diet. *Ann Surg* 222:243-54, 1995.

Small Volumes of Enteral Feedings Normalise Immune Function in Infants Receiving Parenteral Nutrition

Okada Y, Klein N, van Saene HKF, et al (Univ of College London; Royal Children's Hosp of Alder Hey, Liverpool, England)

J Pediatr Surg 33:16-19, 1998 8–21

Introduction.—Total parenteral nutrition (PN) can improve the survival rate of newborn infants, but prolonged duration of total PN increases the risk of infection. Researchers tested the hypothesis that the addition of small enteral feedings during PN would improve the bactericidal activity of newborn infants.

Methods.—Study subjects were 10 infants younger than 6 months who required PN for postoperative gut dysfunction and 9 control infants receiving normal enteral diet. The infants were studied after a mean of 31.1 days of PN with no enteral feeding (total PN) and after a mean of 4.7 days from the addition of small volumes of enteral feeding to PN. Controls had no gastrointestinal anomalies, were not receiving antibiotics, and were studied before minor operations. An *in vitro* whole blood model was used to measure host bactericidal activity against coagulase-negative staphylococci (CNS). Bacterial killing was calculated after a 45-minute bacterial challenge using the Miles-Misra technique. After 2 hours of bacterial challenge, tumor necrosis factor-α (TNF-α) was measured by enzyme-linked immunosorbent assay.

Results.—Patients on PN differed from controls in having smaller body weight, a result of their impaired nutritional status. And as a consequence of PN-related liver dysfunction, infants on PN had higher levels of serum

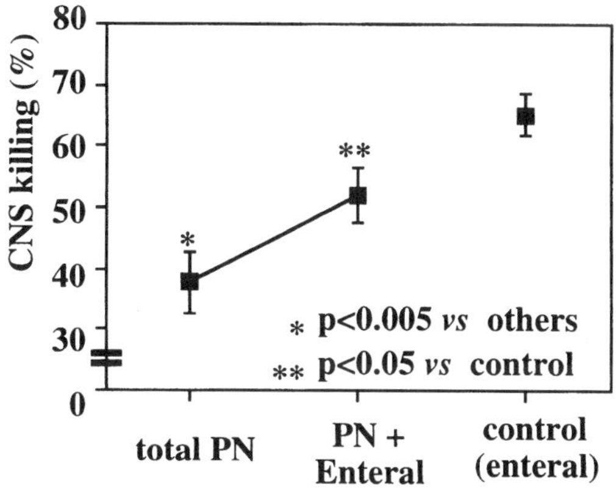

FIGURE 1.—Bactericidal activity against CNS (CNS killing). Data are expressed as mean ± SEM. *Abbreviation: CNS*, coagulase-negative staphylococci. (Courtesy of Okada Y, Klein N, van Saene HKF, et al: Small volumes of enteral feedings normalise immune function in infants receiving parenteral nutrition. *J Pediatr Surg* 33:16-19, 1998.)

total bilirubin and serum alkaline phosphatase than control infants. The lowest levels of CNS killing were observed in infants receiving total PN with no enteral feeding (Fig 1). With the addition of small enteral feedings, CNS killing increased significantly and almost approached the values in normal controls. During total PN, TNF-α production was lower in patients than in controls; TNF-α production was normalized when a small enteral feeding was added to the PN diet.

Conclusion.—Infants receiving PN are at high risk of infection, and there is a significant correlation between duration of total PN and impaired bactericidal activity. The introduction of small volumes of enteral feed can prevent these problems. Thus, stimulation of the gastrointestinal tract may produce beneficial effects on immune status and help to reduce the risk of infectious complications.

Nutritional Support and Infection: Does the Route Matter?

Minard G, Kudsk KA (Univ of Tennessee, Memphis)

World J Surg 22:213-219, 1998 8–22

Introduction.—Total parenteral nutrition (TPN), introduced in 1968, has become the preferred route of nutritional support for many patients. Although a life-saving option for those with severe inflammatory bowel disease, short gut syndrome, and other diseases, TPN may not benefit other patient populations. The enteral route of nutrition has a number of advantages over TPN, including cost, safety, and support of the gut and immune system. Researchers compared the enteral and parenteral routes.

Early Studies.—A 1980 study of patients in a pediatric burn unit suggested the benefit of enteral nutrition on immune function. Patients receiving a high-protein enteral formula had fewer days of bacteremia and days on systemic antibiotics. The survival rate was lower in controls (56% vs. 100%), and all deaths were attributed to infection. Most of the nutrition in study patients was provided via the enteral rather than the parenteral route. In a study of rats given an intraperitoneal *Escherichia coli*-hemoglobin adjuvant injection, 48-hour survival was 60% in the enteral group and 20% in the parenteral group.

Studies of Infection.—Most clinical evidence comparing early enteral feeding with parenteral nutrition has come from studies of patients undergoing celiotomy for abdominal trauma. Results have generally shown a decrease in infectious complications with the use of early enteral nutrition. Results have been inconsistent, however, from enteral feeding studies of patients with severe head injury. A recent area of interest has been the importance of enteral diet composition. "Immune-enhancing" components apparently reduce the infection rates.

Rationale for the Benefit of the Enteral Route.—One hypothesis to explain the increased infection rate in parenterally fed patients is that IV nutrition induces immunosuppression. But the mechanisms through which patients are put at risk for pneumonia and intra-abdominal abscess after trauma or elective surgical procedures are more important than whether TPN is immunosuppressive. Metabolic and immunologic deterioration of the gut barrier may occur in conditions such as infection, chemotherapy, and TPN. The use of enteral versus parenteral nutrition may decrease the permeability of the gut. In addition, enteral nutrition may affect intestinal immunoglobulin.

Discussion.—It is clear that enteral feeding improves the clinical outcome of critically ill and injured patients. Intravenous nutrition, associated with an increased risk of infection, apparently blunts the immunologic response within the intraperitoneal cavity.

Enteral Nutrition Is Superior to Parenteral Nutrition in Severe Acute Pancreatitis: Results of a Randomized Prospective Trial

Kalfarentzos F, Kehagias J, Mead N, et al (Univ of Patras, Greece)

Br J Surg 84:1665-1669, 1997 8–23

Introduction.—The provision of early aggressive nutritional support is of greatest importance in severe acute pancreatitis. Total parenteral nutrition (TPN) is administered to improve nutritional status and avoid pancreatic stimulation. Because TPN is associated with certain disadvantages, including metabolic and electrolyte disturbances, this study evaluated enteral feeding (EF) for its use in severe acute pancreatitis.

Methods.—The efficacy, tolerance, clinical outcome, and cost of EF was compared with that of TPN in a group of 38 patients. All had severe necrotizing pancreatitis. Eighteen patients received EF through a nasoenteric tube with a semi-elemental diet, and 20 were administered TPN through a central venous catheter. The success of nutritional support was determined by nitrogen balance, calculated by subtracting nitrogen losses

TABLE 3.—Patient Morbidity

	Enteral Feeding (n = 18)	Total Parenteral Nutrition (n = 20)
Artificial nutrition-related complications		
No. of patients with catheter-related sepsis	0	2
No. of patients with hyperglycaemia > 200 mg/dl	4	9
Pancreatitis-related complications		
No. of patients with infected pancreatic or peripancreatic necrosis	1	4
No. of patients with abscess formation	1	0
No. of patients with acute pseudocysts	0	1
No. of patients with pancreatic fistula	0	2
Non-pancreatitis-related complications		
Blood culture-positive sepsis	1	3
Urinary tract infection	1	2
Pneumonia/ARDS	2	4
Total no. of patients with septic complications	5 (6)	10* (15)
Total no. of patients with any complication	8 (10)	15† (27)

Abbreviation: ARDS, adult respiratory distress syndrome.
Values in parentheses are total number of complications.
*P <0.01.
† <0.05 (Kruskal-Wallis test)
(Courtesy of Kalfarentzos F, Kehagias J, Mead N, et al: Enteral nutrition is superior to parenteral nutrition in severe acute pancreatitis: Results of a randomized prospective trial. *Br J Surg* 84:1665-1669, 1997. Blackwell Science Ltd.)

plus an estimated stool and obligatory nitrogen loss of 2 g from the total nitrogen administered during a 24-hour period.

Results.—Both enteral and parenteral nutrition were well tolerated. The 2 groups did not differ significantly in ICU support, use of antibiotics, days on artificial nutritional support, and hospital stay. Nitrogen balance was comparable in the 2 groups during the course of the study and improved progressively in both with nutritional support. Compared with those receiving TPN, patients in the EF group had fewer total complications and were at lower risk of septic complications (Table 3). Total parenteral nutrition cost 3 times as much as enteral nutrition, and the cost difference was even greater when the increased rate of complications with TPN was considered.

Conclusion.—Enteral feeding and TPN were comparable in efficacy when administered to patients with acute severe pancreatitis, but EF was associated with significantly fewer complications and cost much less than TPN. The enteral route is recommended for nutrition support in this clinical setting.

▶ Recommendations for using enteral nutrition have become less rigid through the years. Who would have thought 10 years ago that tube feedings would be feasible in patients with severe acute pancreatitis? The difficulty is often not the administration of nutrients, but rather gastrointestinal access. We probably should use the combination of enteral and parenteral nutrition more than we do. I suspect some surgeons discontinue the use of tube feedings if they can't advance the rate above 40 or 50 mL/per hour. Instead, we should probably add one liter of TPN each day.

TABLE.—Key Clinical Trials Evaluating the Use of Nutrition Support in Trauma Patients

Study/Author	Study Group	Conclusions
Moore et al.[1]	Major blunt or penetrating trauma	Early enteral nutrition is superior to parenteral nutrition in reducing major septic morbidity.
Alexander et al.[2]	Children with burns	Patients receiving a high nitrogen enteral diet have better hepatic synthetic function, fewer days of bacteremia, and higher rates of survival than similar children receiving a normal diet.
Kudsk et al.[3]	Major blunt or penetrating trauma	Early enteral nutrition is superior to parenteral nutrition in reducing major post-injury septic complications, such as pneumonia and sepsis.
Moore et al.[4]	Meta-analysis	Early enteral nutrition is superior to parenteral nutrition in reducing major post-trauma septic complications.
Grahm et al.[5]	Head injury patients	Enteral nutrition is equivalent or superior to parenteral nutrition when nutrient intake is controlled.
Norton et al.[5]	Head injury patients	Patients with severe head injury are candidates for parenteral nutrition if they cannot tolerate enteral nutrition because of ileus or a high risk of aspiration.

The recommendation that to use the enteral route preferentially for nutritional support is based on cost data and on studies mainly in injured patients who demonstrate the superiority of enteral over parenteral nutrition (see Table).

W.W. Souba, M.D., Sc.D.

References

1. Moore F, Moore E, Jones T, et al: TEN versus TPN following major abdominal trauma—reduced septic morbidity. *J Trauma* 29: 916-923, 1989.
2. Alexander J, MacMillan B, Stinnett J, et al: Beneficial effects of aggressive protein feeding in severely burned children. *Ann Surg* 192: 505-517, 1980.
3. Kudsk K, Croce M, Fabian T, et al: Enteral versus parenteral feeding: Effects on septic morbidity following blunt and penetrating abdominal trauma. *Ann Surg* 215: 503-513, 1992.
4. Moore F, Feliciano D, Andrassy R, et al: Early enteral feeding, compared with parenteral, reduces postoperative septic complications: The results of a meta-analysis. *Ann Surg* 216: 172-183, 1992.
5. Grahm T, Zadrosny D, Harrington T: The benefits of early jejunal hyperalimentation in the head injured patient. *Neurosurgery* 19: 367-373, 1986.
6. Norton JA, Ott LG, McClain C, et al: Intolerance to enteral feeding in the brain-injured patient. *J Neurosurg* 68: 62-66, 1988.

Clinical Impact of Abnormal Gut Flora in Infants Receiving Parenteral Nutrition

Pierro A, van Saene HKF, Jones MO, et al (Inst of Child Health, London; Univ of Liverpool, England)
Ann Surg 227:547-552, 1998 8–24

Introduction.—Surveillance cultures of the throat and gut are recommended means of identifying neonates at high risk of infection. They have a low positive predictive value, however, and are considered labor inten-

TABLE 4.—Sepsis and Septicemia During Parenteral Nutrition

	Abnormal Flora (n = 41)	Normal Flora (n = 53)	p
Total days at risk*	2,676	617	
Sepsis			
Patients	12 (29%)	3 (6%)	0.005
Episodes	40	3	
Rate of septic episodes (episodes/day)†	0.015	0.005	0.028
Septicemia			
Patients	9 (22%)	1 (2%)	0.005
Episodes	23	1	
Rate of septicemic episodes (episodes/day)†	0.009	0.002	0.045

*Days at risk of sepsis and septicemia = number of days on parenteral nutrition.
†Rate of septic or septicemic episodes = number of episodes divided by the number of days at risk.
(Courtesy of Pierro A, van Saene HKF, Jones MO, et al: Clinical impact of abnormal gut flora in infants receiving parenteral nutrition. *Ann Surg* 227:547-552, 1998.)

sive and expensive. Because infection rates during parenteral nutrition (PN) in infancy can be high, investigators sought to determine whether carriage of abnormal flora is associated with a prolonged duration of PN and an increased incidence of sepsis and septicemia.

Methods.—The prospective study enrolled 94 infants from February 1992 through January 1994. All were receiving PN, started at a mean of 4 days after delivery because of anomalies of the gastrointestinal tract. Eighty-six infants received PN through a central venous line and 8 through a peripheral line. Parenteral nutrition was prepared under strict aseptic conditions and checked regularly for sterility. Throat and rectal swabs were taken on day 1 of PN, then twice weekly.

Results.—Abnormal flora were detected in 41 (44%) of the infants; the remaining 53 infants stayed free of abnormal microorganisms. The abnormal and normal flora groups were similar in gestational age, birth weight, sex ratio, number of operations, use of central venous catheters, and indications for PN. Mean duration of PN was significantly longer in the abnormal group (30 days) than in the normal group (9 days). Infants carrying abnormal bacteria had a significantly higher rate of sepsis and septicemia and of septic and septicemic episodes than those with normal flora (Table 4). Among infants with abnormal flora, *Pseudomonas* and *Enterobacter spp* predominated. The abnormal carrier state occurred after a median of 14 days from starting PN. Sepsis developed after a median of 27 days and septicemia after a median of 39 days.

Conclusion.—Neonates who are receiving long-term PN should have surveillance cultures of the throat and rectum at least once a week. This practice can identify those with abnormal flora, a subset with a high risk of infection. The incidence of both sepsis and septicemia is negligible in infants with normal flora while on PN.

Introduction of Enteral Feeding in Neonates on Extracorporeal Membrane Oxygenation After Evaluation of Intestinal Permeability Changes

Piena M, Albers MJIJ, Van Haard PMM, et al (Univ Hosp, Rotterdam, The Netherlands; Diagnostic Centre SSDZ, Delft, The Netherlands)
J Pediatr Surg 33:30-34, 1998 8–25

Background.—Venoarterial extracorporeal membrane oxygenation (VA-ECMO) is used to provide neonates with partial heart–lung bypass for life-threatening, reversible cardiopulmonary failure. Enteral nutrition is often withheld from these patients receiving ECMO. Intestinal integrity and the effect of minimal enteral nutrition was evaluated in patients receiving ECMO using the sugar absorption test (SAT).

Methods.—From January 1996 to February 1997, 16 neonates were admitted to Sophia Children's Hospital in Rotterdam, The Netherlands, for ECMO therapy. In 7 of these patients, enteral feeding was initiated between the third and ninth day of ECMO. SAT was performed on the first urine specimen collected and was repeated every other day.

Results.—Of the 16 patients in the study group, 13 had increased lactulose/L-rhamnose ratios consistent with increased intestinal permeability. D-xylose excretion percentages were normal in 11 patients. 3-O-methyl-D-glucose excretion percentages were decreased in 15 of 16 patients. The introduction of enteral nutrition did not result in significant changes to any of these parameters in any of the patients receiving ECMO.

Conclusions.—Intestinal integrity was compromised in the majority of neonates receiving ECMO therapy, as assessed by the SAT. Introduction of enteral feeding did not cause a further deterioration of intestinal integrity. This study does not provide support for the practice of withholding enteral nutrition in critically ill neonates receiving ECMO therapy.

Prospective, Randomized Trial on the Effect of Cyclic Versus Continuous Enteral Nutrition on Postoperative Gastric Function After Pylorus-preserving Pancreatoduodenectomy

van Berge Henegouwen MI, Akkermans LMA, van Gulik TM, et al (Univ of Amsterdam; Univ of Utrecht, The Netherlands; Univ of Leiden, The Netherlands)
Ann Surg 226:677-687, 1997 8–26

Introduction.—Delayed gastric emptying after pancreatoduodenectomy has been attributed to a number of pathophysiologic mechanisms. Another potential contributor to this complication is the administration of continuous enteral nutrition through a needle catheter jejunostomy. The infusion of nutrients causes a delay in gastric emptying through activation of gastroduodenal feedback mechanisms. Researchers hypothesized that administering enteral nutrition in a cyclic pattern could suppress this mechanism.

TABLE 5.—Parameters for Gastric Function and Incidence of DGE in All Patients (n=57)

	Continuous Enteral Nutrition (n = 30)			Cyclic Enteral Nutrition (n = 27)			
	Median	Mean	Range	Median	Mean	Range	p
Nasogastric intubation (days)	5.5	9.1	1-65	4	6.7	1-25	0.82
Enteral nutrition (days)	9	10.3	1-28	8	9.3	0-27	0.60
First day of normal diet	11	15.7	5-68	9	12.2	5-38	0.04
Hospital stay (days)	17	21.4	9-73	14	17.5	10-46	0.04
Number of patients with DGE		7 (23%)			7 (26%)		0.82

DGE = delayed gastric emptying; defined as gastric stasis, requiring nasogastric intubation for 10 days or more, or the inability to tolerate a regular (solid) diet on or before the 14th postoperative day.

(Courtesy of van Berge Henegouwen MI, Akkermans LMA, van Gulik TM, et al: Prospective, randomized trial on the effect of cyclic versus continuous enteral nutrition on postoperative gastric function after pylorus-preserving pancreatoduodenectomy. *Ann Surg* 226:677-687, 1997.)

Methods.—Patients enrolled in the study underwent pylorous-preserving pancreatoduodenectomy (PPPD) from September 1995 to December 1996. Fifteen of 72 patients operated or during this period did not meet study criteria, leaving 57 for inclusion. All patients received a needle catheter jejunostomy at the end of the operation for postoperative nutritional support. Enteral nutrition was started on the first postoperative day, with 30 patients randomized to continuous enteral nutrition (CON) and 27 to cyclic enteral nutrition (CYC). The 2 groups were compared for the incidence of delayed gastric emptying, days of nasogastric intubation and jejunal catheter feeding, days until normal diet, and hospital stay.

Results.—The median age of the entire study group was 64. The 2 treatment groups were similar in patient characteristics, preoperative laboratory factors, and histopathologic diagnosis. No differences were found between CON and CYC groups in number of days of nasogastric intubation, days of enteral nutrition, or incidence of delayed gastric emptying (25% overall). Both the number of days until normal diet and hospital stay were shorter for CYC patients (Table 5). Compared with CON patients, plasma cholecystokinin levels were lower in CYC patients both before and after feeding.

Conclusion.—In these patients who had undergone PPPD, cyclic enteral feeding was associated with a more rapid return to a normal diet and a shorter hospital stay compared to continuous enteral feeding. These effects are probably partly from an inhibition of humoral (CCK-mediated) feedback mechanisms.

► In adults as well as children, the clinical significance of abnormal gut flora is not fully understood. It is well established, however, that the simplest and best way to maintain normal gut ecology is to feed via the gastrointestinal tract. Numerous studies, primarily in animals, demonstrate that enteral nutrition increases gut mucosal mass, brush border enzyme activity, barrier integrity, and intestinal immune surveillance. Total parenteral nutrition, on the other hand, leads to a reduction in these indices. While healthy patients may tolerate long-term TPN reasonably well, a superimposed insult, such as a septic event, may result in deleterious consequences.

Despite its benefits, enteral nutrition is not used in all eligible patients with a functional gut. Gastric retention, diarrhea, and abdominal distention can limit the physician's willingness to use enteral feeding. The feeding route is more important than the nutrition amount provided, and the outcome correlates with the enteral protein intake in the injured patient. Thus, even if luminal nutrition cannot meet the patient's calorie and nitrogen requirements, the enteral feeding route should be used unless contraindicated (for example, by bowel obstruction, intractable diarrhea, an inadequate bowel surface area, or feeding intolerance). As discussed earlier, the enteral and parenteral routes may be used simultaneously to meet nutritional requirements.

W.W. Souba, M.D., Sc.D.

9 Growth Factors and Wound Healing

Introduction

The body's response to many surgical diseases is profound, frequently necessitating hospitalization and a relatively long period of care. Because of the morbidity, mortality, and costs associated with such critical diseases, a variety of therapeutic strategies have been proposed to modify the catabolic process. The intent of these therapies is to diminish the magnitude of the stress response or improve the body's ability to respond to the stress state.

One approach that appeared to have promise in its infancy was the use of cytokine antagonists to modify the production of cytokines after injury or inflammation. This research, which has principally focused on the use of cytokine monoclonal antibodies, has not been successful to date in the clinical arena. A second approach has been to enhance anabolism and immune function through the provision of specific nutrients. In this field, several nutrients have been studied, namely glutamine, arginine, nucleic acids, and specific fatty acids. Further research is needed in this area.

A third approach has been the attempt to enhance anabolism through the administration of anabolic agents or growth factors. The present explosion in biotechnology capabilities has allowed, for the first time, the production of growth factors in large quantities. Before the genetics revolution, these peptides could only be isolated in small amounts—quantities that were prohibitive to the conduct of clinical studies. Today, these compounds can be synthesized in megadoses by genetically engineered "smart bacteria."

The role of growth factors in wound healing and in the general field of modifying the catabolic response continues to be an active area of research and a field with tremendous commercial potential. Because wound complications are a major cause of morbidity, mortality, and prolonged hospitalizations, any therapy that could prevent wound complications or speed the healing of wounds has the potential to reduce costs by decreasing length of hospital stay or accelerating recovery.

A variety of cell types are involved in wound healing, including platelets, macrophages, endothelial cells, and fibroblasts, and their role is attributable in large part to their ability to release growth factors. Growth factors can be categorized as a subclass of cytokines that specifically stimulate the migration and proliferation of cells and the synthesis of new tissues. Growth factors are involved in all three phases of wound healing (inflammation, proliferation, remodeling) and also have the ability to regulate many other functions within the cell, including protein synthesis. Growth factors are essential to wound healing, and their roles include: (1) attracting cells (e.g., macrophages, which occupy a key position in immune function) to wound environment; (2) regulating the synthesis of collagen and connective tissue; (3) angiogenesis; (4) tissue remodeling.

Surgeons are well aware of the risk factors associated with impaired wound healing (smoking, diabetes, anemia, steroids, obesity, radiation, chemotherapy, and malnutrition). Growth factors have the potential for accelerating wound repair as they participate in the regulation of cell growth. They should be viewed as the next major advance in caring for the catabolic patient. To date, numerous studies have demonstrated the ability of growth factors to favorably alter the biochemical indices of wound healing and anabolism. Unfortunately, their impact on more meaningful end points has been more difficult to establish. Benefit from these agents must be directly translated into improvements in clinical outcome if these compounds are to be accepted in widespread practice. Thus, the development of carefully designed protocols must occur in order to determine desirable end points to evaluate the real benefits of these agents.

Willey W. Souba, M.D., Sc.D.

Basic Research With Clinical Applicability

Hypoxia Increases Human Keratinocyte Motility on Connective Tissue

O'Toole EA, Marinkovich MP, Peavey CL, et al (Northwestern Univ, Chicago; Stanford Univ, Calif)

J Clin Invest 100:2881-2891, 1997 9–1

Objective.—Healing of skin wounds depends on the migration of keratinocytes from the wound margins, resulting in re-epithelialization. This migration process is enhanced in a hypoxic environment. Keratinocyte motility was measured in response to extracellular matrix and growth factors to examine the effect of hypoxia on human keratinocyte migration over connective tissue components.

Methods.—Human keratinocytes were cultured in a low (0.2% or 2%) and normal (9% or 20%) oxygen environment. Keratinocyte migration was assessed under both conditions. Relative expression of the lamellipodia-associated proteins—ezrin, radixin, and moesin—was determined by means of Western immunoblot analysis. Levels of laminin-5, a keratinocyte motility inhibitor, were determined using immunofluorescence. The profile of cell-surface integrins was determined by means of fluorescent-activated cell sorting analysis. Expression of 92-kd type IV collagenase was analyzed with zymography and immunoblotting, and band intensity was measured with densitometry.

Results.—Keratinocyte migration increased 1.5 to 2.0 times, and expression of the lamellipodia-associated proteins was enhanced in a hypoxic environment compared with normoxic conditions. Production of laminin-5 was decreased under hypoxic but not normoxic conditions. Under hypoxic conditions, the mean track length of motile keratinocytes increased by approximately 40% compared with identical cells migrating under normoxic conditions. The profile of cell-surface integrins was unchanged. Hypoxia did not affect protein synthesis but did induce increased expression of 92-kd type IV collagenase.

Conclusion.—Under hypoxic conditions, keratinocyte migration may be initiated by promoting lamellipodia formation, enhancing collagenase expression, or inhibiting production of laminin-5.

Keratinocyte Growth Factor Promotes Healing of Left-sided Colon Anastomoses

Egger B, Tolmos J, Procaccino F, et al (Harbor-Univ of Calif Los Angeles, Torrance; Amgen Inc, Thousand Oaks, Calif; Univ of Bern, Switzerland)

Am J Surg 176:18-24, 1998 9–2

Introduction.—Leakage from the colonic anastomosis is a significant cause of morbidity and mortality after colorectal surgery. Experimental models show the systemic application of keratinocyte growth factor (KGF) promotes mucosal healing. Other studies suggest KGF may act by accelerating host reparative processes, inducing potent protective mechanisms;

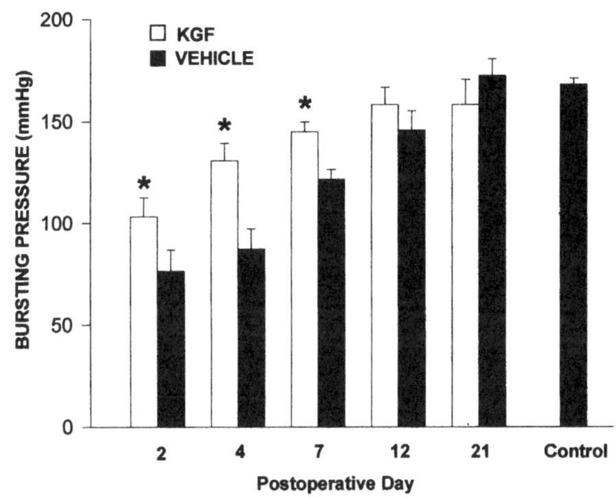

FIGURE 3.—Bursting pressure (mm Hg) of left-sided colonic anastomosis in keratinocyte growth factor (KGF)-treated and vehicle-treated animals. Bursting pressure of colonic anastomosis was significantly higher on postoperative day 2, 4, and 7 in KGF-treated (□) rats compared with vehicle-treated (■) animals. Bursting pressure measured on day 12 and 21 was not at the anastomotic site. (Courtesy of Egger B, Tolmos J, Procaccino F, et al: Keratinocyte growth factor promotes healing of left-sided colon anastomoses. *Am J Surg* 176:18-24. Copyright 1998, with permission from Excerpta Medica Inc.)

or both. This study examined in a rat model the reparative effect of exogenous KGF on healing of colonic anastomotic wounds.

Methods.—Sixty animals were divided into 2 surgical groups of 30 each for colonic anastomoses and 8 served as nonsurgical controls. The rats underwent laparotomy, division of the left colon, and sigmoido-sigmoidostomy. Vehicle or KGF (5 mg/kg) were administered intraperitoneally 12 hours before surgery, then once daily until sacrifice at periods ranging from 2 to 21 days after surgery.

Results.—All animals survived the surgical intervention and lived until sacrificed. The administration of KGF significantly increased anastomotic bursting pressure by 34% on postoperative day 2, by 49% on day 4, and by 19% on day 7 (Fig 3). When compared with vehicle-treated animals, those treated with KGF showed a thickening of the mucosal layer throughout the entire colon, an indirect sign of the induction of epithelial proliferation.

Conclusion.—Exogenous KGF significantly improves and promotes the healing of colonic anastomoses. Treatment with KGF may particularly benefit patients at greatest risk for the complication of anastomotic leakage, those with diabetes and those requiring steroid therapy.

▶ The observation that hypoxic conditions favor wound healing may seem counterintuitive. However, human keratinocytes migrating on connective tissue matrices exhibit accelerated motility when subjected to a low oxygen environment. This determination agrees with the fact that keratinocytes at the margins of skin wounds are in a hypoxic climate. The mechanism by which hypoxia stimulates keratinocyte migration is unclear, and its role in stimulating the elaboration of KGF requires further study. Interestingly, impaired wound healing in diabetic rats and in rodents treated with steroids is associated with decreased expression of KGF. The relationship between these findings and tissue oxygenation also needs additional investigation.

W.W. Souba, M.D., Sc.D.

Metalloproteinase Inhibitors and Wound Healing: A Novel Enhancer of Wound Strength

Witte MB, Thornton FJ, Kiyama T, et al (Johns Hopkins Med Institutions, Baltimore, Md; Univ of Florida, Gainesville)

Surgery 124:464-470, 1998 — 9–3

Introduction.—The strength of a wound depends on the amount and quality of newly synthesized and deposited collagen and on the degradation of preformed collagen. The role of collagen breakdown in wound healing is not fully understood. Researchers hypothesized that inhibition of collagenase activity would improve wound healing by enhancing wound collagen deposition.

Methods.—The role of collagenases (metalloproteinases [MMPs]) in wound healing was investigated using GM6001, a novel inhibitor of

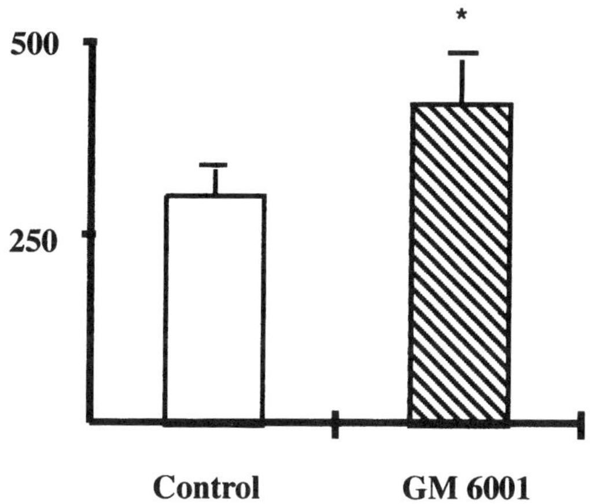

FIGURE 1.—The effect of GM6001 treatment on wound fresh breaking strength. Values are mean ± SEM in grams. **P* < .05 by Student's *t* test. (Courtesy of Witte MB, Thornton FJ, Kiyama T, et al: Metalloproteinase inhibitors and wound healing: A novel enhancer of wound strength. *Surgery* 124:464-470, 1998).

MMPs. Twenty male Sprague-Dawley rats were randomized to either GM6001 (100 mg/kg body weight) or 2 mL saline subcutaneously. The dorsal skin incision model with implantation of polyvinyl alcohol sponges was used. Animals were killed 10 days after the operation and examined for fresh wound breaking strength, scar and sponge hydroxyproline content, and collagen type I gene expression in sponges. Also investigated were the inflammatory response and the wound fluid cytokine (tumor necrosis factor-α [TNF-α] and transforming growth factor-β1 [TGF-β1]) profile.

Results.—Administration of GM6001 versus vehicle (mean 422 vs. 302 g) significantly increased wound strength. Scar collagen content did not differ between the 2 groups. The fresh wound breaking strength was significantly higher in the GM6001 group (Fig 1) compared to controls. Use of GM6001 significantly decreased the inflammatory infiltrate, the collagen content, and the collagen type I gene expression in the sponge granulomas.

Conclusion.—These experiments represent the first effort to examine the effect of MMP inhibition on wound healing. Mechanical strength was enhanced in incised wounds, without an increase in collagen deposition, and overall granulation tissue formation was reduced in sponge granuloma wounds. Findings suggest MMP inhibitors might play a significant role in clinical wound healing.

Reversal of Impaired Wound Repair in iNOS-deficient Mice by Topical Adenoviral-mediated iNOS Gene Transfer

Yamasaki K, Edington HDJ, McClosky C, et al (Univ of Pittsburgh, Pa; GenVec Inc, Rockville, Md)

J Clin Invest 101:967-971, 1998 9–4

Background.—Nitric oxide (NO) is believed to take part in the normal process of wound repair. The inflammatory component of wound healing suggests that cytokine-inducible, or inflammatory, nitric oxide synthase (iNOS) may play a role. However, the nature of the role played by this isoform remains unclear. The effects of iNOS on the rate of excisional wound closure were studied in mice with targeted disruption of the iNOS gene.

Methods.—Healing of dorsal excisional wounds was compared in iNOS knockout mice vs. wild-type mice. Also studied were wild-type mice receiving continuous infusion of N^6-(iminoethyl)-L-lysine. A reverse transcription polymerase chain reaction assay was used to stay expression of iNOS mRNA after wound healing.

Results.—The iNOS knockout mice showed a 31% delay in wound closure, compared with wild-type mice. This delay was prevented when iNOS knockout mice were given a single application of an adenoviral vector containing human iNOS cDNA (AdiNOS) at the time of wounding. Wild-type mice receiving the iNOS inhibitor showed a wound-healing delay similar to that of the iNOS knockout mice. In wild-type mice, peak iNOS mRNA expression occurred 4 to 6 days after wounding. The plasma clearance rate (PCR) studies also demonstrated the expression of human iNOS in animals treated with AdiNOS.

Conclusions.—The findings confirm the role of iNOS in wound healing, with peak levels observed 4 to 6 days after wounding. Inducible NO production appears to accelerate wound healing by several possible mechanisms. The study opens the way to gene transfer techniques using iNOS as a new approach to promoting wound repair by increasing wound NO levels.

▶ As our knowledge of the biology of wound healing increases, the complexity of the diverse events involved in the process becomes more evident. These two papers point to the role of metalloproteinases (MMPs) and iNOS as key actors in the drama of wound repair. MMPs, a family of proteins of which collagenases are members, break down collagen as part of wound remodeling. The observation that inhibition of MMP activity enhances wound healing even though new collagen synthesis is diminished suggests that simultaneously collagen turnover is decreased or collagen maturation (or crosslinking) is increased. iNOS-deficient states, such as diabetes, and steroid treatment are also associated with impaired wound healing. Increased NO production from upregulation of iNOS expression could promote wound healing by stimulating angiogenesis, collagen synthesis, or both.

W.W. Souba, M.D., Sc.D.

Tissue Markers As Predictors of Postoperative Adhesions
Ivarsson M-L, Bergström M, Eriksson E, et al (Göteborg Univ, Sweden)
Br J Surg 85:1549-1554, 1998 9–5

Introduction.—Postoperative adhesions, the main cause of small bowel obstruction, remain an unsolved surgical problem. The formation of postoperative adhesions has been associated with a decreased capacity to degrade intra-abdominally deposited fibrin. Researchers sought to determine if adhesion tissue has reduced plasminogen activation compared with peritoneum, and whether patients in whom extensive adhesions develop have reduced peritoneal plasminogen activation compared with others.

Methods.—Study participants were 12 women and 9 men with a mean age of 66. All were scheduled for abdominal surgery and had previously undergone abdominal surgery. Indications for the present surgery were mainly colonic and gastric resections. Peritoneal biopsies were taken and previously formed adhesion tissue was sampled from 10 of the patients. Adhesion formation was scored into 3 different categories (0, I, and II) based on their quantity, quality, and extent in relation to previous surgery. The fibrinolytic capacity of peritoneum was determined in tissue extracts.

Results.—Adhesions had developed in all patients, with 13 categorized in group I and 8 in group II. Levels of plasminogen activator inhibitor (PAI) type 1 and tissue-type plasminogen activator (tPA)/PAI complex were increased in peritoneal samples from patients with severe adhesions compared with those with less severe adhesions. The fibrinolytic capacity of adhesion tissue was reduced, as indicated by significant decreases in tPA activity and increases in PAI-1 levels. An increased level of tPA/PAI complex compared with unaffected peritoneum, reflected this finding (Fig 2).

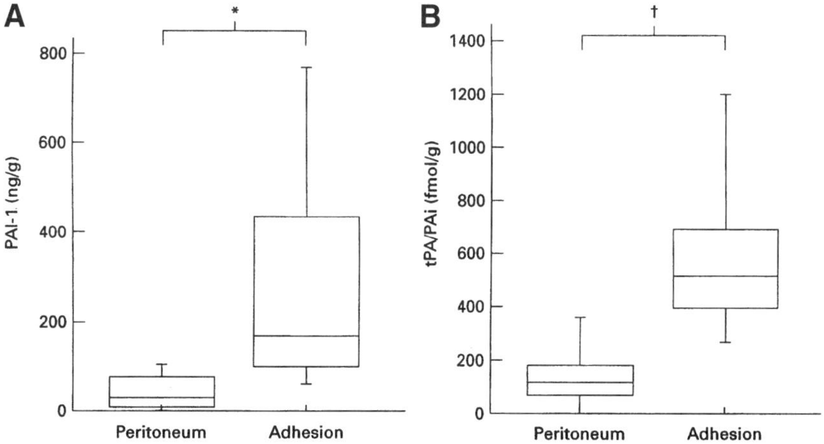

FIGURE 2.—Expression of a plasminogen activator inhibitor (PAI) type a and b tissue-type plasminogen activator (tPA)/PAI complex in adhesion tissue and peritoneum from the same patients. Values are median (horizontal bars) with interquartile range (boxes) and 10-90th centile (error bars). *P = 0.01, †P = 0.008 (Wilcoxon signed rank test). (Courtesy of Ivarsson M-L, Bergström M, Eriksson E, et al: Tissue markers as predictors of postoperative adhesions. *Br J Surg* 85:1549-1554, 1998. Blackwell Science Ltd.)

Conclusion.—Postoperative adhesions had a reduced potential to degrade fibrin, largely because of an increased expression of PAI-1. Patients with an increased tendency to develop extensive adhesions also apparently have a reduced peritoneal capacity to degrade fibrin, primarily because of an overexpression of PAI-1.

Reduction of Adhesion Formation in Rabbits by Intraperitoneal Administration of Lazaroid Formulations

Rodgers KE, Girgis W, St Amand K, et al (Univ of Southern California, Los Angeles)

Hum Reprod 13:2443-2451, 1998 9–6

Objective.—Reducing or preventing adhesion formation would decrease postoperative morbidity and mortality. Various formations of lazaroids, 21-aminosteroids and 2-methylaminochroman compounds have exhibited a protective effect against tissue damage, ischemia, or both, probably by inhibiting lipid peroxide reactions and reducing production of reactive oxygen metabolites. The effect of various lazaroid formulations on the formation of adhesions was investigated in 3 animal models.

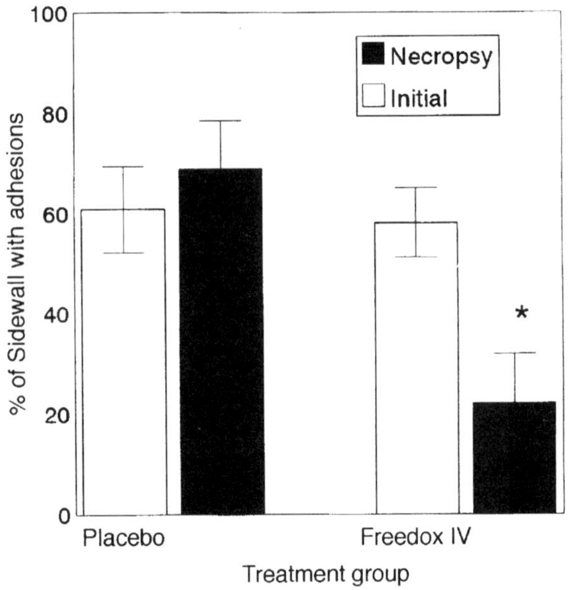

FIGURE 8.—The percentage of the area of sidewall injury that was involved in adhesion formation (no treatment) and reformation (necropsy) following lazaroid administration (25 mg presurgery and 25 mg postsurgery). These results represent mean ± SEM of data from 10 rabbits per group. *$P \leq 0.05$ compared with control. (Courtesy of Rodgers KE, Girgis W, St Amand K, et al: Reduction of adhesion formation in rabbits by intraperitoneal administration of lazaroid formulations. *Hum Reprod* 13:2443-2451. Copyright 1998, European Society for Human Reproduction and Embryology, by permission of Oxford University Press.)

Methods.—Sidewall, double uterine horn, and adhesion reformation surgical models were used to test adhesion formation in rabbits. Adhesion reformation was tested in the sidewall model by lysing existing adhesions 1 week after the initial surgery. Three experiments were performed. First, the nonsteroidal 2-methylaminochroman derivative PNU83,836E was administered at concentrations of 0.06 and 0.6 mg/mL via Alzet pump for 1, 2, 3, and 7 days postoperatively to the site of injury. Second, the antioxidant 21-aminosteroid PNU74006F (tirilazad) or PNU83,836E was administered as a bolus at the end of surgery. In the third, PNU74006F was administered as a bolus before and after surgery. The extent of adhesion formation was assessed at necropsy.

Results.—Adhesion formation was significantly reduced in all 3 experiments. PNU83,836E administered at concentrations of 0.06 and 0.6 mg/mL via Alzet pump reduced adhesions in a dose-response relationship beginning as soon as 24 hours after administration. PNU74006F administered as a bolus before surgery significantly reduced adhesions, even in the absence of bolus administration after surgery. Maximum efficacy was achieved with administration of 1.5 mg before surgery and 3 mg after surgery. Adhesion reformation was significantly reduced by administration of lazaroids (Fig 8).

Conclusion.—Preoperative and postoperative administration of lazaroids significantly reduces adhesion formation in these animal models.

► In patients with a proclivity to form postoperative adhesions, the adhesion tissue may have a reduced ability to degrade fibrin secondary to an increased expression of plasminogen activator inhibitor type 1 (PAI-1). The clinically relevant question is whether we can identify preoperatively these patients and whether therapies that inhibit PAI-1 are feasible. Lazaroids, on the other hand, exert their mechanism of action by inhibiting lipid peroxidation reactions as well as the production of reactive tissue metabolites. Thus, lazaroids could act to block the inhibition of fibrinolyis–deposited fibrin would be more rapidly cleared and the amount of fibrin available for adhesion formation would be diminished.

W.W. Souba, M.D.

Reperfusion Injury Delays Healing of Intestinal Anastomosis in Rat

Kuzu MA, Köksoy C, Kale IT, et al (Univ of Ankara, Turkey)

Am J Surg 176:348-351, 1998 9–7

Objective.—Ischemic bowel disease results in high morbidity and mortality, and revascularization may further induce local tissue injury. The effect of reperfusion injury on the healing of intestinal anastomosis following reperfusion of ischemic intestines was investigated in the rat.

Methods.—Male Wistar rats (n = 102) were divided into 3 groups: in group I (n = 23) the superior mesenteric artery (SMA) and collateral vessels were isolated but not occluded (control group); in group II (n =

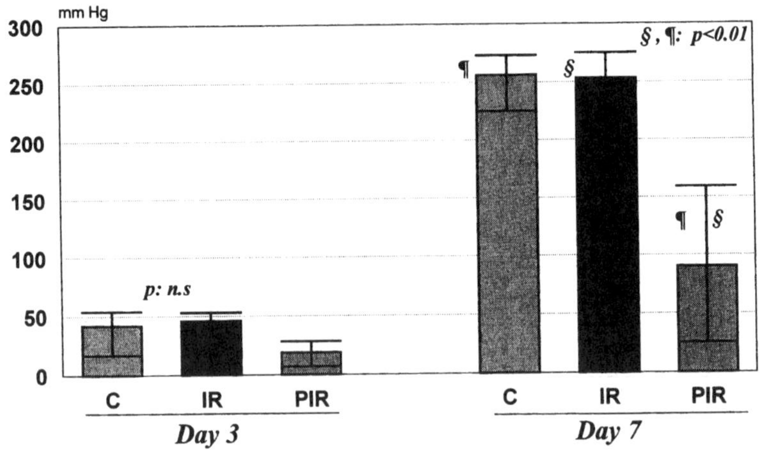

FIGURE.—Anastomotic bursting pressures (median-interquartile range) on the third and seventh postoperative day is shown. C=control anastomosis; IR=ischemia reperfusion; PIR=profound ischemia reperfusion. (Courtesy of Kuzu MA, Köksoy C, Kale IT, et al: Reperfusion injury delays healing of intestinal anastomosis in rat. *Am J Surg* 176:348-351. Copyright 1998, with permission from Excerpta Medica Inc.)

32), the SMA was occluded for 30 minutes; in group III (n = 47), the SMA and collateral vessels were occluded for 30 minutes. After arterial flow was restored, all groups underwent a 3-cm ileal resection with primary anastomosis, 10 cm proximal to the ileocecal valve. Abdominal wound healing, intraabdominal adhesions, anastomotic complications, and anastomotic bursting pressure were determined 3 and 7 days after surgery.

Results.—There was 1 (4%) death in group I, 4 (12.5%) in group II, and 22 (47%) in group III. There was significantly more anastomotic dehiscence in group III (47%) compared with groups I (9%) and II (16%). group III also had significantly more anastomotic adhesions than groups II and I, and group II had significantly more adhesions than group I. Median bursting pressures on days 3 and 7 were 42 and 250 mm Hg in group I, 46 and 253 in group II, and 19 and 90 in group III, respectively. Median bursting pressure in group III on day 7 was significantly lower than for the other groups (Figure).

Conclusion.—Reperfusion injury delays intestinal healing in relation to the extent of ischemic injury resulting in a significantly lower bursting pressure at the anastomosis in animals with more profound ischemic injury.

Protection From Reoxygenation Injury by Inhibition of *rac*1

Kim K-S, Takeda K, Sethi R, et al (NIH, Bethesda, Md; GenVec Incorporated, Rockville, Md; Johns Hopkins School of Medicine, Baltimore, Md; et al)

J Clin Invest 101:1821-1826, 1998 9–8

Introduction.—Reperfusion injury of ischemic tissue appears to be associated with a burst of reactive oxygen species (ROS) formation occurring with reoxygenation. However, there are few data on the pathways of ROS generation under these conditions. Most attempts to limit ROS-associated postischemic tissue damage have focused on the use of antioxidants. Inhibition of the guanosine triphosphate-binding protein *rac*-1 was used in this gene transfer study to inhibit the ROS burst after tissue reoxygenation.

Methods and Results.—Experiments were performed using rat primary vascular smooth muscle cell cultures, placed in a hypoxia chamber and subsequently reoxygenated. The intracellular ROS burst occurring with reoxygenation was inhibited by adenoviral-mediated gene transfer of the dominant negative *rac*-1 gene product N17-*rac*-1, but not the dominant negative *ras* gene N17-*ras* (Fig 4). Under direct oxidant stress, both control cells and N17-rac-1–expressing cells showed equivalent increases in intracellular ROS levels, followed by cell death. N17-*rac*-1 expression acted by blocking production of oxygen radicals, and did not scavenge ROS forming in response to reoxygenation. N17-*rac*-1 expression protected against reoxygenation-induced cell death in other types of cells as well, including fibroblasts, endothelial cells, and ventricular myocytes.

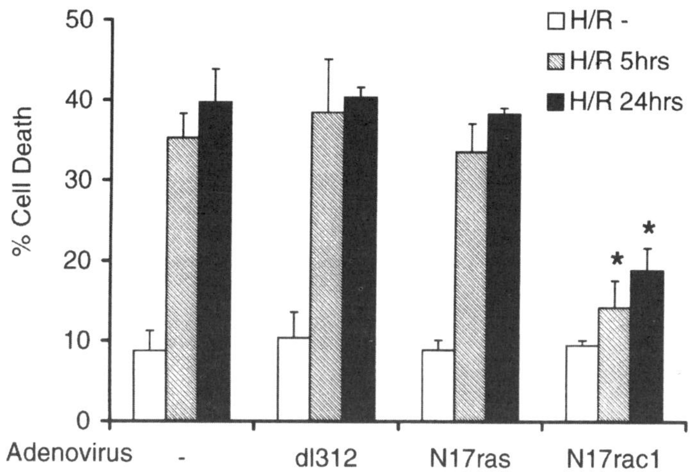

FIGURE 4.—N17*rac*1 expression inhibits cell death. Percentage of nonviable vascular smooth muscle cells under normoxic conditions (*H/R*−) or after 16 h of hypoxia followed by 5 or 24 hours of reoxygenation (*H/R*+). Viability was determined by a fluorescent live/dead assay as described. Cells were infected with 100 moi of the indicated adenovirus for 24 h before being made hypoxic. Results are from one of two similar experiments, each performed in triplicate. (Courtesy of Kim K-S, Takeda K, Sethi R, et al: Protection from reoxygenation injury by inhibition of *rac*1. *J Clin Invest* 101:1821-1826, 1998. Reproduced from The Journal of Clinical Investigation by copyright permission of The Rockefeller University Press.)

Conclusions.—Reoxygenation injury appears to require the activation of *rac* proteins, but not *ras* proteins. Gene transfer to inhibit *rac*-dependent pathways protects against reoxygenation-induced cell death. The findings may open a new approach to preventing reperfusion injury in ischemic tissues.

► While ischemia alone can produce tissue injury at an anastamotic suture line, the reperfusion injury that follows appears to cause greater damage by exposing hypoxic cells to molecular oxygen. The evidence implicating ROS as mediators of the damage has been substantiated by the observation that various chemical and enzymatic antioxidants can protect against reperfusion damage. The *rac* proteins appear to be required in an intracellular pathway leading to ROS generation after hypoxia/reoxygenation since inhibition of the pathways reduced cell death after reperfusion injury. Whether this bench knowledge can be translated to the bedside remains to be established.

W.W. Souba, M.D., Sc.D.

Wound Healing and Growth Factors in Clinical Practice

Less Collagen Production in Smokers
Jorgensen LN, Kallehave F, Christensen E, et al (Univ of Copenhagen)
Surgery 123:450-455, 1998 9–9

Objective.—There is evidence that smoking may be associated with impaired wound healing. However, these studies have been retrospective in nature and have not considered the social and medical parameters that may confound smoking status. The effects of smoking on healing of a test wound were examined in humans.

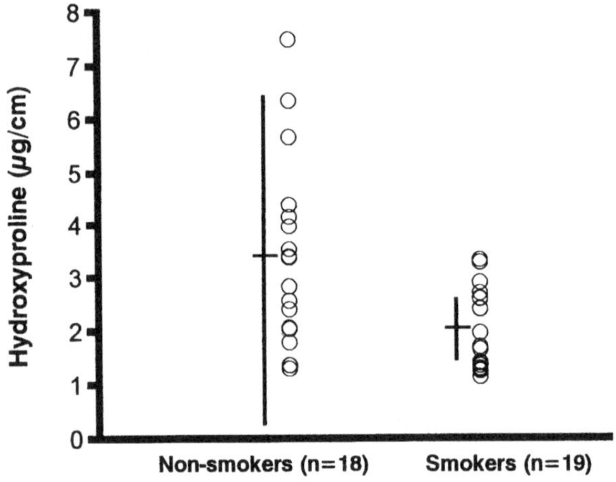

FIGURE 1.—Amount of hydroxyporline accumulated in expanded polytetrafluoroethylene tubing according to group of volunteers. Mean and variance are shown; $P < 0.01$ for comparison between groups, Mann-Whitney test. (Courtesy of Jorgensen LN, Kallehave F, Christensen E, et al: Less collagen production in smokers. *Surgery* 123:450-455, 1998.)

Methods.—The prospective study included 19 volunteers who smoked a median of 20 cigarettes per day and 18 nonsmokers matched for age and sex. Two expanded polytetrafluoroethylene tubes were inserted subcutaneously in the upper arm of each research subject. The response in terms of deposition of total protein and mature collagen, expressed as hydroxyproline, was assessed after a 10-day healing period.

Results.—Median hydroxyproline deposition was 80% higher for nonsmokers than for smokers (Fig 1). Smokers with higher levels of tobacco consumption before and during the study showed lower levels of hydroxyproline deposition. Smokers had impaired deposition of collagenous proteins in particular but not other types of proteins.

Conclusions.—Smokers showed a specific impairment of subcutaneous collagen synthesis. This finding is consistent with reports of impaired wound healing in smokers. Mature collagen is the most important contributor to the strength of operative wounds. Thus, patients should be advised to quit smoking before undergoing surgery.

► Retrospective studies have shown that smokers undergoing reconstructive surgery, colorectal procedures, tibial shaft fracture repairs, and episiotomy repairs are more likely than nonsmokers to have impaired wound healing from necrosis, infection, or dehiscence. The observation, by Jorgensen and colleagues, that collagen production is diminished in smokers also appears to have clinical relevance in patients with hernia. Read[1] reported that subcutaneous fibroblasts from smokers in whom inguinal hernias developed produced less collagen than did fibroblasts harvested from controls.

W.W. Souba, M.D., Sc.D.

Reference

1. Read R: Metabolic factors contributing to herniation: A review. *Hernia* 2:51-55, 1998.

Is Fetal Tissue the Only Factor Responsible for the Properties of Fetal Wound Healing?

Çek DI, Özer K, Perk C, et al (Vakif Gureba Hosp, Istanbul, Turkey; Istanbul Univ, Turkey; Haseki State Hosp, Istanbul, Turkey)

Eur J Plast Surg 21:28-30, 1998 9–10

Objective.—The properties of fetal wound healing are not completely understood. The effect of fetal tissue on fetal type wound healing was investigated by histopathologic analysis of fetal grafts on 10 adult cats.

Methods.—Skin grafts were transferred from fetal cats to the mothers and vice versa. On day 10, 2 incisions were made in the fetal grafts; 1 was sutured and the other was not. Eight to 10 days later, the grafts were removed and examined histopathologically.

Results.—Fetal grafts healed with scar formation regardless of whether they had been sutured. Maternal grafts on the fetuses had less scar formation than fetal grafts on mother cats.

Conclusion.—Healing of fetal grafts on adult cats was the adult type of healing. Scar tissue was found in both the fetal grafts in the adult and maternal grafts in the fetus. Fetal type wound healing is not the result solely of the properties of fetal cells.

▶ The results of this work, performed by surgeons in Turkey, indicate that fetal type wound healing is not solely attributable to the preexisting properties of fetal cells. Other factors, such as amniotic fluid and low oxygen tension, may also play a role. If factors other than cell type can be identified, they may be translatable to adult patients who are candidates for organ transplantation. This might entail a radically different method of controlling tissue rejection than currently targeted.

W.W. Souba, M.D., Sc.D.

Abdominal Adhesiolysis: Inpatient Care and Expenditures in the United States in 1994

Ray NF, Denton WG, Thamer M, et al (MEDTAP, Bethesda, Md; Denton Internatl, Dallas; Med Technology and Practice Patterns Inst, Washington, DC)

J Am Coll Surg 186:1-9, 1998 9–11

Background.—Adhesions after lower abdominal surgery are associated with significant rehospitalization rates and costs. A 1988 study reported that abdominal adhesiolysis prompted almost 282,000 hospitalizations and cost $1.2 billion. One might expect the shift from the open abdominal procedures common in 1988 to today's less invasive techniques (such as laparoscopy) to reduce the incidence of abdominal adhesions and, thus, the need for adhesiolysis and its associated costs. These authors examined this hypothesis by comparing adhesiolysis rates and costs in the United States between 1988 and 1994.

Methods.—The number of hospitalizations for adhesiolysis and the total days of care were estimated from the 1994 National Hospital Discharge Survey, which is conducted by the National Center for Health Statistics. The hospitalization costs were estimated from the 1994 Medical Provider Analysis and Review data, which include discharge records from all U.S. institutions that participate in Medicare. The surgeon costs were estimated from the 1994 Part B Medicare Annual Data file.

Findings.—Adhesiolysis prompted 303,836 hospitalizations in the United States in 1994, compared with 281,982 hospitalizations in 1988. Almost half the adhesiolysis procedures (47%) were performed after obstetric/gynecologic surgery, which accounted for 41,894 days of care and $192.3 million in hospital and surgeon costs. Most of the inpatient days of care (796,119 of the total of 846,415 days) were from adhesiolysis after

TABLE 4.—Comparison of Adhesiolysis Hospitalizations in the United States in 1988 and 1994

Year	Adhesiolysis Hospitalization	Hospitalization Rate (Per 100,000 Persons)	Expenditures (1994 $ Million)* Hospitalization	Surgeon	Total
1988	Primary procedure	22.16	769.8	45.3	815.1
	Secondary procedure	93.35	431.3	190.7	622.0
	Total	115.51	1,201.1	236.0	1,437.1
1994	Primary procedure	22.49	715.2	48.7	764.0
	Secondary procedure	94.85	356.3	205.6	561.9
	Total	117.34	1,071.5	254.3	1,325.9

*Expenditures were calculated based on inpatient cost per day of $1,266 and surgeon cost of $837.

(Courtesy of Ray NF, Denton WG, Thamer M, et al: Abdominal adhesiolysis: Inpatient care and expenditures in the United States in 1994. *J Am Coll Surg* 186:1-9, 1998. Reprinted by permission of the American College of Surgeons.)

digestive system operations (total costs $1.110 billion). Hospitalization rates for either primary or secondary adhesiolysis (per 100,00 persons) were 117.34 in 1988 and 115.51 in 1988 (Table 4). Total costs were $1.236 billion in 1994 and $1.437 billion in 1988. The average length of hospital stay from adhesiolysis was 9.7 days in 1994 and 11.2 days in 1988.

Conclusions.—The number of hospitalizations for abdominal adhesions has increased somewhat since 1988. However, the costs associated with adhesiolysis have decreased by almost 10%, mainly because of a 15% shorter hospital stay in 1994. Based on these data, the current use of laparoscopy was not associated with a decrease in the hospitalization rate for adhesiolysis.

▶ The authors used prevalence-based cost-of-illness methods to estimate inpatient expenditures associated with adhesiolysis in 1994. As previously reported, postoperative adhesions occur most commonly in patients undergoing pelvic surgery or gastrointestinal tract surgery (often colorectal surgery). Readmission of patients with partial small bowel obstruction and subsequent reoperation and lysis of adhesions continues to challenge surgeons. The complication has not diminished in incidence, and it continues to be an expensive proposition.

The cause of postoperative adhesions continues to be an enigma in most patients. It has been postulated that trauma, ischemia, hemorrhage, raw surfaces, and foreign body contamination (e.g., glove powder) may contribute to their formation. Until the etiology of adhesion formation is better understood, postoperative small obstruction secondary to their formation will continue to be a problem. The length of stay associated with managing patients with postoperative adhesions has fallen, but it is still about 9 days.

W.W. Souba, M.D., Sc.D.

The Surgeon as a Risk Factor for Complications of Midline Incisions

Israelsson LA (Sundsvall County Hosp, Sweden)

Eur J Surg 164:353-359, 1998 9–12

Background.—Many factors affect the development of wound infection or incisional hernia after incisions. This study sought to determine the risk factors associated with these complications after midline incisions at 1 hospital.

Methods.—The subjects were 798 patients (530 men and 483 women; mean age, 61 years) who had received a midline laparotomy incision and were available 12 months later for follow-up. All laparotomies were performed by one of 5 junior surgeons (those with <10 years of experience or those on night duty in the emergency department) or 6 senior surgeons. The main outcomes of interest were postoperative wound infection (the discharge of purulent exudate) or an incisional hernia. Variables examined for their association to these outcomes included the patient's age, sex, smoking status, and body mass index; the length of operation; the degree of operative contamination; the units of packed cells used; and the suture length to wound length (SL:WL) ratio.

Findings.—The 5 junior surgeons performed 220 midline laparotomies, and the senior surgeons performed 793. The 2 groups varied significantly in numerous factors, including the age of the patients (senior surgeons operated on younger patients), the degree of wound contamination (senior surgeons operated through cleaner wounds), the SL:WL ratio (4:1 for senior surgeons vs. 5:3 for junior surgeons), and the requirement for packed cells (seniors used more units). Wound infection rates ranged from 0% to 27% and incisional hernia rates ranged from 5% to 26%; the 2 groups did not differ significantly in these outcomes. Multivariate analysis identified 5 predictors of wound infection: young age, overweight, long operation, more wound contamination, and reoperation. Four predictors of incisional hernia were identified (Table 5): older age, overweight, wound infection, and an SL:WL ratio < 4. In fact, 22% of patients with an SL:WL ratio < 4 developed incisional hernia, whereas only 9% of those with a higher ratio did. Data analysis uncorrected for these risk factors identified 2 (senior) surgeons with a significantly higher risk of wound infection and 1 (senior) surgeon with a significantly lower risk; after data

TABLE 5.—Significant Predictors of Incisional Hernia: Results of Multiple Logistic Regression Analysis in 798 Patients

	Regression Coefficient	SE	Odds Ratio	95% CI
Age (years)	0.0219	0.0073	1.0221	1.01 to 1.04
Overweight	0.8953	0.2191	2.4481	1.6 to 3.8
Wound infection	0.9130	0.2888	2.4917	1.4 to 4.4
SL:WL ratio <4	1.0942	0.2174	2.9868	1.9 to 4.6

(Courtesy of Israelsson LA. The surgeon as a risk factor for complications of midline incisions. *Eur J Surg* 164:353-359, 1998.)

were corrected for these risk factors, another surgeon (senior) was found to have a significantly higher rate. Uncorrected data indicated that 2 surgeons (both seniors) had a significantly higher risk of incisional hernia and 2 surgeons (1 junior, 1 senior) had a significantly lower risk. These results were the same when the data were corrected for age, weight, and wound contamination; but factoring in the SL:WL ratio identified only 1 surgeon (senior) with a lower risk.

Conclusion.—The postoperative morbidity rates between these 11 surgeons varied greatly. The suture technique (SL:WL ratio) was the most important determinant in the incidence of incisional hernia. Suture technique also probably affected the incidence of wound infection.

The Association of Intra-abdominal Infection and Abdominal Wound Dehiscence

Graham DJ, Stevenson JT, McHenry CR (Case Western Reserve Univ, Cleveland, Ohio; Cleveland Veteran Affairs Med Ctr, Ohio; MetroHealth Med Ctr, Cleveland, Ohio)

Am Surg 64:660-665, 1998 9–13

Background.—Although abdominal wound dehiscence has traditionally been treated surgically, several studies suggest nonoperative management is possible. These authors examined the risk factors associated with abdominal wound dehiscence to identify prognostic factors that could impact management decisions.

Methods.—Chart review identified 107 patients (85 men and 22 women; mean age, 58 years) who had experienced abdominal wound dehiscence. Factors that could influence the development of dehiscence were examined, including demographic factors, preoperative factors (fever, leukocytosis, wound infection, comorbid diseases), the type of operative procedure preceding the dehiscence, whether the operation was emer-

TABLE 4.—Operative Procedures Preceding Dehiscence

Procedure	No. Infection (n = 43)	Intra-abdominal Infection (n = 47)
Colonic*	10	25
Small bowel	7	6
Gastroduodenal	8	7
Esophageal	5	1
Pancreatic	1	0
Biliary	3	1
Vascular†	6	0
Liver	0	1
Exploratory laparotomy	3	6

*$p < 0.05$.
†$p < 0.01$.
(Courtesy of Graham DJ, Stevenson JT, McHenry CR. The association of intra-abdominal infection and abdominal wound dehiscence. *Am Surg* 64:660-665, 1998.)

gent or elective, the type of incision used, the closure method used, the wound classification, how the dehiscence was treated, and whether signs of systemic infection were present.

Findings.—The most common operations were colon resection (n =41), gastroduodenal procedures (n = 17), small bowel procedures (n =15), and abdominal exploration (n = 11). Most of the patients (93%) had received a midline incision. Of the 17 patients who were managed nonoperatively, 3 (preterminal) patients died. Of the 90 patients who underwent exploratory laparotomy, 43 had no intra-abdominal pathology but 47 (44%) had intra-abdominal infections. Patients with and without intra-abdominal infection could not be distinguished on the basis of demographics, comorbid conditions, or systemic signs of infection. Intra-abdominal infections were significantly more likely in patients undergoing emergency surgery (74% of patients with infection vs. 48% of patients without infection), in patients who had a colonic procedure (55% vs. 25% of those without infection) (Table 4), and in patients whose wound classification was higher (Class III wound, 55% vs. 26% of those without infection). Furthermore, mortality rates were higher when intra-abdominal infections were present (44% vs. 20% in patients without infection).

Conclusions.—Intra-abdominal infection is a well-known risk factor for dehiscence. Overall, 44% of these patients with abdominal wound dehiscence had intra-abdominal infection. Patients with intra-abdominal infection had approximately double the mortality rate of patients without infection. Because of this increased mortality, surgeons must rule out intra-abdominal infection in patients undergoing emergency surgery, a colectomy, or a wound class III procedure before contemplating conservative management.

▶ Only about half of wound dehiscences can be "blamed" on intra-abdominal infection, and most of these midline fascial separations can probably be prevented. Surgical technique is probably key in many of these patients, and several questions come to mind. What kind of suture was used? What kind of closure (interrupted or running) was used? Were the tissue bites 1 cm apart and 1 cm deep in the fascia? Do transverse wounds behave differently than midline wounds? When are retention sutures indicated? All of these technical issues have been discussed in the past.

It is well established that age, obesity, infections, and technique influence the incidence of midline wound complications. Israelsson suggests the suture length to wound length ratio (SL:WL) is also important. If the SL:WL ratio is less than 4, the likelihood of abdominal wall dehiscence increases. This suggests the running midline closure is not snug enough. There must be some upper limit as well—a closure that is too tight will eventually lead to fascial necrosis.

W.W. Souba, M.D., Sc.D.

Modified V-Y Advancement Technique for Mastectomy Closure

Gibbs ER, Kent RB III (Norwood Clinic Inc, Birmingham, Ala)

J Am Coll Surg 187:632-633, 1998 9–14

Background.—The Y-V advancement flap has been used to close musculocutaneous wounds and for reconstructions of skin defects in the lower limb, distal forearm, and dorsal foot. These authors describe its use in the closure of a standard transverse mastectomy incision.

Methods.—The mastectomy is performed with use of the standard bielliptical incision. Then the surgeon retracts the lateral apex of the incision medially, and marks the 2 points superiorly and inferiorly to where the apex is retracted. This retraction results in 2 triangular-shaped portions of the skin (superior and inferior) that will be redundant in the Y-V advancement, and thus, are excised. The surgeon then retracts the lateral apex medially and sutures it to the superior and inferior marks (Fig 4). The surgeon closes the incision in a Y configuration (Fig 5).

Conclusions.—Particularly for patients who are obese and have large breasts, the standard transverse mastectomy incision can laterally leave redundant tissue that can be both cosmetically and functionally bothersome. This modified V-Y advancement eliminates this redundant tissue. However, it should not be used if the patient might seek breast reconstruction.

► I have not used this exact technique before in closing the skin after mastectomy. Generally, I have found that I can fashion a bielliptical incision quite satisfactorily in most patients, even if it means removing excess skin at the time of closure or repairing "dog ears." The technique described by

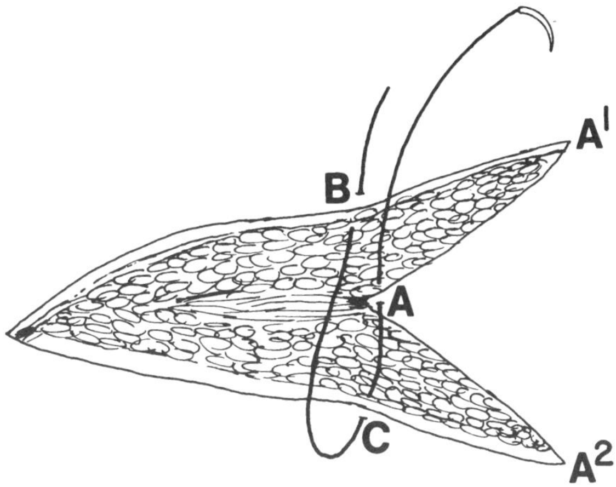

FIGURE 4.—The lateral apex is retracted medially and secured to the superior and inferior skin edges. (Courtesy of Gibbs ER, Kent RB III. Modified V-Y advancement technique for mastectomy closure. *J Am Coll Surg* 187:632-633, 1998. By permission of the American College of Surgeons.)

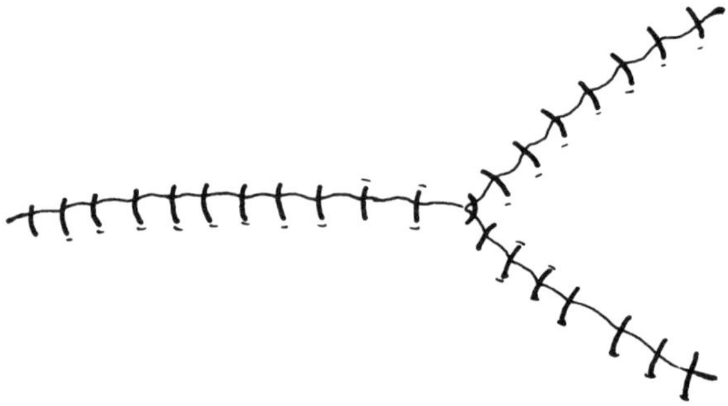

FIGURE 5.—The closure as it appears after completion. (Courtesy of Gibbs ER, Kent RB III. Modified V-Y advancement technique for mastectomy closure. *J Am Coll Surg* 187: 632-633, 1998. By permission of the American College of Surgery.)

the authors appears to be simple and feasible. I wonder about the possibility of necrosis of the apex of skin labeled "A" in Figure 4. As best I can tell, this area would receive its blood supply from that lateral skin flap, which can be quite long.

W.W. Souba, M.D., Sc.D.

10 Gastrointestinal

Introduction

Because of its place and importance in general surgery, surgical gastroenterology remains of seminal interest to the readers of the YEAR BOOK OF SURGERY. For the 1999 edition, the editors have again selected principal contributions that depict representative basic and clinical scientific issues that provide clinical applications for the care of patients. Again, the Editor acknowledges that several important contributions of interest to the readership cannot be included because of space limitations. We continue to recognize the anatomical, pathophysiologic, and technical issues for surgery in patient management; additional articles provided in the Gastrointestinal section include contemporary contributions from basic science that provide physicians the important tools for the future practice of surgical science. The Editor and contributing editors have therefore provided selections that highlight the benchmark clinical trials and translational research that enhance the surgical management of diseases of the gastrointestinal tract.

Kirby I. Bland, M.D.

Esophagus and Stomach

INTRODUCTION

The significant role of gastroesophageal reflux (GER) to general surgeons is underscored by the many papers in the current literature of American and European medical journals. The first diaphragmatic hernia recognition and its successful repair was accomplished by Postempski in 1889. However, it was some 37 years later when Akerland described paraesophageal herniation and suggested this was an uncommon variant of the hiatal hernia. Thereafter, recognition and description of hiatal hernia was completed: type 1, a hiatal hernia in which the GE junction migrates cephalad via the esophageal hiatus; type 2, a rolling hernia (paraesophageal), in which the fundus herniates together with a normal position of the GE junction; type 3, combinations of types 1 and 2, in which both the GE junction and a large portion of the fundus herniate into the left chest. The type 2 variant is rare; the type 3 variants physiologically occur and behave like types 1 and 2 and are commonly classified as paraesophageal. Ellis has previously estimated that paraesophageal herniation accounts for approximately 5% to 10% of all hiatal hernias.

Percutaneous endoscopic gastrostomy (PEG) continues to be the method of choice for the long-term enteral feeding of individuals unable to eat or drink adequately as a result of various maladies. The PEG eliminates the need for gastrostomy or nasogastric tubes, is simple to perform, and is patient- and physician-friendly in management for both patients and outpatients. Some suggest that the PEG method is cost-effective, because it reduces demands on health care resources. Nonetheless, both early and late complications of PEG insertion are real; the most common serious complication is aspiration pneumonitis, which is etiologically related to aspiration of pharyngeal secretions or refluxed gastric acid contents.

Since the first applications of laparoscopic Nissen fundoplication in 1991, this procedure has emerged as the principal surgical therapy for GER, reflected by the hundreds of articles submitted annually on this subject. Previous arguments suggesting that laparoscopic Nissen anti-GER procedures had unacceptably high complication rates and were more laborious and technically difficult have now been largely discounted. Although postoperative side effects occur with both open and laparoscopic approaches, data accumulated in this decade suggest that persistent troublesome solid-food dysphagia is more common after the *laparoscopic* approach (4% to 24%) than was evident with the *open* "floppy" Nissen technique (<3%). The Rosetti-Nissen laparoscopic approach has previously been observed to initiate dysphagia more frequently than its antecedent laparoscopic technique that uses the Toupet-Nissen fundoplication, which requires greater curvature mobilization. Therefore, the majority of international surgeons use the Toupet fundoplication approach when the laparoscopic approach is the preferred method of repair. Abstracts 10–1 and 10–2 query the efficacy of the fundoplication for patients primarily seen initially with atypical symptoms of pulmonary nature, pharyngoesophageal complications, or noncardiac chest pain. These complaints were significantly improved relative to laryngeal symptoms, while less so for pulmonary and chest complaints. Clearly, one cannot exclude the possibility that some of the failures in patients with atypical symptoms are related to a failure of the procedure to control reflux and hence, the reason for the operations for these patients.

In a collective review of over 5,000 patients by Andreollo et al.,[1] the incidence of GER after cardiomyotomy for achalasia *without* an antireflux procedure performed via an open *thoracic* approach was 7.7%. This incidence was significantly lower than the rates observed in cardiomyopathy *without* an antireflux procedure (13.2%), which was also accomplished via an open *abdominal* approach and is similar to the incidence following abdominal cardiomyotomy *with* an antireflux wrap (7.3%). It has been previously suggested that the higher incidence of GER after an open abdominal cardiomyotomy is attributed to undue mobilization of the esophagogastric junction with accompanying damage to supporting ligamentous attachments, particularly the phreno-esophageal membrane. Abstract 10–3 by Kumar and colleagues addresses the technique of laparoscopic cardiomyopathy applied in Dundee, Scotland, to preserve lateral and posterior attachments of the gastroesophageal junction. This important paper addresses the *routine addition* of an antireflux operation but suggests that this added approach is unnecessary for patients undergoing laparoscopic cardiomyotomy, if the surgeon is careful to protect the lateral and posterior esophageal attachments. Refinements in technical approaches with limited laparoscopic cardiomyotomies are effective in relieving dysphagia and are followed by a small and acceptable incidence of GER. This method is to be differentiated from the Italian approach by Bonavina and associates[2] and the approach by Ancona and colleagues[3] which consist of a full 360-degree esophageal mobilization with large myotomy and fundal wrap. Kumar and colleagues suggest that this latter approach for achalasia is unnecessary; the exception is patients with associated diffuse esophageal spasm, because the dual single-stage endoscopic management technique, with long myotomy via the right posterior thorascopic approach and cardiomyotomy via the laparoscopic route, avoids extensive mobilization and disruption of esophageal attachments.

The ideal management of esophageal atresia with tracheoesophageal fistula (TEF) includes division of the fistula and primary repair of the esophagus, preferably with a single operation in the newborn era. Finding a long gap between the esophageal segment and a high upper pouch may preclude surgical repair with primary anastomosis; repair with an anastomosis under tension enhances the risk of anastomotic complications, including GER and recurrent TEF. Healey and associates (Abstract 10–4) more precisely define the ideal approach for the management of infants with long-gap esophageal atresia with TEF and significant respiratory distress syndrome (RDS) and prematurity, or both, and associated cardiac anomalies. Successful anastomosis of the native esophagus was considered the principal outcome measure with recording of the incidence of GER anastomotic complications and survival between primary and delayed repair. This important article suggests that all children with atresia and TEF, regardless of the gap length, can maintain their native esophagus. The principal causes of mortality in this and other studies include the association of severe cardiac anomalies with TEF and atresia. Staged approaches are useful in premature infants with RDS or associated cardiac defects.

Laparoscopic repair of the type 2 rolling esophageal hiatal hernia (paraesophageal) is being performed with increasing frequency. After conventional primary repair, hernia recurrence is reported as low as 8% at 4 years' follow-up by Ellis and associates[4] or as great as 50% when evaluated radiographically. The concept and debate of prosthetic repair of the diaphragmatic defect also remains a controversial issue with the type 2 hernia. Edye and associates (Abstract 10–5) address the laparoscopic repair, which appears to be a durable and acceptable approach in follow-up. The technical discussion provided by these authors has importance to our readers and suggests that complete removal of the sac with adequate crural closure is essential to provide durable long-term satisfactory outcomes.

The next series of abstracts address the development of dysplasia and subsequent adenocarcinoma during the interval of endoscopic surveillance of Barrett's esophagus. Neoplasms are still seen with an increasing frequency, and esophageal carcinoma currently represents the sixth most common neoplasm in the world and is one of the most lethal tumors. The predominant squamous carcinoma cell type predominates worldwide, while in the United States and Europe the incidence of mortality from adenocarcinoma of the esophagus, including the esophagogastric junction, continues to rise, especially among white men in these Western cultures. The triad of articles by Katz and co-workers, Ouatu-Lascar and Triadafilopoulos, and Csendes and colleagues (Abstracts 10–6 to 10–8) suggest that Barrett's may develop dysplasia *without* symptoms of GER. Moreover, should the axiom be true that Barrett's mucosa is less sensitive to acid exposure, as noted by Ouatu-Lascar and Triadafilopoulos, it suggests that complete eradication of any GER symptoms would *not* indicate the conversion to a normal intra-esophageal pH as expected. Taken together, these articles suggest that proper antireflux precautions or surgical conversions with anti-GER techniques, with protection of esophageal mucosa with greater than 90% of acid exposure, are likely to prevent progression of Barrett's to histologic dysplasia. Of great importance is the admonition that patients with histologically confirmed Barrett's mucosa who do not elect, or are prohibited by co-morbid conditions, from undergoing antireflux surgery, should have 24-hour-pH surveillance at two-year intervals. This aggressive surveillance method may allow early detection of dysplastic states, before transformation from in situ to invasive esophageal carcinoma, and may therefore promote early surgical intervention that has an impact on therapeutic outcomes.

The prediction of tumor phenotype aggressiveness and treatment responsiveness by means of tissue analysis is a subject of intense international investigation in molecular biology laboratories. When nonresponsive tumors can be identified, patients may be spared significant toxicity, time, and the expense associated with multidisciplinary therapeutic interventions. The scientific fiction writer H. G. Wells once said, "Every dogma must have its day." The recent redefinition of the adenoma-polyp-carcinoma sequence by Fearon and Vogelstein[5] has allowed a molecular definition that describes the progression and identification of multiple genetic "hits" in neoplasms of the colon and rectum. Moreover, the development and progression of esophageal carcinoma is likewise a multistep initiation process in which specific genetic events appear to follow a temporal sequence, similar to that defined by Fearon and colleagues. The importance of oncogene and tumor suppressor gene alterations may therefore have predictive value for patients with tumors such as esophageal carcinoma. Abstract 10–9 by Ribeiro and co-workers reviewed alterations of the p53 gene to correlate clinical pathological parameters, responses to preoperative chemotherapy or radiotherapy, and outcomes in patients with esophageal carcinoma. The p53 immunopositive tumors were evident in approximately 60% of cases—the typical frequency of the mutation in other solid tumors (e.g., breast carcinoma). The authors confirm the histopathologic/genetic analysis represented a better methodology for determination of p53 mutational damage than immunohistochemistry alone. Further, genetic analysis can be used as a prognostic marker for esophageal carcinoma. This approach, as has been proved in other solid tumor systems, suggests that tumor genotyping of various oncogenes and tumor suppressor genes may define a subset of patients who may respond to chemotherapy and radiotherapy, and it may therefore predict potential benefits from multimodal therapy. As in Abstracts 10–6 and 10–7, such applications of p53 gene sequencing for patients with Barrett's esophagus and dysplasia may have potential surveillance and therapeutic value.

The last article in this section also emphasizes that the tumor suppressor gene p53 produces immunogenic protein which is concomitant with DNA missense mutations, with nuclear accumulation of the p53 protein or both events.[6,7] Moreover, anti-p53 antibody (p53-Ab) has been observed and detected in a subpopulation of patients with a variety of common human neoplasms, including breast, lung, liver, and prostate. Cawley and associates (Abstract 10–10) used enzyme immunoassay and immunoblotting with precipitation assays to verify that the Barrett's esophagus, as well as early esophageal carcinoma, develops p53-Ab that predates clinical diagnosis of the malignancy. Chronic esophagitis may constitute a precursor lesion for the development of squamous carcinoma of the esophagus in endemic geographic areas such as Iran, China, and South Carolina, with changes analogous to Barrett's metaplasia. Therefore, applications of these methodologies may have future clinical applications for identification of high-risk susceptible populations. This work suggests that p53-Ab studies may be appropriate, especially in large populations of patients in whom demonstrable metaplasia of the Barrett's type is evident.

Kirby I. Bland, M.D.

References

1. Andreollo NA, Earlam RJ:. Heller's myotomy for achalasia: Is an added anti-reflux procedure necessary? *Br J Surg* 74:765-769, 1987.
2. Bonavina L, Nosadini A, Bardini R, et al: Primary treatment of esophageal achalasia. Long-term results of myotomy and Dor fundoplication. *Arch Surg* 127:222-226, 1992.
3. Ancona E, Peracchia A, Zaninotto G, et al: Heller Laparoscopic cardiomyotomy with antireflux anterior fundoplication (Dor) in the treatment of esophageal achalasia. *Surg Endosc* 7:459-461, 1993.
4. Ellis FH Jr, Crozier RE, Shea JA: Paraesophageal hiatus hernia. *Arch Surg* 121:416-420, 1986.
5. Fearon ER, Vogelstein B: A genetic model for colorectal tumorigenesis. *Cell* 61:759-767, 1990.
6. Davidoff AM, Iglehart JD, Marks JR: Immune response to p53 is dependent upon p53/HSP70 complexes in breast cancer. *Proc Natl Acad Sci U S A* 89:3439-3442, 1992.
7. Winter SF, Minna JD, Johnson BE, et al: Development of antibodies against p53 in lung cancer patients appears to be dependent upon the type of p53 mutation. *Cancer Res* 53:4168-4174, 1992.

Outcomes of Atypical Symptoms Attributed to Gastroesophageal Reflux Treated by Laparoscopic Fundoplication

So JBY, Zeitels SM, Rattner DW (Massachusetts Gen Hosp, Boston; Harvard Med School, Boston)

Surgery 124:28-32, 1998 10–1

Introduction.—Laparoscopic fundoplication (LF) has emerged as a less invasive alternative to traditional antireflux procedures. This has lowered the threshold for surgery, with the result that more antireflux operations are being performed. Many studies have shown that LF is effective in relieving the typical reflux symptoms of heartburn and regurgitation; however, little is known about its effects on atypical symptoms, such as pulmonary, pharyngolaryngeal, and pain syndromes. The results of LF for patients with atypical symptoms of gastroesophageal reflux were analyzed.

Methods.—One hundred fifty patients who were followed up for at least 1 year after LF were included in the study. Of these, 35 were operated on mainly for atypical symptoms: pulmonary complications in 16 patients, epigastric and chest pain in 12, and pharynoglaryngeal complications in 9. Barium studies revealed that 12 of 27 patients had free reflux and 17 had a hiatal hernia. Pharyngeal symptoms of reflux disease were specificity investigated by dual-probe hydrogen ion concentration testing. Abnormal acid exposure above the cricopharyngeal area was identified in 7 of 7 patients investigated for reflux-induced laryngitis.

Results.—Postoperatively, 9% of patients had persistent dysphagia necessitating dilation. Postoperative questionnaires indicated that accompanying heartburn was relieved in 93% of patients with atypical symptoms. However, just 56% of patients reported improvement in the atypical symptoms for which surgery was indicated. Response rates were 78% for pharyngolaryngeal symptoms, 58% for chest or epigastric pain, and 48% for pulmonary symptoms. Patients whose atypical symptoms were relieved by medications preoperatively were more likely to have a good surgical outcome.

In 2 patients, chest pain was associated with esophageal spasm; reflux was abolished by surgery in both of these patients, but only 1 achieved symptom relief. Postoperative testing in other patients whose atypical symptoms failed to respond to LF also suggested that pathologic reflux was abolished in 14 of 15 cases.

Conclusions.—LF is less effective in relieving atypical symptoms of reflux disease than it is in relieving the typical symptoms of heartburn and regurgitation. Relief of atypical symptoms is more likely for patients whose symptoms were relieved by acid-suppressing drugs. Dual-probe hydrogen ion concentration testing may provide useful information in patients with laryngeal symptoms. Patients undergoing LF for atypical symptoms must be carefully selected and informed regarding the expected results.

The Treatment of Gastroesophageal Reflux Disease With Laparoscopic Nissen Fundoplication: Prospective Evaluation of 100 Patients With "Typical" Symptoms

Peters JH, DeMeester TR, Crookes P, et al (Univ of Southern California, Los Angeles)

Ann Surg 228:40-50, 1998 10–2

Objective.—Laparoscopic Nissen fundoplication, offering success rates exceeding 90%, is becoming the new standard of surgical treatment for gastroesophageal reflux disease (GERD). As a result of this less invasive technique, a growing number of patients are being referred for surgical treatment. The "typical" symptoms of GERD, such as heartburn, regurgitation, and dysphagia, are easily related to the problem of reflux. The postoperative response of atypical symptoms—such as cough, hoarseness, or wheezing—is less reliable. The results of laparoscopic Nissen fundoplication in 100 patients with typical symptoms of GERD were reported.

Technique.—The authors describe their technique of laparoscopic Nissen fundoplication, with modifications including incorporation of the posterior vagus nerve in the fundoplication, extension of the dissection posterior to the gastroesophageal junction and the degree of fundic mobilization, and attention to the geometry of the fundoplication. After hiatal and crural dissection, the esophagus is retracted and the crura approximated using 3 or 4 interrupted 0 silk sutures. A large needle is passed down the left upper 10-mm port to ensure a durable closure. In fundic mobilization, an anterior to posterior orientation is preferred. The posterior pancreaticogastric branches are divided posterior to the upper stomach, continuing until the right crus and caudate lobe are visible from the left side. To create the fundoplication, a Babcock clamp passed through the left lower port is used to grasp the midportion of the posterior fundus, which is passed left to right behind the esophagus. The anterior fundus wall is then brought over the anterior esophageal wall, above the supporting Penrose drain. The anterior and posterior fundic lips are folded around the fundus to meet at the 9-o'clock position, to envelop the esophagus without twisting the fundus. The fundoplication is fixed with a U-stitch and two anchoring sutures of 2-0 silk placed above and below. After the operation has been completed, the stomach should be in its original plane, with the fundoplication suture line facing right anterior and the greater curvature in the left posterior direction.

Results.—This procedure achieved relief of the patients' primary symptoms in 96% of cases. Eighty-three percent of patients considered themselves cured. There were few complications and no deaths. The length of hospital stay decreased from 6.3 days for the first 10 patients to 2.3 days for the last 10 patients.

Conclusions.—Laparoscopic Nissen fundoplication is safe and highly effective in relieving the typical symptoms of GERD. Antireflux surgery may be considered for patients who do not have esophagitis but are dependent on proton pump inhibitors to remain free of symptoms, particularly younger patients and those at risk of severe disease. Routine crural closure avoids the problem of migration of the fundoplication into the chest.

► The success rate of fundoplication in patients with typical reflux symptoms of heartburn and regurgitation is generally reported to be 90% in open surgical series, irrespective of the specific technique used. Peters and colleagues document similar results for laparoscopic fundoplication in this study. Primary symptom reduction was documented in 95% of patients at a mean of 21 months after surgery. Furthermore, these remarkable results were obtained with hospital stays of 48 hours or less. This article documents important technical considerations in the procedure, particularly with reference to the fundoplication itself. As shown in Fig 6 of the original article, a proper fundoplication requires the posterior wall of the fundus and not the anterior wall. The latter results in a wrap, which may cause twisting of the fundus and postoperative symptoms.

This study raises questions of efficacy of the fundoplication in patients primarily with atypical symptoms of pulmonary nature, pharyngolaryngeal complications or non-cardiac chest pain. So et al., in their study of 35 patients with atypical symptoms (Abstract 10–1), found improvement in 78%, 58% and 48% of patients with laryngeal, pulmonary or chest pain symptoms, respectively. Although they provide a less optimistic view of their results, these results are highly encouraging. First, one would not expect all patients with asthma or esophageal spasm to improve with an antireflux procedure. Furthermore, failure to improve in this report was studied with upper gastrointestinal series rather than 24 hour hydrogen ion concentration because of patient refusal. The former test is well documented to be an adequate test to evaluate patients for reflux. Therefore, one cannot exclude the possibility that some of the patient failures with atypical symptoms were due to failure of the procedures to control reflux. In conclusion, it appears that laparoscopic antireflux surgery is an excellent treatment alternative for patients with symptomatic GERD and should be offered to patients with typical and atypical symptoms. The major caveat to this statement is that patients with atypical symptoms must recognize that the success rate for eliminating their atypical symptoms is only 50% to 75%, but 95% for heartburn and regurgitation.

J.F. Amaral, M.D.

Does Laparoscopic Cardiomyotomy Require an Antireflux Procedure?

Kumar V, Shimi SM, Cuschieri A (Univ of Dundee, Scotland)

Endoscopy 30:8-11, 1998 10–3

Introduction.—There is controversy regarding the use of an antireflux wrap after cardiomyotomy for achalasia. The high incidence of gastroesophageal reflux after open procedure has been blamed on undue mobilization of the esophageal junction with damage to the attachments, especially the phrenoesophageal membrane. The Dundee technique limits the mobilization to the anterior wall of the abdominal and thoracic esophagus. Patient outcome was described in a consecutive series of 19 patients treated by laparoscopic cardiomyotomy using the Dundee technique.

Methods.—Patients were prospectively followed up for long-term relief of dysphagia and postoperative incidence of reflux symptoms, with or without esophagitis.

Results.—At a median of 27 months (range, 15-53 months), 12 patients had total relief and 5 had substantial relief from dysphagia (89%). The number of patients experiencing heartburn increased from 4 of 15 to 5 of 15 at a mean follow-up of 27 months. Endoscopically proved esophagitis developed in 1 patient, and was associated with a positive esophageal pH monitoring test.

Conclusions.—The routine use of an antireflux procedure is not justified in patients undergoing laparoscopic cardiomyotomy, as long as the lateral and posterior attachment of the esophagus are kept intact.

▶ Although debate exists, reflux after cardiomyotomy is a well-recognized complication of the procedure, especially when performed transabdominally, and clinical rates of 5% to 10% are common. Furthermore, most experimental models of reflux rely on performance of a cardiomyotomy. Therefore, many believe reflux occurs in 100% of patients after cardiomyotomy, but only a few patients become clinically symptomatic.

In this study, the authors have explored the possibility that the incident reflux is secondary to disruption of the phrenoesophageal ligaments, as has been proposed by those favoring a transthoracic approach. In their technique, they only mobilize the anterior esophagus and perform a short, 3-4 cm myotomy. Postoperatively, they have noted a 6.7% incidence of heartburn, an 11% incidence of failure. An additional 26% of patients had moderate postoperative dysphagia. These results for heartburn compare favorably with those for transthoracic or transabdominal procedures, but postoperative failure or dysphagia may be higher than with the other procedures.

Clearly, this study raises more questions than it answers because of its nonrandomized prospective nature, but it does support myotomy without fundoplication. However, it is hard to believe that complete division of the lower esophageal sphincter (LES) under any circumstances does not lead to reflux. Furthermore, one wonders what the incidence of postoperative paraesophageal hernia formation will be, given a partially anchored LES and open hiatus. Looks like the perfect operation to produce one.

J.F. Amaral, M.D.

Delayed Primary Repair of Esophageal Atresia With Tracheoesophageal Fistula: Is It Worth the Wait?

Healey PJ, Sawin RS, Hall DG, et al (Univ of Washington, Seattle)

Arch Surg 133:552-556, 1998 10–4

Objective.—Management of esophageal atresia (EA) in premature infants with respiratory distress syndrome (RDS) or associated congenital abnormalities is complicated by the fact that these infants may not tolerate lung retraction or long operation time. A long gap may preclude primary anastomosis or carry an increased risk of anastomotic complications, recurrent tracheoesophageal fistula (TEF), or gastroesophageal reflux (GER). The best approach to management of these patients is characterized in a review of a cohort of patients with EA and TEF.

Methods.—Between February 1986 and January 1997, EA or TEF was diagnosed in 118 newborn infants. Of these, 88 had primary repair of EA and TEF within 48 hours of birth and 30 had delayed primary esophageal repair. Delayed repair was performed in 23 children when the proximal pouch was below the thoracic inlet or the RDS resolved. Patient survival, incidence of anastomotic complications, recurrent TEF, and clinically significant GER were determined.

Results.—Of the 19 infants who survived to undergo delayed reconstruction, repair was successful in 18; of these, 3 also underwent an elongating myotomy. Rates of anastomotic stricture (16.6% vs. 12.0%), leak (11.0% vs. 2.3%), recurrent TEF (5.5% vs. 2.3%), GER (22.2% vs. 14.7%), and need for fundoplication (11.1% vs. 2.3%) were similar for both the delayed and primary repair groups. Patients with RDS or cardiac complications were hospitalized between procedures. After 3 months, primary esophageal anastomosis was achievable in all patients with a long-gap EA or an upper esophageal pouch. Three of 10 patients were cared for at home between procedures. Elongation of the upper pouch was not attempted during the interval between procedures. There is some esophageal lengthening that results from tacking the pouch to the vertebral fascia. GER, observed on contrast radiography in all patients, probably contributed to the growth of the distal esophageal segment. Most of the patients who died had severe cardiac lesions.

Conclusion.—All children with EA and TEF can undergo esophageal repair. Almost all of the patients who died had significant cardiac lesions.

► Throughout the world and on the Internet, the same question reverberates regarding delayed primary repair of the esophagus. Over the past decade, this delayed method has become popularized in the face of what were considered disappointing results with esophageal substitution. These authors have presented another set of patients upon which to evaluate the feasibility and outcome of delayed repair. They further extend their observations into the length of time that is required for esophageal elongation before repair, as well as the spectrum of patients who had to remain hospitalized. The complication rate is extremely low, owing to their meticulous attention to the patient's physiology rather than a focus on the defect. What is not answered by this article, and something that we hope will be understood in the future via perhaps a meta-analysis, is an accurate determination of when further esophageal growth can no longer be expected. In other words, should repair uniformly take place after 3 months, or for extremely long-gap patients will further growth occur with nonoperative management? Healthcare providers will need to analyze home care resources to allow more of these infants to go home. This field remains wide open for physical and occupational therapists who will have to deal with long-term swallowing difficulties from delayed feeding and esophageal dysmotility.

T.F. Tracy, Jr., M.D.

Durability of Laparoscopic Repair of Paraesophageal Hernia

Edye MB, Canin-Endres J, Gattorno F, et al (Mount Sinai Med Ctr, New York)

Ann Surg 228:528-535, 1998 10–5

Objective.—Laparoscopic repair of paraesophageal hernia is becoming more common; however, there is little information regarding the duration and long-term benefits of the repair and the benefit of routine inclusion of an antireflux procedure. The primary repair that would minimize hernia recurrence and the results of medium-term follow-up of paraesophageal hernia repair to verify durability and assess the effect of inclusion of an antireflux procedure were presented.

Methods.—Primary esophageal hernia repair was performed laparoscopically in 55 patients by 2 surgeons. Patients were followed for an average of 29 months.

Results.—There were 49 patients (average age, 68 years) available for follow-up. The first 25 patients did not undergo sac excision. Type III or IV hernia was found in 38 patients (76%) and fundoplication in 22 (44%). A 360-degree Nissen fundoplication was performed in 30 patients and a partial Toupet fundoplication in 7. Hernia recurred in 5 patients within 2 months of surgery, and 3 underwent open revision. Two patients had small type I recurrences at follow-up that were treated with medication. Two patients had persistent dysphagia requiring repeated esophageal dilations for 1 and hiatal parahernia repair for the other. A total of 11 patients (22%) had mild-to-moderate reflux, and 15 were taking acid-reducing medications. Thirteen of the latter patients had undergone 360-degree fundoplication.

Conclusion.—Laparoscopic repair of paraesophageal hernia was durable in most patients. Inclusion of an antireflux procedure had no effect on the incidence of reflux symptoms. Morbidity was low, with only 2 patients experiencing dysphagia.

► Laparoscopic repair for paraesophageal hernias is becoming common, despite the fact that data on long-term results is lacking. The authors have concluded that because very few patients had dyspeptic complaints in a mean follow-up of 29 months after repair, the laparoscopic repair for paraesophageal hernia was durable. The lack of a postsurgical reflux, however, should not be construed as sufficient to exclude recurrence. Postoperative barium swallows were not obtained in this cohort of patients. The strength of this article is in the description of the operative procedure, where complete removal of the sac and adequate crural closure are emphasized. These technical points should decrease recurrence rates.

W.G. Cioffi, M.D.

The Development of Dysplasia and Adenocarcinoma During Endoscopic Surveillance of Barrett's Esophagus

Katz D, Rothstein R, Schned A, et al (VA Med Ctr, White River Junction, Vt; Univ of Wisconsin, Madison; Dartmouth Hitchcock Med Ctr, Lebanon, NH; et al)

Am J Gastroenterol 93:536-541, 1998 10–6

Background.—Most esophageal adenocarcinomas probably arise from premalignant Barrett's esophagus. Improved management of Barrett's esophagus may have a significant impact on esophageal carcinoma, which has a poor prognosis and is increasing in incidence. Dysplasia is the best available indicator of malignant potential in Barrett's epithelium, but little is known about the natural history of this finding. The development of dysplasia in Barrett's esophagus, including the associated risk factors, was examined.

Methods.—One hundred two patients with endoscopically diagnosed Barrett's esophagus associated with specialized columnar epithelium were included in the study. All patients underwent 2 or more upper gastrointestinal endoscopic surveillance examinations between 1970 and 1994. Specimens showing any degree of atypia were blindly reviewed by two pathologists to determine the grade of dysplasia. The time to initial diagnosis of dysplasia was calculated, and associated risk factors were assessed.

Results.—Total follow-up was 563 patient-years, with a median of 4.8 years per patient. Three cases of adenocarcinoma were detected after 4 or more years of follow-up. Another case of adenocarcinoma of the cardia was detected incidentally. Low-grade dysplasia developed during follow-up in 19 patients, and high-grade dysplasia developed in 4. Dysplasia was more likely to develop in patients with dyspepsia. There were no cases of dysplasia among patients who had undergone antireflux surgery.

Conclusions.—This follow-up study found a 7% rate of low-grade dysplasia developing within 2 years in patients with nondysplastic Barrett's esophagus. High-grade dysplasia and adenocarcinoma took more than 2 years to develop. Antireflux surgery may have a protective effect against progression to dysplasia. However, the study included only a small number of patients who underwent antireflux surgery; furthermore, proton pump inhibitors were used only during the latter part of follow-up.

Complete Elimination of Reflux Symptoms Does Not Guarantee Normalization of Intraesophageal Acid Reflux in Patients With Barrett's Esophagus

Ouatu-Lascar R, Triadafilopoulos G (Palo Alto Veterans Affairs Health Care System, Calif; Stanford Univ, Calif)

Am J Gastroenterol 93:711-716, 1998 10–7

Introduction.—Various treatments for Barrett's esophagus may lead to partial regression, with the development of areas of squamous tissue within the Barrett's epithelium. Experimental evidence suggests that proliferation of Barrett's epithelium increases in response to short pulses of acid exposure, indicating the importance of powerful acid-suppressive therapy. Sensitivity to acid is reduced for patients with Barrett's esophagus, which may make symptoms an unreliable indicator of the degree of acid reflux. Intraesophageal hydrogen ion concentration (pH) monitoring was used to compare reflux symptoms with the degree of normalization of acid reflux.

Methods.—Thirty patients with reflux symptoms and Barrett's esophagus were included in the study. All received treatment with lansoprazole, 15 to 30 mg/day, to eliminate their symptoms. During this period when the patients were asymptomatic and receiving medication, they underwent ambulatory 24-hour pH monitoring. The study definition of acid reflux was a reduction in pH in the distal esophagus to 4.0 or less. Esophageal manometry was performed as well.

Results.—Forty percent of patients had pathologic reflux, despite the absence of symptoms. The recorded reflux was bipositional and moderately severe, with a mean DeMeester score of 52.8. The remaining 60% of patients had normal esophageal pH, with a DeMeester score of 4.5. The incomplete elimination of reflux was related to inadequate acid suppression by the medication. Dual-channel recordings showed that acid exposure was greater in the distal esophagus than in the proximal esophagus. Patients with and without continued acid reflux were similar in terms of pretreatment symptoms, lansoprazole dosage necessary to achieve asymptomatic status, length of Barrett's esophagus, presence of hiatal hernia, lower esophageal sphincter resting tone and length, and esophageal peristaltic function.

Conclusions.—In patients with Barrett's esophagus, elimination of symptoms does not necessarily mean elimination of esophageal acid reflux.

To achieve complete acid suppression, these patients should undergo 24-hour ambulatory pH studies for titration to high-dose proton pump inhibition.

Long-term Results of Classic Antireflux Surgery in 152 Patients With Barrett's Esophagus: Clinical, Radiologic, Endoscopic, Manometric, and Acid Reflux Test Analysis Before and Late After Operation

Csendes A, Braghetto I, Burdiles P, et al (Univ of Chile, Santiago, José Joaquín Aquirre Hosp, Santiago, Chile)

Surgery 123:645-657, 1998 10–8

Objective.—Nissen fundoplication and Hill's posterior gastropexy with calibration of the cardia have been the classic open surgical procedures for patients with gastroesophageal reflux. Reported success rates are high, but little is known about the outcomes of patients with Barrett's esophagus. The late results of open antireflux surgery in patients with Barrett's esophagus were studied, including clinical and laboratory results.

Methods.—One hundred fifty-two patients with Barrett's esophagus were included in a prospective study. Forty-nine percent of the patients had uncomplicated Barrett's esophagus; this group had specialized columnar epithelium covering at least 3 cm of the distal esophagus, but no stricture, ulcer, or dysplasia. The remaining 51% of the patients had strictures or ulcers, though none had dysplasia or adenocarcinoma. The patients were followed up for more than 100 months.

Results.—On preoperative radiologic studies, most patients had hiatal hernia and free reflux, with dilation of the gastroesophageal junction. Standard acid reflux was positive in all 123 patients in whom it was performed. There was 1 postoperative death. At late follow-up, the surgical failure rate (i.e., Visick grade III or IV) was 54% in patients with uncomplicated Barrett's esophagus and 64% in those with complicated Barrett's esophagus. Three to 6 percent of patients had severe endoscopic recurrence with no clinical signs. For the complicated group, recurrences started early and became progressively more frequent in the years after surgery. Low-grade dysplasia occurred at least 7 years after surgery, always in association with a symptomatic recurrence. There were 4 cases of adenocarcinoma occurring 7 years after surgery, all in patients with complicated Barrett's esophagus.

Conclusions.—This prospective study documents a high failure rate among patients with Barrett's esophagus undergoing classic antireflux surgery. These patients may need more aggressive surgery than bile diversion procedures. Antireflux surgery in patients with Barrett's esophagus reduces, but does not eliminate, acid and alkaline reflux. Because these patients also have impaired esophageal clearance, a small number of reflux episodes may produce more damage than the appearance of dysplasia or adenocarcinoma.

► Is Barrett's esophagus an indication for antireflux surgery? The article by Katz and colleagues (Abstract 10–6) sheds light on this important question in an era of increasing esophageal carcinoma. Although the authors fail to prove a protective effect for antireflux surgery because of the methodologic flaws they discuss, their results are impressive. As shown in Fig 2 of the original article, patients who had a prior antireflux procedure had a zero risk for development of dysplasia, whereas more than 40% without surgery developed dysplasia. In my opinion, these data certainly argue that Barrett's esophagus should be an indication for antireflux surgery until proved otherwise rather than vice versa.

In this regard, antagonists will argue that patients with Barrett's who have undergone antireflux surgery can still develop dysplasia and adenocarcinoma. Indeed, Csendes et al. (Abstract 10–8) show in their study of this very question that 54% of patients with uncomplicated Barrett's and 64% of patients with complicated Barrett's develop dysplasia late after the operation, giving support to this argument. However, what is more important is that all these patients were surgical failures when studied with a 24-hour hydrogen ion concentration (pH), that is, the 24 pH failed. Therefore, they had no protection from acid or alkaline reflux. Interestingly, the authors attribute their results to delayed clearance of the esophagus in Barrett's and some undisclosed mechanism that makes patients more susceptible to failure. Actually, their results show by manometry that their operation at 5 years was not as effective as those with reflux than in those without. Why it failed, however, may have something to do with the Barrett's, since such a rate of failure is not typical with antireflux surgery in general.

A final and important point raised by Csendes is that patients with Barrett's may develop dysplasia without symptoms of reflux. Indeed, Ouatu-Lascar and Triadafilopoulos document in their study (Abstract 10–7) that patients with Barrett's esophagus are less sensitive to acid exposure than patients without Barrett's esophagus and that complete eradication of symptoms does not signal a normal intraesophageal pH.

Taken together, these studies suggest a properly functioning fundoplication that prevents greater than 10% acid exposure is likely to prevent progression of Barrett's to dysplasia. Furthermore, patients with Barrett's esophagus who do undergo antireflux surgery should not only undergo endoscopic but also 24 pH surveillance at 2-year intervals. Therefore, until someone proves otherwise, my patients with Barrett's esophagus will all be offered this treatment plan.

J.F. Amaral, M.D.

p53 Sequence Analysis Predicts Treatment Response and Outcome of Patients With Esophageal Carcinoma

Ribeiro U Jr, Finkelstein SD, Safatle-Ribeiro AV, et al (Univ of Pittsburgh, Pa; Univ of Chicago)

Cancer 83:7-18, 1998 10–9

Introduction.—The ability to predict biological aggressiveness and treatment response by tissue analysis in patients with esophageal carcinoma could be invaluable. Whether alterations of the p53 gene correlate with clinicopathologic parameters, response to preoperative chemotherapy/radiotherapy, and survival was determined in 42 patients with esophageal carcinoma by using topographic genotyping.

Methods.—Tumor specimens underwent histopathologic/genetic analysis of p53 on formalin-fixed, paraffin-embedded tissues. Tissue specimens underwent immunohistochemical staining for p53 protein, then topographic genotyping via polymerase chain reaction amplification and direct sequencing of p53 exons 5-8. All patients were treated with chemotherapy and radiotherapy.

Results.—Seventeen of 42 tumors (40.5%) contained p53 point mutational change in exons 8, 5, 7, and 6, respectively, in 5, 5, 4, and 3 patients, respectively. Eight tumors were weakly immunopositive and had no genotype mutation, suggesting hyperexpression of normal wild-type p53. Genotyping detected 2 immunonegative tumors with deletion-type mutations (exons 5 and 6). Tissue samples obtained before and after chemotherapy/radiotherapy showed fidelity in p53 mutational genotype in all patients. The presence of a p53 point mutation was positively associated with pTNM stage and residual disease in the resected specimen. Survival of patients with p53 mutations was significantly lower, compared with patients with no p53 mutations (overall survival, 21.6 months vs. 40 months; disease-free survival, 14.1 months vs. 38 months).

Conclusions.—Histopathologic/genetic analysis is superior to immunohistochemistry alone in determining p53 mutational change. It may be used as a prognostic marker for esophageal carcinoma. The p53 genotyping may help define a subset of patients who may respond to chemotherapy/radiotherapy and may predict which patients may benefit from multimodality therapy.

► In this paper, p53 analysis was performed on 42 tumors from patients with potentially resectable esophageal carcinoma. In 59.5% of the patients, the tumors were p53 immunopositive. The presence of a p53 point mutation positively correlated with the pTNM stage and residual disease in the resected specimen. Moreover, survival of patients with p53 mutations was significantly lower than that without mutations; the overall survival was 21.6 months vs. 40 months and the disease-free survival, 14.1 months vs. 38 months. The authors concluded that histologic and genetic analysis is a better determinant of p53 mutational damage than immunohistochemistry alone, and can be used as a prognostic marker for esophageal carcinoma.

Taken together, these 2 papers (Abstracts 10–9 and 10–10) clearly demonstrate the role of p53 mutational changes as an important determinant in the development and possible response to chemotherapy for patients with esophageal carcinoma. It may very well be that p53 genotyping will define a subset of patients who will respond to chemotherapy and radiation therapy, and may predict potential benefits from multimodality therapy.

A very useful outcome of these studies will be to apply p53 sequence analysis to patients who have been previously resected or who have Barrett's esophagus and severe dyplasia. These results would suggest that those patients with p53 point mutations and the presence of p53 in the resected specimens would likely mandate more intensive and closer follow-up postoperatively.

H.H. Simms, M.D.

Anti-p53 Antibodies in Patients With Barrett's Esophagus or Esophageal Carcinoma Can Predate Cancer Diagnosis

Cawley HM, Meltzer SJ, De Benedetti VMG, et al (Natl Cancer Inst, Bethesda, Md; Univ of Maryland, Baltimore; German Cancer Research Ctr, Heidelberg, Germany)

Gastroenterology 115:19-27, 1998 10–10

Introduction.—The p53 tumor-suppressor gene is the most frequently altered gene in human cancer. It sometimes produces immunogenic protein that is usually concomitant with either missense mutations in the highly conserved regions of the DNA, nuclear accumulation of p53 protein, or both. Most trials of p53 have focused on patients with late-stage neoplastic disease. There is a relationship between p53 mutation, p53 protein accumulation, and p53 antibody (Ab) in esophageal cancer. It is possible that p53-Ab appears before diagnosis of cancer. Because esophageal cancer is usually detected late, this may help identify high-risk patients. The prevalence and timing of p53-Ab in the plasma were determined in 88 serially endoscoped men with Barrett's metaplasia, squamous cell carcinoma, or adenocarcinoma of the esophagus, or with neither cancer nor Barrett's metaplasia.

Methods.—Venipuncture was performed at the time of endoscopy. Serum samples underwent enzyme immunoassay, immunoblotting, and immunoprecipitation assays for p53 antibodies; polymerase chain reaction, denaturant gradient gel electrophoresis, and sequencing for p53 mutations; and immunohistochemistry of p53 protein.

Results.—Of 88 patients; p53 antibodies were found in 4 patients with Barrett's esophagus, including 1 with dysplasia that later progressed to adenocarcinoma; and 10 patients with cancer (8 squamous, 2 adenocarcinoma). Of 10 patients with cancer, 2 had antibodies before cancer diagnosis (1 squamous, 1 adenocarcinoma). Six patients with antibody-positive cancer had p53 mutations. Two patients with cancer and 1 patient with Barrett's esophagus who were antibody-positive had p53 overexpression in esophageal tissues.

Conclusions.—Clinical diagnosis of malignancy may be predated by the presence of p53 antibodies in patients with Barrett's esophagus and esophageal cancer.

► In this article, the authors have investigated these p53 antibodies to detect mutational changes in patients with Barrett's esophagus. The study was performed in 88 serially endoscoped patients: 36 with Barrett's metaplasia, 23 with esophageal squamous or carcinoma, 10 with esophageal adenocarcinoma, and 19 with esophagitis or normal esophagus. The authors have demonstrated p53 antibodies were detected in 4 patients with Barrett's esophagus, including one with dysplasia that later progressed to adenocarcinoma, and in 10 patients with cancer 2 of whom had antibodies before cancer was diagnosed. Six antibody-positive cancer patients had p53 mutations, whereas 2 patients with cancer or Barrett's esophagus with antibodies had p53 protein overexpressed in esophageal tissue. The authors have concluded that patients with Barrett's esophagus or esophageal cancer can have p53 antibodies develop that may predate the clinical diagnosis of malignancy.

H.H. Simms, M.D.

► Cawley and associates of the National Cancer Institute reiterate that anti-p53 antibodies may predate cancer diagnosis in subjects at increased carcinoma risk for liver, lung, breast, and prostate neoplasms. This analysis used immunoassay, immunoblotting, and immunoprecipitation assays for the p53 antibody, with PCR to complete immunohistochemistry for p53 protein. The authors conclude that the p53 antibody may predate the clinical appearance of neoplasms in patients with Barrett's esophagus and esophageal carcinoma.

These data were completed using 3 independent laboratory assays in a series of 88 patients who were screened by endoscopy for cancer or Barrett's esophagus; of interest, p53 antibody was evident in only 11 patients with cancer and 4 without same. The p53-antibody positivity was evident in 36% of patients with squamous carcinoma and 27% with adenocarcinoma. Of 36 patients in the series with Barrett's metaplasia, 8% had p53-antibody.

Overall, the prevalence of this mutation in esophageal carcinoma is approximately half of the patients studied. The p53-antibody detection assays therefore achieved a low sensitivity (0.33) and a small positive predictive value of only 73%. with specificity of 93%.

I agree that these prognostic indicators increase the probability that positive results in patients *without* cancer diagnosis may be important evidence of the presence of p53 mutations that connote an increased risk for malignancy. It would appear that future studies of p53-antibody would be useful because this may be a mechanism to identify a subset of tumors with an aggressive phenotype for premalignant or malignant transformation of esophageal diseases. Moreover, these initial data support the application of increasing numbers of studies that confirm risk for large populations of patients who have esophageal metaplasia of the Barrett's type.

K.I. Bland, M.D.

Gallbladder, Bile Ducts, Liver, and Pancreas

INTRODUCTION

The introduction and rapid acceptance of laparoscopic cholecystectomy for cholecystitis in the past decade came after confirming the procedure as being less invasive, giving patients a shorter length of hospital stay, and showing morbidity and mortality equivalent to that of open procedures. Nonetheless, the most serious consequence of laparoscopic or open cholecystectomy, aside from death, is injury to the common ducts. In the 1998 YEAR BOOK OF SURGERY, the article by Savader and associates[1] was reviewed. The subject of biliary duct injury and a definition of its management was further defined by these investigators and is important for the following reasons: (1) laparoscopic procedures exceed those done by the open technique by approximately 4 to 10:1; (2) more than 500,000 cholecystectomies are performed per year in the United States alone, with a complication rate of 0.30% to 0.60%, suggesting that 1,500 to 3,000 operations manifest significant bile duct injury; (3) common duct injuries are technically difficult to treat and will accentuate cost-interventional or surgical procedures, or both; (4) the minimally invasive nature of the laparoscopic approach may broaden indications for cholecystectomy and further increase the total number of procedures performed; (5) therapy of common bile duct injuries often requires postoperative stenting for up to 1 year, with resultant long-term morbidity; and (6) the long-term overall morbidity may be accentuated by nonmonetary issues such as hospitalization time, travel, and loss in quality of life. As a consequence of these considerations, Savader and associates concluded that repair of the laparoscopic cholecystectomy-related bile duct injury costs from 4.5 to 26 times that of the uncomplicated open approach and incurs significant mortality. Moreover, intraoperative recognition of such injuries requires immediate conversion to open procedure for definitive repair to decrease mortality, morbidity, cost, length of hospitalization, and the number of outpatient care days.

Abstract 10–11 by Kiviluoto and associates examined the role of laparoscopic cholecystectomy in acute cholecystitis. This procedure in the acute setting has remained controversial, mainly because of concern for the above outcomes as indicated with regard to bile duct injuries and additional complications. With its first introduction, laparoscopic cholecystectomy was considered contraindicated in acute cholecystitis by Cuschieri et al.[2] and by Reddick et al.[3] Operating surgeons feel comfortable with laparoscopic techniques; more recently, acute (nongangrenous) cholecystectomy was considered an appropriate presentation that could be accomplished with laparoscopic approaches. These authors undertook a randomized comparison of the safety and outcomes of the laparoscopic vs. open cholecystectomy in patients with acute and gangrenous cholecystitis presentations. As with any procedure, technical expertise, competency, and recognition of injury are the salient features to avoid morbidity and mortality. The operator should have a low threshold for conversion to the open technique should potential injury be recognized or exist intraoperatively. Nonetheless, this randomized trial puts to rest the dogma that acute or gangrenous cholecystitis is unsafely performed with the laparoscopic approach.

With the introduction and widespread use of laparoscopic surgery have come the widespread applications of monopolar electrosurgery. Trondsen and coworkers (Abstract 10–12) provide the operator the "take-home" concept that the applications of high-energy sources, at or near the bile ducts or clips near these anatomical structures, are not only contraindicated but impart an increased probability of injury to the patient. Such inadvertent and inappropriate approaches increase morbidity, mortality, and likely will increase costs and litigation.

The early and late results for excision of choledochal cysts and their neoplastic risk are reviewed by Saing and co-workers and Fieber and Nance (Abstracts 10–13 and 10–14). Careful prolonged follow-up and surveillance are essential for children undergoing choledochal cyst excision with hepaticojejunostomy because various complications, including anastomotic stricture, cholangitis, and intrahepatic stone formation, are evident with the procedure. In addition to these complications, choledochal cysts are prone to development of biliary cirrhosis, portal hypertension, rupture, pancreatitis, as well as carcinoma. Abstract 10–14 evaluated an extensive series (n = 106) of patients with choledochal cysts. Neoplastic transformation has previously been observed in 2.5% to 26% of cases. There is a propensity for malignancy to occur anywhere in the biliary tract or the gallbladder or pancreas, concurrent with choledochal cysts. This pathogenetic basis postulated by the authors follows the contiguous relationship of other organ system cancers to the origin of the cyst. Endoscopic retrograde cholangiopancreatography (ERCP), CT scan, and genetic markers may allow investigators to define patients at risk and the early surveillance information essential for diagnosis of transformation to malignant states. We would disagree that the empiric application of biliary pancreaticoduodenectomy should be considered a prophylactic measure for such presentations. Moreover, the abdominal organ cluster resection and transplantation appears to be a radical departure, rather than a solution (palliation) for this rare neoplasm.

The rare disorder of Byler's disease (progressive, familial, intrahepatic cholestasis) was studied by Hollands and co-workers (Abstract 10–15). While most cases of hepatocellular cholestasis in infants are initiated by hepatitis, inborn errors of bile acid synthesis, drugs, total parenteral nutrition, or alpha-1 antitrypsin deficiency,[4] Byler's disease is a less-common variant of hepatocellular cholestasis. As reported by Poley,[5] Byler's disease occurs with an incidence of 1 in 90,000 births and an inheritance that is autosomally recessive with variable penetrance. Hollands and co-workers describe a terminal ileal exclusion technique first developed for patients who had previously undergone cholecystectomy. Previously, surgical therapy has included partial biliary diversion and orthotopic liver transplantation. Moreover, partial biliary diversion has been accomplished by cholecystojejunal-cutaneous conduits, cutaneous cholecystoappendicostomy[6] and by ileal bypass.[7] Results of partial biliary diversion have been promising for ameliorating pruritis and for possibly reversing progressive liver disease. Clearly, ileal exclusion or bypass has offered some advantages over liver transplantation and cutaneous biliary diversions. In this article, 80% of children so treated with ileal exclusion have had relief from their pruritis and self-mutilation, with no evidence of diarrhea. This terminal ileal bypass procedure offers a stoma-free, completely reversible "biliary" diversion. Unequivocally, these results will require long-term follow-up before the procedure is advocated as the primary therapy for Byler's disease.

Allan O. Whipple[8] provided intellectual insight into the physiologic events of variceal bleeding in the 1940s when nonselective portosystemic shunts were introduced. In 1967, Dean Warren and Robert Zeppa[9] introduced the concept of *selective* variceal decompression by means of the distal splenorenal shunt. These innovations followed the often ill-fated and technically difficult approaches that were antecedent to these shunts, including side-to-side portocaval, end-to-side portocaval, and proximal splenorenal shunts. Thereafter, in 1973, Sugiura and Futagawa[10] reported on a large series of patients treated with esophagogastric devascularization that had been combined with splenectomy. Thus, surgery has been the principal definitive management of the entity since the 1940s, until the 1970s when endoscopic sclerotherapy was introduced.

Transient obstruction of the ampulla of Vater by biliary calculi is considered the etiology of gallstone pancreatitis. The management of suspected common bile duct stones co-existing with pancreatitis, remains controversial. Fan et al.[11] have previously recommended urgent ERCP in all cases to reduce the incidence of cholangitis. deVirgilio and associates[12] had previously demonstrated that performing preoperative ERCP in all patients with gallstone pancreatitis is unnecessary because only 7% had clinical evidence of cholangitis. In such a setting, urgent ERCP may be limited only to patients with clinical evidence of cholangitis. The latter procedure can be performed with no mortality and only limited complications. In Abstracts 10–16 and 10–17, it is evident that cholangitis is an uncommon accompaniment of gallstone pancreatitis, and the best clinical predictor of persistent common bile duct stones continues to be the serum total bilirubin.

In modern practice, the majority of patients with pancreatitis of gallstone origin would be afforded ERCP prior to intraoperative cholangiography to delineate anatomy of the ducts, and to perform sphincterotomy with extraction of common bile duct stones. This procedure is perhaps best performed within the first 48 hours of scheduled elective cholecystectomy. An additional bench research analysis for the role of cytokines is included by Dunn and associates (Abstract 10–17), to define the pathogenesis of acute pancreatitis. The sequence of events that surround activation of acute pancreatitis remains obscure and complex. This study is the first that demonstrates increased NF-κB activity is evident in acute pancreatitis. Moreover, this study suggests an increase in both tumor necrosis factor α and NF-κB over a similar time course in pancreatic tissue after the induction of acute pancreatitis. This and other studies continue to address the mechanisms for induction of pancreatitis by inhibition of this or other cytokines to see if such interventions correlate with clinical improvement in pancreatitis. These and other genetic modifications, which inhibit the cytokine cascade, may offer potential therapeutic interventions for the therapy of this highly morbid and potentially lethal malady.

To address the issues of chronic pain associated with chronic pancreatitis, McHale and associates (Abstract 10-18) presented the results of surgical attempts to relieve this chronic state. Pseudocyst drainage, sphincteroplasty, or Peustow pancreaticojejunostomy procedures were considered for patients with anatomic pathology causing duct dilatation. The application of these techniques vs. denervation procedures in the absence of duct dilatation suggests that surgical management provided marked relief for 68% of patients. While neither procedure was considered superior to the other, such approaches may be offered to patients with refractory chronic pancreatitis who require traditional narcotic and pain management sequences for their ill-fated outcomes. Long-term follow-up of prospective data for these approaches is essential to provide clinicians with firm recommendations for the management of chronic pancreatitis.

Kirby I. Bland, M.D.

References

1. Saveder SJ, Lillemoe KD, Prescott CA, et al: Laparoscopic cholecystectomy-related bile duct injuries: A health and financial disaster. *Ann Surg* 225:268-273, 1997.
2. Cuschieri A, Dubois F, Mouiel J, et al: The European experience with laparoscopic cholecystectomy. *Am J Surg* 161:385-387, 1991.
3. Reddick EJ, Olsen D, Spaw A, et al: Safe performance of difficult laparoscopic cholecystectomies. *Am J Surg* 161:377-381, 1991.
4. Whitington PF: Chronic cholestasis of infancy. *Ped Clin NA* 43:1-26, 1996.
5. Poley JR: Progressive familial intrahepatic cholestasis with cirrhosis and fatal outcome (Byler disease), in Anderson CM, Burke V, Gracey M (eds): *Paediatric Gastroenterology*. Oxford, Blackwell Scientific, 1987, pp 550-551.
6. Gauderer MWL, Boyle JT. Cholecystoappendicostomy in a child with Alagille syndrome. J Pediatr Surg 32:166-167, 1997.
7. Whitington PF, Whitington GI: Partial external diversion of bile for the treatment of intractable pruritus associated with intrahepatic cholestasis. *Gastroenterology* 95:130-136, 1988.
8. Whipple AO: The problem of portal hypertension in relation to the hepatosplenopathies. Ann Surg 122:449-475, 1945.
9. Warren WD, Zeppa R, Fomon JJ: Selective transsplenic decompression of gastroesophageal varices by distal splenorenal shunt. *Ann Surg* 166:437-455, 1967.
10. Sugiura M, Futagawa S: A new technique for treating esophageal varices. *J Thorac Cardiovasc Surg* 66:677-685, 1973.
11. Fan ST, Lai EC, Mok FP, et al: Early treatment of acute biliary pancreatitis by endoscopic papillotomy. *N Engl J Med* 328:228-232, 1993.
12. de Virgilio C, Verbin C, Chang L, et al: Gallstone pancreatitis: The role of preoperative endoscopic retrograde cholangiopancreatography. *Arch Surg* 129:909-913, 1994.

Randomised Trial of Laparoscopic Versus Open Cholecystectomy for Acute and Gangrenous Cholecystitis

Kiviluoto T, Sirén J, Luukkonen P, et al (Helsinki Univ Central Hosp)
Lancet 351:321-325, 1998 10–11

Introduction.—Laparoscopic cholecystectomy (LC) is the surgical approach of choice for elective cholecystectomy. Its use in acute cholecystitis is controversial. Opinions about LC for acute cholecystitis have been based on retrospective investigation. The safety and outcome of LC vs. open cholecystectomy (OC) in patients with acute cholecystitis were evaluated.

Methods.—Sixty-three patients with acute cholecystitis were randomly assigned to OC or LC (31 and 32 patients, respectively). Patients were followed up for hospital mortality and morbidity, length of hospital stay, and length of sick leave from work. For suspected bile duct stones, patients in the LC group underwent preoperative endoscopic retrograde cholangiography; patients in the OC group underwent intraoperative cholangiography.

Results.—Forty-eight percent and 59%, respectively, of patients from the OC and LC groups were older than 60 years. Both groups had 13 patients with gangrene or empyema and 1 patient with perforation of the gallbladder causing diffuse peritonitis. Five patients (16%) in the LC group were converted to OC because of severe inflammation that distorted the anatomy of Calot's triangle. There were no deaths or bile duct lesions in the LC or OC groups. Postoperative complications were significantly higher in the OC than LC group. Seven (23%) and 6 (19%) patients, respectively, had major and minor complications after OC, compared with 1 (3%) minor complication after LC. The postoperative hospital stay was significantly shorter in the LC than OC group. The mean length of sick leave was shorter for patients in the LC than OC group (13.9 vs. 30.1 days).

Conclusions.—Laparoscopic cholecystectomy in patients with acute and gangrenous cholecystitis is technically demanding. In experienced hands, this can be a safe and effective procedure without increasing mortality or morbidity. A moderately high conversion rate is to be expected. The complication rate for OC in patients older than 60 years was comparable with earlier patient series. Patients in the LC group had no major complications, even though both groups had similarly high proportions of patients older than 60 years.

► Initial descriptions of LC relegated acute cholecystitis to treatment with the open approach. The reasons for this were, primarily, the surgeons' lack of experience, and secondarily, difficulty with anatomy. Those who treat acute cholecystitis via the laparoscopic approach, however, usually find the procedure easier on the patient and the surgeon, when compared with the open approach.

This well-designed randomized study by Kiviluoto and co-workers confirms the superiority of LC for acute cholecystitis over the open approach. Significant benefits were observed in all parameters evaluated. Furthermore, the procedure did not take any longer when performed via the laparoscopic approach. The higher incidence of conversion experienced by these authors is likely to diminish as surgeons gain more experience with the laparoscopic approach. Furthermore, it is not a reason not to attempt the procedure laparoscopically. Given these results, acute cholecystitis should be stricken from the lists of relative or absolute contraindications to laparoscopy. Furthermore, surgeons can no longer tell their patients that this procedure is not as safe as the open approach, but only that they themselves are not as comfortable with the procedure, or that they lack enough experience.

J.F. Amaral, M.D.

An Experimental Study of Effects of Monopolar Diathermy on the Bile Ducts

Trondsen E, Rosseland AR, Bakka A, et al (Univ of Oslo, Norway; Central Hosp of Akershus, Norway; The Natl Hosp, Norway; et al)

Eur J Surg 164:297-303, 1998 10–12

Introduction.—There is concern that monopolar diathermy may cause bile duct strictures after laparoscopic cholecystectomy. Monopolar diathermy current is believed to be spread diffusely in the tissue from the active electrode to the neutral plate, with increases in temperature being directly proportional to the square of the density of the current. This usually produces only a local effect. Temperature rises with duration of diathermy application. Electricity follows the path of least resistance, and at 1 MHz, conductivity (siemens/m) is 1.4 in bile, 0.3 in liver, and 0.02-0.07 in fat. Unexpected damage to tissue by monopolar diathermy has been reported several centimeters away from the diathermy application site in isolated segments of small bowel in earlier trials. The effect of monopolar diathermy on the bile ducts was assessed in 18 pigs to determine whether diathermy current energy could be distributed along channels of high current conductivity that could increase temperature in the bile duct at a distance from the site of application, or could affect the nutritional vessels of the bile duct.

Methods.—Animals underwent laparotomy with application of diathermy using only the coagulation mode at standard sites along the cystic duct, bile ducts, and a cystic duct containing a metal clip at 3-12 times of 5 seconds' duration at each site. Temperatures were noted at standard measurement points on the bile ducts. Twelve pigs were sacrificed after 3 weeks. Bile ducts were examined for late changes.

Results.—Temperature increases of 4-6°C were observed during 6 of 330 diathermy applications along the cystic duct; 4-18°C in 8 of 126 applications along the common bile duct; and 4-11°C at the clip in 9 of 54 applications. No macroscopic or microscopic changes in the bile ducts were detected.

Conclusions.—Monopolar diathermy caused unexpected distant increases in the temperature of the bile duct walls and at a clip on the cystic duct. This may have occurred because diathermy current energy was distributed along channels of high current conductivity.

▶ The introduction and widespread use of laparoscopy in general surgery have brought heightened awareness of the risks of monopolar electrosurgery. Two areas where electrosurgery has been implicated in postoperative complications with regularity are bile duct injuries during laparoscopic cholecystectomy and hiatal stenosis during laparoscopic Nissen fundoplication. Trondsen and colleagues have investigated whether injuries to the bile ducts may be the result of electric current distributed along the ducts from a distant site. Although they were unable to document rises in temperatures high enough to cause thermal damage to the bile ducts, increases in temperature of the bile duct by as much as 18°C were observed at sites distant to the application. This study reinforces the concept that the pathway the current takes through the body is neither constant nor predictable. In addition, it lends credence to the possibility that injuries can occur at a distant site if the conditions are correct. Finally, the "take-home message" of this important paper is: do not use energy of any type near or on the bile ducts. It is not only unnecessary, but it risks significant injury.

J.F. Amaral, M.D.

Early and Late Results of Excision of Choledochal Cysts

Saing H, Han H, Chan KL, et al (Univ of Hong Kong)

J Pediatr Surg 32:1563-1566, 1997 10–13

Introduction.—Previous reports have described the complications, including anastomotic strictures, intrahepatic stone formation, and cholangitis, after initial drainage procedures for choledochal cysts in children. However, there are few data on the late results after choledochal cyst excison with hepaticojejunostomy. The late results of choledochal cyst excision in 84 patients were reported.

Methods.—Definitive surgery was performed in 79 of 84 patients with choledochal cysts. Internal drainage procedures were performed in 38 patients treated between 1965 and 1972. Subsequently, 41 patients underwent cyst excision and hepaticojejunostomy using a 40-cm Roux limb without an antireflux valve. Cyst excision was done primarily in 39 patients, and secondarily after choledochojejunostomy in 2. Mean follow-up was 8.5 years.

Results.—Internal drainage procedures carried significant morbidity and mortality. In contrast, cyst excision provided excellent results in most cases, with 93% of patients doing well at follow-up. Three patients had intrahepatic stones 2-11 years after cyst excision; these were asymptomatic in 1 case. Additional surgery was required in all 3 cases. There was no mortality among the children managed with cyst excision.

Conclusions.—Good long-term results were reported after choledochal cyst excision in children. Membranous stenoses are thought to play a major role in the development of congenital intrahepatic duct dilation and subsequent intrahepatic stone formation. Stricture and stone formation can develop many years after cyst excision; stones can also form without symptoms and without initial cholangitis. Very high anastomoses are recommended for the prevention of anastomotic strictures.

Choledochal Cyst and Neoplasm: A Comprehensive Review of 106 Cases and Presentation of Two Original Cases

Fieber SS, Nance FC (Saint Barnabas Med Ctr, Livingston, NJ; Univ of Medicine and Dentistry of New Jersey, Newark)

Am Surg 63:982-987, 1997 10–14

Objective.—More than 3,000 cases of cystic dilation of the biliary tree have been reported in the literature. Complications of choledochal cysts include cholangitis, biliary cirrhosis, portal hypertension, lithiasis, rupture, and carcinoma. One hundred six cases of choledochal cysts associated with neoplasms have been identified. The relationship between choledochal cyst and primary neoplasm in situ or in the biliary tract, gallbladder, or pancreas was analyzed.

Findings.—The 106 cases from the literature, as well as 2 new cases, were reviewed. The estimated incidence of choledochal cysts was 1 per 13,000 U.S. hospital admissions. Neoplasm with choledochal cyst was most likely to occur in the second to fourth decades of life. Of the reported cases, the choledochal cyst was the primary site of adenocarcinoma in 31% of cases. Of the extracystic sites, 43% involved cholangiocarcinoma and 7% anaplastic carcinoma. In 68 cases, neoplasms were identified at the initial laparotomy. Resection was performed in 30 patients; 20 of these patients survived for longer than 1 year, including 7 patients who underwent biliary pancreaticoduodenostomy. Elective surgery was performed in 38 patients with "pristine" choledochal cysts; of these 28 underwent internal drainage. In 3 patients, carcinoma of the biliary tract developed decades after choledochocystoduodenostomy.

Conclusions.—Patients with choledochal cysts may have neoplasia develop anywhere along the biliary tract or in the gallbladder or pancreas. Patients with choledochal cysts and neoplasia have a high incidence of an anomalous relation at the pancreaticobiliary duct junction. The malignancy is noted at the initial laparotomy in nearly two thirds of cases.

▶ Despite the true rare incidence of choledochal cysts, the fascination with this congenital anomaly continues. Both of these articles (Abstracts 10–13 and 10–14) give individual important pieces of information. The early outcome from cyst excision is excellent, with only recurrent cholangitis and technical problems leading to leakage as the most disconcerting. Drainage procedures have a higher incidence of complications because of significant anatomic variants, or the presence of periportal inflammatory disease that inhibits appropriate cyst excision. The clear association of cysts with intrahepatic and high extrahepatic strictures and membranes needs to be emphasized and sought after via cholangiography. These associated anomalies will lead to further jaundice and further biliary obstruction and subsequent stone formation. They are highly plausible sources for the etiology of cholangiocarcinoma as noted in the accompanying review of 106 cases of associated choledochal cysts and neoplasm. In that report, the majority of cases of associated tumors remained adenocarcinomas, and in only 31% of those cases was the primary site of the carcinoma within the choledochal cyst. Certainly, this condition has extensive anatomical and cellular molecular implications throughout the biliary tract. This acknowledgment may bring further interesting observations, as we are now in an era of earlier cyst excision resulting from the extreme sensitivity of fetal ultrasound and the subsequent neonatal diagnosis of choledochal cysts.

T.F. Tracy, Jr., M.D.

Ileal Exclusion for Byler's Disease: An Alternative Surgical Approach With Promising Early Results for Pruritus

Hollands CM, Rivera-Pedrogo FJ, Gonzalez-Vallina R, et al (Miami Children's Hosp, Fla)

J Pediatr Surg 33:220-224, 1998 10–15

Background.—Progressive familial intrahepatic cholestasis (PFIC)—also called Byler's disease—is an uncommon cause of hepatocellular cholestasis. Affected children have intermittent, painless jaundice. Intense pruritus that is disproportionate to the degree of hyperbilirubinemia can lead to self-mutilation by scratching. Good results have been achieved with liver transplantation and cutaneous biliary diversion procedures, both of which have their complications. Ileal exclusion or bypass procedures offer some important potential advantages over these approaches. The results of ileal exclusion in 5 patients with PFIC were reported.

Methods.—A standardized approach to terminal ileal exclusion was developed in 5 children with PFIC, diagnosed by the presence of characteristic histologic findings and chronic cholestasis in the absence of any defined metabolic or anatomical abnormality. The length of the small intestine was approximated using Siebert's graph of the relationship between crown-heel length and small-bowel length. A low estimate was derived by calculating the midpoint between the mean and 1 SD below the mean. Fifteen percent of this length was bypassed. The procedure resulted in a stapled, side-to-side, functional, end-to-end ileocolonic anastomosis performed just distal to the ileocecal valve.

Results.—An average of 16 months postoperatively, 4 of 5 patients were largely free of pruritus and self-mutilation. Two were completely free of pruritus, whereas 2 scratched only when under stress. All 4 patients were free of diarrhea. The fifth patient had initial relief, followed by progression of her liver disease.

Conclusions.—Promising early results are reported with this terminal ileal exclusion procedure for patients with PFIC. The procedure offers good relief from pruritus with a stoma-free "biliary diversion" that is completely reversible. Longer follow-up is needed, including evaluation of the effects on growth and development, liver function, and liver histology.

► Progressive familial intrahepatic cholestasis has had devastating consequences for these children who persistently scratch and mutilate themselves. The outstanding results that have been accomplished through varying biliary cutaneous conduits have resulted in some dramatic successes along with the associated problems of stoma management. The use of ileal exclusion, especially as outlined in this article, is an attractive first step in management, and it does not burn any bridges toward eventual biliary cutaneous diversion. The attractive calculations that have been presented for exclusion of 15% of the small bowel is a very sound basic science presumption; however, in the face of failure, cutaneous conduits may prove to be more efficacious.

T.F. Tracy, Jr., M.D.

Gallstone Pancreatitis: A Prospective Study on the Incidence of Cholangitis and Clinical Predictors of Retained Common Bile Duct Stones

Chang L, Lo SK, Stabile BE, et al (Univ of Californina, Los Angeles)

Am J Gastroenterol 93:527-531, 1998 10–16

Introduction.—Although some studies recommend urgent endoscopic retrograde cholangiopancreatography (ERCP) in all cases of gallstone pancreatitis to reduce the incidence of cholangitis, the authors of this report do not find this to be necessary. A prospective study was conducted to define the incidence of cholangitis in gallstone pancreatitis and to identify clinical factors predictive of persistent common bile duct (CBD) stones in patients without cholangitis.

Methods.—Diagnosis of gallstone pancreatitis was based upon the presence of upper abdominal pain and tenderness, amylase elevation more than 3 times the upper limit of normal (>330 U/L), ultrasound documentation of gallstones at admission, and the absence of alcohol abuse, hypercalcemia, hypertriglyceridemia, or medications known to cause pancreatitis. Urgent ERCP was limited to patients with evidence of cholangitis, clinically defined as temperature elevation (> 38.6°C), elevated bilirubin, right upper quadrant pain, and documentation at ERCP of purulent drainage from the ampulla. One hundred twenty-two consecutive patients were evaluated for the presence of CBD stones as determined by elective ERCP or intraoperative cholangiography (IOC).

Results.—Patients had a mean age of 37 years and a mean amylase of 1,742. Cholangitis was present in 4 (3%), including 3 with cholangitis on admission. All underwent urgent ERCP without complications. These 4 patients and 18 others were excluded from analysis of CBD stone predictors. The remaining 100 patients underwent elective ERCP or IOC. Persistent CBD stones were present in 21. Multivariate analysis determined the best predictor of CBD stones to be serum total bilirubin on hospital day 2. A serum total bilirubin level greater than 1.35 mg/dL had a sensitivity of 90.5% and a specificity of 63%. Variables not predictive of CBD stones included age, gender, mean APACHE II score, amylase level, and the presence of CBD dilation on ultrasound.

Conclusion.—Because cholangitis is uncommon in patients with acute gallstone pancreatitis, urgent ERCP is not indicated for all cases. Cholangitis can be readily treated by urgent ERCP once it is recognized. Serum total bilirubin on hospital day 2 is the best clinical predictor of persistent CBD stones.

▶ In this study, the aim was to define the incidence of cholangitis in gallstone pancreatitis and to identify clinical predictions of persistent common bile duct stones. One hundred twenty-two consecutive patients with acute gallstone pancreatitis were prospectively evaluated for the presence of common bile duct stones by elective ERCP or intraoperative cholangiography. Only 3% of the patients had cholangitis, and all underwent urgent ERCP successfully. Fifteen percent of the patients without a cholangiogram were excluded, and the 100 remaining patients constituted the bulk of the patients in this study. Twenty-one percent had persistent common bile duct stones, and multivariate analysis demonstrated that serum total bilirubin on hospital day 2 was the best predictor of common bile duct stones. Importantly, age, gender, mean APACHE II score, amylase, and the presence of common bile dilatation on ultrasound were not predictive of common bile duct stones.

In this article, the authors have concluded that in patients with gallstone pancreatitis, cholangitis is uncommon and the best clinical predictor of persistent common bile duct stones is the level of serum total bilirubin on hospital day 2. This article confirms the clinical suspicion of many practitioners involved in hepatobiliary surgery that in patients with gallstone pancreatitis, cholangitis is uncommon. Further, it is suggested that either intraoperative cholangiography or elective ERCP are equally beneficial at identifying common bile duct stones. However, modern clinical practice is such that in most patients with gallstone pancreatitis, provided that there is no cholangitis, elective ERCP rather than intraoperative cholangiography is first performed to delineate the anatomy of the duct, perform a sphincterotomy, and remove any common bile duct stones. In this article, the authors did not address the important issue of the timing of ERCP followed by surgery. Results in our own institution suggest that ERCP should be performed within 48 hours of scheduled elective laparoscopic cholecystectomy after resolution of the episode of gallstone pancreatitis. One other analysis that was not mentioned in this study is the presence of a dilated common bile duct that apparently was not determined by multivariate analysis. Other studies conclude that a persistently dilated common bile duct is highly suggestive of either recently passed or persistent common bile duct stones.

H.H. Simms, M.D.

Therapeutic Modification of Nuclear Factor κB Binding Activity and Tumor Necrosis Factor-α; Gene Expression During Acute Biliary Pancreatitis

Dunn JA, Li C, Ha T, et al (East Tennessee State Univ, Johnson City)
Am Surg 63:1036-1044, 1997 10–17

Background.—Cytokines play a proven pathogenic role in acute pancreatitis, particularly overproduction of tumor necrosis factor-α (TNF-α) in several organs. However, studies using anticytokine antibodies to treat pancreatitis have not given consistent results. Nuclear factor (NF)-κB is a transcriptional activator that acts as a pleiotropic regulator of genes involved in stress and inflammation. A treatment that would modify NF-κB binding and TNF-α gene overexpression was tested in an animal model of acute pancreatitis.

Methods.—The study used a model of reversible acute biliary pancreatitis in male Sprague-Dawley rats. At intervals of 0 to 30 minutes and of 1 to 24 hours after induction of pancreatitis or sham operation, the animals were killed for analysis of the pancreas. This included electrophoretic mobility shift assay to assess NF-κB binding activity and reverse transcription–polymerase chain reaction to measure TNF-α gene expression. In further studies, the free-radical blocker amobarbital, 60 mg/kg was given intraperitoneally 3 hours before induction of pancreatitis to block activation of NF-κB.

Results.—By 4 hours after induction of pancreatitis, NF-κB binding activity was significantly increased. This increase lasted for up to 24 hours after induction. Levels of TNF-α messenger RNA were maximal at 24 hours. Amobarbital pretreatment prevented both activation of NFκB and overexpression of the TNF-α gene. The severity of pancreatitis, as judged by amylase and clinical recovery, was significantly reduced in mice treated with amobarbital.

Conclusion.—In this animal model of acute pancreatitis, amobarbital treatment to prevent the activation of NF-κB prevents overexpression of the inflammatory cytokine TNF-α. This treatment also appears to reduce the clinical severity of pancreatitis. The findings could have implications for the treatment of acute pancreatitis, although the effects of modulating NF-κB activity after the induction of pancreatitis will have to be determined.

► In a model of acute biliary pancreatitis in Sprague-Dawley rats, NF-κB binding was determined by electrophoretic mobility shift assay, and TNF-α gene expression was assayed using reverse transcription–polymerase chain reaction. The authors have demonstrated that NF-κB binding activity was markedly higher after pancreatitis induction and TNF-α messenger RNA levels peaked at 24 hours. Most importantly, when amobarbital was used to block NF-κB activation 3 hours before induction of pancreatitis, the activation of NF-κB and over-expression of the TNF-α gene was prevented with a significant decrease in the severity of pancreatitis as assessed by amylase and clinical recovery.

This paper is important because it is one of the first to demonstrate that preventing the activation of NF-κB eliminates the induced overexposure to inflammatory cytokines and also offers the possibility of intervention affecting clinical outcome. Obviously one of the drawbacks of this manuscript is that the blockade of NF-κB activation in this model involves pretreatment. Therefore, future studies need to address the issue of how often after the induction of the pancreatitis NF-κB activation could be inhibited and still result in a salutory effect with regard to clinical outcome.

H.H. Simms, M.D.

Surgical Management of Chronic Pain From Chronic Pancreatitis

McHale A, Buechter KJ, Cohn I Jr, et al (Louisiana State Univ, New Orleans)

Am Surg 63:1119-1123, 1997 10–18

Objective.—Intractable pain is the major clinical problem in patients with chronic pancreatitis. The authors have developed a new algorithm for the management of the pain of chronic pancreatitis, including an initial surgical attack on ductal hypertension, if present, followed by denervation procedures. They report their 3-year experience with this approach.

Methods.—Patients with chronic pancreatitis who required high-dose narcotics or hospitalization for pain control were evaluated according to the study algorithm. Surgery, including Puestow's procedure, pseudocyst drainage, or sphincteroplasty, was performed to correct any anatomical abnormality that was causing ductal dilation. For patients without ductal dilation, or those with recurrent postoperative pain, denervation procedures (i.e., splenopancreatic flap, thoracoscopic sympathectomy, or resection) were performed. The patients were observed for an average of 26 months.

Results.—A total of 44 operations in 37 patients were carried out solely in an attempt to control the pain of chronic pancreatitis. The patients were 23 men and 14 women; 70% had chronic alcoholic pancreatitis. Surgery provided pain relief in 68% of the patients, with no single procedure proving more effective than the others. The pain recurrence rate was 32% with decompressive surgery and 27% with denervation procedures.

Conclusions.—The authors report good results with an algorithm of surgical management for patients with pain and chronic pancreatitis. The algorithm is based on the hypothesis that the pain of chronic pancreatitis is caused by ductal hypertension or is neurally mediated. The pain improvement rate of 68% compares favorably with that reported by other studies, although follow-up is short so far. The results of thoracoscopic sympathectomy are promising.

▶ In this article, the authors have addressed the issue of the optimal surgical procedure for the typical problem of pain control after chronic pancreatitis. In this study, 37 patients underwent 44 operations solely in an attempt to control pain. The operative procedures were dictated by the evidence of any anatomical disease that caused ductal dilatation. If ductal dilatation was demonstrated with endoscopic retrograde cholangiopancreatography (ERCP) or abdominal CT scan, then a Peustow's procedure, pseudocyst drainage, or sphincteroplasty was performed. If there was no evidence of ductal dilatation, or if pain recurred postoperatively, denervation procedures (splenopancreatic flap, thoracic sympathectomy, or resection) were performed. Of note, the follow-up average for these patients was significant at 26 months. Pain recurrence was generally equivalent with both decompressive and denervation procedures averaging approximately 35% to 40%. In general, 68% of patients had significant relief of their pain. These authors clearly demonstrate that no one procedure is superior to another; therefore, I would agree with their suggestions that the initial approach for the treatment of chronic pain from pancreatitis be based on the anatomical pathoses demonstrated by either abdominal and pelvic CT scan or ERCP. One drawback to this article is that the morbidity and mortality of the various procedures is not pointed out; therefore, it is not completely possible to compare operative results between decompressive and denervation procedures.

H.H. Simms, M.D.

Abdomen and Small Bowel

INTRODUCTION

Since the adoption of staging laparotomy in the 1960s for individuals with Hodgkin's disease, and for some patients with non-Hodgkin's lymphoma, innovative techniques have been used for planning radiotherapy fields and avoiding of overtreatment of the abdomen in early-stage disease. With the introduction of advanced and high-quality CT scanning, as well as access to histology with CT-directed biopsy, a reduction in the role of laparotomy has been evident. Recently, the increased application of combination modality therapy has afforded the patients improved morbidity and decreased mortality for this lymphatic neoplastic disorder. With the introduction in the late 1980s of minimal-access surgery with laparoscopy, significant approaches to the evaluation of oncologic diseases and their management has occurred. For lymphoma, laparoscopy or peritoneoscopy have been used for many years to direct liver biopsy for specific sites.[1] Mann and co-workers (Abstract 10–19) review the extensive experience for the application of laparoscopic procedures on patients with suspected or known lymphoma and define the role of laparoscopy. While laparoscopy is increasingly used as a staging method for other epithelial and mesenchymal tumors, it is evident that this technique has evolved sufficiently to provide tissue samples of suspected lymphoma for diagnostic purposes. This approach should be considered "state-of-the-art" when percutaneous biopsy is not technically possible and when chromosomal or genetic analysis is essential for treatment decisions, as well as when CT approaches with percutaneous biopsy are inadequate or unreliable.

The important contribution by Soballe and associates (Abstract 10–20) confirms the significant increase in infectivity of incisions when the coagulation current of monopolar surgery is used in contrast to the cold-steel scalpel. Infectivity implies that the use of coagulation current reduces the required bacterial inoculum for infection as much as a 1,000-fold. While any technical error in general surgery has the potential to increase morbidity and increase the length of hospital stay, this finding has considerable implications in the current era of cost-containment because abdominal infections significantly increase hospital stays. This study and that of Trondsen and co-workers (Abstract 10–12) reiterate the importance of judicious use of electrosurgery in the operating room at lower powers, at lower current amperage, and remote from organs in which potential injury may initiate significant irreversible damage with dire consequences (i.e., the biliary ductal system).

Multiple articles in this section deal with the consequences of systemic inflammation following laparoscopy/laparotomy and the inflammatory response initiated with acute mesenteric ischemia, reperfusion injury, and the consequences of massive small-bowel resection. There are increasing applications of laparoscopic surgery for intra-abdominal diseases complicated by inflammatory disorders; the successful therapy of appendicitis, perforated duodenal ulcer, and diverticulitis have been reported with laparoscopic approaches that have low morbidity and mortality.[2-6] Further, the physiological effects of pneumoperitoneum and the theoretical concern of elevated intra-abdominal pressure to promote bacteremia in systemic inflammatory responses of laparoscopic surgery continue to be debated. The physiologic consequences of this systemic insult have been minimally studied and remain controversial. These processes relative to effects on peripheral leukocyte populations, pro-inflammatory tumor necrosis factor (TNF-α) plasma levels, and the ex vivo secretion of peripheral blood mononuclear cells have been carefully studied in rat models. The consequences of these physiologic events bear importance in that, in the rodent model the inflammatory response was significantly greater in the *open* laparotomy group than that in the *laparoscopic* group. The utility of the laparoscopy technique affords the organism some protection over laparotomy for inflammatory conditions and may also contribute to the reduction in physiologic insult with this minimally invasive approach. Future research will clarify these physiologic events in humans.

The presence of an adynamic ileus after major abdominal surgery is characterized by the absence of bowel sounds and evidence of loss of neuromuscular motility initiated by neuronal inhibition after sympathetic overreactivity. Simple bowel trauma, infection, intestinal evisceration, etc., are considered the common etiologic processes to initiate adynamic ileus. It is evident that molecular biology will now define the mechanisms for this physiologic observation. Clearly, incremental surgical manipulation (laparotomy, eventration, "running," and compression of the bowel) enhance resident phagocytes and cause a progressive increase in neutrophil infiltration with a decrease in bethanechol-stimulated contraction. These molecular and cellular events occur as a response to minimal trauma in which resident macrophages set in place an inflammatory cascade, which may be a cause of dysfunction of the intestinal muscularis. Defining these molecular events will therefore allow mechanisms to abate the duration of the ileus or inhibit its onset, and may thereafter decrease length of hospital stay and costs incurred with this adverse physiologic event.

Three signal papers (Abstracts 10–21 to 10–23) review the physiologic consequences and adaptive mechanisms that occur after massive intestinal injury and resection. Acute mesenteric ischemia continues to pose a significant surgical challenge, which is based on its pathogenesis: arterial embolism, arterial thrombosis, venous occlusion, and nonocclusive disease, all of which must be differentiated for appropriate treatment. The high mortality (70% to 90%) for patients with acute arterial and functional mesenteric ischemia has changed little in the last decades. The important contribution by Klempnauer and associates (Abstract 10–23) suggests that anticoagulation with vitamin A antagonists for patients with venous thrombosis and arterial embolism, or inhibition of thrombocyte aggregation for patients with arterial thrombosis and nonocclusive mesenteric ischemia, afforded patients a remarkably low risk of recurrent mesenteric ischemia. This and other articles have defined the observation that impaired life expectancy of long-surviving patients is mainly a result of cardiovascular co-morbidity and malignancy. After massive enterectomy, the remnant intestine undergoes compensatory adaptation. Epidermal growth factor (EGF) and human growth hormone (hGH) have each been shown to enhance total length of small intestinal nutrient transport after massive enterectomy. For both infants and adults, molecular and hormonal approaches may enhance survivorship. Fiore and co-workers (Abstract 10–24) and Iannoli and associates (Abstract 10–25) conducted laboratory studies to improve trophic effects on small intestinal enterocytes with interleukin-11 (IL-11) or by the co-infusion of hGH and EGF to enhance intestinal adaptation. The underlying co-morbid factors of the adult have been the principal deterrents to long-term survival. For the infant, the massive physiological and nutritional insult with loss of absorptive capacity of small and large bowel for nutrient support has been the principal process leading to mortality. Increasing applications of the aforementioned technology will clearly be afforded physicians of the next millennium, which, together with small bowel transplantation, may enhance survival in these major physiologic insults.

Advances in neonatal intensive care have improved the survival of infants, leading to viability at or as low as 22 weeks gestational age.[7] These events followed the enormous progress made in respiratory support, including the use of steroid administration, high-frequency ventilation, and surfactant. Nonetheless, survival of the extremely premature and small infant remains marginal, for which intestinal perforations initiate significant mortality. Ein and associates[8] previously described peritoneal drainage as a method for stabilization of the critically ill, low-birth weight infant with intestinal perforation until surgical intervention can be completed on the more "stable" patient. Lessin and associates (Abstract 10–26) demonstrate that the application of peritoneal drainage is an effective therapeutic choice for intestinal perforation in the extremely low birth weight infant (< 750 g). However, this technique must undergo extensive evaluation and prospective studies to determine its worth in the overall management of these micro-premature infants.

The issue of how best to identify (diagnose) the occult patent contralateral processus vaginalis in the child initially seen with a unilateral inguinal hernia has been debated for more than 50 years. The ideal diagnostic tool does not exist; however, proper identification of the occult processus will potentially eliminate unnecessary open inguinal exploration and the need of subsequent contralateral hernia repair. The simplest preoperative diagnostic test remains the physical exam; the "silk glove sign," with palpation of the processus vaginalis over the pubic tubercle, is a method used in the diagnosis of the patent processus vaginalis. The false-positive rate reported by Gilbert and Clatworthy was 33% and a false-negative rate of 53% was evident. Other methods to detect the patent processus include herniography, ultrasound, passage of Bakes choledochal dilator through the open neck of the sac, intraoperative diagnostic pneumoperitoneum, and finally, the most radical (but accurate) measure, routine open exploration of the contralateral groin. The final paper of this series (Abstract 10–27) concludes that in an extensive evaluation of the pediatric population, that contralateral hernia was seen on laparoscopy in excess of one third of the total population. This defect was confirmed to be a patent processus vaginalis or true hernia sac. This benchmark paper suggests that laparoscopy is the ideal tool in the diagnosis of the contralateral patent processus intraoperatively. As in other procedures with precisely defined indications, it is a highly sensitive, specific, and safe diagnostic methodology.

Kirby I. Bland, M.D.

References

1. Glatstein E, Guernsey JM, Rosenberg SA, et al: The value of laparotomy and splenectomy in the staging of Hodgkin's disease. *Cancer* 24:709-718, 1969.
2. Attwood SE, Hill AD, Murphy PG, et al: A prospective randomized trial of laparoscopic vs open appendectomy. *Surgery* 112:497-501, 1992.
3. Geis WP, Kim HC: Use of laparoscopy in the diagnosis and treatment of patients with surgical abdominal sepsis. *Surg Endosc* 9:178-182, 1995.
4. Hansen JB, Smithers BM, Schache D, et al: Laparoscopic vs open appendectomy: A prospective randomized trial. *World J Surg* 20: 17-20, 1996.
5. Tate J, Dawson JW, Chung SC, et al: Laparoscopic vs open appendectomy: prospective randomised trial. *Lancet* 342: 633-637, 1993.
6. Urbano D, Rossi M, De Simone P, et al: Alternative laparoscopic management of perforated peptic ulcers. *Surg Endosc* 8: 1208-1211, 1994.
7. Hack M, Friedman H, Fanaroff AA: Outcomes of extremely low birth weight infants. *Pediatrics* 98: 931-937, 1996.

8. Ein SH, Marshall DG, Girvan D: Peritoneal drainage under local anesthesia for necrotizing enterocolitis. *J Pediatr Surg* 12: 963-967, 1977.

Emerging Role of Laparoscopy in the Diagnosis of Lymphoma

Mann GB, Conlon KC, LaQuaglia M, et al (Mem Sloan-Kettering Cancer Ctr, New York)

J Clin Oncol 16:1909-1915, 1998 10–19

Introduction.—Fine-needle aspiration cytology is not able to provide the architectural information so important in establishing a diagnosis of lymphoma. The recent development of more sophisticated laparoscopy instruments has allowed surgeons to access most parts of the abdominal cavity, including the retroperitoneum, and to obtain biopsy specimens from areas that were previously inaccessible. Few reports have addressed the effectiveness or potential role of laparoscopy in the diagnosis of lymphoma. Laparoscopic procedures were reviewed in patients with known or suspected lymphoma to determine the application and role of laparoscopy in lymphoma.

Methods.—Medical records of 94 patients who underwent 101 laparoscopic procedures between June 1993 and October 1996 were reviewed for demographic and clinicopathologic data.

Results.—Laparoscopy was diagnostic in 85 patients. Procedures were performed in 48 patients at primary presentation, in 21 patients with possible relapse, in 8 patients during the course of treatment, and in 8 patients to assess a liver lesion. In the remaining 16 patients, laparoscopy was used in the staging of possible intra-abdominal disease. Unsuccessful diagnostic procedures had been performed previously in 27 patients. There were no operative deaths. The postoperative complication rate was 8% (8 complications). There was sufficient information in all procedures performed for diagnosis. Diagnoses were Hodgkin's disease in 14 patients, non-Hodgkin's lymphoma in 48 patients, other neoplastic conditions in 6 patients, and benign conditions in 33 patients. There was one false-negative procedure and one nonresult for technical reasons. Ten patients underwent chemotherapy before discharge at a median delay of 3.5 days. The precise diagnosis differed significantly from initial diagnosis in 5 of 24 patients (21%) with recurrent or persistent lymphoma.

Conclusions.—Sufficient tissue samples can be provided by laparoscopy for full diagnostic analysis of suspected lymphoma. Laparoscopy should be considered when percutaneous biopsy is not technically feasible, when chromosomal or genetic analysis is required for treatment decisions, or when results of percutaneous biopsy are not adequate for making therapeutic decisions.

▶ The specific diagnosis of intra-abdominal lymphoma has always been a clinically challenging one. Despite the use of lymphangiography and CT, a specific pathologic diagnosis must be made that often requires evaluation of a large amount of tissue. This tissue is required for determination of tissue architecture, cell markers, and genetic analysis. Unfortunately, fine-needle aspiration (FNA) often falls short of providing enough tissue for analysis. Consequently, repeat procedures or a formal exploratory laparotomy are needed. Mann and colleagues also make a strong case implying that inaccurate information is often used rather than subjecting the patient to a formal laparotomy.

In this paper, these authors present a convincing argument for the adoption of laparoscopy in the setting where FNA has failed to provide enough tissue in a primary lymphoma, and replacement of FNA with laparoscopy in the setting of recurrent lymphoma. Given the emergence of microlaparoscopy, one wonders whether that modality shouldn't replace even FNA biopsy in the initial diagnosis of lymphoma. Under some circumstances, this might even be done under local anesthesia.

J.F. Amaral, M.D.

Electric Cautery Lowers the Contamination Threshold for Infection of Laparotomies

Soballe PW, Nimbkar NV, Hayward I, et al (Uniformed Services Univ of Health Sciences, Bethesda, Md)

Am J Surg 175:263-266, 1998 10–20

Introduction.—Any modification of surgical technique that could reduce the overall incidence of wound infection would improve quality and reduce costs because infectious complications significantly increase hospital stay. Researchers hypothesized that electric cautery, which causes more damage than the scalpel, increases the rate of infectious complications.

Methods.—This experimental study used rats randomized to 1 of 3 incisions: cold knife, electric cutting current, or electric coagulating current. Subcutaneous tissue was inoculated with 0.2 mL normal saline solution containing 0, 10^3, 10^5, 10^7, or 10^9 bacteria. All animals were killed on postoperative day 7, and tissue from the abdominal incision was removed for analysis.

Results.—At all levels of bacterial contamination, electric coagulation produced significantly more tissue necrosis and inflammation than did the cold knife. Coagulation current caused greater inflammation and necrosis than the cutting current until bacterial contamination reached 10^9. In a comparison of the cutting current with the scalpel, no differences were apparent until contamination reached 10^5. Most wounds had abscesses at higher levels of contamination, regardless of the incision method.

Conclusion.—Because electric coagulation current causes more inflammation, necrosis, and abscesses than the scalpel at all bacterial levels, the method should be limited to cases in which there is a need for meticulous hemostasis. The indications for electric cutting current are uncertain, because it is less hemostatic, yet less destructive than coagulation cutting.

▶ Electrosurgery remains a mainstay of operative therapy because of the ease with which hemostasis is obtained and the speed with which tissues are divided. Although electrosurgery is a focal point of surgical care, little teaching is directed during residency training to the risks, physiology, and appropriate use of this modality. Indeed, most surgeons view the risks of electrosurgery as being limited to rare instances of ground pad injuries, insulation failures, or alternate site injuries—problems that can be eliminated with modern-day isolated generators and active electrode and return electrode monitoring.

The article by Soballe and colleagues serves to remind us that the risks and complications of electrosurgery are real and ever-present, and often not considered. These investigators clearly document a significant increase in infectivity of incisions when the coagulation current of monopolar surgery is used vs. a cold steel scalpel. This is directly related to the amount of debris and necrotic tissue produced by electrosurgery. As the figure shows, the use of coagulation current reduces the required bacterial inoculum by as much as 1,000 times. This finding has important implications in an era of cost containment because infection increases hospital stay by 7 to 8 days. Clearly, these data argue for more judicious use of electrosurgery in the operating room at lower powers and, when possible, with the cutting current. Furthermore, it supports the use of less tissue-damaging hemostatic modalities, such as ultrasonic energy or even surgical ligatures and clips. I'll gladly take an extra 15 minutes in the operating room over 7 days in the hospital.

J.F. Amaral, M.D.

Increased Systemic Inflammation After Laparotomy vs Laparoscopy in an Animal Model of Peritonitis

Jacobi CA, Ordemann J, Zieren HU, et al (Univ of Berlin; Univ of Marburg, Germany)

Arch Surg 133:258-262, 1998 10–21

Introduction.—There is concern that elevated intra-abdominal pressure during laparoscopic surgery may promote bacteremia and systemic inflammatory response in patients with intra-abdominal disease complicated by inflammatory processes and peritonitis. The influence of laparotomy and laparoscopy on local and systemic inflammation was assessed in a rat model of peritonitis.

Methods.—Sixty male inbred Wistar rats were injected with a standardized fecal inoculum intraperitoneally. Twenty rats each were randomly assigned to either laparotomy with abdominal closure after 30 minutes, laparoscopy with insufflation of carbon dioxide for 30 minutes, or no further manipulation after stool inoculation (controls). Blood samples were collected perioperatively to determine bacteremia, leukocyte subpopulations, tumor necrosis factor-α (TNF-α) plasma levels, and ex vivo secretion of TNF-α by monocytes. Laparotomy was performed on all animals at day 7 after inoculation to determine the number of intraperitoneal abscesses.

Results.—Bacteremia was significantly higher 1 hour after intervention in the laparotomy and laparoscopy groups, compared with controls. All groups had significant monocytopenia and lymphocytopenia within 1 hour after fecal inoculation, with complete recovery on day 2 in the control and laparoscopy groups only. Intraperitoneal abscess formation was observed at 1 week after inoculation in all 20 rats in the laparotomy group, 15 of 20 rats in the laparoscopic group, and 18 of 20 rats in the control group. Compared with rats in the laparoscopy and control groups, rats in the laparotomy group had a significantly higher mean number of abscesses, as well as significant increases in TNF-α plasma levels and decreases in ex vivo production of TNF-α.

Conclusions.—The incidence of bacteremia and systemic inflammation was increased by laparotomy and laparoscopy in this rat model of peritonitis. The inflammatory response was significantly greater in the laparotomy group than in the laparoscopy group.

▶ This study compares the systemic response to peritonitis in animals treated with laparotomy vs. laparoscopy or no manipulation. It is curious that the investigators proposed that laparoscopy would produce more inflammatory response than the traditional approach. The accumulating body of data in the literature actually favors the opposite hypothesis: i.e., the systemic and local responses should be lower with laparoscopy than with laparotomy. Indeed, that was the case in this study. This is not surprising, given the smaller incisions used in laparoscopy when compared with laparotomy, because numerous data are available implicating the wound as the principal source of inflammatory response and a major contributor to the metabolic response that follows injury and sepsis. Clinically, this study supports increasing utilization of laparoscopy rather than laparotomy in inflammatory conditions such as appendicitis and diverticulitis, especially given the reduced abscess formation in the laparoscopy group compared with the laparotomy group.

J.F. Amaral, M.D.

Surgical Manipulation of the Gut Elicits an Intestinal Muscularis Inflammatory Response Resulting in Postsurgical Ileus

Kalff JC, Schraut WH, Simmons RL, et al (Univ of Pittsburgh, Pa)

Ann Surg 228:652-663, 1998 10–22

Introduction.—There is controversy regarding the extent, location, and duration of postsurgical ileus. Little is known about the underlying cellular mechanisms of this surgical conundrum that causes prolonged hospital stays and discomfort. The cellular and functional consequences of various

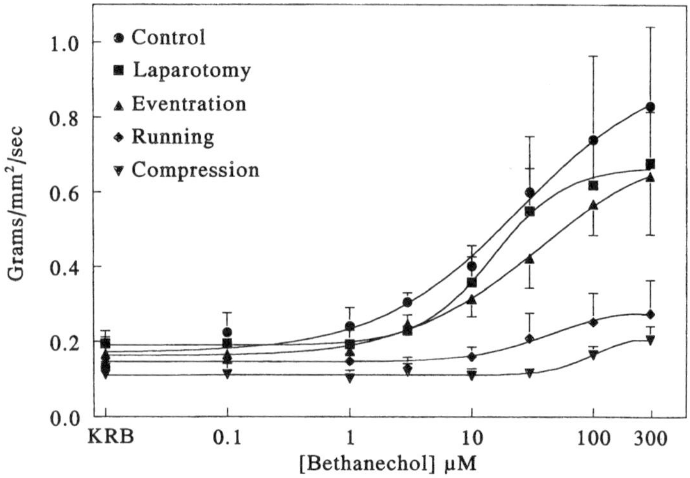

FIGURE 2.—Bethanechol-stimulated dose-response curves of circular muscle contractile activity generated from jejunal muscle after increasing degrees of surgical manipulation. Data are expressed as mean ± SEM. N = 5-7. *Abbreviation*: *KRB*, Krebs-Ringer buffer. (Courtesy of Kalff JC, Schraut WH, Simmons RL, et al: Surgical manipulation of the gut elicits an intestinal muscularis inflammatory response resulting in postsurgical ileus. *Ann Surg* 228:652-663, 1998.)

degrees of mild surgical manipulation were assessed on rat jejunal muscularis externa.

Methods.—Rats underwent incremental degrees of surgical manipulation after general anesthesia. Animals were placed in 1 of 5 groups: control: no anesthesia or surgery; laparotomy: abdomen was left open under a moist tent gauze for 10 minutes; eventuation: small intestine eventuated to the left and kept on a moist cotton gauze for 10 minutes; running: entire small bowel was gently inspected along its entire length; and compression: small bowel run along entire length and made to pass into the cecum by an aboral compression of the gut lumen. Animals were sacrificed either immediately, at 24 hours, or at 7 days. Muscularis infiltrates were characterized immunohistochemically on postoperative days 1 and 7. Circular muscle activity was determined by mechanical and intracellular recording techniques in vitro.

Results.—Surgical manipulation created a rise in resident phagocytes that stained for the activation marker lymphocyte function-associated antigen. Incremental degrees of manipulation produced a progressive increase in neutrophil infiltration and a drop in bethanechol-stimulated contractions (Fig 2). A rise in macrophages, monocytes, dendritic cells, T cells, natural killer cells, and mast cells was observed with compression.

Conclusion.—These findings show for the first time that clinically relevant and commonly performed surgical manipulation of the gut—but not laparotomy per se—causes failure of gut circular muscle function 24 hours later. The resident network of unactivated muscularis macrophages activate immediately and within 24 hours cause extravasation of several leukocyte populations in the rat muscularis. Postoperative ileus may be caused by an inflammatory response to motion that causes muscle dysfunction.

▶ This article deals with the pathophysiologic mechanisms that lead to ileus after abdominal surgery. In a rat model, increasing degrees of surgical manipulation were used including laparotomy, eventration, running of the small bowel, and compression of the bowel. Postoperatively, muscular infiltrates were characterized immunohistochemically, and circular muscle activity was assessed.

The results demonstrated that surgical manipulation caused a marked increase in resident phagocytes with further incremental degrees of manipulation, causing a progressive increase in neutrophil infiltration and a decrease in bethanechol-stimulation contractions. The results also showed significant increases in macrophages, monocytes, and other inflammatory cells with compression of the bowel. The authors have concluded that their data support the hypothesis that the degree of gut paralysis to cholinergic stimulation is proportional to the degree of trauma and the extent of cellular infiltration, and that postsurgical ileus is a result of an inflammatory response to minimal trauma, which may be set in motion by resident macrophages.

This article has been written in an attempt to investigate the mechanisms of postsurgical ileus and supports the contention that many of our mentors taught us, i.e., that absolute gentleness is required when handling the intestinal tract. An unanswered question: Is there a synergistic response between manipulation of the bowel and an already existing inflammation, such as peritonitis, that would result in an even further reduction in muscularis stimulated contraction? The authors are to be congratulated for pursuing this work. Further studies in this regard would be extremely helpful.

H.H. Simms, M.D.

Long-term Results After Surgery for Acute Mesenteric Ischemia

Klempnauer J, Grothues F, Bektas H, et al (Hannover Med School, Germany)

Surgery 121:239-243, 1997 10–23

Objective.—Acute mesenteric ischemia carries a high mortality rate. Although aggressive surgical treatment is recommended, there have been few studies that have examined the long-term results after surgery. Results of a retrospective analysis of the outcomes and rehabilitation statuses of patients who were discharged from the hospital after successful surgical intervention for acute mesenteric ischemia are reported.

Methods.—Of the 90 patients who underwent surgical intervention between 1972 and 1993 for acute mesenteric ischemia, 31 survived. A questionnaire was sent to the 16 patients still alive at the time of the study. Information on the 15 who had subsequently died was obtained from the family physician. Actuarial patient survival was calculated using the Kaplan-Meier method and compared.

Results.—The type of mesenteric ischemia in patients discharged from the hospital included arterial embolism (n = 5), arterial thrombosis (n = 5), venous thrombosis (n = 19), and nonocclusive disease (n = 2). Survival at 2 and 5 years was 70% and 50%. Only 1 patient died from recurrent mesenteric ischemia. The remainder died from myocardial infarction (n = 4), congestive heart failure (n = 2), stroke (n = 2), malignant disease (n = 3), gastrointestinal bleeding (n = 2), and liver failure (n = 1). Four of 19 patients had short bowel syndrome after surgery but none required parenteral nutrition. Eight of the 15 living patients had returned to work, 4 had retired, and 3 were unable to return to work.

Conclusion.—Long-term results showed that there was little risk of recurrence of mesenteric ischemia. Deaths occurred primarily from cardiovascular and malignant conditions.

▶ This retrospective review looked at the long-term prognosis of patients after initially successful surgical intervention for acute mesenteric ischemia. Overall mortality rate was 66%. Anticoagulation consisted of vitamin K antagonists in patients with venous thrombosis and arterial embolism or inhibition of thrombocyte aggregation in patients with arterial thrombosis and nonocclusive mesenteric ischemia. Of note, 2- and 5-year survival rates were 70% and 50%, respectively, and related mainly to cardiovascular comorbidity and malignant disease. Only 1 patient died after a recurrent attack of arterial mesenteric thrombosis. Also significant, 20% of the patients had chronic short bowel syndrome after extensive bowel resection, but none require permanent parenteral nutrition. This study clearly demonstrates that with appropriate anticoagulation there is remarkably low risk of recurrent mesenteric ischemia. Our results at this institution would mirror the findings in this publication and strongly support the idea that acute interventions with regard to acute mesenteric ischemia should be provided, except in those patients who have prohibitive comorbid risk factors related to cardiovascular disease or the presence of concomitant malignancy.

H.H. Simms, M.D.

Comparison of Interleukin-11 and Epidermal Growth Factor on Residual Small Intestine After Massive Small Bowel Resection

Fiore NF, Ledniczky G, Liu Q, et al (Indiana Univ, Indianapolis)

J Pediatr Surg 33:24-29, 1998 10–24

Objective.—In animal models of short bowel syndrome, both interleukin-11 (IL-11) and epidermal growth factor (EGF) promote the proliferation and differentiation of small intestinal crypt cells while enhancing bowel adaptation. In mice with major burns, IL-11 treatment preserves small intestine crypt architecture and prolongs survival. Epidermal growth factor has trophic effects on the intestinal mucosa; it also increases brush border enteropeptidase activity and glucose, electrolyte, and glutamine uptake. Interleukin-11 and EGF were compared for their effects on small intestine morphology after massive small bowel resection in rats.

Methods.—Eighty-five percent mid–small bowel resection with primary anastomosis was performed in Sprague-Dawley rats. One group was treated with bovine serum albumin; one with IL-11, 125 μg/kg subcutaneously twice daily; one with EGF, 0.10 μg/g subcutaneously twice daily; and one with both IL-11 and EGF in the above doses. Some animals in each group were killed for examination after 4 days, and the rest after 8 days. The groups were compared for weight, mucosal length, bowel wall muscle thickness, and expression of proliferating cell nuclear antigen in intestinal crypt and smooth muscle cells.

Results.—Rats receiving IL-11 only or IL-11 plus EGF had increased mucosal thickness, compared with animals receiving EGF only or bovine serum albumin. Muscle thickness was significantly increased for animals receiving EGF, with or without IL-11, suggesting that EGF is trophic for the muscularis propria layer.

Conclusions.—Both IL-11 and EGF have a trophic effect on small bowel epithelium through an increase in crypt cell mitotic rate. The action of IL-11 is primarily on enterocytes, whereas EGF enhances both enterocyte and myocyte proliferation. In patients with short bowel syndrome, treatment with IL-11—with or without EGF—might improve small bowel adaptation.

Epidermal Growth Factor and Human Growth Hormone Accelerate Adaptation After Massive Enterectomy in an Additive, Nutrient-dependent, and Site-specific Fashion

Iannoli P, Miller JH, Ryan CK, et al (Univ of Rochester, NY; Emory Univ, Atlanta, Ga)

Surgery 122:721-729, 1997 10–25

Purpose.—Short bowel syndrome after massive enterectomy (ME) is a devastating clinical condition. As long as 40% of the small intestine remains, sufficient compensatory adaptation will occur to permit a transition from parenteral to enteral nutrition. Animal studies have suggested that treatment with human growth hormone (hGH) or epidermal growth factor (EGF) can increase total-length small intestine nutrient transport after ME. The individual and combined effects of hGH and EGF on the adaptation of proximal and distal small bowel after ME were assessed.

Methods.—Seventy percent mid-jejunoileal resection was performed in New Zealand white rabbits. One week later, the animals were started on hGH, 0.2 mg/kg/day; EGF, 1.5 μg/kg/hr; hGH plus EGF; or an equal volume of vehicle. Each treatment continued for 7 days. The effects of the various treatments on transport of glucose, glutamine, alanine, leucine, and arginine were assessed. Other outcome measures included serum insulin-like growth factor-I (IGF-I) concentrations, proximal and distal villus and microvillus heights, and expression of IGF binding protein

(IGFBP)-3 and -4 mRNA in full-thickness proximal and distal gut remnants.

Results.—Animals receiving hGH plus EGF showed 100% upregulation of glucose transport in the proximal remnant. Glutamine uptake increased by 80% and leucine transport by 60%. Alanine and arginine transport in the distal remnant increased by 150% and 400%, respectively. Microvillus height increased in this group by 25% to 35%, both proximally and distally. There were no differences between treatment groups in serum IGF-I levels or gross villus heights. Animals receiving hGH had increased IGFBP-3 mRNA levels in the proximal, but not the distal, intestine. Treatment with EGF had no effect on gut expression of IGFBP-3 or IGFBP-4.

Conclusions.—Treatment with a combination of hGH and EGF accelerates intestinal adaptation after ME in rabbits. The effect is nutrient dependent and site specific, and occurs through enhanced nutrient transport and microvillus hypertrophy. The anabolic actions of hGH occur through generation of IGF-I, thus leading to both endocrine and paracrine effects. Decreased local expression of IGFBP-3 after ME may result in increased availability of free IGF-I, thus facilitating gut adaptation.

▶ Short bowel syndrome in infants and children remains an extremely important clinical challenge with as many multifactorial determinants as there are newborn etiologies of the disease. The devastating problems of necrotizing enterocolitis, gastroschisis, and small bowel atresias along with volvulus present challenges to intestinal adaptation just when growth and gastrointestinal maturation begins. The development and maturation of the gastrointestinal tract in the face of short bowel syndrome must occur with concurrent adaptation to intestinal loss. Both papers (Abstracts 10–24 and 10–25) offer different insights into combination growth factor therapy with a common element of EGF. It is an important contribution to note the differential effects of EGF, especially on its proliferation in both enterocytes and myoctes. The novel addition of IL-11 to these treatment regimens demonstrates significant promise for not only mucosal development but also prevention of bacterial translocation, which contributes to morbidity in short bowel syndrome and its associated liver disease.

Once the gut has matured, the implications of ME are still significant, and adaptation is equally important for survival. The insights provided by combined EGF and hGH supplementation on regulation of IGF-I and its binding protein are significant additions to the mechanisms of adaptation. It is an important significant negative finding that the authors have presented by demonstrating that alterations in intestinal amino acid transport are unrelated to the components in the gut IGF system. Further focus on alterations in transporters during adaptation is bound to occur and provides some interesting challenges to the neonatal models of short bowel syndrome that have maturational challenges to gut transporters, as well as adaptive challenges caused by significant resections of small bowel.

T.F. Tracy, Jr., M.D.

Peritoneal Drainage as Definitive Treatment for Intestinal Perforation in Infants With Extremely Low Birth Weight (<750 g)

Lessin MS, Luks FI, Wesselhoeft CW, et al (Brown Univ, Providence, RI; Hasbro Children's Hosp, Providence, RI)

J Pediatr Surg 33:370-372, 1998 10–26

Introduction.—For critically ill, low–birth weight infants with intestinal perforation, peritoneal drainage was introduced as a means of stabilizing the patient's condition for surgery. However, experience suggests that these infants may show dramatic improvement with peritoneal drainage, permitting survival without surgery. Peritoneal drainage was evaluated as definitive therapy for extremely low birth weight (ELBW) infants with intestinal perforation.

Methods.—The 18-month protocol included 9 ELBW infants (weight less than 750 g) with intestinal perforation. All were treated with peritoneal drainage, achieved via a catheter placed in the right lower quadrant. Once the child's clinical condition improved and peritoneal drainage ceased, the drains were removed.

Results.—Seven of 9 patients survived the initial drainage procedure, and 6 patients were still alive at a mean follow-up of 12 months. Five of these 6 long-term survivors healed without sequelae, with no need for further surgery. One patient had an abdominal wall abscess below the drain site, which required incision and drainage.

Conclusions.—For most ELBW infants with intestinal perforation, peritoneal drainage appears to offer a definitive approach to therapy. This is a new treatment option for a group of premature infants who have high mortality and are major surgical risks.

▶ This article pushes the envelope of management for bowel perforation even further for extremely low birth weight infants (less than 750 g). It joins a host of other significant reports that use primary drainage for necrotizing enterocolitis for newborns less than 1,500 g. The only caution that one must raise relates to the early presentation of intestinal perforation in these "micro-preemies." Many neonatologists and pediatric surgeons feel that early bowel perforation is not caused by the "classic" necrotizing enterocolitis that presents with pneumatosis. In fact, this form of perforation may be distinctly different in the extremely low birth weight infant. Further cautions in the application of this technique relate to decisions regarding the failure of primary drainage and evaluations of infants for subsequent complications such as abscess and stricture. The positive results gained from this study may be based on elements of a scarless type of "fetal healing" after early intestinal perforation.

T.F. Tracy, Jr., M.D.

Laparoscopic Evaluation of the Pediatric Inguinal Hernia—A Meta-analysis

Miltenburg DM, Nuchtern JG, Jaksic T, et al (Baylor College of Medicine, Houston)

J Pediatr Surg 33:874-879, 1998 10–27

Objective.—Most children with inguinal hernia have a unilateral hernia. Most hernias arise from a patent processus vaginalis (PPV). The best method for diagnosing an occult contralateral PPV is controversial. A review and a meta-analysis of the use of diagnostic laparoscopy were performed to determine the efficacy of the technique in infants and children.

Methods.—Thirteen studies were identified, and 4 were excluded. A total of 964 patients (762 boys, 138 girls, 64 unspecified), aged 0 months to 18 years, from 9 studies were included.

Results.—Laparoscopy, performed in 964 patients, revealed a hernia or PPV in 376 and negative findings in 588. On contralateral exploration, 373 hernia sacs or PPVs were found, for a sensitivity of 99.4% and a specificity of 99.5%. Sex, age, and side of hernia had no effect on the sensitivity and specificity of laparoscopy. Laparoscopy required an additional 5 minutes and 45 seconds. There were 2 complications as a result of laparoscopy.

Conclusion.—Laparoscopy is a safe and effective way of diagnosing contralateral PPV in children undergoing inguinal hernia repair.

▶ This is the first meta-analysis of laparoscopy for contralateral groin and inguinal exploration. This specific clinical issue is still the subject of significant fervor and controversy within pediatric surgery, despite large series of patients. Most recent studies indicate only a 16% of incidence of contralateral inguinal hernia; yet this study indicates that more than one third of the patients will have an identifiable inguinal hernia or PPV. Again, what is a hernia and what isn't? It is comforting to note that, for those surgeons who indeed cannot rest with less than a 20% chance that a contralateral hernia will occur (in the face of almost no anesthetic risk for future exploration or repair), laparoscopy is a safe and sensitive tool.

T.F. Tracy, Jr., M.D.

Colon, Rectum, and Anus

Introduction

The diagnosis of acute appendicitis continues to be based principally on clinical findings alone; diagnosis of atypical presentations may be assisted by the use of plain abdominal films, barium enemas, and abdominal sonography. CT has been widely used in adults to diagnose appendicitis, with accuracy equal to or higher than that of US. The use of high-frequency compression sonography in children and adults with acute abdominal pain has improved diagnostic accuracy and outcomes. Rarely is the appendix visualized on routine abdominal sonography. Moreover, acute appendicitis cannot be conclusively confirmed by sonographic techniques that do not use high-frequency linear transducers and careful graded compression. An acceptable finding between the negative appendectomy rate and the perforation rate is central to the ongoing debate and controversy that surround the diagnosis and therapy of appendicitis. The majority of surgeons suggest that the decrease in morbidity and mortality would best be achieved only when exchanged for the higher negative appendectomy rate. Some argue that the practice of indiscriminate appendectomy is unjustified.

In randomized prospective single-center clinical trials, excellent results have been suggested for applications of US in the diagnosis of appendicitis. Recent meta-analyses by Cassina and associates[1] and Orr et al.[2] confirm that the average sensitivity with US is as great as 90% with specificity up to 100%. Clearly, accuracy with applications of any test, including US, is dependent on operator-dependent experience, as well as the consequences for availability and benefit of the investigation. Studies by Sarfati and associates[3] and Ford and co-workers[4] have looked at the clinical consequences of US and noted no clinical benefit relative to perforation, negative appendectomy, or complication rates.

Balthazar and associates (Abstract 10–28) suggest that the judicious application of CT imaging in individuals with equivocal clinical presentation suspected of appendicitis may enhance improvement in preoperative diagnosis. Moreover, Horwitz and colleagues (Abstract 10–29) suggest that the technique (open vs. laparoscopic) in the pediatric population remains highly controversial. It would appear that the laparoscopic appendectomy should be avoided for children who have complicated appendicitis because of the frequency of postoperative abdominal abscess. As with any new approach, verification with prospective analysis, including morbidity reduction and cost implications, is essential for prospective recommendations.

Levitt and colleagues (Abstract 10–30) find a beneficial use for the usually troublesome appendix, performing an appendicostomy to create a conduit for antegrade enemas. They report 95% fecal continence in children after this procedure.

The association between the Peutz-Jeghers syndrome and an increased risk for carcinoma remains controversial. While early reports did not demonstrate predisposition to cancer in this syndrome, more recent studies describe an increased risk for both gastrointestinal and extraintestinal neoplasms.[5-8] Distinctive but uncommon neoplasms associated with the syndrome include sex-cord tumors with annular tubules, the rare Sertoli's cell tumor associated with sexual precocity, and adenoma malignum of the cervix. The signal paper by Boardman et al. (Abstract 10–31) addresses the controversial issue in these patients with juvenile polyposis. The relative risk for breast and gynecologic cancer suggests a particularly elevated incidence. Virtual colonoscopy combining spiral volumetric CT scanning of the air-insufflated colon with computer-aided visualization tools enables a *noninvasive assessment* of the colonic mucosa. This new method of colon examination, in which computer-aided 3-D visualization of spiral CT simulates fiberoptic colonoscopy, may have future diagnostic applications. This evolving technology must be evaluated relative to the "gold standard" colonoscopy to determine its overall worth as a diagnostic, screening, and follow-up procedure (Abstract 10–32).

With increasing pressures to affect the cost of health care by reduction of resource uses and length of hospital stay, the report by Bradshaw and associates (Abstract 10–33) has particular clinical and financial interest. The application of standardized perioperative protocols contributed to early return of bowel function with reduced length of hospital stay for patients undergoing colon surgery. These and similar studies will be used in multiple organ systems in routine clinical surgery to enhance the reduction of perioperative stay, thereby influencing fiduciary and clinical outcomes of invasive procedures.

Nicholls and Banerjee (Abstract 10–35) and Cohen and colleagues (Abstract 10–36) deal with pouchitis and reconstruction of pelvic pouches in the management of inflammatory bowel disease. The ileoanal anastomosis with pouch creation is the current therapeutic choice for the majority of patients who face colectomy for chronic ulcerative colitis or familial adenomatosis polyposis (FAP). However, symptomatic inflammation of the pouch occurs in 7% to 40% of patients undergoing this surgical procedure. The majority of complications related to pouchitis have occurred in patients with a history of ulcerative colitis; the complication develops in only a few patients with FAP. The theories of pouchitis include bacterial overgrowth, stasis, ischemia, and underlying co-morbid diseases (indeterminate colitis, "backwash" ileitis, and unrecognized Crohn's disease). Generally, successful management is possible without excision of the pouch for incapacitating and refractory complications. The commitment of the surgeon and the patient to achieve successful outcome is essential, and it is stressed by Cohen and associates (Abstract 10–36). Today, radical reconstructive surgery can be completed where local procedures to effect pouch salvage have failed, and it should be considered as first-line management where factors dictate that local procedures might fail. Therefore, severe pouch-specific complications are best managed successfully by surgeons with special interests in pelvic-pouch surgery and who possess considerable experience dealing with these complications.

Anosphincteric injury occurring secondary to obstetric or operative trauma is considered a cause for fecal incontinence in the majority of patients facing corrective surgery. History and physical examination may be unrevealing or demonstrate decreased resting or squeeze pressure in patients with obstetric trauma; anatomical and physiologic evaluation of the sphincter should include anorectal manometry, anal electromyography, pudendal nerve motor latency, and transanal US. Transanal US, combined with decreased anal pressures, correctly identifies all intact sphincters and 90% of known anal sphincteric injuries (Abstract 10–37). Restoration of anal sphincter function by single-stage dynamic graciloplasty using a modified (split-sling) technique restored function of an insufficient or excised anal sphincter in the report by Rosen et al. (Abstract 10–34). This single-stage procedure using a single wrap in a modified technique was applied mainly in patients following abdominoperineal resection to alleviate the problems and pitfalls that have arisen during the learning curve of this new procedure.

The annoying and incapacitating problem of chronic anal fissure has been addressed by Maria and co-workers (Abstract 10–38) in a double-blind, placebo-controlled study. Sphincterotomy continues to be the most widely applied therapy for this condition, but it often permanently weakens the internal sphincter and may therefore anatomically and physiologically progress to anal deformity and incontinence. The effective therapy with local infiltration of the botulinum toxin into the internal anal sphincter has promise for long-term control of this significant, common, and underdiagnosed malady.

Agachan and associates (Abstract 10–39) suggest that the optimal surgical therapy for management of rectal prolapse remains intensely controversial. More than 130 different procedures that have been described to treat rectal prolapse have been documented in the last 2 decades; no consensus for operative choice exists.[9] The description and application of multiple operative approaches with variable outcomes signal the difficulty or the apparent absence of quality and functional outcomes with one specific surgical technique. Surgical tradition has maintained that *recurrence rates* represent the standard evaluation criterion for prolapse operations; recent emphasis is also placed upon *functional outcomes*. While perineal operations remain appropriate for elderly or high-risk patients with prolapse, perineal rectosigmoidectomy remains the preferred procedure because it is well-tolerated, technically simple, and can be combined with the levatoroplasty while providing low recurrence rates and acceptable morbidity. Agachan and associates compared two procedures (perineal rectosigmoidectomy with levatoroplasty and Delorme's procedure) with that of perineal rectosigmoidectomy alone. The addition of the levatoroplasty to perineal rectosigmoidectomy was observed to have the superior outcome in the therapy of rectal prolapse. This safe procedure provides better short-term functional outcomes than either of the simpler techniques and should be considered the gold standard by which we compare future therapies for rectal prolapse.

General surgeons have been advised, since the experiences of World War II and the Vietnam War, that isolated rectal trauma is best managed by fecal diversion to diminish morbidity and mortality. This has been applied subsequently for the management of open pelvic fractures.[10,11] The appreciated mortality of open pelvic fractures is significant, up to 70% of patients so affected, with approximately 2 to 5 times the mortality of closed pelvic fractures. For 30% to 50% of such cases, mortality is attributed principally to the pelvic fracture, of which one third have concurrent development of sepsis from infectious sources within the pelvis. Modern principles of wound care related to open pelvic fractures have suggested that diversion of the fecal stream would hypothetically protect internal mechanical hardware and enhance wound repair. Moreover, while transmural rectal injury with functional distal sphincteric obstruction logically suggests that diversion is of value, the necessity of fecal diversion in the absence of proven transmural rectal trauma is principally unproven. Woods and co-workers (Abstract 10–40) provide a case-control analysis from a university-based, tertiary care level I trauma center, which includes an experience with 60 cases along with an additional 186 patients amenable to analysis. The authors conclude that this technical addition to protect open fractures was not associated with a lower incidence of abdominopelvic infectious complications. In contrast, diversion may protect a select group of individuals with extensive soft tissue injury and posterior wounds. We agree that this benchmark study calls for a national prospective multicenter trial that carefully evaluates selective management incorporating fecal diversion with this injury.

Kirby I. Bland, M.D.

References

1. Cassina P, Rothlin M, Largiader F: Die effizienz der chirurgischen grunddiagnostik beim akuten bauchschmerz. *Chirurg* 67:254-260, 1996.
2. Orr RK, Porter D, Hartman D: Special contributions: ultrasonography to evaluate adults for appendicitis: decision making based on meta-analysis and probabilistic reasoning. *Acad Emerg Med* 2:644-650, 1995.
3. Sarfati MR, Hunter GC, Witzke DB, et al: Impact of adjunctive testing on the diagnosis and clinical course of patients with acute appendicitis. *Am J Surg* 166:660-665, 1993.
4. Ford RD, Passinault WJ, Morse ME: Diagnostic ultrasound for suspected appendicitis: Does the added cost produce a better outcome? *Am Surg* 60:895-898, 1994.
5. Giardiello FM, Welsh SB, Hamilton SR, Oferhaus GJ, Gittelsohn AM, Booker SV, et al. Increased risk of cancer in the Peutz-Jeghers syndrome. *N Engl J Med* 316: 1511-1514, 1987.
6. Spigelman AD, Murday V, Phillips RK: Cancer and the Peutz-Jeghers syndrome. *Gut* 30:1588-1590, 1989.
7. Young RH, Welch WR, Dickerson GR, Scully RE. Ovarian sex cord tumor with annular tubules; review of 74 cases including 27 with Peutz-Jeghers syndrome and four with adenoma malignum of the cervix. *Cancer* 50:1384-1402, 1982.
8. Srivatsa PJ, Kenney GL, Podratz KC: Disseminated cervical adenoma malignum and bilateral ovarian sex cord tumors with annular tubules associated with Peutz-Jeghers syndrome. *Gynecol Oncol* 53:256-264, 1994.
9. Goldberg SM, Gordon PH: Operative treatment of complete prolapse of the rectum, in Wajarian JS, Delaney JP (eds): *Surgery of the Gastrointestinal Tract.* New York, Intercontinental Medical Books, 1974, pp 423-429.
10. Ganchrow MI, Lavenson GS, McNamara JJ. Surgical management of traumatic injuries of the colon and rectum. *Arch Surg* 100:515-520, 1970.
11. Trunkey D, Hays RJ, Shires GT. Management of rectal trauma. *J Trauma* 13:411-415, 1973.

Appendicitis: The Impact of Computed Tomography Imaging on Negative Appendectomy and Perforation Rates

Balthazar EJ, Rofsky NM, Zucker R (New York Univ)
Am J Gastroenterol 93:768-771, 1998 10–28

Introduction.—Clinical examination and laboratory tests followed by surgery are the accepted diagnostic approach to appendicitis, despite a negative appendectomy rate of 20%. The rate is only 10% in men, but 25% to 45% in women of childbearing age. New approaches to decreasing the negative appendectomy rate have been studied, including laparoscopy, sonography, and abdominal CT. However, little information's available on how these tests affect the diagnosis and clinical course of acute appendicitis. The impact of abdominal CT on the negative appendectomy rate and perforation rate was assessed in a retrospective study of hospital patients admitted from July 1993 to June 1995.

Methods.—The study included 146 patients clinically suspected of having acute appendicitis. The patients were 69 females, including 54 women of childbearing age, and 77 males. The average age was 38 years. All patients underwent emergency abdominal CT examination. One hundred twenty-two patients had surgery.

Findings.—The negative appendectomy rate was 4%, while the perforation rate among patients undergoing surgery was 22%. Among women of childbearing age, the negative appendectomy rate was 8% and the perforation rate 19%. Abdominal CT had an accuracy of 96%, sensitivity of 96%, specificity of 97%, and positive and negative predictive value of 99% and 88%, respectively. Eighteen of the 24 patients in whom surgery was avoided were women of childbearing age.

Conclusions.—In patients with clinically suspected acute appendicitis, emergency abdominal CT can help in making the preoperative diagnosis. The result is a significant reduction in the risk of negative appendectomy, with no increase in the risk of appendiceal perforation. Abdominal CT may be especially helpful in patients with equivocal clinical findings and in women of menstruating age.

▶ This paper is a retrospective analysis on 146 consecutive patients who presented to the New York-Tisch Medical Center over a 2-year period and underwent CAT scan examination before institution of therapy. The negative appendectomy rate was 4% in 122 patients operated on with a perforation rate of 22%. As one can see from Table 1 in the original article, the sensitivity, specificity and overall accuracy of the test is around 96%, with an excellent positive predictive value of 99% and an acceptable negative predictive value of 82%. This report is similar to others in the recent literature, emphasizing the superiority of CT scan vs. ultrasound in cases in which the diagnosis of appendicitis is equivocal. Of course, most surgeons believe that appendicitis remains a clinical diagnosis, and that there is no substitute for a thorough history and physical examination in the management of this condition. The danger of these reports on CT diagnosis of appendicitis is for our younger colleagues-in-training, as well as for emergency room physicians or other primary-care physicians, to abuse imaging techniques to diagnose this condition. Obtaining a CT scan is not only expensive but may lead to an unnecessary delay in treatment. Nonetheless, in equivocal cases, especially in nonpregnant women, the greatest value of abdominal CT scan in the diagnosis of appendicitis lies in its negative predictive value. A reliable patient with a CT scan negative for appendicitis can probably be discharged without incurring any of the costs of hospitalization or observation, and in the majority of cases will do well. The use of any imaging test should always be part of the overall diagnostic process and represent an addition rather than a replacement of the more traditional history and physical examination method.

V.E. Pricolo, M.D.

Should Laparoscopic Appendectomy Be Avoided for Complicated Appendicitis in Children?

Horwitz JR, Custer MD, May BH, et al (Univ of Texas-Houston; Texas A&M Univ, Temple)

J Pediatr Surg 32:1601-1603, 1997 10–29

Purpose.—Recent studies have suggested that performing laparoscopic appendectomy in adult patients with perforated or gangrenous appendicitis may increase the risk of infectious complications. Most comparisons of open vs. laparoscopic appendectomy have not focused on the results in complicated cases, or excluded such cases altogether. The results of open vs. laparoscopic appendectomy in children with complicated appendicitis were assessed.

Methods and Findings.—Fifty-six children who had surgery for complicated appendicitis were retrospectively studied. Appendectomy was performed by laparoscopy in 27 cases and open surgery in 22. The postoperative complication rate was 43% overall: 56% with laparoscopic appendectomy vs. 18% with open appendectomy. Intra-abdominal abscess developed in 14 patients, or one fourth of the entire series. The rate of this complication was 41% after laparoscopic appendectomy vs. 9% after open appendectomy.

Conclusions.—Laparoscopic appendectomy in children with complicated appendicitis is associated with a high incidence of complications, including postoperative intraoperative abscess formation. Laparoscopic appendectomy should be avoided in such cases; if complicated appendicitis is discovered at laparoscopy, the operation should be converted to an open one. In equivocal cases, the operation could start with gasless laparoscopy, followed by a standard laparoscopic procedure if the patient has simple, acute appendicitis.

▶ The rush to incorporate laparoscopy for many pediatric surgical conditions is tempered by reports such as this. For many years, it has been difficult to justify up to 3 incisions adding up to 2 cm vs. a 2-cm simple muscle-splitting incision in the right lower quadrant. For advocates of the open procedure, they must acknowledge that sometimes the dissection and the mission become more extensive, certainly in complicated appendicitis. Does laparoscopy allow better operative control, limiting the incision, and afford for better operating clarity? This may not be the appropriate question as raised by these authors. This series represents clear evidence in adults that laparoscopy for complicated appendicitis does lead to higher incidences of abscess and infection. Further studies will potentially bear this out and will require prospective evaluation, as suggested by the authors. Tertiary care children's hospitals will most likely be the sites of these studies, with up to 60% of their patients being seen initially with complicated appendicitis.

T.F. Tracy, Jr., M.D.

Continent Appendicostomy in the Bowel Management of Fecally Incontinent Children

Levitt MA, Soffer SZ, Peña A (Long Island Jewish Med Ctr, New Hyde Park, NY; Albert Einstein College of Medicine, Bronx, NY)

J Pediatr Surg 32:1630-1633, 1997 10–30

Introduction.—Fecal incontinence is a common problem in children, affecting many patients with anorectal malformations, spina bifida, or Hirschsprung's disease. If nothing is done, the child will suffer social and psychologic consequences; diverting colostomy can be done, but then the family must carry the burden of ostomy care. A bowel management program including enemas can be effective but is unpleasant, especially for older children. A previous surgical report described the use of the appendix as a conduit by which to administer an antegrade enema. Experience with a modified continent appendicostomy technique for the management of children with fecal incontinence was reported.

> *Technique.*—The original technique of Malone et al. involved dividing the appendiceal base, inverting it, and reimplanting it into the cecum by an antireflux technique. The modified technique was made simpler by plicating the cecum around the appendix. This created a 1-way valve mechanism while leaving the appendix in its original position. An inconspicuous umbilical stoma was created by mobilization of the cecum and exteriorization of the umbilicus. Cecal wall tissue was used to create a neoappendix if the appendix had been previously removed.

Experience.—This procedure was used in 20 patients with fecal incontinence. Nineteen were children, aged 3-16 years; most had a history of anorectal malformations. All patients but 1 were rendered completely clean 24 hours a day, with no episodes of soiling. A neoappendix was created in 8 cases. In 16 patients, the stoma was made at the umbilicus. Most of the children were able to perform catheterization by themselves. There were 5 postoperative complications, including 1 case of stomal atresia.

Conclusions.—Continent appendicostomy offers a new option for the management of children with fecal incontinence. It provides a safe and effective route for enema administration for patients in whom bowel management with rectal enemas has proven effective. The procedure allows patients to remain clean, provides an inconspicuous stoma, and allows children to catheterize themselves. The appendix has proven useful in the management of fecal and urinary incontinence, and should be preserved whenever possible in patients at risk for these problems.

► The advantages of antegrade enemas are tremendous. The postoperative complications are relatively low, and with the rise of a well-designed bowel management team, significant patient satisfaction and compliance can be achieved. This innovation, first popularized in the United Kingdom, will have a very measurable impact on the lives of children and adolescents with control problems. No longer is incidental appendectomy during the time of Hirschsprung's reconstruction or procedures for imperforate anus a recommended practice.

T.F. Tracy, Jr., M.D.

Increased Risk for Cancer in Patients With the Peutz-Jeghers Syndrome

Boardman LA, Thibodeau SN, Schaid DJ, et al (Mayo Clinic, Rochester, Minn)

Ann Intern Med 128:896-899, 1998 10–31

Objective.—Controversy exists as to whether patients with Peutz-Jeghers syndrome are at increased risk of cancer. Other polyposis syndromes are known to predispose to cancer. The occurrence of cancer in a group of patients with Peutz-Jeghers syndrome was analyzed in a retrospective cohort study.

Methods.—A review of Mayo Clinic files identified 34 patients with Peutz-Jeghers syndrome seen between 1945 and 1996. The patients were from 31 Peutz-Jeghers kindreds. All patients had confirmed hamartomatous polyps with small-bowel polyposis, melanotic pigmentation, and/or a family history of the disease. Their subsequent cancer experience was assessed by chart review and telephone follow-up interviews. Relative risk ratios for cancer were calculated with the use of Surveillance, Epidemiology, and End Results (SEER) data.

Results.—Fifty-three percent of patients developed noncutaneous cancers during follow-up. A total of 26 cancers were diagnosed including 10 gastrointestinal cancers. Multiple primary cancers occurred in 6 patients. Compared with population data, the relative risk of cancer among patients with Peutz-Jeghers syndrome was 18.5 for women (95% confidence interval, 8.5 to 35.2) and 6.2 for men (95% confidence interval, 2.5 to 12.8). Gynecologic or breast cancer developed in half of the female patients, relative risk (RR) 20.3 (95% confidence interval, 7.4 to 44.2). A distinctive benign genital tract tumor developed in 5 of the women with gynecologic or breast cancers.

Conclusions.—Long-term follow-up reveals a marked predisposition to cancer among patients with Peutz-Jeghers syndrome. The study documents non-gastrointestinal (breast, ovarian, cervical, uterine, thyroid, lung, and prostate) and gastrointestinal cancers (colon, duodenal, and esophageal) in this group of patients. Risk appears to be especially high for women.

Reservation Card for the Year Book

Yes! I would like my own copy of ***Year Book of Surgery***® at the price of **$76.95** (**$85.00** outside the U.S.) plus sales tax, postage, and handling. Please begin my subscription with the current edition according to the terms described below.* I understand that I will have 30 days to examine each annual edition.

Name ______________________________

Address ______________________________

City ______________________ State __________ ZIP __________

Method of Payment

Check (in U.S. dollars, drawn on a U.S. bank, payable to ***Year Book of Surgery***®)

❑ VISA ❑ MasterCard ❑ Discover ❑ AmEx ❑ Bill me

Card number ______________________ Exp. date: __________

Signature ______________________________

Prices are subject to change without notice. PMC-366

Subscribe to the related journal in your field!

Yes! Begin my one-year subscription to ***Surgery*** (12 issues).

Name ______________________

Institution ______________________

Address ______________________

City ______________ State ________

ZIP/PC __________ Country __________

Specialty ______________________
(Students/residents, please list Institution)

Subscription prices (through 9/30/99)

		USA	Canada*	Int'l
Individuals	❑	$142.00	$182.97	$171.00
Institutions	❑	299.00	350.96	328.00
Students, residents	❑	67.00	102.72	96.00

Method of payment

Enclose payment (check or credit card number) and we'll send an extra issue FREE!

❑ Check (in U.S. dollars, drawn on a U.S. bank, and payable to ***Surgery***)

❑ VISA ❑ MasterCard ❑ Discover

❑ AmEx ❑ Bill me Exp. date __________

Card # ______________________

Signature ______________________

*Includes Canadian GST

Individual/student subscriptions must be in the name of, billed to, and paid for by the individual.

Airmail rates available upon request.
Prices subject to change without notice.

J011991YA

*Your Year Book service guarantee:

When you subscribe to the *Year Book*, you will receive advance notice of future annual volumes about two months before publication. To receive the new edition, you need do nothing—we'll send you the new volume as soon as it is available. If you want to discontinue, the advance notice allows you time to notify us of your decision. If you are not completely satisfied, you have 30 days to return any *Year Book*.

NO POSTAGE NECESSARY IF MAILED IN THE UNITED STATES

BUSINESS REPLY MAIL

FIRST-CLASS MAIL PERMIT NO 135 ST LOUIS MO

POSTAGE WILL BE PAID BY ADDRESSEE

SUBSCRIPTION SERVICES
MOSBY, INC.
11830 WESTLINE INDUSTRIAL DRIVE
ST. LOUIS MO 63146-9988

NO POSTAGE NECESSARY IF MAILED IN THE UNITED STATES

BUSINESS REPLY MAIL

FIRST-CLASS MAIL PERMIT NO 135 ST LOUIS MO

POSTAGE WILL BE PAID BY ADDRESSEE

SUBSCRIPTION SERVICES
MOSBY, INC.
11830 WESTLINE INDUSTRIAL DRIVE
ST. LOUIS MO 63146-9988

Want to speed up the process?

To order a *Year Book* or *Advances*, you also may call 1-800-426-4545

To subscribe to a journal today, call toll-free in the U.S.: 1-800-453-4351 or fax 314-432-1158 Outside the U.S., call: 314-453-4351

Visit us at: *www.mosby.com/periodicals*

Mosby, Inc.
Subscription Services
11830 Westline Industrial Drive
St. Louis, MO 63146 U.S.A.

Mosby

Regular screening for colon, breast, and cervical cancer is indicated in patients with Peutz-Jeghers syndrome.

▶ This interesting report from the Mayo Clinic addresses the controversial issue of an increased risk of cancer in patients with juvenile polyposis. This retrospective cohort study in 34 patients with Peutz-Jeghers syndrome identifies a total of 10 cases of gastrointestinal cancer and 16 cases of extraintestinal cancer. As one can see from the 2 tables, the onset of these cancer cases is well beyond the pediatric age group, ranging anywhere between age 32 and 57 for the gastrointestinal cancer cases, and between 23 and 66 for the extraintestinal cancer cases. The overall relative risk for development of cancer in this series of Peutz-Jeghers patients was 9.9% (95% CI, 5.7 to 16.2). For men, the relative risk was 6.2, significantly lower than for women, in whom it was 18.5. In all patients, the relative risk for gastrointestinal cancer was 50.5. This risk was also greater for women (150.9) than for men (30.3). In this long-term follow-up study of a cohort of 34 patients with the Peutz-Jeghers syndrome, a marked predisposition for both gastrointestinal and extraintestinal cancer is emphasized. Similar observations have been reported by other authors, and we have observed similar findings in our institution in cases of juvenile polyposis. The risk for intestinal carcinoma was obviously greater when an adenomatous component was identified in the excised polyp. The association with cancer in such cases is not expected to be significantly different than any other adenomas.[1] In this study, women in affected families seem to have a greater susceptibility for the development of cancer, especially breast and gynecologic cancers. The important implication of this risk mandates regular screening in these patients for at least colonic, breast and cervical carcinoma.

V.E. Pricolo, M.D.

Reference

1. Coburn MC, Pricolo VE, DeLuca FG, et al: Malignant potential in intestinal juvenile polyposis syndromes. *Ann Surg Oncol* 2:386-391, 1995.

Detection of Colonic Polyps in a Phantom Model: Implications for Virtual Colonoscopy Data Acquistion

Beaulieu CF, Napel S, Daniel BL, et al (Stanford Univ, Calif)

J Comput Assist Tomogr 22:656-663, 1998 10–32

Background.—By combining spiral volumetric CT scanning with computer-assisted visualization tools, 3-dimensional CT colonography—also called virtual colonoscopy—provides a noninvasive means of assessing the colonic mucosa. The objective of virtual colonoscopy is accurate detection of precancerous polyps measuring 1 cm or greater. The effect of CT acquisition parameters on polyp detectability and sizing during virtual colonoscopy was analyzed in a phantom study.

Methods.—The model used segments of plastic tubing with spherical plastic beads, ranging in diameter from 2.5 to 10.0 mm, randomly attached to the inner wall. The tubes were sealed and immersed in water and scanned at various collimation/pitch settings in orientations perpendicular and parallel to the scanner gantry. Reconstruction intervals of 0.5 to 5.0 mm were used to create image sets for each acquisition. Bead detection in transverse cross-sections was assessed in blinded fashion. The reviewers used source CT images for acquisitions obtained with the tube oriented perpendicular to the gantry and orthogonal reformatted images for scans oriented parallel to the gantry. The effects of scan acquisition and reconstruction parameters on clinical lesion detectability were evaluated.

Results.—Regardless of tube orientation, collimator/pitch settings, and reconstruction intervals, all beads measuring 4 mm or larger were correctly detected. However, for 5 mm collimation/pitch 2 scans oriented parallel to the gantry, detection of 2.5-mm beads was only 78% to 94%. With increasing collimation and pitch, the beads appeared to become elongated in the direction of the slice. Approximately three-fourths of this elongation was related to increasing the collimation from 3 to 5 mm, while the rest resulted from doubling the pitch from 3 to 5 mm.

Conclusions.—In this phantom model of virtual colonoscopy, a CT collimation setting of 5 mm with a pitch of up to 2 appears effective for the detection of high-contrast lesions measuring as little as 4 mm. At narrower collimation/lower pitch settings, accuracy of lesion size and geometry may decrease. This model does not address the importance of CT artifacts associated with increasing pitch, which may affect clinical judgments that are based on the findings of virtual colonoscopy.

► This intriguing contribution from the Department of Radiology and Statistics at Stanford University Medical Center addresses the issue of development of new technology in the detection of colorectal diseases. Virtual colonoscopy has received much attention as a new method that may offer a less-invasive way of detecting colorectal conditions, colorectal lesions, and in particular, carcinoma. The article offers a detailed description of the physics and technological background required for the phantom construction, CT acquisition and reconstruction, as well as image processing and review for detection. The CAT scanning reconstruction at 5 mm collimation up to pitch 2 appears to be adequate for detection of lesions as small as 4 mm. However, lesion size and geometry may be important variables in the ability to detect lesions at different settings. It appears that colonoscopy at this time remains the gold standard for the detection of colorectal diseases, in particular, small mucosal lesions that may otherwise be missed. This technical development is certainly of great interest, but it appears that further large sample studies are required in comparison with colonoscopy to further assess its reliability.

V.E. Pricolo, M.D.

Standardized Perioperative Care Protocols and Reduced Length of Stay After Colon Surgery

Bradshaw BGG, Liu SS, Thirlby RC (Virginia Mason Med Ctr, Seattle)

J Am Coll Surg 186:501-506, 1998 10–33

Background.—Critical pathways and standard order sets have been used as part of efforts to reduce lengths of the hospital stays while improving quality of care. In a randomized trial, the authors found that perioperative epidural bupivacaine or morphine/bupivacaine was associated with earlier return of bowel function after elective colon resection. All subjects in this study were treated under a standardized perioperative protocol, which included ketorolac, early nasogastric tube removal, early feeding with a low-fat liquid diet, and ambulation on the first day after surgery. The contribution of this perioperative protocol to early return of bowel function and hospital discharge was assessed.

Methods.—The case-control study included 36 trial patients treated on the standardized perioperative protocol and the same number of control patients treated off protocol. All patients underwent colorectal surgery performed by the same surgeons during the same calendar year. The 2 groups were comparable in the type of surgery and anesthesia. The hospital courses of patients treated on protocol were compared to those treated off protocol.

Results.—Time to removal of the nasogastric tube was 2.2 days in the control group vs. 1.0 day in the study group. Average time to starting an oral diet was 2.9 days in the control group, who usually started on clear liquids; the study patients started on a specific liquid diet 1 day postoperatively. From return of bowel sounds through flatus and bowel movements, patients treated under the standardized perioperative protocol had return of bowel function about 1 day sooner. Time to discharge was also about a day sooner in the study group vs. the control group.

Conclusions.—By eliminating variations in anesthesia and postoperative care, a standardized perioperative protocol like the one evaluated in this study appears to shorten the time to return of bowel function and time to hospital discharge in patients undergoing elective colon resection. The study protocol appears to have reduced the length of stay without compromising patient outcomes. The protocol's effect on outcomes appears to be independent of anesthetic technique.

▶ This well-designed study addresses the hypothesis that critical pathways may shorten length of stay after colon surgery. Thirty-six study patients were compared with 36 control patients undergoing colorectal surgery by the same surgeons during the same calendar year to determine whether a standardized perioperative protocol would lead to earlier return of bowel function and allow for earlier discharge from the hospital. The patients enrolled in the critical pathway study could be discharged 1 day sooner than control patients.

This study addresses several important aspects of reducing length of stay after colorectal surgery in a time where the pressures to reduce the costs of health care have led hospital administrations to emphasize reduction of resources and decreased hospital length of stay. A few years ago, it appeared that laparoscopic colon and rectal surgery may facilitate this process. The omission of a nasogastric tube in the postoperative period, the initiation of feeding without waiting for flatus or bowel movement, and cautious analgesic protocols have all contributed to shortening of hospital stay. In our institution, we have implemented a similar critical pathway after colon and rectal surgery, and we are observing similar results, especially when otherwise, a large group of surgeons and residents in a teaching setting would create a tremendous variability in postoperative management orders. The main advantage of the standardization of perioperative care is the reduction in such variability. The most important caveat in this process, of course, is to allow room for judgment, and allow progression in the critical pathway based on achievement of certain goals by the patient, for example, reduced pain level, ability to ambulate, presence of bowel sounds, and presence of flatus. In our institution, our preference is then to implement the interventions not based on the postoperative "day," but rather on the postoperative "phase." The shortest length of stay we've observed in patients who underwent a colonic resection with a laparoscopic technique has been 72 hours. In patients after a traditional colon resection with a longer incision and no laparoscopic dissection, the length of stay in the best possible scenario has been 96 hours. It is also of paramount importance to prepare patient families or any other support group at home, such as visiting nurses, to anticipate discharges from the day of admission, or even at the time of the preoperative office visit.

V.E. Pricolo, M.D.

Restoration of Anal Sphincter Function by Single-Stage Dynamic Graciloplasty With a Modified (Split Sling) Technique

Rosen HR, Novi G, Zoech G, et al (Danube Hosp, Vienna)
Am J Surg 175:187-193, 1998 10–34

Introduction.—"Dynamic graciloplasty" refers to the use of electrostimulation to transform fast-twitching type II muscle fibers into slow-twitching type I fibers, thus providing skeletal muscles with the capacity for tetanic contraction. This technique has given promising results in the treatment of patients with fecal incontinence or those who have undergone excision of the anal sphincter. The results of dynamic graciloplasty were seen in 28 patients.

Methods.—The 5-year experience included 16 men and 12 women (median age, 53.5 years) who had fecal incontinence or had undergone abdominoperineal resection (APR) of the anal sphincter. Twelve patients underwent APR with synchronous graciloplasty to restore the excised sphincter. Six underwent total anorectal reconstruction after previous

APR. Four patients had acquired fecal incontinence, and 6 had congenital atresia. In a 1-stage procedure, the muscle was transposed and the stimulation electrodes and pulse generator implanted. The neosphincter was wrapped with a modified split-sling technique. This was followed by controlled neuromuscular stimulation to transform the muscle, performed over 8 weeks in the early part of the experience and 4 weeks in the latter part.

Results.—There were no postoperative deaths. Early in the experience, 4 patients had rectal injury, most often caused by overstimulation causing extensive tension of the muscle sling. Median resting pressure increased from 27.5 mm Hg before surgery to 42.8 mm Hg after graciloplasty, with no further change after muscle transformation. Median squeeze pressure increased from 39.2 to 89.3 mm Hg. Ninety percent of patients had congenital or acquired incontinence for solids or liquids or solids alone. In contrast, only 55.5% of patients with APR had satisfactory outcomes, defined as continence for solids or liquids, solids alone, or with occasional episodes for liquids. Defecation disorders were the major functional problem for patients who had undergone APR, necessitating enemas for treatment.

Conclusions.—With the 1-stage technique used in this study, dynamic graciloplasty can achieve continence within 7 weeks in patients with an insufficient or excised anal sphincter. The muscle wrap must be placed under correct tension to avoid direct injury to the rectum. To address this issue, the authors have created a modified intraoperative anal manometry device to provide objective data on the pressures created by the neosphincter. To achieve satisfactory results with dynamic graciloplasty, patients must be carefully selected and informed about potential postoperative problems with this last-resort technique.

▶ This interesting contribution from our Austrian colleagues reports their experience over a 6-year period with 28 patients treated with dynamic graciloplasty. A significant number of patients had an absent anus, either because of congenital atresia or because of previous abdominoperineal resection. The functional results are outstanding, considering that patients who underwent operation for congenital atresia achieved satisfactory continence scores in 90% of cases, and patients operated on after abdominoperineal resection had a satisfactory functional outcome in about half of the cases. Interestingly, the main problem in this latter group of patients was defecation disturbance that necessitated local treatment with enemas. The technique of dynamic graciloplasty continues to remain a valuable addition to the armamentarium of the advanced colon and rectal surgeon, who is dealing with the challenges of incontinence or elimination of a permanent stoma. We are currently involved in a multicenter trial of implanting an artificial bowel sphincter, which may become a valuable alternative to dynamic graciloplasty in the near future.

V.E. Pricolo, M.D.

Pouchitis: Risk Factors, Etiology, and Treatment

Nicholls RJ, Chir M, Banerjee AK (St Mark's Hosp, Middlesex, England; Royal Halifax Infirmary, West Yorkshire, England)

World J Surg 22:347-351, 1998 10–35

Objective.—Up to 40% of patients undergoing ileoanal anastomosis with pouch creation will develop pouchitis. This is an inflammation of the pouch, causing such symptoms as crampy abdominal pain, fever, rectal bleeding, and diarrhea, and occurring in either intermittent attacks or as a chronic pouchitis syndrome. The findings of a systematic review of the literature on pouchitis are reported, focusing on the etiology, diagnosis, and treatment.

Etiology.—Pouchitis probably results from a combination of genetic, immune, microbial, and toxic mediators. There is evidence to support various etiologies, including causes involving bacteria, stasis, ischemia, and underlying disease. Some of these studies may offer insights into the pathogenesis of inflammatory bowel disease. Pouchitis is most common in patients with a history of ulcerative colitis, affecting few patients operated on for familial adenomatous polyposis.

Diagnosis.—Patients typically present with sudden malaise and diarrhea. Extraintestinal manifestations may also occur. Acute pouchitis quickly improves with metronidazole treatment; chronic pouchitis does not respond to conventional anti-inflammatory drugs. Pouchitis may be divided into 3 subtypes: acute, acute relapsing, and chronic unremitting. The differential diagnosis includes outflow obstruction, infection, and Crohn's disease. The diagnosis is made by the combination of symptoms and the histologic confirmation of acute inflammation. The severity of the symptoms may be correlated with the histologic and endoscopic changes observed. The histologic findings include chronic inflammation and villous atrophy, colonic metaplasia, and "diversion" changes.

Treatment.—Treatment focuses on relieving diarrheal symptoms while replacing lost iron and vitamins. The usual dosage of metronidazole is 200 mg orally 3 times daily; this is effective in about 80% of patients. Other reported treatments include topical 5-aminosalicylic acid, topical or systemic steroids, and binding resins, such as kaopectate. Surgery is not commonly performed. Simple defunctioning does not alleviate the inflammation; temporary ileostomy is unlikely to be reversed later. Only about 1% of patients require pouch excision.

Discussion.—Pouchitis is a common complication of ileoanal anastomosis with pouch creation among patients with ulcerative colitis, though rare among those with polyposis. The diagnosis of pouchitis should be made carefully and should not be applied to patients with poor pouch function or with Crohn's disease. Most attacks of pouchitis will respond to treatment with metronidazole. In chronic cases, other functional abnormalities may be present and are potentially debilitating.

► This interesting review by Dr. Nicholls, a co-author in the first clinical series on ileoanal anastomosis from England in 1976, addresses the much-debated issues surrounding pouchitis. Restorative proctocolectomy with ileal pouch-anal anastomosis remains the definitive treatment of choice for ulcerative colitis and familial adenomatous polyposis. The likelihood of developing pouchitis is often very difficult to estimate and, as one can see from Table 1 in the original article, there are several theories surrounding its possible etiology. In this scholarly review, the different theories and data regarding pathophysiology of this condition are well discussed. The issue of the definitive diagnosis is also relevant, because it is a common occurrence for patients who have undergone this operation to be labeled with a diagnosis of "pouchitis" for any event that may lead to increased frequency of bowel movements, which may be related to various other conditions (infectious diarrhea, outflow obstruction, Crohn's disease). The differential diagnosis and definitive determination by a careful clinical history, physical examination, as well as endoscopy of the pouch with biopsy, is of critical importance. The different management options are reviewed and generally successful management is the rule, with pouch excision necessary in only approximately 1% of patients with pouchitis.

V.E. Pricolo, M.D.

Reconstructive Surgery for Pelvic Pouches

Cohen Z, Smith D, McLeod R (Univ of Toronto)

World J Surg 22:342-346, 1998 10–36

Background.—For patients with ulcerative colitis, restorative proctocolectomy with ileo–-pouch-anal anastomosis is the surgical treatment of choice. It is also used selectively in patients with familial adenomatous polyposis. Leakage from the ileo–pouch-anal anastomosis can be a difficult-to-manage complication, which in some cases resists all attempts at local repair. A more radical reconstructive approach for salvage of the pelvic pouch is described.

Patients.—The experience included 24 patients with septic complications after ileo-pouch-anal anastomosis that did not improve with local reconstructive surgery. The patients were 19 women and 5 men, mean age, 28 years. Twenty-two had ulcerative colitis, and 10 were referred for reconstructive surgery from other centers. The patients averaged nearly 3 local salvage procedures over a mean of 35-months before radical reconstruction was done. Twelve of the 19 female patients had an anastomotic vaginal fistula.

Reconstruction and Outcomes.—In 14 patients, the existing pouch was used for revision surgery; in 10 patients, the initial pouch was excised and a second pouch created. Just 2 of the 24 reconstructed pouches had to be removed. The success rate of radical reconstruction was greater than 75%. Four patients still had an ileostomy, although 2 of these were awaiting closure of loop ileostomy. Functional outcome was assessable in 18 patients, 13 (72%) of whom had normal daytime continence and 17 (94%) of whom had sexual function. All 18 patients were satisfied or very satisfied, although functional assessment suggested that only 13 had satisfactory function.

Conclusions.—Radical reconstructive surgery has an important role to play in patients with ileo-pouch-anal anastomosis complications in whom attempts at local pouch repair have failed. This approach might also be useful for patients in whom first-line management seems likely to fail. Good results depend on commitment by both the surgeon and patient. Severe complications like those in this series can be managed successfully by experienced surgeons with a specific interest in pouch surgery.

▶ This report from the Toronto Colorectal Group reviews 24 patients who required a more radical reconstructive approach for salvage of a pelvic pouch after local procedures had failed, and complications had developed. This procedure still enjoys an excellent rate of satisfaction among patients with ulcerative colitis and familial polyposis, despite a complication rate around 40% reported by all institutions with a large experience with this procedure. The various surgical approaches, ranging from revision to redo of the pouch, are analyzed in this article which reports a greater than 75% success rate using a reconstructive approach. It is essential for surgeons embarking on these complex procedures to make a long-term commitment to providing patients with all possible options to maintain an acceptable quality of life, which was the reason for choosing this procedure in the first place.

V.E. Pricolo, M.D.

Diagnosing Anal Sphincter Injury With Transanal Ultrasound and Manometry

Sentovich SM, Blatchford GJ, Rivela LJ, et al (Beth Israel Deaconess Med Ctr, Boston; Creighton Univ, Omaha, Neb)

Dis Colon Rectum 40:1430-1434, 1997 10–37

Background.—Various techniques are used in an attempt to understand the origin of fecal incontinence in women, particularly anorectal manometry and transanal ultrasound. Both tests provide useful information for the diagnosis of anal sphincter injury. The value of anorectal manometry and transanal ultrasound in diagnosing anal sphincter injury was assessed.

Methods.—The study included 20 asymptomatic nulliparous women and 20 asymptomatic parous women, all of whom underwent anorectal manometry and transanal ultrasound. Also studied were 31 incontinent women who later underwent sphincteroplasty for surgical verification of anal sphincter injury. Computerized manometry was used to assess mean maximum resting and squeeze pressures, sphincter length, and vector symmetry for all patients. The transanal ultrasound scans were read without knowledge of the history, physical examination, and manometry findings.

Results.—Manometry revealed higher resting and squeeze pressures in asymptomatic nulliparous women than in asymptomatic parous women. Pressures were higher in both groups of asymptomatic women than in the incontinent women. The incontinent women also had significantly reduced anal sphincter length and vector symmetry index. Of incontinent women with confirmed anal sphincter injury, 90% had decreased resting and squeeze pressures consistent with sphincter injury. In contrast, only 42% of this group had decreased anal sphincter length and vector symmetry. One hundred percent of confirmed sphincter injuries were demonstrated by transanal ultrasound. However, ultrasound also gave a 10% false-negative rate among asymptomatic nulliparous women without anal sphincter injuries. False-negative diagnoses were particularly likely when scanning proximal to the distal 1.5 cm of the anal canal.

Conclusions.—Manometry demonstrates reduced resting and squeeze pressures in 90% of patients with surgically confirmed anal sphincter injury. Decreased anal sphincter length and vector symmetry index are less reliable findings. Transanal ultrasound is excellent at depicting known sphincter injuries, but is prone to false-positive results in the distal 1.5 cm of the anal canal. Used in women with reduced anal pressures, transanal ultrasound can correctly identify all intact sphincters and 90% of injured sphincters.

▶ This study compares the results of manometry testing as well as endoanal ultrasonography in a group of 20 asymptomatic nulliparous women and 20 asymptomatic parous women, with results obtained in 31 incontinent women who subsequently underwent anal sphincteroplasty. As one can see from Table 4 in the original article, the combination of manometry and transanal ultrasonography is extremely valuable in predicting sphincter injury in these 3 groups of women. It is also our experience in the anorectal physiology laboratory in our institution that the combination of these 2 tests is necessary. In fact, they provide adequate assessment of anosphincteric injury from a morphologic as well as from a functional point of view. Only by obtaining combined information from both these tests, can one plan the most satisfactory operative intervention.

V.E. Pricolo, M.D.

A Comparison of Botulinum Toxin and Saline for the Treatment of Chronic Anal Fissure

Maria G, Cassetta E, Gui D, et al (Università Cattolica del Sarco Cuore, Rome; Centro S Giovanni di Dio, Fatebenefratelli, Brescia, Italy)
N Engl J Med 338:217-220, 1998 10–38

Purpose.—Patients with chronic anal fissure have tearing of the lower half of the anal canal, possibly related to severe constipation or straining at stool. Internal anal sphincter contraction serves to maintain the fissure. Surgical sphincterotomy, the most common treatment, is done to relieve symptoms and promote healing. However, it also weakens the internal sphincter, possibly leading to complications, such as anal deformity and incontinence. A preliminary study suggested that local infiltration of botulinum toxin may be effective. A double-blind, placebo-controlled trial of this treatment alternative is reported.

Methods.—The study included 30 consecutive patients with symptomatic chronic anal fissure. The 15 patients in the treatment group received 2 injections of botulinum toxin A, for a total of 20 U in a volume of 0.4 mL. The control group received saline injections. The results were assessed for fissure healing with scar formation and symptomatic improvement.

Results.—After a follow-up of 2 months, fissures had healed in 73% of patients receiving botulinum toxin vs. 13% of those receiving saline. Symptom relief was achieved in 87% of the treatment group vs. 27% of the control group. Both groups showed no significant change in maximal voluntary pressures from baseline. Patients receiving botulinum toxin injections had a 25% reduction in resting anal pressure, whereas the control group showed no change.

Ten of the control patients went on to receive botulinum toxin injections, while 3 underwent sphincterotomy. Seven of the 10 patients treated with botulinum toxin had fissure healing, while the other 3 went on to surgery. Four patients from the original treatment who had persistent fissures were retreated with botulinum toxin, 25 U. Retreatment produced fissure healing within 2 months in all patients. Temporary flatus incontinence was a problem after botulinum toxin injection for 1 patient in the control group. No relapses occurred through 16 months of follow-up.

Conclusions.—As an alternative to sphincterotomy, patients with chronic anal fissure may be effectively treated with local infiltration of botulinum toxin. This treatment is simple, inexpensive, and does not require anesthesia. It may be especially valuable for patients at risk of incontinence.

▶ This contribution by a group of investigators from the departments of surgery and neurology of the Catholic University in Rome addressed the annoying issue of chronic anal fissure. In this article, patients were assigned to a double-blind, placebo-controlled study to undergo evaluation of botulinum toxin. The treated patients received 20 units of botulinum toxin A, while the control group received saline. As one can see from the tables included, and from the results, the treated group had a greater decrease in maximal voluntary pressure but a less-pronounced change in resting pressures. Incontinence was remarkably rare and transient, and noticed only in 1 patient who experienced temporary flatus and incontinence after treatment with botulinum toxin and after failing to respond to saline in the control group. There were no relapses after an average 16-month follow-up. Local infiltration of botulinum toxin appears to be an effective treatment for chronic anal fissure, as reported by other international studies. The main alternative to this treatment, which is currently under investigation, is application of nitroglycerine ointment. We are participating in a multicenter clinical trial to establish the optimal dosage and frequency of application of nitroglycerine ointment. Although according to this article, the perianal injections were easily performed, painless and did not cause any local or systemic complications, application of an ointment may be more acceptable to patients.

V.E. Pricolo, M.D.

Comparison of Three Perineal Procedures for the Treatment of Rectal Prolapse

Agachan F, Reissman P, Pfeifer J, et al (Cleveland Clinic Florida, Fort Lauderdale, Fla)

South Med J 90:925-932, 1998 10–39

Objective.—Despite the many different operations proposed, there is still no consensus as to the optimal surgical technique for management of rectal prolapse. The emphasis in assessing the results has recently shifted from recurrence rates to functional outcomes. The short-term outcomes of 3 surgical procedures for the treatment of rectal prolapse were compared.

Methods.—The analysis included 61 patients undergoing 1 of 3 perineal procedures for correction of full-thickness rectal prolapse during a 6-year period. The procedures were perineal rectosigmoidectomy, perineal rectosigmoidectomy with levatoroplasty, and Delorme's procedure. The patients were 55 women and 6 men, mean age, 75 years. The 3 techniques were compared for morbidity, mortality, short-term recurrence rates, and subjective function. In addition, continence was assessed using a standard incontinence scoring system, accounting for frequency and type of incontinence.

Results.—Sixteen deaths occurred from comorbid conditions during follow-up of 3 to 42 months. Median hospital stay was about 5 days with each procedure. The short-term recurrence rate was 13% after perineal rectosigmoidectomy, 5% after perineal rectosigmoidectomy with levatoroplasty and 38% after Delorme's operation. On a scale of 0 to 20, mean postoperative incontinence scores in the 3 operations were 7, 5, and 11, respectively. The 3 procedures also differed significantly in mean resection length, coloanal anastomotic stricture, and leakage. However, the 3 procedures had similar results on anal manometric studies both preoperatively and postoperatively, and no significant manometric changes were observed.

Conclusions.—For patients with rectal prolapse, perineal rectosigmoidectomy with levatoroplasty is a safe procedure that produces better short-term functional outcomes than perineal rectosigmoidectomy or Delorme's procedure. The addition of levatoroplasty improves incontinence outcomes while reducing the short-term recurrence rate. The results suggest that Delorme's procedure is indicated only for patients with minimal rectal prolapse, in whom perineal rectosigmoidectomy is impossible.

▶ This review of the Cleveland Clinic, Florida's experience with the treatment of rectal prolapse over a 7-year period compares patients who underwent 1 of 3 procedures: Delorme's procedure, perineal rectosigmoidectomy, or perineal rectosigmoidectomy with levatoroplasty. A thorough clinical and physiologic assessment was carried out before and after treatment. Results were assessed additionally with an incontinence scoring system. As one can see from the table, the lowest recurrence rate and the best and lowest incontinence scores were obtained when a levatoroplasty was added to the perineal rectosigmoidectomy. Perineal rectosigmoidectomy with a levatoroplasty is a safe procedure that appears to provide better short-term functional outcome than either perineal rectosigmoidectomy alone or Delorme's operation. The role of a Delorme's procedure appears to be limited to cases of minimal length of prolapse, where a perineal rectosigmoidectomy would be technically impossible.

V.E. Pricolo, M.D.

Open Pelvic Fracture and Fecal Diversion

Woods RK, O'Keefe G, Rhee P, et al (Univ of Washington, Seattle)

Arch Surg 133:281-286, 1998 10–40

Objective.—Approximately one third to one half of the deaths observed during repair of open pelvic fracture result from sepsis developing from an infectious source within the pelvis. Therefore, mandatory fecal diversion has been advocated, although the need for such diversion has not been proved. The infectious complications in patients who underwent diversion and those who did not were compared retrospectively in a case-control study.

Methods.—Between July 1987 and December 1993, 60 patients with open pelvic fracture were treated with (group 1, N = 19) or without (group 2, N = 41) fecal diversion. An additional 186 patients amenable to analysis were found in a literature review and were included in the study. Infection rates were compared between groups.

Results.—Abdominopelvic infections developed in 5 diverted patients (27%) and in 7 nondiverted patients (17%). After controlling for Injury Severity Score, Glasgow Coma Scale Score, initial vital signs, pelvic injury pattern and severity, and time to skeletal fixation, the differences were not significant. Mechanical instability was the only variable associated with infection, according to stepwise regression analysis. Combining information from this series of patients with the additional 186 cases found in the literature resulted in a composite series of 246 patients. Of the composite group, 46 of the 171 diverted patients (27%) and 22 of the 75 nondiverted (29%) had infectious complications.

Conclusion.—These results do not support fecal diversion as a technique for reducing the incidence of infectious complications in patients with an open pelvic fracture.

▶ This article challenges the dictum that open pelvic fractures require fecal diversion in an attempt to decrease infection-related morbidity. Although this study has multiple flaws that include its nonrandomized nature, the authors present a convincing argument that diversion of the fecal stream is not associated with a lower incidence of abdominopelvic infection complications. The data suggest that, rather than blind performance of diversion in all patients, management should be individualized. Cautious interpretation of the conclusions, however, is warranted, and this article should serve as an impetus for a randomized trial of diversion in open pelvic fractures, given the potential morbidity of the initial exploration and subsequent ostomy closure.

W.G. Cioffi, M.D.

11 Oncology

Introduction

This year has seen maturation of many clinical trials that will help the practicing surgeon in the care of his patient. Similarly, new technology, new surgical techniques, and advancements in tumor markers and prevention and calculation of risk have been seen.

Many of the clinical trials are large multicentered prospective studies. They help define the parameters for treatment and frequently help define parameters for more conservative approaches. Examples are the 8-year follow-up of the National Surgical Adjuvant Breast and Bowel Project B-17 trial and the primary chemotherapy trial with similar follow-up from Milan. Similarly, large clinical experiences have helped to define the likelihood of tumor spread. HER2/neu overexpression and lymphatic vessel invasion were commonly associated with palpable breast cancers and more likely to show nodal metastases. In rectal cancer, differentiation, tumor size, and depth of penetration were associated with a significant increase in positive lymph nodes if aneuploidy was also present. Of course, both of these studies would suggest that patients have further, more aggressive adjuvant treatments. In a similar fashion, parameters are being determined for prognosis of patients with hereditary nonpolyposis colorectal carcinoma.

Clinical trials have also been done to help define parameters for better care. An example is the very large institutional analysis of 5-year survivors with periampulary adenocarcinoma. Similarly, treatment-related factors affecting outcome with breast conserving therapy for ductal carcinoma in situ is presented. Some trials have been performed in very rare tumors such as retroperitoneal soft tissue sarcomas. Here, incomplete resection as well as grade and size were found to be important in disease-specific survival.

Another issue touched upon by several groups was the improved results from specialized centers. This was seen in the treatment of pancreatic cancers where facilities that perform pancreaticoduodenectomies at high volume are associated with a marked decrease of in-hospital mortality rates. Similar results were found in the study for soft tissue sarcoma. Regional specialized centers and subspecialty surgeons may be overtly supported as managed care contracting organizations begin to follow outcomes benchmarking.

Surgeons are always interested in alternative and new technology. This year saw studies that defined parameters for stent placement in the palliative treatment of acute colorectal obstruction, comparisons between small and large colonic J-pouches after coloanal anastomoses, and use of positron emission tomography and CT in detecting recurrent and metastatic colorectal cancers.

Because surgeons are often the primary caregiver of the newly diagnosed oncology patient, assessment of risk in family members is going to take an increasingly important role. Not only will it be important for surgeons to familiarize themselves with specific risks (such as cancer risk among women with cosmetic breast implants), but also to estimate hereditary risk. Although a mutlidisciplinary genetic counseling team is most appropriate in fully explaining risks to patients, the surgeon often will be the initial interface and therefore have an increasingly important role in defining who requires genetic counseling and further analyse an often difficult and emotional set of circustances for the patients or family member.

This past year has seen further advances in the understanding of tumor biology, whether this be the association of impaired interleukin-12 production with a defective antitumor response or tumor angiogenesis and its effect on the mode of metastasis.

Several selections this past year have dealt with 2 other important areas where cancer surgeons play an important role: prevention strategies such as alteration of dietary intake to modify colonic epithelial cells, and postsurgical surveillance utilizing colonoscopy. Once again, a comprehensive approach is necessary, with analysis of benefit and risk as well as cost playing an important role before changing behaviors.

In cancer surgery, there is a tendency toward more conservative approaches. This is important in the treatment of breast cancer or in the selection of patients with rectal cancer in an attempt to preserve a functional rectum. Each of these areas involves not only careful patient selection and paying close attention to meticulous technique, but also involvement of multimodality therapy that may reduce the risk of recurrence and improve overall survival.

Surgeons who treat cancer are constantly striving to provide better care, often with less mutilating surgeries and improved outcome. There has been an explosion of clinical trials offering alternatives to standard surgical paradigms (for example, sentinel lymph node biopsy techniques). A better understanding of the basic tumor biology will not only help to predict risk but define better treatment modalities and appropriate surveillance. Fortunately, surgeons will continue to be at the center of all of these advances.

Timothy J. Eberlein, M.D.

Breast

Lumpectomy and Radiation Therapy for the Treatment of Intraductal Breast Cancer: Findings From National Surgical Adjuvant Breast and Bowel Project B-17

Fisher B, Dignam J, Wolmark N, et al (Allegheny Univ, Pittsburgh, Pa)
J Clin Oncol 16:441-452, 1998 11–1

Introduction.—Since 1985, the standard treatment for women with intraductal carcinoma in situ has been lumpectomy with radiation, but an updated clinical trial had not been conducted. After 8 years, a study was conducted to follow up this information and to evaluate the worth of radiation therapy after lumpectomy.

Methods.—Eight hundred and eighteen women with localized intraductal carcinoma in situ were randomly assigned either to lumpectomy plus radiation at 50 Gy or to lumpectomy. So that resected specimen margins were histologically tumor-free, tissue was removed. There was a mean follow-up time of 90 months, with a range of 67 to 130 months. Central clinical, mammographic, and pathologic assessments were used to determine size and method of tumor detection. Estimates were also made of event-free survival and survival, relative risk for event-specific end points,

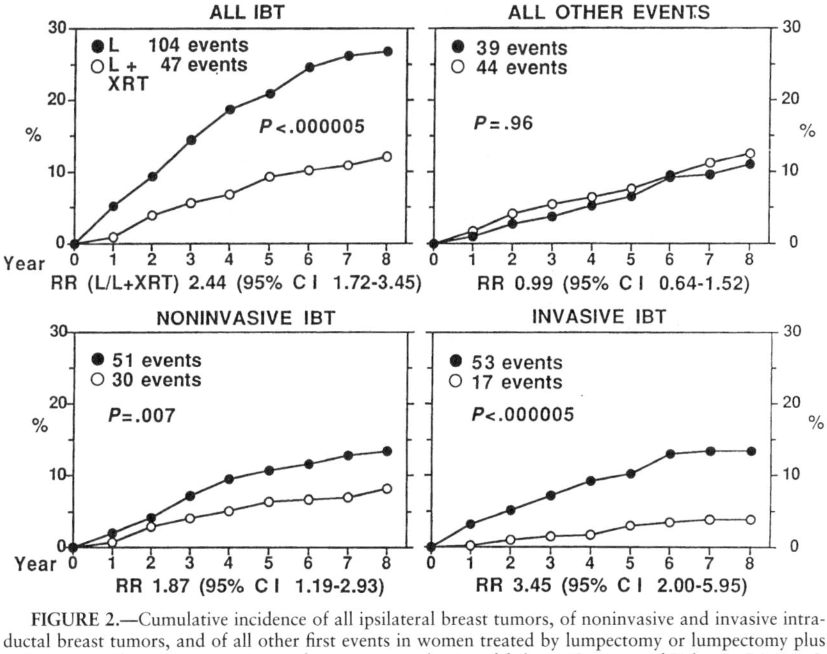

FIGURE 2.—Cumulative incidence of all ipsilateral breast tumors, of noninvasive and invasive intraductal breast tumors, and of all other first events in women treated by lumpectomy or lumpectomy plus radiation. P values are comparisons of average annual rates of failure. (Courtesy of Fisher B, Dignam J, Wolmark N, et al: Lumpectomy and radiation therapy for the treatment of intraductal breast cancer: Findings from National Surgical Adjuvant Breast and Bowel Project B-17. *J Clin Oncol* 16:441-452, 1998.)

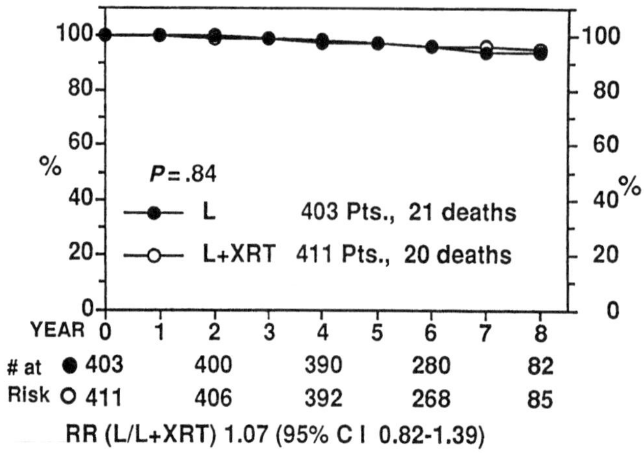

FIGURE 4.—Survival of women treated by lumpectomy (L) or lumpectomy and radiation therapy (L+XRT). (Courtesy of Fisher B, Dignam J, Wolmark N, et al: Lumpectomy, and radiation therapy for the treatment of intraductal breast cancer: Findings from National Surgical Adjuvant Breast and Bowel Project B-17. *J Clin Oncol* 16:441-452, 1998.

average annual rates of occurrence for specific events, and cumulative probability of specific components of event-free survival.

Results.—After 5 to 8 years of follow-up, the benefit of lumpectomy plus radiation was virtually unchanged and was due to a reduction in invasive and noninvasive ipsilateral breast tumors. In both treatment groups, the incidence of locoregional and distant events remained similar (Fig 2). Breast cancer was only infrequently related to deaths. The incidence of invasive ipsilateral breast tumor decreased from 13.4% to 3.9%, and the incidence of noninvasive ipsilateral breast tumor decreased from 13.4% to 8.2%, in both treatment groups.

Conclusion.—For women with localized, mammographically detected intraductal carcinoma-in-situ, lumpectomy plus radiation is more beneficial than lumpectomy alone, as was evidenced by 8 years of follow-up (Fig 4). Both groups benefited from radiation when patients were evaluated according to the mammographic characteristics of their intraductal carcinoma in situ.

▶ This study, previously presented, is a randomization of lumpectomy vs. lumpectomy and radiation therapy for localized intraductal carcinoma in situ (DCIS). This article now gives 8-year follow-up data. The results have not significantly changed since the last publication. As seen in Figure 4, overall survival is not different between the groups. However, as seen in Fig 2, there is a significant reduction in incidence of noninvasive ipsilateral breast tumor, as well as ipsilateral invasive tumor.

Approximately 33% of the patients were aged 49 years or younger. This indicates that DCIS is detected in younger women. Although the detection of DCIS in these patients is not reflected by increasing their overall survival as a result of mammography, assessment is important not only because of its impact on reduction in mortality but also because of its contribution to quality-of-life attained through breast preservation.

Data are not yet available to identify which patients do not need to be treated with radiation therapy. This article gives further impetus to the management of this type of tumor with breast conservation and argues against treatment of this group of patients with mastectomy.

T.J. Eberlein, M.D.

Primary Chemotherapy in Operable Breast Cancer: Eight-Year Experience at the Milan Cancer Institute

Bonadonna G, Valagussa P, Brambilla C, et al (Istituto Nazionale Tumori, Milan, Italy)

J Clin Oncol 16:93-100, 1998 11–2

Introduction.—As part of a multidisciplinary approach for locally advanced inoperable disease, primary chemotherapy for breast cancer has been introduced to achieve prompt tumor response using only a few chemotherapy cycles. Mastectomy was the surgical treatment of choice after drug response. Two consecutive prospective nonrandomized studies were begun in women with large but operable cancers. The 8-year experience, which had the aims of decreasing the size of the primary tumor, avoiding mastectomy, and allowing for effective local and distant control, is reported.

Methods.—In a 2-year period, 231 women with operable breast cancers measuring 3 cm or more were enrolled. The women were tested with 5 different regimens in 7 consecutive groups of 33 patients each. For 3 or 4 cycles, the different drug regimens (cyclophosphamide, methotrexate, and fluorouracil; anthracycline- or mitoxantrone-containing combinations; or doxorubicin alone) were delivered at full dose. In another trial, during a 5-year period 310 women with primary tumors measuring 2.5 cm or more in diameter were enrolled. This study involved 3 cycles of single-agent anthracycline delivered as primary chemotherapy. After chemotherapy, the women had breast-sparing surgery in the presence of objective tumor

TABLE 4.—Essential Results at Surgery

Tumor Diameter, cm (Clinical, at Diagnosi)	No. of Patients	Pathologic Complete Remission: Gross No.	%	Microscopic No.	%	pT1 0.1-2.0 cm No.	%	Quadrantectomy No.	%
2.5-4.0	292	14	5	8	3	158	54	267	91
4.1-5.0	160	16	10	5	3	73	46	136	85
>5.0	84	10	12	1	1	20	24	52	62
Total	536	40	7	14	3	351	47	455	85

(Courtesy of Bonadonna G, Valagussa P, Brambilla C, et al: Primary chemotherapy in operable breast cancer: Eight-year experience at the Milan Cancer Institute. *J Clin Oncol* 16:93-100, 1998.)

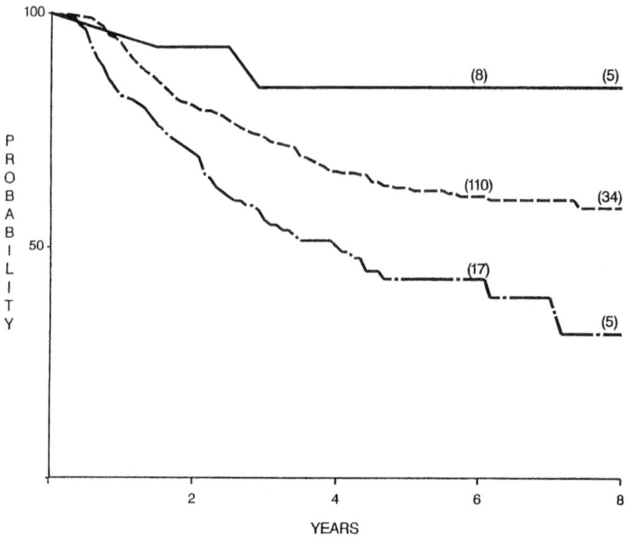

FIGURE 3.—Eight-year relapse-free survival after primary chemotherapy and surgery relative to the degree of response to primary chemotherapy (univariate analysis, P = .0001; multivariate analysis, P = .034). *Solid line* complete tumor disappearance on microscopic examination; *dashed line*, partial responder; *dotted line*, minor response or no change. (Courtesy of Bonadonna G, Valagussa P, Brambilla C, et al: Primary chemotherapy in operable breast cancer: Eight-year experience at the Milan Cancer Institute. *J Clin Oncol* 16:93-100, 1998.)

remission. Women at high risk of disease relapse had additional postoperative chemotherapy, and they were followed up for a median of 65 months.

Results.—The 2 trials had fairly comparable characteristics. Breast-sparing surgery was performed on 85% of women after primary chemotherapy. Surgical specimens failed to show any residual neoplastic cell in 3% or 14 patients (Table 4). The significant variables that influenced the 8-year relapse-free survival were the histologically assessed extent of axillary node involvement and the degree of response to primary chemotherapy (Fig 3). The cumulative risk of local relapse as first event alone was 6.8% in women subjected to a breast-conserving approach.

Conclusion.—In women with tumors of more than 5 cm, primary chemotherapy can be safely administered and can allow breast-sparing surgery in a high fraction of patients (62%). Properly conceived, large, randomized studies with more effective and newer drug regimens are warranted to effectively assess the long-term results of this approach.

▶ This article reports 2 prospective but nonrandomized studies at the Milan Cancer Institute. While 85% of the patients who received primary chemotherapy could be treated with breast-sparing surgery for tumors greater than 5 cm, only 62% received breast-sparing surgery. Thus, breast-sparing surgery was achieved in a high proportion of patients. As has been previously reported, tumor size and nodal status were important in predicting 8-year relapse-free survival. However, unique to analysis of these data was the correlation between survival and degree of response to chemotherapy. The risk of local recurrence was 6.8%.

As larger randomized trials with different chemotherapeutic agents begin, we will be able to identify whether a survival advantage exists with up-front chemotherapy. In the meantime, women can be offered a choice of up-front chemotherapy, to enhance their ability to be treated with breast sparing surgery without the likelihood of increasing risk of local recurrence. If improved pathologic complete remission occurs with newer regimens of primary chemotherapy, and if this translates into improved survival when compared to that produced by the classic postoperative chemotherapy regimens, then our overall strategy for the management of operable breast cancer will require a further departure from our traditional breast-sparing regimens.

T.J. Eberlein, M.D.

Predicting Axillary Nodal Positivity in 1,787 Patients With Invasive Breast Carcinoma

Silverstein MJ (The Breast Ctr, Van Nuys, Calif)
Breast J 4:324-329, 1998 11–3

Introduction.—For women with breast cancer, the main prognostic factor for survival is still axillary lymph node status. Some means of predicting the presence or absence of axillary lymph node involvement before surgery could avoid axillary dissection in select low-risk patients. This study assessed tumor size (T category of the thyroid node metastasis [TNM] classification) and lesion palpability for their relationship to nodal positivity, survival, and other prognostic factors.

Methods.—The study included 1,787 women with invasive breast cancer who underwent axillary lymph node dissection over 18 years at 1 cancer center. The breast cancers were stratified by method of diagnosis

TABLE 4.—Laboratory and Pathologic Findings: 1,787 Patients

	Nonpalpable	Palpable	P Value
Number of patients	375	1,412	
Positive axillary nodes	50 (13%)	592 (42%)	0.00001
Favorable histology	56/375 (15%)	96/1,492 (7%)	0.00001
ER positive	190/240 (79%)	734/1,046 (70%)	0.005
PR positive	160/240 (67%)	612/1,031 (59%)	0.04
Her2-neu overexpression	80/170 (47%)	63/227 (28%)	0.0001
Lymph/Vasc invasion	44/350 (13%)	360/1,310 (27%)	0.00001
Diploid	89/167 (53%)	206/459 (45%)	0.06
Low S-phase (<6.1)	95/152 (63%)	210/432 (49%)	0.003
High nuclear grade (nuclear grade = 3)	93/375 (25%)	529/1,412 (37%)	0.00001

(Courtesy of Silverstein MJ: Predicting axillary nodal positivity in 1,787 patients with invasive breast carcinoma. *Breast J* 4:324-329, 1998. Reprinted by permission of Blackwell Science, Inc.)

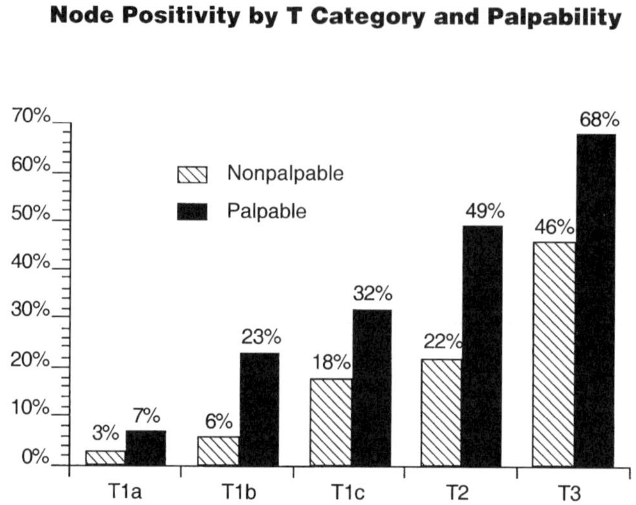

FIGURE 2.—Axillary node positivity by T category and palpability. The differences in nodal positivity between palpable and nonpalpable T1b-T2 lesions are significant (all P values 0.003 or less). The difference between T3 lesions is not significant because there are too few nonpalpable T3 lesions. (Courtesy of Silverstein MJ: Predicting axillary nodal positivity in 1,787 patients with invasive breast carcinoma. *Breast J* 4:324-329, 1998. Reprinted by permission of Blackwell Science, Inc.)

(i.e., nonpalpable lesions detected by mammography vs. palpable lesions detected by clinical examination). The cancers were also categorized by T category, according to the tumor, node, metastasis (TNM) classification of the American Joint Committee on Cancer. The sizes of nonpalpable lesions that could not be visualized by the pathologist were determined using a combination of microscopic and mammographic measurements. The stratified groups were then compared for laboratory findings and breast-cancer–specific survival (Table 4).

Results.—Thirty-six percent of axillary lymph node dissections revealed metastases. Forty-two percent of palpable cancers were associated with axillary metastases compared with 13% of nonpalpable cancers. The risk of nodal positivity increased with each increment in T category; within each category, risk was higher for palpable than for nonpalpable lesions (Fig 2). Palpable cancers were less likely to be estrogen receptor– and progesterone receptor–positive, less likely to have a favorable histologic pattern, and less likely to be diploid. They were more likely to have a high S-phase fraction, to have a high nuclear grade, and to be associated with lymphatic tumor emboli or vascular invasion. Patients with palpable lesions and invasive disease had a 10-year Kaplan-Meier survival rate of 75% compared with 90% for patients with nonpalpable lesions. Lesion palpability was a poor prognostic factor for patients with node-negative disease but did not affect the survival rate for patients with node-positive disease.

Conclusions.—Among women with invasive breast cancer, the rate of axillary lymph node positivity is greater for patients with palpable lesions than for those with nonpalpable lesions. Palpability is a poor prognostic sign. Outcome prediction and treatment selection should not be performed on the basis of T category only. The TNM classification might be improved by including palpability in the T category.

▶ Several studies have shown that the larger the tumor size, the more likely it is that there will be positive axillary lymph nodes. This very interesting study shows that starting with T1b lesions, there is a significant difference in risk of axillary nodal positivity between palpable and nonpalpable tumors (see Fig 2). It is interesting that nonpalpable lesions were statistically more likely to be estrogen receptor positive and progesterone receptor positive. Nonpalpable lesions also had a greater chance of being diploid with a low S-phase. Palpable lesions were much more likely to overexpress Her2-neu or to show lymphatic tumor vascular invasion. Palpable lesions also had a higher risk of nuclear grade (see Table 4). Thus, having a palpable lesion carried a worse prognosis. As more early detection is undertaken (and lesions are found mammographically), this may explain the increased survivability in breast cancer. In the meantime, a palpable lesion, especially with other correlative poor risk features (even if otherwise staged to be small) might be a candidate for adjuvant chemotherapy.

T.J. Eberlein, M.D.

Ductal Carcinoma In Situ Detected in the Mammographic Era: An Analysis of Clinical, Pathologic, and Treatment-Related Factors Affecting Outcome With Breast-Conserving Therapy

Vicini FA, Lacerna MD, Goldstein NS, et al (William Beaumont Hosp, Royal Oak, Mich; Med College of Wisconsin, Milwaukee)

Int J Radiat Oncol Biol Phys 39:627-635, 1997 11–4

Background.—Although we do know that breast-conserving therapy (BCT) in patients with ductal carcinoma in situ (DCIS) is as useful as mastectomy, we do not know which treatment factors will optimize results. These authors examined various clinical, pathologic, and treatment-related factors to determine which factors had the most effect on outcome.

Methods.—BCT was used to treat 107 breasts with DCIS in 105 women who ranged from 36 to 79 years of age. Every patient underwent preoperative mammography, definitive breast irradiation (median dose, 50.4 Gy; range, 43.1-56.0 Gy), and excisional biopsy. Reexcision of the primary tumor site occurred in 70 cases (65%) because of uncertain, positive, or close (≤2 mm) margins. A booster dose of irradiation was used in 99 patients (93%), for a medial total dose of 60.4 Gy (range, 59.1-71.8 Gy). Histologic specimens from 86 cases (80%) were reviewed for DCIS tumor size, DCIS dispersion, DCIS architecture, DCIS nuclear grade, the presence or absence of cancerization of lobules (COL) by DCIS cells, and where COL was found in relation to tumor margins.

TABLE 4.—Local Recurrence Correlated With Various Histologic Features (Univariate Analysis)

Histologic Feature	All Failures p-value	TR/MM p-value
Final Margin	0.134	0.021
Negative (n = 82)		
Close/positive (n = 24)		
Slides with COL near margin*	0.167	0.037
Lobules with COL near margin†	0.227	0.065
DCIS Pattern of Involvement‡	0.446	0.058
Tumor size	0.423	0.080
Histologic subtype	0.387	0.100
Comedo		
Noncomedo		
Highest nuclear grade (I vs. II/III)	0.598	0.237
Predominant nuclear grade (I vs. II/III)	0.384	0.143
COL degree	0.761	0.247
Present vs. Absent		
Moderate/ marked		
Necrosis (Central)	0.938	0.882
Present vs. Absent		
Stromal reaction	0.643	0.217
Mitoses, ≤3/HPF	0.627	0.546
Lymphocytic infiltrate	0.971	0.748
Calicifications with DCIS	0.078	0.184
Residual DCIS in Reexcision	0.846	0.509

*Number of slides with at least 1 focus of COL within one-half low-power field of the margin.
†Number of lobules involved by DCIS cancerization within one-half low-power field of the margin.
‡Dispersed *vs.* mass.
Abbreviations: TR/MM, true recurrence/marginal mass; *COL*, cancerization of lobules; *DCIS*, ductal carcinoma in situ; *HPF*, high-power field.
(Courtesy of Vicini FA, Lacerna MD, Goldstein NS, et al: Ductal carcinoma in situ detected in the mammographic era: An analysis of clinical, pathologic, and treatment-related factors affecting outcome with breast-conserving therapy. *Int J Radiat Oncol Biol Phys* 39:627-635, 1997. Reprinted with permission from Elsevier Science.)

Findings.—During a median 78 months of follow-up, recurrences developed in 10 of the breasts; local controls rates at 5 and 10 years were 91.2% and 89.8%, respectively. In 7 of these 10 cases, the local recurrence was due to invasive ductal carcinoma, whereas in the other 3 cases the recurrence was due to pure DCIS. Mastectomy was performed in these 10 patients, and at a median of 30.6 months after surgery, 9 patients remained disease free. The 1 patient with a recurrence after mastectomy had invasive disease and died of metastases to a distant site. No clinical, pathologic, or treatment-related factors were associated with the development of ipsilateral breast disease. However, when the analysis was limited to recurrences within or immediately adjacent to the site of the lumpectomy, the margin status and the extent of COL near the margin were significantly associated with disease recurrence (Table 4).

Conclusions.—As found in other studies, local control and overall survival are generally excellent when BCT is used to treat DCIS detected by mammography. Disease recurrence is most associated with cancerous cells or COL near the tumor margin. Thus, a more complete surgical plan with greater tumor resection margins could lead to improved outcomes in these patients.

▶ This is another relatively small study of 105 patients treated with breast-conserving therapy with a median follow-up of 78 months. Ten patients had recurrence. Three of the recurrences were DCIS and 7 had invasive carcinoma. This is a slightly higher than usual incidence of invasive recurrence, especially after radiation therapy. In fact, in the NSABP study (Abstract 11–1), the increase in survival was primarily due to reduction in invasive carcinomas subsequent to treatment. As can be seen in Table 4, margin of excision is also important as well as the pattern of DCIS and the amount of tumor at or near the margin. This work is similar to the findings of the Joint Center for Radiation Therapy in Boston,[1] which showed that patients with close margins who received radiation therapy were equally well treated as were patients with widely negative margins. However, the greater the number of foci of tumor at the margins was associated with an increased risk of local occurrence. It will be important to continue to follow these patients for a longer period because with ductal carcinoma in situ treatment may only delay recurrence.

T.J. Eberlein, M.D.

Reference

1. Gage I, Schnitt SJ, Nixon AJ, et al: Pathologic margin involvement and the risk of recurrence in patients treated with breast-conserving therapy. *Cancer* 78:1921-1928, 1996.

Use of Breast-Conserving Surgery for Treatment of Stage I and Stage II Breast Cancer

Guadagnoli E, Weeks JC, Shapiro CL, et al (Harvard Med School, Boston; Dana-Farber Cancer Inst, Boston; Meyers Primary Care Inst, Worcester, Mass; et al)

J Clin Oncol 16:101-106, 1998 11–5

Introduction.—Breast conservation surgery has been identified as an appropriate primary therapy for most women with stage I or II breast cancer. Nevertheless, the method appears to be underused at smaller hospitals and for women who are older, less educated, poorly insured, members of minorities, and rural dwelling. The practice of breast-conserving surgery was studied in 2 states (Massachusetts and Minnesota) reported to differ significantly with respect to surgical treatment of breast cancer.

Methods.—Thirty hospitals in Minnesota and 18 in Massachusetts participated in the study. Hospital records were searched for patients seen with stage I or II disease between September 1993 and September 1995. Data abstractors documented patients' clinical status, diagnostic work-up, and primary treatment. Income and education were also defined for each patient. Three to 5 months after diagnosis, patients were contacted to determine whether their surgeon discussed alternative surgical treatments and their reason for choosing the surgery they received.

Results.—Most patients were 60 years or older, white, diagnosed with stage I disease, and had no history of breast or other cancer. Surgeons were predominantly male (90% in Massachusetts and 87% in Minnesota), board-certified, and had 20 years or greater of experience. The patients' median household income, as determined by residence zip code, was less than $40,000 for 55% of those from Massachusetts vs. 67% for those from Minnesota. More women in Massachusetts, however, lived in areas where fewer residents had a high school education. Overall, the rate of breast-conserving surgery was higher than previously reported in both states (74% in Massachusetts and 48% in Minnesota among those eligible for the surgery). Among those who underwent mastectomy, 27% in Minnesota and 15% in Massachusetts reported that their surgeon did not discuss breast-conserving surgery. More women in Minnesota (74% vs. 62%) chose mastectomy on their surgeon's recommendation. The rate of breast-conserving surgery in Massachusetts was highest for women treated at teaching hospitals.

Conclusions.—Rates of breast-conserving surgery for early-stage breast cancer varied considerably between Massachusetts and Minnesota. It has yet to be determined whether these variations are the result of patient choice or surgeon preference.

▶ I have included this study comparing patients with early-stage breast cancer in Massachusetts and in Minnesota. The popularization of breast-conserving therapy is certainly making an impact in that the rate of breast-conserving surgery in both states was higher than previously reported. However, more women underwent mastectomy in Minnesota and more of those women reported that the surgeon did not discuss breast-conserving surgery with them. Treatment in teaching hospitals was associated with breast conservation, and treatment of older women was associated with mastectomy.

Continued education of surgeons regarding the indications and limitations of breast-conserving surgery is necessary. Only when surgeons understand these limitations will the comfort level with breast-conserving surgery increase more uniformly.

T.J. Eberlein, M.D.

Complications of Axillary Lymph Node Dissection for Carcinoma of the Breast: A Report Based on a Patient Survey

Warmuth MA, Bowen G, Prosnitz LR, et al (Duke Univ, Durham, NC)

Cancer 83:1362-1368, 1998 11–6

Objective.—The majority of breast cancer patients undergo removal of axillary lymph nodes for purposes of staging. Because the majority of

TABLE 2.—Significant Predictor Variables

Symptom	Predictor Variables	Predicted Probability of Symptom	Univariate *P* Value	Multivariate *P* Value
Pain	Age (yrs)			
	<40	0.46	0.001	—
	40-49	0.37		
	50-59	0.30		
	60-69	0.24		
	>70	0.18		
Numbness	Age (yrs)			
	<40	0.50	0.003	0.004
	40-49	0.42		
	50-59	0.36		
	60-69	0.30		
	>70	0.24		
	Smoking		0.009	0.012
	No	0.30		
	Yes	0.44		
Arm Limitation	Tamoxifen			
	No	0.04	0.016	—
	Yes	0.12		
Arm Swelling	Age (yrs)			
	<40	0.27	0.001	0.004
	40-49	0.20		
	50-59	0.14		
	60-69	0.10		
	>70	0.07		
	BSA			
	1.6	0.10	0.003	0.008
	1.7	0.13		
	1.8	0.15		
Inflammation and/or infection in the arm or breast	RT			
	No	0.05	0.01	—
	Yes	0.28		

Abbreviations: BSA, body surface area; *RT*, radiation therapy.

(Courtesy of Warmuth MA, Bowen G, Prosnitz LR, et al: Complications of axillary lymph node dissection for carcinoma of the breast: A report based on a patient survey. *Cancer* 83:1362-1368, 1998 © 1998, American Cancer Society. Reprinted by permission of Wiley-Liss, Inc., a subsidiary of John Wiley & Sons, Inc.)

women with negative nodes now undergo adjuvant therapy, the benefits of lymph node dissection are being reinvestigated. The risks and benefits of axillary lymph node dissection, including an assessment of morbidity resulting from this procedure, were evaluated in a cross-sectional survey of women diagnosed with breast cancer more than 2 years previously to determine the prevalence of patient-perceived long-term complications after lymph node dissection and the factors that may predict complications.

Methods.—A 6-page self-administered questionnaire was mailed to 432 women, aged 27 to 82 years, in the tumor registry at Duke University Medical Center in Durham, North Carolina, who had surgery for stage I or II breast cancer and were disease-free. Participants were asked about their symptoms of breast, chest, or axillary pain: that is, numbness or tingling of the chest, breast, axilla, or arm; limitation of shoulder or arm motion; and arm swelling. They were asked to rate on a 7-point Likert scale the severity of each symptom and its effect on daily activities within the previous 2 weeks.

Results.—Of the 330 respondents, 85% had undergone mastectomy, 80% had negative nodes, 33% had adjuvant chemotherapy, 50% had received tamoxifen, 17% had received adjuvant chemotherapy and radiation therapy, and 26% had radiotherapy. At least 1 symptom was reported by 55% of respondents including numbness or tingling (35%), pain (30%), arm swelling (15%), limited arm movement (8%), and infection or inflammation (9%). Most symptoms did not significantly interfere with daily activities. Age and type of adjuvant therapy predicted different symptoms (Table 2).

Conclusion.—Two to 5 years after lymph node dissection, women were still experiencing symptoms of pain, numbness, or tingling, most of which were mild. Women undergoing radiation therapy were significantly more likely to have experienced infection or inflammation, whereas women undergoing tamoxifen therapy were significantly more likely to have arm or shoulder movement limitations.

▶ Four-hundred and thirty-two patients underwent a survey following axillary lymph node dissection. Mild symptoms could be seen as far out as five years following axillary lymph node dissection. As is seen in Table 2, using multivariate models, younger age and history of smoking were associated with persistent numbness. Upper-extremity limitation of movement was associated with adjuvant tamoxifen. Arm swelling was associated with both younger age and greater body surface area. Radiation therapy clearly increased the risk of infection or inflammation of the arm or breast.

I have found that preserving the intercostal brachial nerve and sparing all of the fat and tissue around the axillary vein minimizes the risk of numbness and arm swelling, even in young patients and/or smokers.

T.J. Eberlein, M.D.

Underlying Pathology in Mammary Paget's Disease

Yim JH, Wick MR, Philpott GW, et al (Washington Univ, St Louis)

Ann Surg Oncol 4:287-292, 1997 11–7

Background.—Though mammary Paget's disease has long been recognized, there is ongoing debate over its cause and treatment. Mastectomy has been the standard therapy, but recent studies have recommended radiotherapy with no resection. The breast findings, disease stage, and outcomes of patients with mammary Paget's disease were correlated in a retrospective study.

Methods.—The review included clinical, mammographic, and pathologic data from 38 women with mammary Paget's disease. The median age of patients was 38. All patients had histologically confirmed Paget's disease; 17 had a palpable mass and 21 did not. All patients but 2 underwent

TABLE 4.—Multifocal Disease Identified by Mammography

	No Mass (n = 11)	Mass (n = 14)*
Identified multifocal lesion(s)	4 (36%)	9 (64%)
Missed multifocal lesion(s)	7 (64%)	5 (36%)
Missed multifocal invasive cancer	2 (18%)	3 (21%)†

*Two mammograms were unavailable or not performed.
†One lesion not identified on mammogram was palpable.
(Courtesy of Yim JH, Wick MR, Philpott GW, et al: Underlying pathology in mammary Paget's disease. *Ann Surg Oncol* 4:287-292, 1997).

mastectomy, with histopathologic evaluation of the entire breast and of lymph nodes for evidence of carcinoma.

Findings.—Ninety-two percent of patients had underlying carcinoma, either ductal carcinoma in situ, invasive ductal cancer, or both. This included 85% of patients with no palpable mass. Seventy-three percent of patients had multifocal disease. Mammography failed to detect the multifocal lesions in 64% of patients with no palpable mass. Patients with a palpable mass were significantly more likely to have invasive cancer, multifocal lesions, and positive lymph nodes (Table 4). They also had a worse survival rate (Fig 1).

Conclusions.—Most patients with mammary Paget's disease have underlying multifocal carcinoma, including invasive lesions. This underlying disease is frequently missed by both clinical examination and mammography. Though breast-conservation therapy may be possible for some

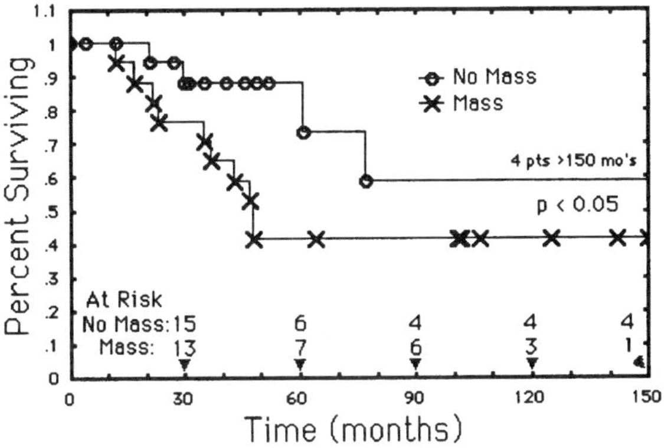

FIGURE 1.—Kaplan-Meier survival curves of patients with mammary Paget's disease with or without palpable mass. Number of patients at risk in each group, based on length of follow-up, is listed at bottom for every 30 months. *P* is less than 0.05 by F test. (Courtesy of Yim JH, Wick MR, Philpott GW, et al: Underlying pathology in mammary Paget's disease. *Ann Surg Oncol* 4:287-292, 1997).

patients with Paget's disease, it is difficult to select appropriate candidates whose disease can be completely excised without mastectomy.

▶ Management of patients with mammary Paget's disease is controversial. These authors, who retrospectively reviewed 38 patients with Paget's disease either with or without a palpable mass, identify the breast findings associated with disease stage and outcome. Patients without a palpable mass had ductal carcinoma in situ, and only 4 patients had additional invasive ductal carcinoma. In contrast, patients with a palpable mass and Paget's disease had a much higher incidence of invasive cancer, positive axillary lymph nodes, and multifocal disease. Mammography missed multifocal lesions in a very high proportion of patients with no palpable mass. In patients in whom a mass was palpable, mammography missed lesions in other areas of the breast almost a third of the time (see Table 4). In this relatively small study, patients with a palpable mass, and Paget's disease had a worse survival rate than did patients with no palpable mass (see Fig 1). Thus, depending on whether a palpable mass is present, treatment of Paget's disease should take into account the underlying pathology and recognize that there is a substantial risk of unidentified discontiguous disease in the breast.

T.J. Eberlein, M.D.

Mitosin (a New Proliferation Marker) Correlates With Clinical Outcome in Node-Negative Breast Cancer

Clark GM, Allred DC, Hilsenbeck SG, et al (Univ of Texas, San Antonio)
Cancer Res 57:5505-5508, 1997 11–8

Background.—Tumor proliferation rate, an important prognostic factor in breast cancer, is usually measured in terms of S-phase fraction (SPF) by flow cytometry. However, flow cytometry is not a good approach for use in formalin-fixed, paraffin-embedded tumor specimens or in small breast cancers. Immunohistochemical (IHC) analysis of cell cycle–related antigens seems to be a better approach to the evaluation of small archival tissue samples. Expression of mitosin—a 350 kD nuclear phosphoprotein expressed in the late G_1, S, G_2, and M phases but not in the G_0 phase of the cell cycle—by IHC was studied in archival specimens as a prognostic factor for breast cancer.

Methods.—The pilot study used the monoclonal antibody 14C10, which is 1 of several newly developed antibodies to mitosin, to measure mitosin expression by IHC in a series of 386 archival specimens of node-negative breast cancer. The results were correlated with flow cytometric measurements of SPF, as well as with other clinicopathologic features and patient outcome. The median duration of patient follow-up was 78 months.

Results.—The median number of mitosin-positive cells was 7%, with a range of 1% to 47%. Mitosin was strongly and positively correlated with

TABLE 3.—Univariate and Multivariate Analyses of DFS (353 Patients With 92 Recurrences) and OS (353 Patients and 79 Deaths) Using Mitosin as a Dichotomous Variable (Cutpoint >9%)

	Disease-free Survival			Overall Survival		
Variable	Univariate *P*	Multivariate *P*	Relative Risk (95% Confidence Interval)	Univariate *P*	Multivariate *P*	Relative Risk (95% Confidence Interval)
Tumor size (cm)	0.0014	0.0022	2.1 (1.3-3.4)	0.0124	0.0139	1.9 (1.1-3.1)
Mitosin	0.0161	0.0222	1.6 (1.1-2.4)	0.8336	0.9276	
ER	0.4947	0.1041		0.5323	0.1545	
Patient age (yr)	0.5690	0.1672		0.2220	0.1591	
PgR	0.9902	0.2152		0.6323	0.8778	

(Courtesy of Clark GM, Allred DC, Hilsenbeck SG, et al: Mitosin (a new proliferation marker) correlates with clinical outcome in node-negative breast cancer. *Cancer Res* 57:5505-5508, 1997.)

SPF, and negatively correlated with estrogen receptor level, progesterone receptor level, and patient age. There was no relationship between mitosin and overall survival. However, on univariate analysis, patients with more than 9% mitosin-positive cells had a 5-year disease-free survival rate of 68% compared with 84% for patients with lower levels of mitosin expression. On multivariate analysis, which included the effects of estrogen receptor, progesterone receptor, patient age, and SPF, the only independent predictors of recurrence were tumor size larger than 2 cm and high-mitosin expression (Table 3). Relative risks for these factors were 2.47 and 1.72, respectively.

Conclusions.—In node-negative breast cancers, mitosin expression by IHC may be a better prognostic indicator than SPF measured by flow cytometry. The results of this pilot study must be validated in additional clinical studies, however. Immunohistochemistry for mitosin is also simpler and less expensive than SPF, which may lead to wider use of tumor proliferation as a prognostic factor for breast cancer.

► Mitosin is a direct participant in mitotic-phase progression. Therefore, it makes an attractive potential target for the quantitative assessment of proliferation by immunohistochemistry of routine archival tumor tissue. This study looked at 386 node-negative patients. It was designed to determine if a relationship exists between mitosin S-phase fraction and other standard prognostic factors with clinical outcome.

Table 3 demonstrates that, with respect to disease-free survival, mitosin, in fact, was a predictor for outcome next to tumor size. However, with respect to overall survival, mitosin was not a predictor of outcome. This would certainly suggest, but does not prove, that mitosin, which can be assessed by immunohistochemistry, could potentially replace S-phase fraction (which is more labor intensive and expensive) as a prognostic factor in breast cancer.

T.J. Eberlein, M.D.

Guidelines for Sentinel Node Biopsy and Lymphatic Mapping of Patients With Breast Cancer

Cox CE, Pendas S, Cox JM, et al (Univ of South Florida, Tampa; Maimonides Med Ctr, Brooklyn, NY)
Ann Surg 227:645-653, 1998 11–9

Objective.—Because of the dramatic increase in the prevalence of breast cancer anticipated in the coming decades, improved breast care methods need to be developed. Lymphatic mapping is a technique that can predict individual tumor behavior with greater accuracy and sensitivity and lower morbidity. The outcomes of 466 consecutive patients after sentinel lymph node (SLN) mapping were prospectively reviewed.

Methods.—Between April 1994 and November 1997, 466 consecutive breast cancer patients underwent intraoperative lymph node mapping using Lymphazurin blue dye and filtered technetium-labeled sulfur colloid. An SLN was defined as any blue or hot node with a 10:1 ex vivo gamma probe ratio of SLN to non SLN. Sentinel lymph nodes were excised and submitted for pathologic evaluation. An SLN was defined as cytokeratin-positive if it had a defined cluster of positive-staining cells that could be confirmed histologically with hematoxylin and eosin stains.

Results.—Fine-needle aspiration or stereotactic core biopsy was used to diagnose 195 cases and excisional biopsy to diagnose 227 cases. An SLN was not identified in 26 cases which were diagnosed by fine needle aspiration (n = 15) or excisional biopsy (n = 11). Nodal excision was performed in these 26 patients and 4 showed evidence of metastatic disease. There was 1 skip metastasis where the SLN was negative but higher nodes were positive. Of the 844 SLNs excised, 169 (20%) were positive for metastatic disease in 105 (23.8%) patients. An average of 1.92 nodes per patient were excised. There were 233 hot and blue nodes, 339 hot nodes, and 272 blue nodes. The number of positive nodes increased with tumor size.

Conclusion.—A combination of blue dye and radiolabeled sulfur colloid accurately identified SLNs. Approximately 24% of patients had metastatic disease in the lymph glands. The remaining patients can successfully be treated as outpatients. Process and procedure guidelines are included.

▶ This article describes a study of 466 consecutive patients with newly diagnosed breast cancer. These patients underwent lymphatic mapping using either vital blue dye or filtered technetium-labeled sulfur colloid. This is one of the largest series of breast cancer patients using these techniques. In this series, blue dye sensitivity was not as high as that reported by other authors. These authors believe that it takes more time and expertise, as well as focus, to use a blue dye technique. Massaging of the breast is also necessary to ensure that the blue dye flows in the lymphatics. Using a combination of both techniques, however, these authors successfully identified a sentinel lymph node in 94.4% of the patients. There was only one false negative patient in the entire 466.

These authors are now routinely using polymerase chain reaction analysis of the lymph node. Thus, patients who are demonstrated by sentinel node mapping and by polymerase chain reaction analysis to have completely negative nodes may be candidates for not having adjuvant chemotherapy.

Another question often raised is about how the technique is learned and how steep the learning curve is. These authors currently use a 2-day course taught at their institution. The course, however, requires that the pathologist, nuclear medicine, specialist and radiologist as well as the surgeon participate, because it is a true multidisciplinary approach. Without this multidisciplinary approach, sentinel lymph node biopsy would be difficult to perform.

T.J. Eberlein, M.D.

Use of Paravertebral Block Anesthesia in the Surgical Management of Breast Cancer: Experience in 156 Cases

Coveney E, Weltz CR, Greengrass R, et al (Duke Univ, Durham, NC)

Ann Surg 227:496-501, 1998 11–10

Introduction.—The most common surgical procedures used in the treatment of breast cancer are modified radical mastectomy and lumpectomy with axillary dissection. Typically, general anesthesia is used for both procedures, and inpatient hospitalization is required. Recovery room stay and hospitalization may be prolonged after general anesthesia because of nausea, vomiting, and pain. Researchers report their 2-year experience with the regional anesthesia technique of a paravertebral block for operative treatment of breast cancer.

Methods.—During the study period, a paravertebral block was employed in 156 procedures (145 patients), and general anesthesia was used in 100 procedures (100 patients). Patients were scheduled to undergo surgery on an ambulatory basis or to be admitted overnight; they were discharged when they were able to tolerate oral intake and when oral analgesics achieved adequate pain control. Paravertebral block and general-anesthesia groups were compared for anesthetic effectiveness and complications; inpatient experience with postoperative pain, nausea, and vomiting, and length of stay.

Results.—The 2 anesthesia groups did not differ significantly in the mean age of patients, the number of axillary dissections performed with each anesthetic method studied, or mean operative times and operative blood loss for a modified radical mastectomy and for wide local excision with axillary dissection. Surgery was successfully completed in 85% of the cases with a paravertebral block alone; supplemental anesthesia was needed in the remaining cases, and 9% of the patients required general anesthesia. There were 4 (2.6%) complications in the paravertebral block group. The need for medication for nausea and vomiting was greater in the general anesthesia group (39%) than in the block group (20%), and significantly more patients in the former group required narcotic analgesia

(98% vs. 25%). Discharge within the day of surgery was possible for more patients who had paravertebral block (96% vs. 76%).

Conclusion.—Patients undergoing major operations for breast cancer had minimal complications and a low rate of conversion to general anesthesia when paravertebral block was used. Nausea, vomiting, and postoperative pain were less than in those who were given an anesthetic, and hospital stay was shortened.

▶ This is a retrospective analysis of 145 consequtive patients undergoing breast cancer operations. The authors used paravertebral blocks. As has been previously demonstrated with high thoracic epidural anesthesia, these authors also showed a reduction in nausea and vomiting, as well as a reduction in the length of stay. As with high thoracic epidural anesthesia, these authors found that the success of paravertebral blocks was correlated with the experience of the anesthesiologist. Clearly, this type of anesthestic as well as high thoracic epidural anesthetic, which may be somewhat technically easier on the patient, can improve patient satisfaction, reduce the need for narcotic, and shorten the length of stay. Our experience with high thoracic epidural, anesthesia, in fact, demonstrates that the vast majority of patients are able to be treated strictly as outpatients. This type of anesthetic, especially high thoracic epidural, has also been used by plastic surgeons for such breast surgery as augmentation or reduction, again with very satisfying results.

T.J. Eberlein, M.D.

Cancer Risk Among Women With Cosmetic Breast Implants: a Population-Based Cohort Study in Sweden

McLaughlin JK, Nyrén O, Blot WJ, et al (Internatl Epidemiology Inst, Rockville, Md; Karolinska Inst, Stockholm; Natl Cancer Inst, Bethesda, Md)

J Natl Cancer Inst 90:156-158, 1998 11–11

Introduction.—Epidemiologic data have not confirmed a suspected increase in breast cancer in women who have cosmetic breast implants. Results of a large national systematic follow-up of a population-based cohort of Swedish women was presented to examine the occurrence of cancers of the breast and other organs in recipients of breast implants.

Findings.—A total of 3,473 women with breast implants were followed for an average of 10 years (maximum, 29 years). Women in this cohort tended to be young (median age, 30 years at the time of cosmetic breast implant surgery). The number of implant recipients in whom some form of cancer developed was 74, compared with an expected 70.3. The most common type cancer was breast cancer. It occurred less often than expected (18 vs. 25). A higher incidence of cervical cancer and a significantly higher incidence of lung cancer than was expected was observed. (Table 2).

Discussion/Conclusion.—These data are in agreement with earlier findings that suggest that the risk of breast cancer among women with silicone

TABLE 2.—Standardized Incidence Ratios and 95% Confidence Intervals for Selected Cancer Sites Among Women With Cosmetic Breast Implants

Cancer	Observed	Expected	SIR	95% CI
Total	74	70.3	1.1	0.8-1.3
Digestive tract	8	8.6	0.9	0.4-1.8
Large bowel	3	4.5	0.7	0.1-2.0
Other	5	4.1	1.2	0.4-2.8
Lung	7	2.6	2.7	1.1-5.6
Skin	5	5.8	0.9	0.3-2.0
Breast	18	25.0	0.7	0.4-1.1
Reproductive system	18	13.9	1.3	0.8-2.0
Cervix	10	5.3	1.9	0.9-3.5
Ovary	6	4.6	1.3	0.5-2.8
Other	2	4.0	0.5	0.1-1.8
Brain	4	3.5	1.1	0.3-2.9
Lymphohematopoietic system	5	3.7	1.4	0.4-3.2
Hodgkin's disease	0	0.6	0.0	0.0-6.1
Non-Hodgkin's lymphoma	1	1.6	0.6	0.0-3.5
Multiple myeloma	1	0.4	2.6	0.1-14.6
Leukemia	3	1.1	2.7	0.6-7.8
Other	9	7.3	1.2	0.6-2.3

Note: Observed numbers of cancers among women in the cohort were compared with those expected based on age and calendar-specific Swedish cancer rates. Standardized incidence ratios (*SIRs*) were calculated as the ratios of observed to expected numbers of cancers, with 95% confidence intervals (*CIs*) for the SIRs calculated under Poisson assumptions. (Breslow NE, Day NE: Statistical methods in cancer research. Vol II. The design and analysis of cohort studies. *IARC Sci Publ* 82:1-406, 1987.)

(Courtesy of McLaughlin JK, Nyrén O, Blot WJ, et al: Cancer risk among women with cosmetic breast implants: A population-based cohort study in Sweden. *J Natl Cancer Inst* 90:156-158, 1998. Reprinted by permission of Oxford University Press.)

breast implants is not increased, but may even be decreased. The nonsignificant reduction in the incidence of breast cancer may be explained by concomitant risk factors of lower age at first pregnancy and decreased glandular density of recipients.

▶ This is the finding of a large national systematic follow-up of women in Sweden who received cosmetic breast implants (*not* immediate reconstruction after treatment of malignancy). This is a follow-up to a report published in 1995. It has larger number and longer follow-up.

As seen in Table 2, there is a slightly increased risk of diagnosis of cancer subsequent to implant surgery. Breast cancer was, in fact, the most common malignancy diagnosed; however, the likelihood of breast cancer was lower in the observed patient population than was expected. Only 1 patient was given a diagnosis of a connective tissue cancer.

This study does show a higher-than-expected number of cervical and lung cancers detected; however, this is consistent with the prevalence of risk factors in this patient population, for example, smoking and sexual activity. The study shows a statistically nonsignificant reduction in the incidence of breast cancer that may be the result of a lower age at first pregnancy and/or a decreased glandular density. These findings suggest that breast implants are unlikely to pose a carcinogenic risk.

T.J. Eberlein, M.D.

Overestimation of Hereditary Breast Cancer Risk

Iglehart JD, Miron A, Rimer BK, et al (Duke Univ, Durham, NC)

Ann Surg 228:375-384, 1998 11–12

Objective.—There are misconceptions and confusion about hereditary ovarian and breast cancers. The Specialized Program of Research Excellence (SPORE) in Breast Cancer at Duke University asked eligible women to estimate their probability of carrying a breast cancer gene.

Methods.—Two educational interventions were offered in a randomized fashion to women interested in genetic counseling and possible testing for the breast cancer genes, *BRCA1* and *BRCA2*. A baseline survey was mailed to participants. Participants were randomly allocated to receive either standard print materials about breast or ovarian cancer genetics and genetic testing or educational materials addressing individual preference for quantitative or qualitative risk estimates and carrier probability. Participant estimates were compared with those of experts, using a statistical model, and with testing results.

Results.—The responses of 200 participants were not correlated with the responses of experts or results of the statistical model. Women with breast cancer tended to assume that they carried the gene for breast cancer and significantly overrated their risk of breast and ovarian cancer. Of 100 women tested, 21 were found to have mutations of the *BRCA1* or *BRCA2* genes (Fig 5). Many women with a relative having breast cancer tended to overestimate their risk. Fifteen percent of women screened who had a high calculated probability of carrying the *BRCA1* or *BRCA2* gene had negative screening results.

Conclusion.—Women with a history of breast cancer tend to overrate their hereditary risk. Better education and counseling is necessary to bring perceptions in alignment with probabilities. A certain percentage of high-risk women had negative screening results.

▶ This is a very interesting paper that provided genetic testing free of charge. Estimates of risk of developing cancer were given by participants and compared to those estimates given by a panel of experts using a statistical model. As can be seen in Figure 5, subjects' assessments of hereditary factors were routinely overestimated in women with a family history of cancer. This study emphasizes the important need for education and counseling before obtaining genetic testing, as well as after genetic testing, to help place the test results in their proper context.

T.J. Eberlein, M.D.

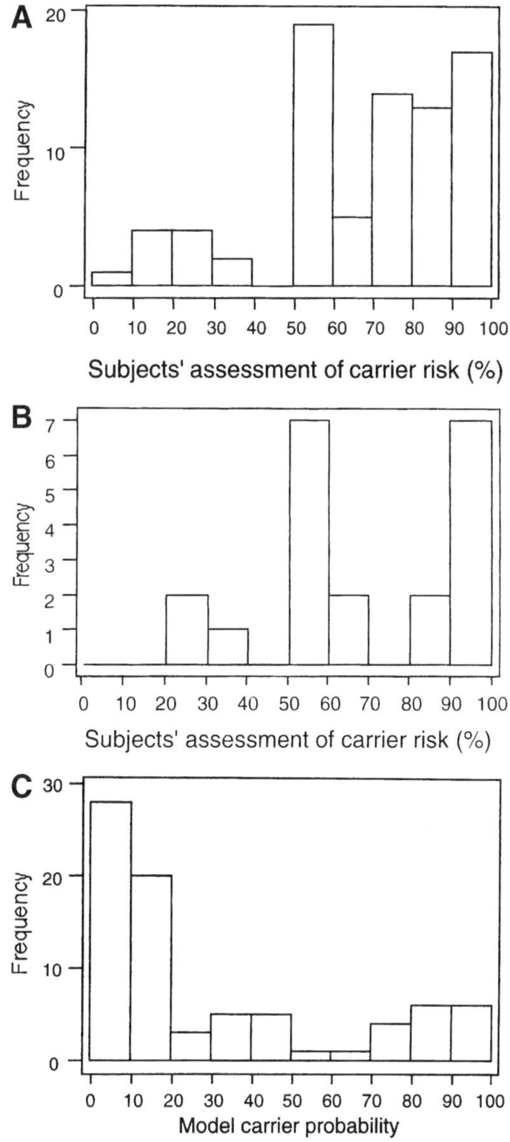

FIGURE 5.—Risk estimates among 100 women who were screened for *BRCA1* and *BRCA2* mutations. **A** is a frequency histogram for the self-estimates of women whose test results were negative for a mutation (excluding inconclusive results). **B** shows a frequency histogram for the self-estimates of women who had a mutation in either gene. C shows the distribution of carrier probability estimates provided by BRCAPRO among women who had negative screening results for *BRCA1* and *BRCA2* mutations (excluding inconclusive results). (Courtesy of Iglehart JD, Miron A, Rimer BK, et al: Overestimation of hereditary breast cancer risk. *Ann Surg* 228:375-384, 1998).

Colorectal

Dissemination of Tumor Cells in Patients Undergoing Surgery for Colorectal Cancer

Weitz J, Kienle P, Lacroix J, et al (Univ of Heidelberg, Germany)
Clin Cancer Res 4:343-348, 1998 11–13

Introduction.—Metastatic disease develops in nearly 30% to 50% of patients with resectable malignant colorectal tumors. Preoperative or intraoperative dissemination of metastatic tumor cells is probably an early event in tumor progression and is not detectable by conventional staging techniques. The extent of preoperative and intraoperative tumor cell dissemination was assessed in 65 patients with histologically confirmed colorectal adenocarcinoma.

Methods.—Three blood samples were obtained from patients: after anesthesia induction, after resection of the tumor, and 24 hours after surgery. Eighteen patients undergoing colorectal resection and 6 patients undergoing liver resection for benign diseases acted as controls. Blood samples were evaluated for RNA extraction, assessment of cytokeraton-20 (CK-20) by reverse transcription–polymerase chain reaction (RT-PCR), and sequencing of PCR products.

Results.—It was possible to detect 10 colorectal cancers cells in 10 mL of blood. Circulating tumor cells were seen in 24 of 58 patients with colorectal resections (correlated to the tumor stage) (Table 1) and 6 of 7 patients who underwent hemihepatectomy for liver metastasis. Circulating tumor cells were observed during surgery or during and after surgery in 8 of 58 patients with colorectal resection and 5 of 7 patients with hemihepatectomy.

Conclusions.—The presence of circulating tumor cells during surgery or during and after surgery (and not before surgery) indicates that hemato-

TABLE 1.—Correlation Between Tumor Cell Detection (Pre-, Intra-, or Postoperatively) and Tumor-Node-Metastasis Status in Patients Undergoing Resection of Primary Colorectal Cancer*

		A. Tumor		
T_1	T_2	T_3	T_4	*P*
0/4	3/11	15/33	6/10	0.027
0%	27%	45%	60%	
		B. Node		
N_0	N_1	N_2	N_3	*P*
9/32	4/12	4/6	7/8	0.001
28%	33%	67%	88%	
		C. Metastasis (stage)		
Stage I	Stage II	Stage III	Stage IV	*P*
1/11	6/19	7/16	10/12	<0.001
9%	32%	44%	83%	

*Ps were calculated with the Cochran-Armitage trend test.

(Courtesy of Weitz J, Kienle P, Lacroix J, et al: Dissemination of tumor cells in patients undergoing surgery for colorectal cancer. *Clin Cancer Res* 4:343-348, 1998.)

genic tumor cell dissemination is a common and early event in colorectal cancer. Surgery augments the release of tumor cells into the circulation. Long-term follow-up of this cohort will give data on the prognostic relevance of circulating tumors cells and may lead to new therapeutic concepts for perioperative prophylaxis.

▶ I have chosen this article simply because of the prevalence of studies that show the presence of circulating malignant cells at the time of evaluation of cancer patients. This particular study used RT-PCR assays. The authors were able to detect as few as 10 colorectal cancer cells in 10 mL of blood. Although there is no long-term follow-up, there was clearly a correlation between tumor cell detection and tumor size, nodal metastasis, and clinical stage (Table 1). The presence of these circulating tumor cells does not necessarily predict subsequent metastatic disease because implantation seems to be very inefficient. There is some evidence that circulating tumor cells may be destroyed (perhaps through an antibody-mediated lysis). This study does verify that preoperative and intraoperative tumor cell dissemination is a frequent event in colorectal cancer. Long-term studies are needed to provide data on the prognostic relevance of these circulating tumor cells and may be a basis for selection of patients for adjuvant therapies.

T.J. Eberlein, M.D.

Tumor Angiogenesis and Mode of Metastasis in Patients With Colorectal Cancer

Tanigawa N, Amaya H, Matsumura M, et al (Fukui Med School, Japan)

Cancer Res 57:1043-1046, 1997 11–14

Introduction.—The inverse relationship between tumor vascularity and patient survival has been demonstrated in tumors from a variety of sites, but little is known of the significance of tumor vascularity in colorectal cancer. Clinical data and primary tumors specimens from 133 patients with colorectal cancer were analyzed to determine the importance of tumor vascularity as a predictor of survival and mode of metastasis.

Methods.—All patients had undergone tumor resection and regional lymph node dissection for adenocarcinoma of the colon or rectum. Stage I disease was present in 12% of cases, stage II in 30%, stage III in 35%, and stage IV in 23%. For 2 years after surgery, 81 patients younger than 70 and with stage II, III, or IV disease were treated with tegafur. Primary tumors were immunostained for CD34 antigen, blood vessels within 5 microscopic fields at ×200 were counted, and a mean count was assigned. The patients' clinical characteristics were compared with microvessel counts.

Results.—Fifty-eight (44%) patients died at a median of 26 months after surgery. The remaining 75 patients have survived for a median of 72 months. Half of the patients were found to have lymph node metastases at

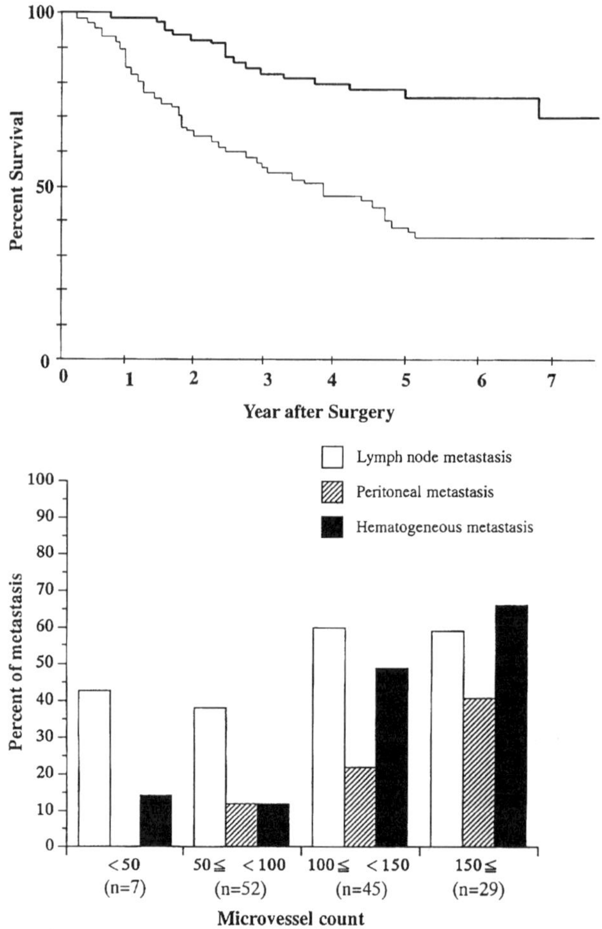

FIGURE 1.—A, overall survival curves for patients with colorectal cancer. Survival of 67 patients with hypovascular tumors (microvessel count < 105, *dark line*) was significantly greater than that of 66 patients with hypervascular tumors (microvessel count ≥ 105, *light line*). $P < 0.00001$ by generalized Wilcoxon test. B, metastatic disease among 133 patients in relation to microvessel count in progressive 50-vessel increments. The incidence of lymph node metastasis does not change regardless of vessel counts. The prevalence of hematogenous metastasis increased as vessel counts increased, whereas such a trend was less remarkable in peritoneal metastasis. (Courtesy of Tanigawa N, Amaya H, Matsumura M, et al: Tumor angiogenesis and mode of metastasis in patients with colorectal cancer. *Cancer Res* 57:1043-1046, 1997.)

surgery. Peritoneal metastases occurred in 21% of patients and hematogenous metastases in 37%. The mean intratumoral microvessel count was 96 mean square deviation for the survivors and 133 mean square deviation for those who had died of disease recurrence after surgery, a significant difference. Hypervascular tumors were more likely to have poorly differentiated tumor histology, lymphatic vessel invasion, penetration into the serosa, and metastases. There was a statistically significant difference in the survival rate in favor of the hypovascular group (Fig 1).

Conclusions.—Patients with colorectal cancer should have angiogenesis graded by pathologists because tumor vascularization may be an important prognostic factor. In this series of patients, vessel count was the most important factor in multiple logistic regression analyses and correlated significantly with hematogenous metastasis.

▶ This is a study involving the analysis of 133 patients. These patients underwent tumor resection for andenocarcinoma of the colon or rectum. They did not receive chemotherapy or radiation therapy before surgery. All had resection plus lymph node dissection. The primary tumors were then immunostained for CD34 antigen to highlight endothelial cells. As seen in Figure 1, patients with hypervascular tumors (microvessel count ≥ 105) had a significantly worse prognosis. Metastatic disease, especially as manifested by the prevalence of hematogenous metastasis, increased as vessel count increased. Routine grading of angiogenesis by pathology may be an important prognostic factor in patients with colorectal cancer and serve as a focus for identifying patients in need of adjuvant therapy. These tumors in this patient population may also be ideal for a study of antiangiogenesis factors.

T.J. Eberlein, M.D.

Impaired Interleukin-12 Production Is Associated With a Defective Anti-Tumor Response in Colorectal Cancer

O'Hara RJ, Greenman J, Drew PJ, et al (Univ of Hull, East Yorkshire, England; Castle Hill Hosp, East Yorkshire, England)

Dis Colon Rectum 41:460-463, 1998 11–15

Objective.—The overall 5-year survival rate for patients with colorectal cancer is less than 40%. Interleukin-12 (IL-12) is known to induce cell-mediated immunity. The adequacy of production of IL-12 was investigated in patients with colorectal cancer and the levels as they relate to disease stage were assessed.

Methods.—Preoperative IL-12 levels were measured in *Staphylococcus aureus* Cowans Strain 1–stimulated peripheral blood mononuclear cells from patients with colorectal cancer undergoing elective surgery (n = 28) and from age-matched patients undergoing elective hernia surgery (n = 14). Interleukin-12 expression was determined using a solid-phase enzyme-linked immunosorbent assay. All tumors were staged by a pathologist blinded to assay results.

Results.—Production of IL-12 was significantly lower in colorectal cancer patients than in controls (6.63 pg/mL vs. 17.3 pg/mL). Patients with node-negative tumors had significantly higher IL-12 levels than patients with node-positive tumors (11.4 pg/mL vs. 0.96 pg/mL). Median IL-12 levels were 6.93 pg/mL for Dukes stage A, 12.7 pg/mL for Dukes stage B, and 0.96 pg/mL for Dukes stage C tumors. Median IL-12 levels were 25.4

pg/mL for stage T1 tumors, 6.93 pg/mL for T2, 5.90 pg/mL for T3, and 6.32 pg/mL for T4.

Conclusions.—Compared with controls, IL-12 production is significantly lower in patients with colorectal cancer, especially in those with advanced disease, suggesting a defective Th1 response.

▶ Interleukin-12 is a cytokine produced by antigen-presenting cells. It is important in that it favors an immune response dominated by Th1 helper lymphocytes. These lymphocytes produce γ-interferon and IL-2, which are cytokines that augment an immune response. In contrast, many patients with malignancy tend to have an immune response profile predominated by the Th2 type of lymphocytes that produce IL-4 and IL-10 (which tend to suppress the immune response). Therefore, it is not surprising that in patients with colorectal cancer, IL-12 production is impaired. Levels of IL-12 were particularly low in patients with Dukes C disease and/or patients with node-positive disease. These findings raised the possibility that patients such as those with Dukes stage C colorectal cancer may benefit from exogenous IL-12 treatment. Unfortunately, in preliminary clinical trials, IL-12 has not had significant enough impact to reverse the level of Th2 lymphocytes and thereby make immune recognition more efficient.

T.J. Eberlein, M.D.

Prognostic Factors After Cryotherapy for Hepatic Metastases From Colorectal Cancer

Seifert JK, Morris DL (Univ of New South Wales, Sydney, Australia)
Ann Surg 228:201-208, 1998 11–16

Objective.—Although hepatic cryoablation has been used for local ablation in some patients with nonresectable liver metastases from colorectal cancer, the tumor recurs in most patients, and they die of their disease. Prognostic factors that might improve patient selection were retrospectively analyzed.

Methods.—Between April 1990 and May 1997, 195 patients were treated with hepatic cryotherapy. Of these, 116 (85 men), aged 31 to 85, had liver metastases from colorectal cancer. Complications were recorded and prognostic factors influencing survival were analyzed statistically.

Results.—One patient with heart disease died during the perioperative period. The morbidity rate was 27.6%. There were 43 patients alive at a median follow-up of 20.5 months. Median survival was 26 months. Survival at 1, 2, 3, and 5 years was 82.4%, 55.7%, 32.3%, and 13.4%, respectively. According to multivariate regression analysis, serum carcinoembryonic antigen level before surgery, diameter of cryotreated lesions, untreated extrahepatic disease at laparotomy, nodal involvement at primary resection, radicality of cryotreatment, poor differentiation of the primary tumor, and metachronous development of liver metastases were independent prognostic factors of poor prognosis (Table 3).

TABLE 3.—Covariates With Independent Prognostic Significance in Cox-Regression

Variable	B	SE	Sig	Exp(B)
Preoperative serum CEA level [ng/ml]			.0003	
< = 5 *vs.* 5.01–100	−.2518	.2066	.2230	.7774
< = 5 *vs.* >100	.5072	.2531	.0451	1.6606
< = 5 *vs.* unknown	.8803	.2750	.0014	2.4117
Diameter of cryotreated liver metastases [cm]			.0096	
< = 3 *vs.* 3.1–5	.3852	.2866	.1789	1.4700
< = 3 *vs.* >5	.5427	.2964	.0671	1.7206
< = 3 *vs.* unknown	−.5230	.6138	.3942	.5928
Extrahepatic disease at laparotomy			.0427	
No *vs* yes, not treated	1.1550	.5204	.0264	3.1741
No *vs.* yes, resected	−.4136	.4357	.3425	.6613
Histological differentiation of the primary			.0470	
Poor *vs.* unknown	−.1683	.3435	.6242	.8451
Poor *vs.* well/moderate	−.3875	.2179	.0753	.6788
Nodal involvement at primary resection			.0001	
No *vs.* yes	.9375	.2485	.0002	2.5536
No *vs.* unknown	−.2190	.3556	.5380	.8033
Radicality of treatment			.0136	
R0 *vs.* R1	.5826	.3058	.0568	1.7907
R0 *vs.* R2	.0233	.2522	.9264	1.0236
Time of diagnosis of liver metastases				
Meta-*vs.* synchronous	−.9260	.3041	.0023	.3961

Note: n = 116 patients.

Abbreviations: CEA, carcinoembryonic antigen; *B,* β regression coefficient; *SE,* standard error; *Sig,* significance; *Exp(β),* exponent β.

(Courtesy of Seifert JK, Morris DL: Prognostic factors after cryotherapy for hepatic metastases from colorectal cancer. *Ann Surg* 228:201-208, 1998).

Conclusion.—The prognostic factors identified should improve patient selection for cryotherapy for hepatic metastases from colorectal cancer.

▶ Hepatic cryotherapy has been used increasingly as a treatment for nonresectable liver metastases from colorectal cancer. The safety of this procedure is now well established. This article begins to identify factors that are associated with cryotherapy and that may be important in prognosis. As seen in Table 3, low preoperative serum carcinoembryonic antigen, the diameter of the cryo-treated liver metastases, and whether the liver metastases were diagnosed at the same time as or subsequent to primary resection were important. Completeness of cryotherapy is very important. These authors believe that failure to achieve normal levels of carcinoembryonic antigen after cryotherapy is caused by either unrecognized extrahepatic disease or by failure to eradicate all hepatic disease. This article further confirms the safety and efficacy of cryotherapy, which, when combined with regional chemotherapy, can offer improved survival.

T.J. Eberlein, M.D.

Colorectal Carcinoma Survival Among Hereditary Nonpolyposis Colorectal Carcinoma Family Members

Watson P, Lin KM, Rodriguez-Bigas MA, et al (Creighton Univ, Omaha, Neb; Roswell Park Cancer Inst, Buffalo, NY)

Cancer 83:259-266, 1998 11–17

Introduction.—Patients with hereditary nonpolyposis colorectal carcinoma (HNPCC) reportedly have a better prognosis than patients with sporadic colorectal carcinoma (CRC). It is not known whether this is because of differences in stage at diagnosis. Stage and survival were assessed in a retrospective cohort of HNPCC family members in whom CRC developed, and compared with the same factors in an unselected hospital series of patients with sporadic CRC.

Methods.—Two hundred seventy-four members of 98 HNPCC families were compared with an unselected series of 820 patients with CRC. The TNM system of the American Joint Committee on Cancer and the International Union Against Cancer was used to stage all patients. Median follow-up for patients with HNPCC was more than 10 years; for patients with CRC, it was 8.5 years. Survival from diagnosis to death was calculated for both groups.

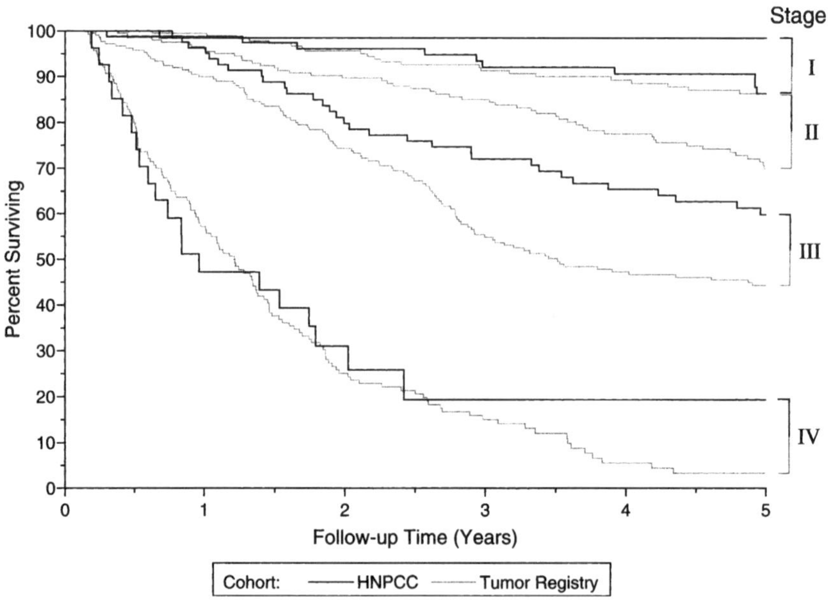

FIGURE 1.—Five-year Kaplan-Meier curves for hereditary nonpolyposis colorectal carcinoma (*HNPCC*) and tumor registry (TR) cases are plotted separately for each stage, with individual adjustment for non–colorectal carcinoma (CRC) deaths in the TR cases (adjusted survival). Five-year curves are presented to maximize resolution during the first 5 years, when most CRC deaths occur. Ten-year curves (not shown) show that the HNPCC survival advantage in stages I–III is consistent during years 5-10. (Courtesy of Watson P, Lin KM, Rodriguez-Bigas MA, et al: Colorectal carcinoma survival among nonpolyposis colorectal carcinoma family members. *Cancer* 83:259-266. Copyright 1998, American Cancer Society. Reprinted by permission of Wiley-Liss, Inc., a subsidiary of John Wiley & Sons, Inc.)

Results.—Patients with HNPCC had significantly lower stage disease and significantly lower distant metastases, compared with patients with CRC. Regardless of adjustment for younger age, a stage-stratified survival analysis revealed that patients with HNPCC had a significant overall survival advantage (Fig 1).

Conclusions.—Patients with HNPCC had a lower disease stage at diagnosis, compared with patients with CRC. Patients with HNPCC survived longer than unselected patients with same-stage tumors. When adjusted for age and stage, the estimated death rate for patients with HNPCC was about two thirds the rate of that for unselected patients with CRC.

▶ This very interesting study shows that patients with HNPCC had a lower stage disease at diagnosis than unselected CRC patients, primarily because of rarer distant metastases at the time of diagnosis (Fig 1). This lack of distant metastases was seen even when controlling for tumor depth. Interestingly, there was no significant difference between HNPCC patients and other CRC patients in the distribution of tumor classification or in the proportion of lymph node–positive cases. Perhaps the improved survival is a biological property. This may be hinted at in the histology, because HNPCC patients frequently have poorly differentiated carcinomas, but these tend to be very much like the undifferentiated type of carcinoma seen in the general population. A peritumoral lymphoid response seems to be predictive of a favorable prognosis. This lymphoid response tends to be more prevalent in HNPCC patients.

T.J. Eberlein, M.D.

Benefits of Colonoscopic Surveillance and Prophylactic Colectomy in Patients With Hereditary Nonpolyposis Colorectal Cancer Mutations

Syngal S, Weeks JC, Schrag D, et al (Harvard Med School; Harvard School of Public Health, Boston)

Ann Intern Med 129:787-796, 1998 11–18

Objective.—Genetic testing makes it possible to identify carriers of a mutation for hereditary nonpolyposis colorectal cancer, but the optimal management of such patients is unclear. Choosing between cancer risk-reduction strategies involves weighing the high risk of cancer, surgical and procedure-associated risks, and the health-related quality of life associated with prophylactic colectomy, endoscopic surveillance, and having cancer. A decision analysis was developed to assess the outcomes of various preventive strategies for patients carrying the genetic mutation.

Methods.—A Markov model was constructed with use of the decision analysis program DATA to compare strategies by following a hypothetical cohort of patients, aged 25, testing positive for the mutation, by tracking the annual incidence of polyps, colorectal cancer by stage, and mortality. Outcomes were life expectancy and quality-adjusted life expectancy.

Results.—All interventions significantly increased life expectancy by 13.5 to 15.6 years and quality-adjusted life expectancy by 10.9 to 14.0 years. The benefit of colectomy compared with surveillance decreased with the age of the patient. There was little benefit to a colectomy performed at diagnosis. The quality-adjusted life expectancy benefit compared with surveillance was highest for immediate prophylactic proctocolectomy (3.1 years) and lowest for subtotal segmental resection at diagnosis (0.3 year).

Conclusion.—For patients who are carriers of a mutation for hereditary nonpolyposis colorectal cancer, surveillance is an acceptable alternative to prophylactic surgery. Whereas prophylactic surgery provides the longest life expectancy, such a decision is a deeply personal one.

▶ This is a decision analysis model looking at patients with hereditary nonpolyposis colorectal cancer. Optimal management for patients with elevated risk of cancer in carriers of this mutation is unknown. Options, of course, are immediate prophylactic colectomy, delayed colectomy based on age, presence of an adenoma, or the diagnosis of colorectal cancer, as well as endoscopic surveillance. Proctocolectomy with an ileoanal anastomosis or a subtotal colectomy with an ileorectal anastomosis was the surgical procedure of choice. All reduction strategies led to large gains in life expectancy for carriers of a mutation for hereditary nonpolyposis colorectal cancer. Colonoscopic surveillance, however, was effective in reducing risk of cancer in carriers of a mutation.

As genetic testing becomes more prevalent, prophylactic surgery will certainly be an option. However, this article is included because it shows that an alternative to prophylactic surgical procedures (in this case, colonoscopic surveillance) is a viable and important option. This article also underscores the importance of genetic counseling before a decision is made for intervention. Obviously, any decision of such importance is highly personal but would benefit from professional counseling.

T.J. Eberlein, M.D.

Initial Clinical Experience With Colonic Stent Placement

Wholey MH, Levine EA, Ferral H, et al (Louisiana State Univ, New Orleans)

Am J Surg 175:194-197, 1998 11–19

Purpose.—There is growing interest in the use of self-expandable metallic stents for the treatment of patients with colonic strictures and occlusions. Stent placement permits colonic decompression and bowel preparation before a single-stage procedure and may serve as an elective primary anastomosis without the need for temporary colostomy. An experience with the use of colonic stents for the treatment of colonic obstruction is reported.

Patients.—Stents were placed in 10 patients with acute colonic obstruction. There were 6 men and 4 women, mean age 65 years. The cause of the obstruction was benign in some patients and malignant in others; in 3 patients with extensive metastases, treatment was considered palliative only. Five lesions were located in the descending colon and 5 in the rectosigmoid colon. In each patient a self-expanding metallic stent was placed under fluoroscopic guidance. The results were assessed by clinical follow-up until stent removal or death.

Results.—The technical success rate was 100%. In 9 of the 10 patients, clinical decompression was achieved within 6 hours. Standard mechanical bowel preparation and elective resection of obstructions were performed in 6 patients, whereas stent placement was considered palliative in 4 patients. Stent migration occurred in 4 cases; 1 patient died of procedure-related causes. Stents migrating to the rectum were easily reached and replaced under fluoroscopic guidance. None of the patients had perforations.

Conclusions.—Encouraging results are reported with the use of metallic stents to relieve acute colonic obstruction. Stent placement is a minimally invasive procedure that requires little patient preparation and provides rapid relief of symptoms. Stents can be used for stabilization and bowel preparation before elective single-stage surgery, or they may remain in place for long-term palliation. If the gastrointestinal tract can tolerate stents on a long-term basis, they may be useful for such indications as strictures caused by inflammatory bowel disease.

▶ This is a small series of 10 patients who underwent colonoscopic stent placement with a self-expanding metallic stent deployed under fluoroscopic guidance. The object was to avoid the necessity for colostomy. One patient underwent a colostomy for a failed decompression because of inspissated barium, and that patient died. However, all of the other patients avoided colostomy and did well. I have had personal experience with this technique and have found it to be valuable, especially in a setting of metastatic recurrent cancer causing low colonic obstruction. We were able to successfully avoid operation and avoid the necessity for colostomy. This technique requires careful patient selection and excellent technical skill on the part of the endoscopist. Thus, it is not for the faint of heart. As more endoscopists become more familiar with this technology, laparotomy and palliative colostomy can be avoided in a number of patients.

T.J. Eberlein, M.D.

Acute Colorectal Obstruction: Stent Placement for Palliative Treatment—Results of a Multicenter Study

De Gregorio MA, Mainar A, Tejero E, et al (Hosp Clínico Universitario, Zaragoza, Spain; Hosp Central del Insalud de Soria, Spain; Clínica La Zaruela, Madrid; et al)

Radiology 209:117-120, 1998 11–20

Objective.—Metallic stents have been used for palliative treatment of malignant diseases of the biliary tract and the esophagus. Because surgery is not an option for all patients with neoplastic large-bowel obstruction, a new procedure was developed using large-caliber metallic stents for treating those obstructions. The effectiveness of this method was assessed.

Methods.—In a prospective trial, colonic stents were placed into 24 patients (8 women), aged 60 to 98 years, with acute large-bowel obstruction. Placement was palliative in 9 and performed as an emergency procedure to permit tumor staging in 15. A total of 26 stents were placed with fluoroscopic guidance. Plain radiographs were taken at 24, 48, and 72 hours, expansion and patency were assessed at 1 and 3 months, and patients were followed at 6-month intervals thereafter for an average of 8.4 months for patients who lived and 6.3 months for patients who died.

Results.—Bowel obstruction resolved within 24 hours in 23 patients. One patient with an incomplete stent opening required a colostomy for colonic decompression. Five patients had minor complications, including 3 with minimal abdominal pain and 2 with mild rectal bleeding. Two patients had poorly positioned stents and only 1 could be corrected with a new prosthesis. A new colonic obstruction that developed in 1 patient at 7 months as a result of occlusive ingrowth of tumor into the stent was treated with placement of another stent. Two patients who experienced fecal impaction at the proximal end of the stent were treated with cleansing enemas. The 6-month mortality rate was 24%.

Conclusion.—Colorectal stent placement was successful for the palliative treatment of acute colorectal obstruction in patients with disseminated neoplastic disease.

► Although this study has only 24 patients with acute colonic obstruction, it is a multicenter trial. Complications to this stent placement were mild bleeding, abdominal pain, poor positioning, and in 1 patient, because a new prosthesis could not be reimplanted, an emergency surgery was necessary. It is important that patients be maintained on stool softeners, because they can suffer from fecal impactions at the proximal end of the stent. Thus metallic stents can be used for palliative treatment of malignant colorectal obstruction in patients with disseminated disease and in those who are a poor surgical risk. Newer stents that could prevent tumor in-growth might even improve on these results.

T.J. Eberlein, M.D.

Prospective, Randomized Study Comparing Clinical Results Between Small and Large Colonic J-Pouch Following Coloanal Anastomosis

Lazorthes F, Gamagami R, Chiotasso P, et al (Purpan Hosp, Toulouse, France; Univ of California, San Diego)

Dis Colon Rectum 40:1409-1413, 1997 11–21

Introduction.—Coloanal anastomoses have benefited patients with rectal tumors, but postoperative disturbances in bowel function occur in up to 50% of patients. These disturbances are caused in part by reduction of

TABLE 3.—Postoperative Functional Outcome

	3 Months		6 Months		12 Months		24 Months	
	Small Pouch (n = 18)	Large Pouch (n = 21)	Small Pouch (n = 17)	Large Pouch (n = 22)	Small Pouch (n = 14)	Large Pouch (n = 17)	Small Pouch (n = 10)	Large Pouch (n = 10)
Mean frequency of bowel movements in 24 hours (SEM)	2.55 ± (1.38)	3.00 ± (1.89)	2.35 ± (1.11)	2.00 ± (1.51)	1.80 ± (1.14)	2.00 ± (1.63)	1.80 ± (1.31)	1.88 ± (1.69)
Urgency	5 (28)	4 (19)	1 (6)	2 (9)	1 (7)	2 (17)	0 (0)	0 (0)
Continence								
Complete fecal continence	9 (50)	10 (48)	12 (71)	14 (63)	8 (57)	12 (70)	7 (70)	6 (60)
Incontinent to gas	2 (11)	1 (4)	2 (12)	1 (5)	1 (7)	0 (0)	0 (0)	2 (20)
Minor leakage	4 (22)	8 (38)	1 (6)	6 (27)	4 (29)	4 (24)	3 (30)	2 (20)
Incontinent to stool	3 (17)	2 (10)	2 (11)	1 (5)	1 (7)	1 (6)	0 (0)	0 (0)
Laxative use	1 (6)	0 (0)	3 (18)	3 (14)	2 (15)	0 (0)	1 (10)	2 (20)
Enema use	2 (12)	0 (0)	1 (6)	1 (6)	1 (8)	3 (18)	0 (0)	2 (20)

Numbers in parentheses refer to percent of the total in each group.

(Courtesy of Lazorthes F, Gamagami R, Chiotasso P, et al: Prospective, randomized study comparing clinical results between small and large colonic J-pouch following coloanal anastomosis. *Dis Colon rectum* 40(12):1409-1413, 1997.)

the neorectal capacity. For more than a decade, the authors have successfully used the colonic J-pouch to improve functional outcome and compensate for reduced capacity. The clinical outcome of the small 6-cm and the large 10-cm colonic J-pouch anastomosis was compared.

Methods.—Fifty-nine consecutive patients with rectal carcinoma were recruited for the study, and 47 were randomly assigned to either the small-pouch group (n = 23) or the large-pouch group (n = 24). Half of the patients in each group had the abdominotranssphincteric technique performed, and half underwent low anterior resection with either stapled or handsewn coloanal anastomosis. The pouch-anal anastomoses were stapled in 95% of the small-pouch and in 80% of the large-pouch groups. Eleven patients in each group received a course of preoperative radiotherapy, and 1 from each group received adjuvant postoperative radiotherapy. Bowel function was evaluated after colostomy closure at 3, 6, 12, and 24 months.

Results.—The 2 groups were similar in age, gender, and clinical characteristics. One patient given a large pouch had cirrhosis and bleeding esophageal varices and died in the hospital. A rectovaginal fistula developed in 1 patient in the small-pouch group. At each of the follow-up periods, evaluable patients from the 2 groups did not differ statistically in mean defecation frequency, urgency, or continence. Two years after surgery, only 1 patient (10%) in the small-pouch group needed a laxative for occasional constipation. In contrast, 3 patients (30%) in the large-pouch group required a laxative and/or enema for bowel evacuation (Table 3).

Conclusions.—The optimum size for a colonic pouch in relation to clinical function after colonic anastomosis had not been examined in patients with long-term follow-up. Findings in this series indicate that a small reservoir provides functional results similar to those of a large reservoir, without the subsequent need for laxatives and/or enemas.

▶ There is improving consensus that reconstruction with a J-pouch after coloanal anastomosis is preferable to straight colonic reconstruction. However, controversy still exists as to the size of this pouch. In this paper, the authors compare a 6-cm J-pouch with a 10-cm J-pouch. The numbers in this study are relatively small; however, at 2 years of follow-up, 3 of the patients with the large pouch required laxative or enema or both for bowel evacuation. Only 1 of the patients with a small pouch required this intervention. The time of follow-up of function of these J-pouches may have a bearing on interpretation. The value of this particular study is seen in Table 3, which shows that there is some variability with respect to postoperative functional outcome depending on the time of follow-up. This may also explain the variance in other studies that have been done comparing large and small pouches.

This question will be more definitively answered with a larger, prospective randomized trial.

T.J. Eberlein, M.D.

Detection of Recurrent and Metastatic Colorectal Cancer: Comparison of Positron Emission Tomography and Computed Tomography

Ogunbiyi OA, Flanagan FL, Dehdashti F, et al (Washington Univ, St Louis)

Ann Surg Oncol 4:613-620, 1997 11–22

Objective.—Approximately one third of patients with colorectal cancer who undergo curative resection have a recurrence within 2 years. Because 20% to 30% of these patients can be cured by surgical resection, accurate staging is very important. Although recent studies have demonstrated the difficulty of distinguishing scar from tumor by computed tomography (CT), whole-body fluoro-2-deoxy-D-glucose (FDG) positron emission tomography (PET) has been used successfully for tumor staging. Results of the use of FDG-PET for staging recurrent and metastatic colorectal cancer, a comparison of FDG-PET and CT results, and the impact of FDG-PET on the clinical management of patients with these cancers are reported.

Methods.—Between January 1991 and January 1995, 58 patients (25 women), aged 23 to 81 years, were evaluated by CT and FDG-PET for recurrent (n = 47) or metastatic disease (n = 11). Results were retrospectively compared with surgical and pathologic findings, clinical course, and autopsy results.

Results.—Forty patients had recurrent disease, 11 had advanced disease, and 7 were disease free. Patients were followed-up for at least 12 months or until death. Recurrent disease was diagnosed in 21 of 47 patients. FDG-PET identified 19 of these patients and CT 12 (P = 0.008) for sensitivities and specificities of 91% and 100% and 52% and 80%, respectively (Table 2). Hepatic metastases were diagnosed in 23 of 58 patients and identified in 22 by FDG-PET and in 17 by CT (P = 0.02) (Table 3). Respective sensitivities and specificities were 95% and 100% and 74% and 85%. FDG-PET results altered the management of 10 of 23 patients with hepatic metastases.

Conclusion.—FDG-PET was significantly more sensitive and specific in detecting recurrent and metastatic disease in patients with colorectal cancer and identifying patients for curative surgery.

TABLE 2.—Local Pelvic Recurrence—PET and CT Results Compared to Final Diagnosis (n = 47)

	Histopathologic and Clinical Follow-up	
	Disease	No Disease
PET positive	19	0
PET negative	2	26
CT positive	12	5
CT negative	9	21

(Courtesy of Ogunbiyi OA, Flanagan FL, Dehdashti F, et al: Detection of recurrent and metastatic colorectal cancer: Comparison of positron emission tomography and computed tomography. *Ann Surg Oncol* 4:613-620, 1997.)

TABLE 3.—Hepatic Metastases—PET and CT Results Compared to Final Diagnosis (n = 58)

	Histopathologic and Clinical Follow-up Disease	No Disease
PET positive	22	0
PET negative	1	35
CT positive	17	5
CT negative	6	30

(Courtesy of Ogunbiyi OA, Flanagan FL, Dehdashti F, et al: Detection of recurrent and metastatic colorectal cancer: Comparison of positron emission tomography and computed tomography. *Ann Surg Oncol* 4:613-620, 1997.)

► It is difficult to evaluate patients with suspected recurrent or advanced primary colorectal cancer. The current diagnostic methods are not sensitive enough to differentiate resectable disease from disseminated metastases in all cases. This study uses PET with FDG. This radiopharmaceutical takes advantage of the increase in glycolysis that occurs in tumor cells; therefore theoretical detection of these lesions is made more accurate. The study shows in Table 2 with respect to local pelvic recurrence that PET scanning was 100% accurate in detecting disease but had several false-negative results. In contrast, CT had a sensitivity of 52% and specificity of 80%. Similarly with hepatic metastases (Table 3), PET scanning was far superior to CT results. FDG-PET is becoming the standard in both detecting disease and documenting the extent of disease, thereby helping select suitable patients for curative surgery. By more accurately predicting resectability, PET offers a more cost-effective and efficient means to manage such patients.

T.J. Eberlein, M.D.

Colon

Postsurgical Surveillance of Colon Cancer: Preliminary Cost Analysis of Physician Examination, Carcinoembryonic Antigen Testing, Chest X-ray, and Colonoscopy

Graham RA, Wang S, Catalano PJ, et al (New England Med Ctr, Boston; Dana Farber Cancer Inst, Boston; Univ of Pennsylvania, Philadelphia)

Ann Surg 228:59-63, 1998 11–23

Background.—After surgery for colon cancer, patients are monitored to detect recurrent or metachronous disease. There is little information on the actual cost of such monitoring. The relative and absolute costs of monitoring patients after surgical resection for primary colon carcinoma were determined. These costs included physician examination, carcinoembryonic antigen assessment, chest radiographs, and colonoscopy.

Methods.—Of 1,356 patients who underwent surgical resection for primary colon carcinoma, 421 had recurrent disease and were included in this study. The cost of each test was based on 1995 Medicare reimbursement: $65 for physician examination, $28 for carcinoembryonic antigen assessment, $46 for film and interpretation of chest radiographs, and $409 for colonoscopy, including 1-hour facility fee and physician fee. Follow-up was defined as time to recurrence, or up to 5 years in patients who did not have recurrent disease. Patients were divided into 3 disease groups: nonrecurrent disease, recurrent but not resectable disease, and recurrent but resectable disease with curative intent. The mean cost of each test in detecting recurrent but resectable disease was determined.

Results.—Of 421 patients with recurrent disease, 96 had recurrent but resectable disease (group 3) and underwent surgical resection. For these 96 patients, recurrent disease was first identified by carcinoembryonic antigen assessment in 30 patients, chest radiographs in 12 patients, colonoscopy in 14 patients, and other testing in 40 patients. Of these latter 40 patients, 24 had symptoms. Routine physician examination did not identify resectable recurrent disease in any patient. The total cost of physician examination was just over $418,600. For carcinoembryonic antigen assessment, the total cost was $170,880, the detection rate was 2.2%, and the cost per recurrence was nearly $5,700. For chest radiographs, the total cost was about $120,935, the detection rate was 0.9%, and the cost per recurrence was nearly $10,080. For colonoscopy, the total cost was about $641,345, the detection rate was 1.0%, and the cost per recurrence was just over $45,800.

Discussion.—These results show that carcinoembryonic antigen assessment was the most cost-effective test for identifying potentially curable disease in patients after surgical resection for primary colon carcinoma. Physician visits were useful for evaluating symptoms, but routine physician examination did not improve detection of recurrent disease.

► This is a study of almost 1,400 Eastern Cooperative Oncology Group patients who underwent surgical resection for colon carcinoma. The patients were divided into three specific disease categories: nonrecurrent, recurrent but nonresectable, and recurrent but resectable with an intent to cure the patient. The cost of each test was then calculated for each of the three groups. It was interesting that physician visits were effective in evaluation of symptoms; however, if the patient had symptoms, then resection for cure was not possible. Carcinoembryonic antigen measurement was the most cost-effective test for detecting potentially curable recurrent disease. Several issues connected with this study deserve emphasis. The first is that since the study represents a multi-institution cooperative group, it probably reflects clinical practice in the real world. The authors emphasize the importance of surveillance testing being concentrated in the first 5 years in patients with colon cancer. Finally, the authors establish a rank order of cost effectiveness for follow-up testing in patients with colon cancer: CEA testing > chest x-ray > colonoscopy > physical examination. Twenty percent or more of the patients with early detection can be cured if adequately resected. Therefore, surveillance follow-up and its cost-effectiveness in this era of managed care practice are both important for the practicing surgeon.

T.J. Eberlein, M.D.

Randomized Trial of Surgery Versus Surgery Followed by Adjuvant Hepatic Arterial Infusion With 5-Fluorouracil and Folinic Acid for Liver Metastases of Colorectal Cancer

Lorenz M, for the German Cooperative on Liver Metastases (Johann Wolfgang Goethe Univ, Frankfurt am Main, Germany)

Ann Surg 228:756-762, 1998 11–24

Background.—Liver metastases develop in 40% to 50% of patients with colorectal cancer. The five-year survival rate after curative resection is only 25% to 30%, with 60% of patients developing intrahepatic recurrence at a median of 9 to 12 months. Postoperative intra-arterial infusion of 5-fluorouracil (5-FU) was used in an attempt to reduce intrahepatic recurrence and improve survival in patients undergoing resection of liver metastases from colorectal cancer.

Methods.—Two hundred twenty-six patients with colorectal liver metastases, stratified for number of metastases and primary tumor site, were included in the randomomized, multicenter trial. The patients' median age was 61 years. All underwent resection of the hepatic metastases. In addition, the adjuvant therapy group received postoperative 5-FU, given by hepatic arterial infusion at a rate of 1,000 mg/m²/day for 5 days as a continuous 24 hour infusion. This group also received a short infusion of folinic acid, 200 mg/m²/day for 5 days. The main outcome measure was survival. This report describes the findings at the first planned interim analysis, at which there were 219 evaluable patients.

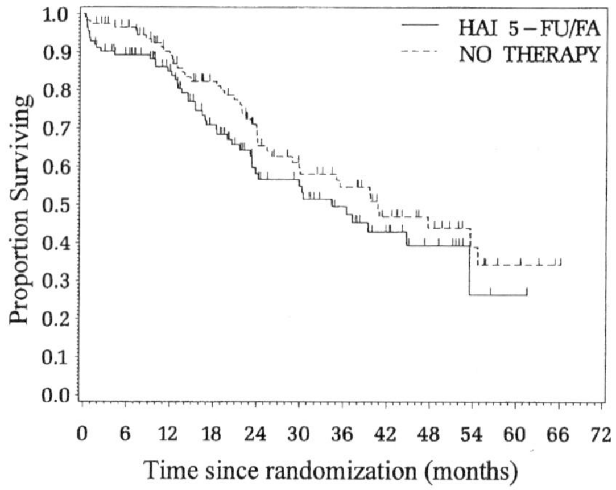

Patients at risk (| censored)

HAI 5 – FU/FA	113	91	76	57	38	32	24	16	9	2	1	0	0
NO THERAPY	113	100	81	67	49	39	33	22	15	8	4	1	0

FIGURE 1.—Cumulative overall survival after liver resection by treatment group ("intention to treat"): resection only vs. adjuvant hepatic arterial infusion with 5-FU/folinic acid (HAI 5-FU/FA) for 5 days every 28 days for 6 months (p = 0.1519). (Courtesy of Lorenz M, for the German Cooperative on Liver Metatases: Randomized trial of surgery versus surgery followed by adjuvant hepatic arterial infusion with 5-fluorouracil and folinic acid for liver metastases of colorectal cancer. *Ann Surg* 228:756-762, 1998.)

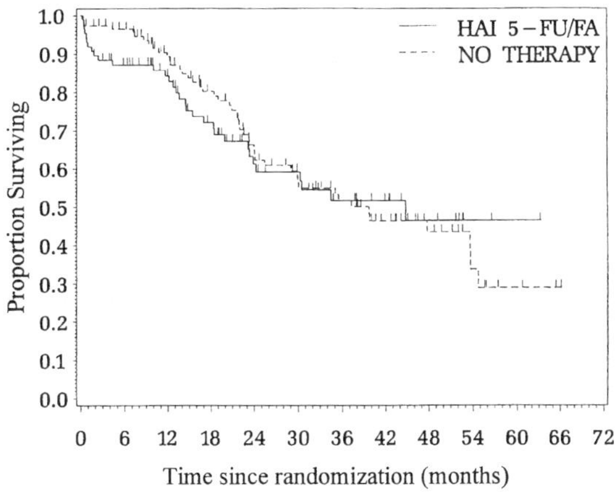

Patients at risk (| censored)

HAI 5-FU/FA	87	70	58	45	30	25	18	14	7	2	1	0	0
NO THERAPY	114	102	82	66	48	38	32	22	15	7	3	1	0

FIGURE 2.—Cumulative overall survival after liver resection by treatment group ("as treated"); resection only vs. adjuvant hepatic arterial infusion with 5-FU/folinic acid (HAI 5-FU/FA) for 5 days every 28 days for 6 months. (Courtesy of Lorenz M, for the German Cooperative on Liver Metastases: Randomized trial of surgery versus surgery followed by adjuvant hepatic arterial infusion with 5-fluorouracil and folinic acid for liver metastases of colorectal cancer. *Ann Surg* 228:756-762, 1998.)

Results.—Curative resection was achieved in 89% of patients. At interim analysis, 91 patients had died, and median survival was similar between groups: 34.5 months for the adjuvant therapy group and 40.8 months for the control group (Fig 1). Median survival time to progression was 14.2 and 13.7 months, respectively. On "as-treated" analysis, median survival was 44.8 months with adjuvant therapy vs. 39.7 months in the control group, while median survival time to progression was 44.8 vs. 23.3 months (Fig 2). However, the advantages of adjuvant therapy did not translate into a significant difference in survival. One-fourth of the cycles of adjuvant 5-FU were associated with grade III or IV toxicity, mainly stomatitis and nausea; nearly three-fourths of patients were affected.

Conclusions.—For patients undergoing resection of colorectal cancer metastases to the liver, adjuvant hepatic arterial infusion of 5-FU/folinic acid does not appear to be beneficial, even on as-treated analysis. The confidence interval is consistent with a possible 15% reduction or a 100% increase in risk of death with adjuvant therapy. This study was terminated at the first planned interim analysis. Adjuvant intra-arterial therapy for colorectal liver metastases should be limited to controlled trials.

► Surgical therapy of hepatic metastases due to colorectal cancer has been shown to provide long-term survival; however, anywhere from 60% to 75% of patients will have recurrence. While many of these patients will recur with liver and systemic disease, some patients will clearly recur in liver parenchyma only. Only a highly selected minority of patients would be candidates for reresections. The rationale of this study is to minimize the risk of recurrence utilizing hepatic artery infusion of chemotherapy. Two hundred twenty-six patients were included in the study. This report consists of a planned interim analysis. Figure 1 shows the cumulative overall survival by intention to treat; there is no statistical difference. Figure 2 simply shows the overall survival when the study cohort was analyzed "as treated." Adjuvant therapy showed a very insignificant increase in survival, however, median survival time to progression to the liver was nearly doubled with adjuvant therapy. Nonetheless, patient accrual was terminated because of the conclusion that hepatic artery infusion would not show significant improvement in survival. The authors speculate that the reason for this lack of significant survival advantage may be a result of the length of treatment (6 months) or perhaps to the selection of drugs (although 5-FU is among the most active chemotherapeutic agents in this disease). Additionally, there were significant technical complications leading to early cessation of treatment. There were also relatively significant toxicities that could be explained by reduced hepatic extraction of 5-FU after liver resection. Nonetheless, the authors conclude that further adjuvant intra-arterial therapy should be performed only in a controlled setting. We will await other verifying studies.

T.J. Eberlein, M.D.

Modulation of Abnormal Colonic Epithelial Cell Proliferation and Differentiation by Low-Fat Dairy Foods: A Randomized Controlled Trial

Holt PR, Atillasoy EO, Gilman J, et al (Columbia Univ, New York)

JAMA 280:1074-1079, 1998 11–25

Objective.—Higher dietary levels of calcium and vitamin D appear to inhibit the colonic epithelial cell proliferation that precedes the development of colon cancer. In a randomized, single-blind, controlled study, the effect of dairy food supplementation was tested in patients with previous colonic adenomas, who were at higher risk of colon cancer.

Methods.—Patients either maintained their conventional diets (n = 33) or received a diet containing low-fat dairy products with 1200 mg or less calcium (n = 37). In addition, patients were stratified by age into 2 groups, those 60 years and older and those younger than 60 years. Patients had nutritional assessments and dietary monitoring at baseline and at 6-month intervals. Rectosigmoid biopsies were performed twice at baseline (1 month apart) and at 6 and 12 months. Cell proliferation and morphometric studies were performed.

Results.—Eleven patients were dropped from the study. Whereas proliferation patterns at 6 and 12 months for control patients were similar to patterns found at baseline, numbers of proliferating cells were significantly decreased for the diet group as measured by labeled thymidine uptake in epithelial cells. The diet group, but not the control group, also had a significantly reduced cytokeratin AE1 expression and significantly reduced acidic mucin scores compared with baseline values.

Conclusion.—Results of this small study suggest that increasing daily calcium intake reduces proliferative activity of colonic epithelial cells and normalizes markers of cellular differentiation in patients at increased risk of colon cancer.

▶ This is a relatively small, randomized, single-blind, controlled study of outpatients who were subjected to a low-fat dairy product containing varying degrees of calcium. Using a large number of cellular proliferative and cytokeratin measures, these authors showed that the diet contributed toward normalization of colonic epithelial cells.

Calcium was the major nutrient change in the diet of these patients. This study, because of its very small size, however, did not identify whether or not calcium supplementation would alter recurrence of colonic adenoma. Also, this study does not prove that calcium, in fact, was responsible for the various biomarker changes observed in the study. Larger studies will be necessary to verify this study; however, it appears that dietary calcium supplementation may not only be important in reducing the risk of osteoporosis but also may reduce the risk of colonic neoplasia.

T.J. Eberlein, M.D.

Confirmation That Chromosome *18q* Allelic Loss in Colon Cancer Is a Prognostic Indicator

Ogunbiyi OA, Goodfellow PJ, Herfarth K, et al (Washington Univ, St Louis; VA Med Ctr, St Louis)

J Clin Oncol 16:427-433, 1998 11–26

Introduction.—Because half of all patients with colorectal cancer die of metastatic disease, adjuvant therapy has become increasingly important. Chemotherapy and/or radiation therapy can benefit patients likely to have recurrence, but prognostic factors predictive of recurrence need to be identified. Tumor specimens from patients who had undergone potentially curative surgery for adenocarcinoma of the colon were examined to determine the prognostic value of *18q* loss of heterozygosity (LOH).

Methods.—Paired primary tumor and normal tissue specimens were obtained from 151 patients who had undergone curative surgery between 1985 and 1990. Tumor DNA was prepared using tissues with neoplastic cellularity of 65% or greater. Polymerase chain reaction was used to assess allelic loss of 5 chromosome *18q* microsatellite markers in the tumors. Tumors were designated LOH positive when the relative intensity of the 2 alleles in the tumor DNA differed from the relative intensity in normal tissue by a factor of 3. The relationship between allelic loss and disease-free and disease-specific survival was analyzed.

Results.—Twenty-five patients were excluded from analysis because they were lost to follow-up, had noninformative data, or had replication error–positive tumors in which it is difficult to determine allelic loss. Sixty-seven of the remaining 126 tumors exhibited LOH. Chromosome

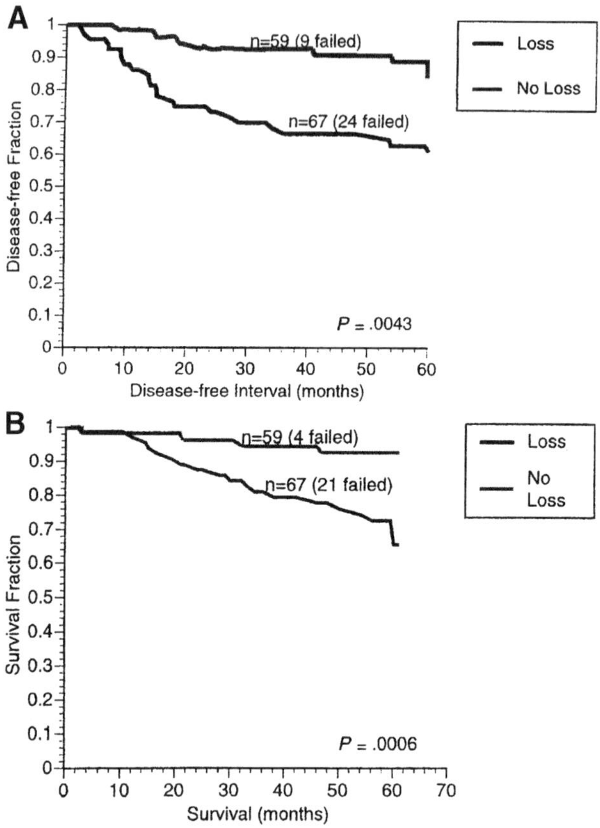

FIGURE 3.—Kaplan-Meier life-table analysis of overall (A) disease-free and (B) disease-specific survival of patients with adenocarcinoma of the colon, according to chromosome *18q* loss of heterozygosity. (Courtesy of Ogunbiyi OA, Goodfellow PJ, Herfarth K, et al: Confirmation that chromosome *18q* allelic loss in colon cancer is a prognostic indicator. *J Clin Oncol* 16:427-433, 1998.)

18q allelic loss was a negative prognostic indicator, both of disease-free and disease-specific survival (Fig 3), and in patients with both stage II and stage III disease.

Conclusions.—Chromosome *18q* allelic loss provides prognostic information in patients with colon cancer who have undergone curative surgery. This finding was a negative prognostic indicator for both disease-free and disease-specific survival, and for colon cancer patients as a whole as well as those with stage II and stage III disease.

▶ Previous studies have shown allelic loss of chromosome *18q* or loss of expression of the punitive tumor-suppressor gene *deleted in colorectal cancer* (DCC) can identify stage II colon cancer patients that have an unfavorable prognosis. This study looked at 126 tumors and found that 67 had loss of heterozygosity. As seen in Figure 3, loss of heterozygosity of *18q* was associated with a reduced disease-free and disease-specific survival. Somewhat different from other studies, these authors showed reduction in survival, even for stage III patients.

Loss of heterozygosity is a phenomenon seen in developing tumors, which eliminates both copies of a tumor-suppressor gene. There is biological evidence that *18q* carries a colonic tumor-suppressor gene. Thus, allelic loss of *18q* may certainly be of important prognostic value in colorectal cancer. These findings may make it useful in selecting patients, especially patients with stage II disease, for adjuvant chemotherapy after curative resection. There is now sufficient evidence to consider a randomized prospective clinical trial of adjuvant chemotherapy in patients with stage II colon cancer and *18q* allelic loss.

T.J. Eberlein, M.D.

Surgery for Recurrent Colon Cancer: Strategies for Identifying Resectable Recurrence and Success Rates After Resection

Goldberg RM, and the Southwest Oncology Group (Mayo Clinic, Rochester, Minn; et al)

Ann Intern Med 129:27-35, 1998 11–27

Background.—After surgery for colon cancer, follow-up testing is recommended to identify resectable recurrence. However, there is little information on the efficacy or outcomes of such testing or on optimal strategies for testing.

Methods.—In a retrospective cohort study, 1,247 patients with resected stage II or stage II colon cancer were evaluated. Patients had postoperative chemotherapy plus follow-up or had follow-up alone. The relation between follow-up testing and salvage surgery was determined, as well as outcome and surgical mortality.

Results.—Recurrence of colon cancer was seen in 548 patients. Salvage surgery was performed in 222 patients curative-intent surgery was performed for hepatic recurrence in 28 patients, pulmonary metastasis in 20 patients, local recurrence in 24 patients, and recurrence at other sites in 37 patients. Curative-intent surgery was preceded by follow-up testing in 36 patients, elevated carcinoembryonic antigen (CEA) level in 41 patients, and presence of symptoms in 27 patients. Median follow-up after curative-intent surgery was more than 5 years. The disease-free survival rate at 5 years was 23%. Patients who had recurrence within 1 year after curative-intent surgery had a poorer prognosis, but those who had recurrence more than 3 years after curative- intent surgery had a more favorable prognosis (Fig 2). The only significant independent predictor of disease-free survival was a solitary lesion (Fig 3). The surgical mortality rate was 2%. Curative-intent surgery was performed in 15 patients with second primary colorectal cancer; 12 patients survived and were free of disease.

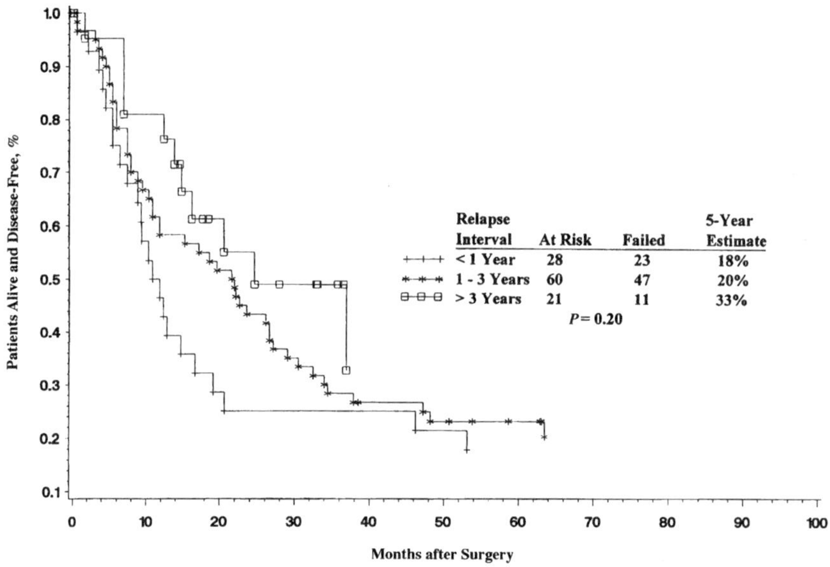

FIGURE 2.—Disease-free survival after curative-intent salvage surgery by relapse interval. (Courtesy of Goldberg RM, and the Southwest Oncology Group: Surgery for recurrent colon cancer: Strategies for identifying resectable recurrence and success rates after resection. *Ann Intern Med* 129:27-35, 1998.)

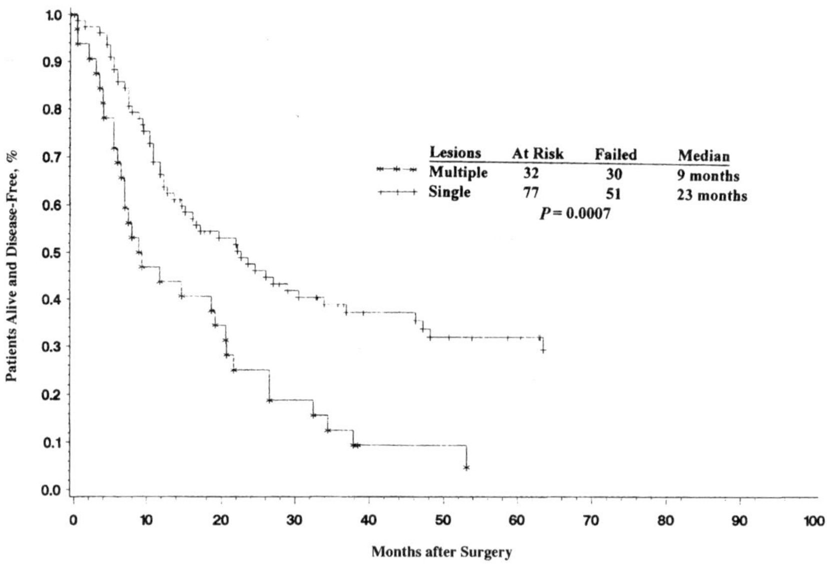

FIGURE 3.—Disease-free survival after curative-intent salvage surgery by number of lesions. (Courtesy of Goldberg RM, and the Southwest Oncology Group: Surgery for recurrent colon cancer: Strategies for identifying resectable recurrence and success rates after resection. *Ann Intern Med* 129:27-35, 1998.)

Discussion.—These results suggest that long-term, disease-free survival can be achieved after second operations for colon cancer that are prompted by follow-up testing or the presence of symptoms.

▶ This study looked at 548 patients with recurrent colon cancer. Patients underwent physical examination, blood work, chest x-ray examination, colonic examination, and monitoring of CEA levels. The estimated 5-year disease-free survival rate in this study is approximately 23%. As seen in Figure 2, the longer the interval between primary treatment and relapse, the greater the likelihood of cure. Similarly, as seen in Figure 3, patients who have multiple areas of recurrence are less likely to benefit from surgery than patients with a single area of recurrence. One caveat worth noting in this study is that curative salvage surgery was particularly effective when the cancer recurred during years 2 and 3 after initial surgery. This was particularly true in patients who had fluorouracil plus levamisole. Furthermore, this study emphasizes the importance of annual examinations for 3 to 5 years.

T.J. Eberlein, M.D.

Rectal

Characteristics of Rectal Carcinomas That Predict the Presence of Lymph Node Metastases: Implications for Patient Selection for Local Therapy

Zenni GC, Abraham K, Harford FJ, et al (Loyola Univ, Maywood, Ill; Hines VA Hosp, Ill)

J Surg Oncol 67:99-103, 1998 11–28

Objective.—Whereas 5% of patients with rectal cancer can be cured with local therapy, this treatment does not identify regional lymph node

TABLE 1.—Rectal Carcinoma Tumor Characteristics Versus Nodal Status

	Total (%)	Lymph Node (%) Negative 78 (59)	Positive 55 (41)	p*
Size (largest diameter) (133 pts.)				
≤3 cm	27 (20)	19 (70)	8 (30)	NS
>3 cm	106 (80)	59 (56)	47 (44)	
Wall penetration (133 pts.)				
T1	10 (8)	9 (90)	1 (10)	
T2	35 (26)	26 (74)	9 (26)	<0.001
T3	88 (66)	43 (49)	45 (51)	
Differentiation (133 pts.)				
Well	50 (38)	42 (84)	8 (16)	
Moderate	61 (46)	32 (53)	29 (47)	<0.0001
Poor	22 (16)	4 (18)	18 (82)	
Ploidy (129 pts.)				
Diploid	88 (68)	58 (66)	30 (34)	<0.02
Aneuploid	41 (32)	17 (41)	24 (59)	

*Chi-square test, significant at $P < 0.05$.

Abbreviations: Pts, patients; *NS,* not statistical.

(Courtesy of Zenni GC, Abraham K, Harford FJ, et al: Characteristics of rectal carcinomas that predict the presence of lymph node metastases: Implications for patient selection for local therapy. *J Surg Oncol* 67:99-103, 1998. Reprinted by permission of Wiley-Liss, Inc., a subsidiary of John Wiley & Sons, Inc.)

TABLE 2.—Probability of Nodal Metastasis in Rectal Carcinoma by Logistic Regression

Differentiation	Penetration	Ploidy	Probability
Well	T1	D	0.06
	T2	D	0.11
	T2	A	0.20
	T3	D	0.18
	T3	A	0.31
Moderate	T1	D	0.21
	T2	D	0.32
	T2	A	0.50
	T3	D	0.46
	T3	A	0.64
Poor	T2	D	0.65
	T3	D	0.77
	T3	A	0.88

Abbreviations: T1, mucosal and submucosal penetration; *T2,* incomplete muscularis propria penetration; *T3,* penetration through the muscularis propria; *D,* diploid; *A,* aneuploid.

(Courtesy of Zenni GC, Abraham K, Harford FJ, et al: Characteristics of rectal carcinomas that predict the presence of lymph node metastases: Implications for patient selection for local therapy. *J Surg Oncol* 67:99-103, 1998. Reprinted by permission of Wiley-Liss, Inc., a subsidiary of John Wiley & Sons, Inc.)

metastases. Attempts have been made to define the characteristics of rectal tumors that would identify those patients who would be good candidates for local treatment. Results of a retrospective study of the prognostic value of DNA ploidy, degree of differentiation, depth of wall penetration, and tumor size as predictors of nodal spread are presented.

Methods.—Charts of 133 patients (37 women), aged 29 to 92 years, with adenocarcinoma of the rectum were reviewed. The relationship between tumor variables and nodal status was assessed with the 2-tailed chi-square test, and the role of the combination of tumor characteristics as predictors of the presence or absence of nodal metastases was subjected to logistic regression analysis.

Results.—There were 10 T1 tumors (8%), 35 T2 tumors (26%), and 88 T3 tumors (66%) (Table 1). Most tumors were larger than 3 cm. Positive nodes were found in 55 patients (41%). The incidence of positive lymph nodes significantly increased with depth of tumor penetration, as the tumor became less-well differentiated, and with aneuploidy. Degree of differentiation was significantly and independently correlated with depth of penetration and with DNA ploidy. Logistic regression analysis determined no correlation between tumor size and lymph node status (Table 2). Patients with aneuploid tumors were significantly more likely to have nodal metastases than patients with diploid tumors.

Conclusion.—Increasing degree of differentiation, depth of tumor penetration, and ploidy status were predictors of nodal metastases. Aneuploidy significantly increased the likelihood of lymph node metastasis.

► This VA series of 133 patients with rectal cancer was retrospectively reviewed. The purpose of the study was to identify potential predictors of lymph node metastases. As seen in Table 1, penetration of the wall, poor differentiation, and especially aneuploidy characteristic of the tumor predicted lymph node metastases. It is interesting that depth of wall penetration and differentiation were not as helpful in predicting lymph node metastases when considered alone, since nearly one third of the patients with well-differentiated and moderately differentiated tumors had regional lymph node metastases. The use of ploidy in combination with the other traditional criteria provided the best prediction of probability of positive lymph nodes. Thus, any combination of degree of differentiation, tumor size, and depth of penetration meant a significant increase in positive lymph nodes if aneuploidy was present (Table 2). The use of criteria such as these may well help to predict favorable outcome for patients and therefore select candidates for local treatment. Alternatively, in the presence of aneuploidy, especially with poorly differentiated and deeper lesions, patients would be better treated with more radical surgery.

T.J. Eberlein, M.D.

Conservative Management of Rectal Adenocarcinoma by Radiotherapy

Maingon P, Guerif S, Darsouni R, et al (Centre Georges-Francois-Leclerc, Dijon, France)

Int J Radiat Oncol Biol Phys 40:1077-1085, 1998 11–29

Introduction.—The authors' hospital has a long and extensive experience with radiotherapy for the conservative management of rectal adenocarcinoma. They have reported a 5-year survival rate of 74%, with a 4.5% local failure rate and a 3.8% nodal failure rate. This report analyzes their experience with radiotherapy for low rectal cancers.

Methods.—The 20-year analysis included 151 patients with low rectal adenocarcinomas managed with curative intent by radiotherapy alone. There were 78 males and 73 females, mean age 71. According to Dijon clinical staging, 34% of tumors were stage T1A, 15% were stage T1B, 25% were stage T2B, and 8% were stage T3. Recent experience included rectal US examination, the results of which were compared with those of CT scanning and MRI, when performed. Sixty-nine percent of patients received intracavitary contact radiation, 30% received brachytherapy, and 22.5% received external radiotherapy. The results were analyzed in terms of pelvic tumor control, survival, toxicity, and sphincter function. Mean follow-up was 65 months.

Results.—Ninety-three percent of patients had a complete response. The local failure rate was 28%, including 2 local failures that occurred in the pelvic lymph nodes after intracavitary radiation. Local failure was more likely in patients with tumors larger than 3 cm and in those with altered mobility. With the addition of external radiotherapy, the chances of local control were improved for patients whose prognosis was poor and salvage surgery was possible in 39 patients with recurrent tumors. Including the results of salvage therapy, the experience showed a local control rate of 82%, with unlimited follow-up. The actuarial 5-year survival rate was 57%, with a specific survival rate of 66%. Local control and survival rates were unaffected by tumor differentiation or distance between the anal margin and the inferior level of the lesion. About 4% of patients had severe, grade 3, late effects. The sphincter preservation rate was 84%, with 98% of these patients having normal sphincter function.

Conclusions.—For patients with clinical stage IA tumors, intracavitary contact x-ray therapy is the procedure of choice for rectal adenocarcinoma. For patients with larger tumors, outcomes are significantly better with the addition of external radiotherapy. Patients can be selected for treatment on the basis of clinical staging and transrectal US. For selected patients with small rectal adenocarcinomas, radiotherapy may be an appropriate alternative to mutilating surgery.

▶ This is a study of 151 patients who received radiotherapy alone for rectal adenocarcinoma. Local failure was observed in 28% of the patients. Size significantly influenced the risk of local failure. Nearly half of the patients with tumors of more than 3 cm had recurrence; the recurrence rate was reduced if the tumor size was less than 3 cm. Alteration of mobility correlated with higher risk of local failure. Toxicity included acute proctitis, diarrhea, minimal rectal bleeding, and pain. There were three cases of rectal necrosis after treatment with external radiation. Sphincter preservation was obtained in 84% of the patients, with 98% of those patients having normal sphincter function. Late severe damage was noted in 10 patients. Transrectal US and specific clinical staging will allow selection of patients. Radiotherapy alone may be used in highly selected cases if the tumor is small, mobile, and properly staged and if the patient is followed up carefully. This therapy, although not popular in a majority of patients, will certainly increase our armamentarium for preserving sphincter function in patients with rectal adenocarcinoma.

T.J. Eberlein, M.D.

Prospective Evaluation of Local Excision for Small Rectal Cancers

Bleday R, Breen E, Jessup JM, et al (Harvard Med School, Boston)

Dis Colon Rectum 40:388-392, 1997 11–30

Introduction.—Because of the morbidity and mortality associated with abdominoperineal resection (APR), local excision is considered as an alternative in patients with small rectal cancers. Some retrospective series have reported good results after local excision when strict selection criteria are followed. A prospective registry of patients eligible for local excision of rectal cancer was reviewed for outcome and recurrence.

Methods.—Eligible patients had histologically documented adenocarcinoma, with tumors less than 4 cm in diameter, involving less than 40% of the bowel wall circumference, and a proximal margin within 10 cm of the dentate line. Tumors were also required to be limited to the bowel wall with no evidence of distant metastases. Local excision was done by a transanal, transsphincteric, or transcoccygeal approach. Free margins

TABLE 4.—Patterns of Failure

TNM	Degree of Differentiation	Margin Status	Lymphatic Invasion	Mucin-Producing	Months to Recurrence	Salvage
T1,NX	Moderate	Negative	Yes	No	37.9	APR
T1,NX	Well	+ Proximal	Yes	No	35.6	Colostomy
T3,NX	Moderate	Negative	No	Yes	7.1	APR
T3,N2	Poor	+ Radial	Yes	Yes	16.9	APR

Abbreviation: APR, abdominoperineal resection.

(Courtesy of Bleday R, Breen E, Jessup JM, et al: Prospective evaluation of local excision for small rectal cancers. *Dis Colon Rectum* 40:388-392, 1997.)

were confirmed by frozen section. The depth of tumor invasion into the bowel wall determined the need for adjuvant therapy. Patients with T1 lesions were observed; those with T2 lesions received postoperative chemoradiation. In the case of T3 lesions, adjuvant therapy was recommended, although radical excision vs. observation was counseled in some cases. Follow-up consisted of colonoscopy at 1 year, then at least every 2 years until 5 years after surgery.

Results.—Forty-eight patients with an average age of 63 years were followed up. A fecal fistula developed in 3 of 15 patients who had undergone a transsphincteric or a transcoccygeal resection. At a mean follow-up of 40.5 months, the local recurrence rate was 8%. Three of 4 patients with recurrences were salvaged with APR; 1 remains disease-free, 1 has distant recurrence, and 1 died of distant recurrence. Local recurrences developed in 3 of the 5 patients whose tumors had lymphatic invasion of cancer cells. Locoregional recurrences were found in both patients with positive margins on the final pathology of resected specimens (Table 4).

Conclusions.—In selected patients with small rectal cancers, local excision can be performed with minimum morbidity and a low (8%) recurrence rate. Further therapy, including APR, should be considered in cases with lymphatic invasion or positive margins. Patients with both T2 or T3 cancers appear to benefit from adjuvant chemoradiation. There were no significant complications or fecal fistulas in the group of 33 patients resected by a transanal approach.

▶ This is not a randomized study but, in fact, a retrospective analysis of a prospective registry of patients. These patients underwent transanal transsphincteric or transcoccygeal technique. Patients that had T2 and T3 tumors underwent multimodality therapy. Eight percent of the patients had local recurrence; positive margins and the presence of lymphatic invasion correlated with the eventual development of local recurrence (Table 4). Three of the four patients were treated with a salvage APR.

This local recurrence rate is comparable with that of historical controls receiving APRs for similarly staged patients. It is interesting that the patients who had T2 lesions (and were all treated with postoperative chemoradiation) failed to develop any local recurrence. In the patients with larger T3 tumors (once again treated with chemoradiation), positive margins and lymphatic invasion were associated with local recurrence. Follow-up of this study is 40.5 months and, therefore, with a longer-term follow-up, more local recurrence may be seen.

Unfortunately, we are restricted to subset analysis to identify those patients who do poorly with local excision or local excision plus chemoradiation, because a definitive prospective trial randomly assigning patients to local excision or APR is not feasible.

T.J. Eberlein, M.D.

Role of p53 and p21/WAF1 Detection in Patient Selection for Preoperative Radiotherapy in Rectal Cancer Patients

Fu C-G, Tominaga O, Nagawa H, et al (Univ of Tokyo; Second Military Med Univ, Shanghai, Peoples Republic of China)

Dis Colon Rectum 41:68-74, 1998 11–31

Introduction.—Preoperative radiation can decrease tumor bulk in patients with rectal carcinoma, changing a fixed and unresectable tumor to one that is mobile and resectable. Not all tumors are radiosensitive, however, and this quality may be related to the expression of tumor suppressor genes p53 and p21 (also known as WAF1). Biopsy samples from patients with primary rectal carcinoma were analyzed histochemically for p53 and p21 expression. Findings were examined for their relationship to histopathologic changes after radiation and other clinical features.

Methods.—Formalin-fixed, paraffin-embedded, preradiation and postradiation biopsy samples were obtained from 49 cases of primary rectal carcinoma. Patients were 34 men and 15 women with a mean age of 56 years. All tumors were locally advanced, 32 were well differentiated, 13 were moderately differentiated, and 4 were mucinous carcinomas. In all cases the total radiation dose was 50 Gy. Patients were followed up for a mean of 54.7 months. Specimens were evaluated according to the positive tumor cell percentage and the staining intensity.

Results.—The overall expression of p53 and p21/WAF1 was 49% and 28.6%, respectively. Information of p53 and/or p21 status before radiotherapy was found to be an independent factor predictive of an effect of radiation on tumors of the rectum. Eighteen tumors (36.7%) demonstrated obvious histopathological effects of radiation. None of the 4 mucinous carcinomas were radiosensitive, and more tumors in the moderate (53.9%) group than in the well-differentiated (34.4%) group were histopathologically radiosensitive (not a statistically significant difference). Most of the p53(+) or p21(−) tumors were radioresistant, whereas the majority of p53(−) or p21(+) tumors were radiosensitive. Radioresistant p53(+) and p21(−) tumors were reduced significantly less in bulk after radiation, had more local recurrence and more distant metastases, and were associated with a shorter 5-year survival rate. The likelihood of radioresistance was increased (Table 3) when tumors were both p53(+) and p21(−).

TABLE 3.—The Relationship Between Radiosensitivity and the Combination of p53 and p21 Staining

	Staining Status			
Pathologically	p53(−) and p21(+)*	p53(+) and p21(−)*	p53(+) and p21(+)	p53(−) and p21(−)
Radioresistant	1	21	2	7
Radiosensitive	10	1	1	6

*P < 0.001 (Fisher's exact test).
Abbreviations: (−), negative staining; (+), positive staining.
(Courtesy of Fu C-G, Tominaga O, Nagawa H, et al: Role of p53 and p21/WAF1 detection in patient selection for preoperative radiotherapy in rectal cancer patients. *Dis Colon Rectum* 41(1):68-74, 1998.)

Conclusions.—Many recent studies suggest that p53 and p21 status may play important roles in determining tumor radiosensitivity through the apoptosis pathway. Immunohistochemical detection of these tumor suppressor genes in patients with rectal carcinoma may provide selection criteria for preoperative radiotherapy.

▶ This is a study of formalin-fixed, paraffin-embedded biopsy samples of primary rectal carcinoma. They were analyzed by immunohistochemistry for p53 and p21 expression. As identified in Table 3, most of the p53 positive (mutant p53) tumors were p21 negative. On the other hand, the majority of the p21 positive tumors were p53 negative. This may suggest that in human rectal carcinomas, wild-type p53 may also be essential for activation and expression of p21. Wild-type p53 regulates cell transition from G2 to S phase in the cell cycle and induces G1 arrest in response to DNA damage, whereas p53 mutation results in functional abnormalities of p53 products and leads to radioresistance. It is interesting that the authors also looked at bcl-2 staining and could find no correlation in their study. Identification of these genetic abnormalities by immunohistochemistry may help select patients for preoperative radiotherapy.

T.J. Eberlein, M.D.

Outcome After Proctectomy for Rectal Cancer in Department of Veterans Affairs Hospitals: A Report From the National Surgical Quality Improvement Program

Longo WE, Virgo KS, Johnson FE, et al (St Louis Univ; Hines VA Cooperative Studies Program Coodinating Ctr, Hines, Ill; Harvard Med School, Boston)
Ann Surg 228:64-70, 1998 11–32

Background.—The ability to predict risk of perioperative morbidity and mortality may improve planning of surgical treatment. Risk factors predictive of adverse outcomes in patients who have had proctectomy for cancer in Department of Veterans Affairs Medical Centers were determined.

TABLE 2.—30-Day Mortality: Logistic Regression Analysis Results

Variable	Parameter Estimate	p Value	Odds Ratio
Intercept	0.2776	0.8782	
Preoperative BUN (mg/dl)	0.0530	0.0347	1.054
Impaired sensorium (Y/N)	2.0953	0.0041	8.128
Preoperative albumin (g/dl)*	−1.0577	0.0183	0.347
PTT > 25 secs	−1.0761	0.0295	0.341
Model Fit			
Model chi-square =	20.992 (p = 0.0003)		
Hosmer-Lemeshow goodness of fit =	5.9383 (p = 0.6541)		
c Index =	0.755		
R^2 =	3.55		
Maximum Rescaled R^2 =	14.17		

*The normal value of 4.3 was substituted for missing values because albumin was assumed to be normal if no preoperative value was recorded.

(Courtesy of Longo WE, Virgo KS, Johnson FE, et al: Outcome after proctectomy for cancer in Department of Veterans Affairs hospitals. *Ann Surg* 228:64-70, 1998.)

Methods.—Data on all patients registered with the database of the National Veterans Affairs Surgical Quality Improvement Program who underwent proctectomy for rectal cancer between 1991 and 1995 were obtained. This program contains data on more than 287,000 patients; data are collected prospectively and extensively validated. Analysis was made of 68 presurgical and 12 intraoperative independent variables and of 21 dependent variables of specific adverse outcomes. Models predicting 30-day mortality and 30-day morbidity for the 10 most common complications were constructed with the use of stepwise logistic regression analysis.

Results.—Data were obtained on 591 patients, of whom 467 had abdominoperineal resection and 124 had sphincter-saving procedures. At least 1 complication was seen in 30% of the patients. The most common complications were prolonged ileus, urinary tract infection, pneumonia, and deep wound infection. At 30 days, the mortality rate was 3.2%. For the majority of complications, the 30-day mortality rate was significantly higher in patients with complications than in patients with no complications. For the following complications, the 30-day mortality rate was higher than 50%: cardiac arrest requiring cardiopulmonary resuscitation, deep venous thrombosis or thrombophlebitis, coma longer than 24 hours, acute renal failure, cerebrovascular accident, and pulmonary embolism. Analysis showed that a high risk of 30-day mortality was predicted by the following 4 presurgical factors: elevated blood urea nitrogen level, impaired sensorium, low serum albumin concentration, and partial thromboplastin time of 25 seconds or less (Table 2).

Discussion.—These results indicate that mortality rates after proctectomy in Veterans Affairs hospitals are similar to mortality rates reported by other large studies. The majority of postsurgical complications are associated with higher mortality rates at 30 days.

▶ This report from the National Surgical Quality Improvement Program of the Veterans Administration encompasses data from more than 287,000 patients. Although the 30-day mortality rate found in this study (3.2%) was comparable to other reported series, four presurgical factors seemed to predict a high risk of 30-day mortality in this patient population (Table 2). In addition to the preoperative predictors (elevated BUN, impaired sensorium, and low serum albumin), these authors showed high mortality rates for patients with postsurgical acute renal failure, cardiovascular accidents, or pulmonary embolism. As other databases become available in large patient populations, hypothesis testing can be performed and compared with the data of this study. In the meantime, it is hoped that the surgeon would bear in mind these predictors of 30-day death and complication rates. Future studies will generate intervention trials in which modification of certain risk factors will be attempted.

T.J. Eberlein, M.D.

Hepatopancreatic

Statewide Regionalization of Pancreaticoduodenectomy and Its Effect on In-Hospital Mortality

Gordon TA, Bowman HM, Tielsch JM, et al (Johns Hopkins Hosp, Baltimore, Md; Johns Hopkins Univ, Baltimore, Md)
Ann Surg 1:71-78, 1998 11–33

Background.—Pancreaticoduodenectomy is a complex, high-risk procedure that is performed in many hospitals in the United States. The in-hospital mortality rate for pancreaticoduodenectomy was more than 20% before 1980 but has since decreased significantly, to 4% or less in high-volume tertiary care centers. Studies have shown that the mortality rate for this procedure is significantly lower in high-volume tertiary care centers than in low-volume community hospitals. In the state of Maryland the effect of statewide regionalization of pancreaticoduodenectomy on in-hospital mortality rates was examined during a 12-year period.

Methods.—Discharge data were obtained from state hospitals in Maryland for patients who underwent pancreaticoduodenectomy between 1984 and 1995. Hospitals were classified as high-volume or low-volume providers. Surgical volume and mortality rates were analyzed for the entire state and for high-volume and low-volume provider groups. Regression analysis determined whether hospital share of pancreaticoduodenectomy significantly predicted in-hospital mortality after adjustment for study year and patient characteristics. The percentage of decline in statewide in-hospital mortality attributable to a high-volume provider's increasing share was also calculated.

Results.—From 1984 to 1995, 795 pancreaticoduodenectomies were performed in 43 hospitals in Maryland (state residents only). Between 1984 and 1995, the annual share of pancreaticoduodenectomies increased from 20.7% to 58.5% in one center, and the statewide in-hospital mortality rate decreased from 17.2% to 4.9%. After adjustment for study year and patient characteristics, hospital share was still a significant predictor of in-hospital mortality. It was estimated that 61% of the decrease in statewide in-hospital mortality rate for pancreaticoduodenectomy was attributable to the high-volume provider's increasing share of pancreaticoduodenectomy.

Discussion.—These results show that regionalization of pancreaticoduodenectomy to one or more high-volume tertiary care centers can significantly decrease in-hospital mortality rate. Regionalization of high-risk procedures can optimize patient outcome. Further studies are needed to determine the procedures for which regionalization would be most beneficial, as well as the best means of accomplishing regionalization.

► This is a study by the Johns Hopkins group, who over the last decade or more have shown improved survival and reduced morbidity rates as their experience with surgical management of pancreatic cancer increases. This specific study looked at Maryland State Hospital discharge data. These authors show that as pancreaticoduodenectomies are performed at high-volume facilities, they are associated with a marked decrease in in-hospital mortality rates. This would certainly seem to argue for the effectiveness of regionalization of high-risk and potentially high-morbidity procedures such as Whipple operations. This trend toward regional specialization will also be hastened by managed care contracting and outcomes benchmarking by insurers and third-party payors.

T.J. Eberlein, M.D.

Periampullary Adenocarcinoma: Analysis of 5-Year Survivors

Yeo CJ, Sohn TA, Cameron JL, et al (Johns Hopkins Med Institutions, Baltimore, Md)

Ann Surg 227:821-831, 1998 11–34

Background.—In patients with periampullary adenocarcinoma, outcome is related to tumor site, stage, and type of intervention. It has been suggested that resection is not indicated because of the poor outcomes achieved, particularly for patients with primary pancreatic cancers. Most previous reports rely on Kaplan-Meier actuarial 5-year survival rates, which may differ from actual 5-year survival. The 5-year results of pancreaticoduodenectomy for patients with periampullary adenocarcinoma are reported.

Patients and Outcomes.—The 22-year surgical series included 242 patients with periampullary adenocarcinoma who underwent pancreaticoduodenal resection at least 5 years previously. There were 133 men and 109 women, with a median age of 64 years. The primary tumor site was the pancreas in 62% of the patients, the ampulla in 19%, the bile duct in 12%, and the duodenum in 7%. The pancreatic tumors had the lowest rate of node-negative resections and the highest rate of positive surgical margins. The operative mortality rate was about 5% overall but dropped to 2% for the 100 patients most recently operated on.

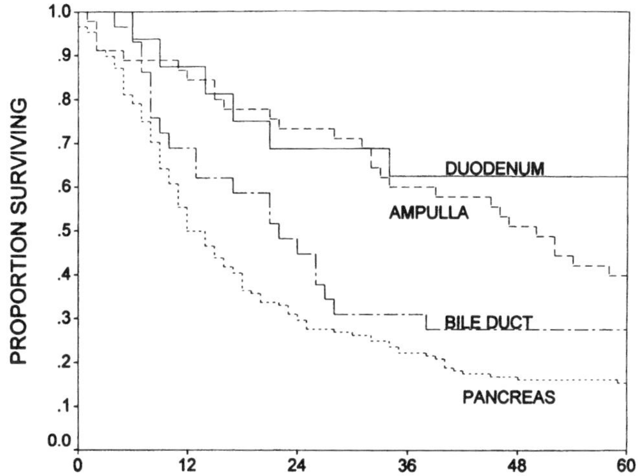

FIGURE 2.—The tumor-specific actual survival curves for the cohort of 242 patients treated by pancreaticoduodenectomy for periampullary adenocarcinoma. (Courtesy of Yeo CJ, Sohn TA, Cameron JL, et al: Periampullary adenocarcinoma: Analysis of 5-year survivors. *Ann Surg* 227:821-831, 1998.)

The actual 5-year survival rate was 28%, with 58 patients surviving for 5 years, 28 for 7 years, and 7 for 10 years. Actual survival at 5 years was 59% for patients with duodenal cancers, 39% for those with ampullary cancers, 27% for those with distal bile duct cancers, and 15% for those with pancreatic cancers (Fig 2). Ten-year actuarial survival was 59% for duodenal cancers, 25% for ampullary cancers, 21% for distal bile duct cancers, and 5% for pancreatic cancers. Characteristics of 5-year survivors included a higher percentage of well-differentiated tumors, 14% vs. 4% for patients who did not survive for 5 years; a higher rate of negative

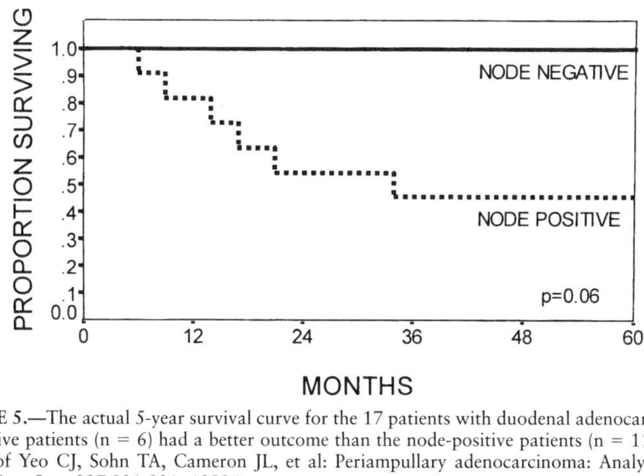

FIGURE 5.—The actual 5-year survival curve for the 17 patients with duodenal adenocarcinoma. The node-negative patients (n = 6) had a better outcome than the node-positive patients (n = 11, P = 0.06). (Courtesy of Yeo CJ, Sohn TA, Cameron JL, et al: Periampullary adenocarcinoma: Analysis of 5-year survivors. *Ann Surg* 227:821-831, 1998.)

resection margins, 98% vs. 73%, and a higher rate of negative lymph nodes, 62% vs. 31% (Fig 5).

Conclusions.—Analysis of the long-term results of pancreaticoduodenectomy for patients with periampullary adenocarcinoma suggests that survival rates are best for patients with duodenal adenocarcinoma and worst for those with pancreatic primary tumors. Other important prognostic factors are resection margins, lymph node status, and tumor differentiation. Patients with periampullary adenocarcinoma are still at risk of death from cancer recurrence beyond 5 years after resection, especially those with pancreatic adenocarcinoma. New diagnostic and therapeutic approaches to periampullary tumors, and pancreatic adenocarcinoma in particular, are needed.

► This is a study of 242 patients who underwent Whipple procedures for periampullary adenocarcinoma at Johns Hopkins University. Therefore, the experience of the authors is unparalleled. As seen in Fig 2, there is a descreasing 5-year survival rate, starting with the duodenum, then the ampulla, the bile duct, and finally the pancreas. Especially for patients with duodenal cancers, aggressive surgical management can result in significant long-term survival. As seen in Fig 5, nodal status is important for each of these histologic types. Similar curves were generated for each of the other histologic types that were presented in the article. Resection margin and degree of tumor differentiation also significantly influenced long-term outcome. Thus, the experience of the surgical team plays an important role in maximizing 5-year survival. This study shows that in patients with pancreatic carcinoma 5-year survival is not equated with cure. In fact, patients can die of recurrent disease after 5 years of survival.

T.J. Eberlein, M.D.

Laparoscopy and Laparoscopic Ultrasonography Avoid Exploratory Laparotomy in Patients With Hepatocellular Carcinoma

Lo C-M, Lai ECS, Liu C-L, et al (Univ of Hong Kong, China)

Ann Surg 227:527-532, 1998 11–35

Objective.—Because surgical resection for hepatocellular carcinoma (HCC) is possible in only 9% to 40% of patients, selection of patients requires assessment of liver function and extent of disease. The value of laparoscopy and laparoscopic US in avoiding laparotomy was assessed prospectively in patients with potentially resectable HCC.

Methods.—Between June 1994 and June 1996, 370 patients had HCC diagnosed. Of the 110 (30%) considered to have potentially resectable disease, 91 (14 women), aged 18-82 years, had laparoscopy with laparoscopic US immediately before a planned laparotomy. Nineteen patients were excluded because of previous abdominal surgery (n = 12), ruptured tumors (n = 4), refusal (n = 2), and instrument failure (n = 1). Unresectability was defined as disease not amenable to curative resection or inadequate size of the liver remnant.

Results.—The median time for laparoscopy with laparoscopic US was 30 minutes. The procedure was successful in all patients. Fifteen patients were found to have unresectable disease by laparoscopy and laparoscopic US. Of the 76 who underwent laparotomy, 67 (RES group) had resection, and 9 were not resectable. Laparoscopy with laparoscopic US avoided laparotomy in 15 (63%) of 24 patients. Laparoscopy failed to detect unresectable disease in 7 of 12 patients with tumors of more than 10 cm in diameter, and in only 2 of 12 patients with tumors of 10 cm or less in diameter, but identified 6 of 7 patients with inadequate liver remnant, 11 of 13 patients with bilobar intrahepatic metastases, and 1 of 1 patients with peritoneal metastasis. The procedure failed to detect main portal vein tumor thrombi in 3 of 5 patients, inferior vena cava tumor thrombi in 1 of 2 patients, and invasion of adjacent organs in 3 of 3 patients. There were no complications after laparoscopic examination. Two laparotomy patients had pneumonia (n = 1) and pleural effusion (n = 1). Laparoscopic patients with unresectable disease had a faster postoperative recovery and were able to begin palliative treatment sooner.

Conclusions.—Laparoscopy with laparoscopic US avoided laparotomy in 63% of HCC patients with inoperable disease. There were no complications, and postoperative recovery was faster.

► Laparoscopy is becoming more important in accurate staging of patients with abdominal malignancy. This study uses laparoscopy and laparoscopic US in patients with HCC. Laparoscopic examination was less effective when the tumor was very large (greater than 10 cm). It also was less sensitive in determining the presence of tumor thrombi in major vascular structures, as well as the potential extent of invasion into adjacent organs. As expected, the avoidance of laparotomy made postoperative recovery faster and easier on the patient.

T.J. Eberlein, M.D.

Prospective Evaluation of Pringle Maneuver in Hepatectomy for Liver Tumors by a Randomized Study

Man K, Fan S-T, Ng IO, et al (Univ of Hong Kong)
Ann Surg 226:704-713, 1997 11–36

Objective.—Although the Pringle maneuver is commonly used to decrease bleeding during hepatectomy, there is the possibility of ischemic injury, particularly in cirrhotic patients. The safety and efficacy of the Pringle maneuver in reducing blood loss during hepatectomy was evaluated in a prospective randomized study.

Methods.—Between July 1995 and February 1997, 100 consecutive patients were randomly allocated to hepatectomy without (n = 50) or with the intermittent Pringle maneuver (n = 50) applied for 20 minutes with a clamp release of 5 minutes. Blood loss was assessed before, during, and

TABLE 2.—Intraoperative Data of Patients With Hepatectomy Using Pringle Maneuver and Control Patients

	Pringle Group (n = 50)	Control Group (n = 50)	p
Major hepatectomy	34	35	
Right hepatic lobectomy	24	21	
Right extended lobectomy	5	9	
Left hepatic lobectomy	4	4	
Left extended lobectomy	1	1	
Minor hepatectomy	16	15	
Left lateral segmentectomy	7	6	
Subsegmentectomy	9	9	
Ischemic time (min)	88 (24-101)	0	
Total blood loss (L)	1.28 (0.33-9.42)	1.99 (0.26-13.9)	0.006*
Blood loss during liver transection ((L)	0.61 (0.09-8.5)	1.41 (0.17-11.4)	0.0002*
Transection surface area (cm^2)	68 (22-130)	60.5 (16-155)	0.064
Blood loss per transection area (mL/cm^2)	12 (3-74)	22 (5-150)	0.0001*
Blood transfusion (L)	0 (0-8.6)	0.6 (0-12.9)	0.02*
Patients without blood transfusion	32	21	0.028*
Liver transection time (min)	138 (33-300)	169 (40-463)	0.162
Liver transection time (min/cm^2)	2 (1-3.6)	2.8 (0.2-6)	0.016*

Note: Values are mean (range).
*Significant value.
(Courtesy of Man K, Fan S-T, Ng IO, et al: Prospective evaluation of Pringle maneuver in hepatectomy for liver tumors by a randomized study. *Ann Surg* 226:704-713, 1997.)

after transection. Arterial ketone body ratio, indocyanine green clearance, and serum transferrin were measured.

Results.—Blood loss during transection and blood loss per square centimeter of transection area was significantly lower for the Pringle maneuver group than for the control group (Table 2). In the Pringle maneuver group, the arterial ketone body ratio 2 hours after surgery and the serum total bilirubin levels on the day of and the day after surgery were significantly higher than in the control group. In a subgroup of cirrhotic patients, postoperative serum transferrin values were higher on postoperative days 1 and 8. There were complications in 13 patients in the Pringle maneuver group and in 15 patients in the control group. There were 2 deaths in the control group and 1 in the Pringle maneuver group.

Conclusion.—The Pringle maneuver, performed during liver transection, is safe and effective in reducing blood loss and results in improved liver function during the early postoperative period.

► This is a randomized study of 100 consecutive patients who were randomly assigned to liver transection under intermittent Pringle maneuver or transection without. This is the first randomized prospective trial evaluating the Pringle maneuver. As seen in Table 2, the Pringle maneuver was beneficial in reducing blood loss and shortening the time of completion of the liver transection. Similarly, the patients in the Pringle category somewhat unexpectedly demonstrated better postoperative liver function. This was likely due to less hemodynamic disturbance as well as retrograde perfusion through the hepatic veins. It is interesting that the patients with cirrhosis seemed to benefit most from the procedure. However, it should be noted that the cirrhotic patients chosen for hepatectomy in this study were those with the most well-compensated liver function. Another emphasis is that the Pringle maneuver used in this study was intermittent and not continuous.

T.J. Eberlein, M.D.

Cryosurgery as a Treatment for Advanced Stage Hepatocellular Carcinoma: Results, Complications, and Alcohol Ablation

Wong WS, Patel SC, Cruz FS, et al (Alhambra Hosp, Calif; Arcadia Radiology Med Group, Calif)

Cancer 82:1268-1278, 1998 11–37

Objective.—Hepatocellular carcinoma is a highly virulent cancer, with a late presentation and a poor prognosis. Cryosurgery has proved effective for the treatment of liver metastases; it is a focal treatment that can spare more uninvolved liver tissue than surgical resection. Cryosurgery, alone or in combination with alcohol ablation, was evaluated as a treatment for advanced-stage hepatocellular carcinoma.

Methods.—The 4-year experience included 12 patients with biopsy-diagnosed hepatocellular carcinoma. There were 9 males and 3 females, mean age 59; 11 of the patients were Asian. The average tumor was 7 cm, in the greatest dimension, with a range of 3-13 cm. Disease stage, according to the TNM staging system, was IVA in 9 patients, III in 2 patients, and II in 1 patient. All underwent a thorough preoperative workup to exclude the presence of extrahepatic disease. The patients then underwent US-guided cryosurgical ablation of their cancer. If they had residual or recur-

TABLE 3.—Pattern of Recurrence and Patient Survival

Patient No.	Pattern of Recurrence/Failure	Survival (mo)	Current Status
1	Recurred in other parts of liver	12	Died
2	Died of liver failure; no known recurrence	9	Died
3	Recurred in other parts of liver	26	Died
4	Disseminated disease in other parts of liver	6	Died
5	Disease free	36	Alive
6	Died of liver failure; no known recurrence	9	Died
7	Died of liver failure; no known recurrence	20	Died
8	Recurred at local site within portal vein	5	Died
9	Disease free	30	Alive
10	Surgically related death	0	Died
11	Disease free after 9 months	9	Alive
12	Disease free after 3 months	3	Alive

(Courtesy of Wong WS, Patel SC, Cruz FS, et al: Cryosurgery as a treatment for advanced stage hepatocellular carcinoma: Results, complications, and alcohol ablation. *Cancer* 82:1268-1278, 1998. Reprinted by permission of Wiley-Liss, Inc., a subsidiary of John Wiley & Sons, Inc.)

rent tumor after cryosurgery, alcohol ablation was performed under CT guidance.

Results.—The tumors shrank in size after cryosurgery. Although the change in size was not significant, biopsies performed in 5 patients showed only dead or scar tissue, and the mass continued to shrink with continued CT follow-up. Three patients had residual tumor, for which they underwent alcohol ablation. Five of 10 patients were alive at 1 year and 3 of 10 were alive at 3 years. Freedom from disease was achieved for 2.5 and 3 years in 2 patients with stage IVA disease; initial tumor sizes were 13 and 8 cm, respectively (Table 3). Bleeding was the main complication, with average blood loss of 700 mL. Injury to the right lung and right hemidiaphragm was common, with nearly every patient experiencing some degree of postoperative atelectasis.

Conclusions.—Cryosurgery appears to be a promising treatment for primary hepatocellular carcinoma. Adjunctive alcohol ablation is used to treat residual tumor and to control recurrences. This approach can effectively control the cancer of the liver, in some cases prolonging the patient's life. The authors have salvaged more than 10% of patients with stage IVA disease in this way; major complications are frequent.

▶ The authors use US-guided cryosurgical ablation of hepatocellular carcinoma, followed by postoperative alcohol ablation for residual or recurrent disease. As expected, bleeding was the major complication and was directly related to the severity of the underlying liver disease. It did not seem to be related to the size or number of cryoprobes used. Injury to the right lung and hemidiaphragm was also a common complication, with nearly every patient having atelectasis. As experience with cryosurgery is increased, this may become an alternative treatment for patients with hepatocellulalr carcinoma.

T.J. Eberlein, M.D.

Hepatic Artery Chemoembolization for Management of Patients With Advanced Metastatic Carcinoid Tumors

Drougas JG, Anthony LB, Blair TK, et al (Vanderbilt Univ, Nashville, Tenn)

Am J Surg 175:408-412, 1998 11–38

Background.—The prognosis for individuals with hepatic metastases from carcinoid tumors is poor. There are few treatment options for patients with advanced metastatic carcinoid tumors whose disease progresses after conventional therapy. The goal of treatment is usually to palliate symptoms, because such patients are seldom candidates for curative resection. The safety and efficacy of hepatic artery chemoembolization as palliative treatment were determined.

Methods.—Intra-artery chemotherapy and hepatic artery chemoembolization were administered to 15 patients with advanced bilobar hepatic carcinoid metastases in whom disease had progressed after treatment with somatostatin analogues. Treatment consisted of 5 days of intra-arterial

5-fluorouracil (1g/m^2), then hepatic artery chemoembolization with adriamycin (60 mg), cisplatin (100 mg), mitomycin C (30 mg), and polyvinyl alcohol (200 µ to 710 µ). Patients were given a consistent dose of octreotide (150 µ to 2,000 µg subcutaneous by every 8 hours) before, during, and after the procedure.

Results.—At baseline and at 3 months, clinical, laboratory, radiographic, and quality-of-life factors were evaluated to determine the effectiveness of treatment. In 8 of 12 patients who had diarrhea, 7 of 12 patients who had flushing, 9 of 12 patients who had abdominal pain, and 4 of 7 patients who had malaise, symptoms improved. A decrease in elevated tumor markers was seen in all patients. At 3 months, biochemical markers had decreased by 60% for 5-HIAA, 75% for chromogranin A, and 50% for neuron-specific enolase. Tomographic evaluation showed tumor liquefaction in 10 of 13 patients. The mean Karnofsky performance status increased from 66 to 84. Thirteen patients died between 1 week and 71 months after treatment. Median follow-up was 16 months.

Discussion.—In these patients with advanced hepatic carcinoid disease, hepatic artery chemoembolization improved symptoms of carcinoid syndrome. The tumor response rate was high, and short-term quality of life improved. Hepatic artery chemoembolization is safe and effective for palliating symptoms in these patients. It is well tolerated and has no apparent long-term complications.

▶ This is a study of hepatic artery chemoembolization. Unfortunately, it is limited to a relatively small number of patients with proven advanced bilobar hepatic carcinoid metastases. Surgical resection in advanced patients with metastatic carcinoid tumors is seldom feasible. Standard chemotherapeutic drugs offer poor response rates. Somatostatin is much more effective and has even been associated with tumor regression. However, patients become increasingly refractory to this therapy. All patients in this series experienced symptomatic relief. However, this was most marked for patients with abdominal pain and incapacitating diarrhea. Hepatic abscess formation was not identified in this series; thus, hepatic artery chemoembolization offers a potentially palliative alternative to patients with advanced metastatic carcinoid tumors.

T.J. Eberlein, M.D.

Soft Tissue Sarcoma

Variable Management of Soft Tissue Sarcoma: Regional Audit With Implications for Specialist Care

Clasby R, Tilling K, Smith MA, et al (St Thomas's Hosp, London)
Br J Surg 84:1692-1696, 1997 11–39

Introduction.—A group of patients with primary soft tissue sarcoma was reviewed for clinical characteristics, management, and outcome. These tumors account for only about 1% of all malignant neoplasms, and there have been wide variations in treatment and uptake of resources.

TABLE 3.—Comparison of Local Recurrence Rate in Patients Undergoing Wide or Marginal Excision

	Wide	Marginal	Total
Local recurrence	19 (14·2)	53 (41·4)	72 (27·5)
No local recurrence	115 (85·8)	75 (58·6)	190 (72·5)
Total	134 (100)	128 (100)	262 (100)

Values in parentheses are percentages. $\chi^2 = 24.33$, 1 d.f., $P < 0.001$.

(Courtesy of Clasby R, Tilling K, Smith MA, et al: Variable management of soft tissue sarcoma: Regional audit with implications for specialist care. *Br J Surg* 84:1692-1696. Copyright 1997, Blackwell Science Ltd.)

Methods.—Cases were obtained by direct notification from consultants and through a review of hospital records and of cancer registry data in the South-East Thames Region for the period between 1986 and 1992. Inclusion criteria were designed to define optimal management of a mass greater than 5 cm in diameter that was situated in subcutaneous or deep soft tissue. The primary aim of surgery was to perform wide excision with 1- to 2-cm margins where possible; the histopathology report was to describe the histologic diagnosis, status of the resection margins, tumor grade, and tumor size. Management of patients was assessed and compared between specialties and between districts within a large region.

Results.—Of the 489 patients identified, 377 were eligible for the study. General surgeons had treated 202 patients (53.6%), orthopedic surgeons 102 (27.1%), and plastic surgeons 19 (5.0%). The remaining 54 patients (14.3%) were treated by a wide variety of other specialists. The time from the first symptoms to the first hospital time differed significantly among districts (range 1 month to 3.3 years), but the time from the first hospital appointment to the first treatment was similar. Only 21.3% of patients underwent optimal investigation, and there was a wide variation among specialties in the use of MRI and CT. Adequate treatment, consisting of wide excision or surgery with radiotherapy, was performed in only 60.0% of cases. Orthopedic surgeons referred half of their patients for adjunctive therapy, whereas the referral rate for general surgeons was 26.2%. Overall, 36.3% of patients received adjunctive therapy. Local recurrence was more common (Table 3) and mortality was increased (Table 4) in patients having marginal vs. wide excision. Variables significant in relation to

TABLE 4.—Comparison of Mortality Rate in Patients Undergoing Wide or Marginal Excision

	Wide	Marginal	Total
Dead	22 (16·3)	53 (42·4)	75 (28·8)
Alive	113 (83·7)	72 (57·6)	185 (71·2)
Total	135 (100)	125 (100)	260 (100)

Values in parentheses are percentages. $\chi^2 = 21.55$, 1 d.f., $P < 0.001$.

(Courtesy of Clasby R, Tilling K, Smith MA, et al: Variable management of soft tissue sarcoma: Regional audit with implications for specialist care. *Br J Surg* 84:1692-1696. Copyright 1997, Blackwell Science Ltd.)

TABLE 5.—Survival Analysis of 377 Primary Soft Tissue Sarcomas Incorporating Local Recurrence as a Variable

Variable	Hazard Ratio*	χ^2	*P*
Age (years)†	1·02 (1·01-1·03)	14·30	0·0002
Recurrence			
None	1·00	35·66	<0·0001
Local	1·62 (0·93-2·84)		
Distant (metastasis)	4·49 (2·72-7·41)		
Tumour size (cm)			
< 10	1·00	36·59	<0·0001
> 10	1·78 (1·04-3·07)		
Not stated	4·85 (2·92-8·04)		
Histology			
Not liposarcoma	1·00	5·29	0·021
Liposarcoma	0·53 (0·29-0·94)		
Presence of mass (months)			
< 12	1·00	11·48	0·0007
> 12	0·37 (0·20-0·71)		

Values in parentheses are 95% confidence intervals.
*A hazard ratio of more than 1 indicates that the variable is positively associated with death.
†Age was measured as a continuous variable.
(Courtesy of Clasby R, Tilling K, Smith MA, et al: Variable management of soft tissue sarcoma: Regional audit with implications for specialist care. *Br J Surg* 84:1692-1696. Copyright 1997, Blackwell Science Ltd.)

survival (Table 5) were age, histology, tumor size, recurrence, and preoperative duration of tumor.

Conclusions.—Many patients with soft tissue sarcoma receive suboptimal clinical examinations and investigations, and inadequate treatment. Appropriate management should include referral to a specialist center.

▶ This is a very interesting study. It analyzes 377 patients with primary soft tissue sarcoma and analyzes their management and compares outcomes between specialties. The findings showed only 60% of the patients seemed to be treated adequately. As is seen in Table 3, marginal excision was associated with a very high recurrence rate (41.4%). Similarly, patients with marginal excisions were associated with a higher mortality rate. Another important finding implicating pathologic review is that only 43% of the cases included tumor grade (obviously an important staging factor). As was documented in this study, there appeared to be, if anything, a delay in diagnosis, indicating that diagnosis of soft tissue sarcoma is often delayed because of the low index of clinical suspicion. While the authors in this study conclude that soft tissue sarcomas are managed most appropriately in specialist centers, their own data indicate that as long as the surgeon is well practiced in sarcoma management, optimal care can result.

T.J. Eberlein, M.D.

Retroperitoneal Soft-Tissue Sarcoma: Analysis of 500 Patients Treated and Followed at a Single Institution

Lewis JJ, Leung D, Woodruff JM, et al (Mem Sloan-Kettering Cancer Ctr)
Ann Surg 228:355-365, 1998 11–40

Objective.—Chemotherapy is not effective for retroperitoneal soft-tissue sarcomas, and use of radiation is restricted because of toxicity to surrounding structures. Disease-specific survival and disease-free survival were analyzed in a large cohort of patients treated and studied prospectively at 1 institution.

Methods.—Between July 1, 1982 and September 30, 1997, 500 patients (214 women), aged 16-88, were treated for retroperitoneal sarcoma at Memorial Sloan-Kettering Cancer Center. Local recurrence, distant metastases, and disease-specific survival were outcome measures. Age at diagnosis, sex, status at diagnosis, tumor, and treatment variables were correlated with outcome.

Results.—There were 278 (56%) patients with primary disease, 119 (24%) with local recurrence, and 103 (20%) with metastases. The median survival was 22 months overall and 40 months for survivors. Median survival was 72 months for patients with primary disease, 28 months for those with recurrent disease, and 10 months for those with metastatic disease. Most tumors were high grade (64%) and larger than 10 cm (60%). The main tumor types were liposarcoma (41%) and leiomyosarcoma (27%). Of 231 patients who underwent resection, 46 (20%) had incomplete resection with gross residual disease. Of 185 patients having complete resection, 136 (74%) had negative margins. Perioperative mortality was 4%. During a median 28-month follow-up, 61 patients had a local recurrence, 30 patients had distant metastases, and 112 died of their disease. Disease-free survival was analyzed for 231 patients with primary disease who underwent resection (Fig 3). Metastasis-free survival in these patients at 2 and 5 years was 88% and 79%, respectively. Disease-specific survival was analyzed in 278 patients with primary disease (Table 5 and Fig 5).

Conclusion.—Stage at diagnosis, high histologic grade, unresectable primary tumor, and positive margins were associated with mortality.

FIGURE 3.—*A*, Kaplan-Meier local recurrence-free survival in patients with primary disease who underwent resection. Of these 231 patients, local recurrence subsequently developed in 61. Local recurrence-free survival was 81% (confidence interval 76% to 86%) at 2 years and 59% (confidence interval 55% to 63%) at 5 years. *B*, Kaplan-Meier disease-specific survival after local recurrence developed in patients with primary disease. Of the patients with primary disease, 231 underwent complete resection. Local recurrence developed in 61 of these patients. Median survival after local recurrence was 28 months, the same as for those (see Fig 2) with local recurrence. *C*, Kaplan-Meier disease-specific survival after local recurrence developed in patients with primary disease, divided by resection of recurrence. Of the 61 patients in whom local recurrence developed, 35 (57%) underwent complete resection. This was significant for predicting subsequent survival (P = 0.01). *D*, rate of complete resection for primary disease and after the first, second, and third local recurrences. The number of patients who underwent complete

(*Continued*)

FIGURE 3 (cont.)

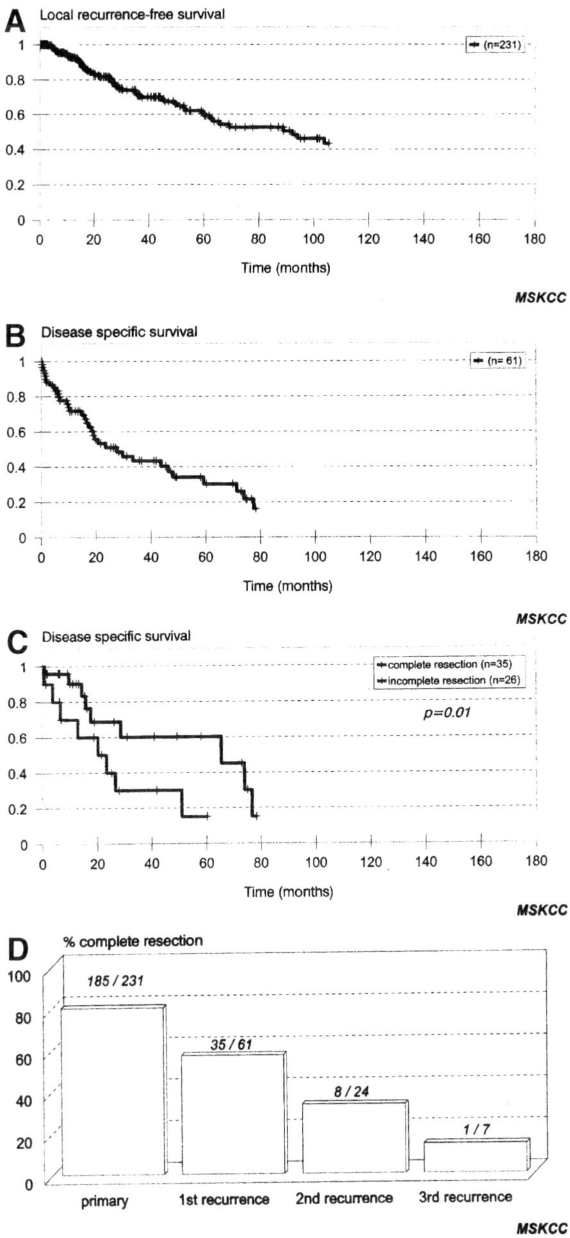

resection, divided by the number of those undergoing attempted resection, is indicated on the curve. The rate of complete resection was 80%, 57%, 33%, and 14%, respectively. (Courtesy of Lewis JJ, Leung D, Woodruff JM, et al: Retroperitoneal soft-tissue sarcoma: Analysis of 500 patients treated and followed at a single institution. *Ann Surg* 228:355-365, 1998).

TABLE 5.—Analysis of Disease-Specific Survival in 278 Primary Retroperitoneal Sarcoma Patients

	n	p Value* (Univariate)	p Value (Multivariate)	Relative Risk† (CI)
Sex		0.6		
Male	170			
Female	108			
Age		0.08		
>50 years	183			
<50 years	95			
Grade		0.001		
High	168		0.001	3.2 (2.0-5.0)
Low	110			
Size		0.2		
>10 cm	196		0.02	1.7 (1.1-2.7)
≤10 cm	80			
Histological subtype		0.08		
Liposarcoma	116			
Others	87			
Leiomyosarcoma	63			
Fibrosarcoma	22			
Surgical resection margins		0.001		
Negative micro & gross margins	136			
Positive micro & negative gross margins	49			
Unresectable	47		0.001	4.7 (2.9-7.5)
Positive micro & gross margins	46		0.001	4.0 (2.5-6.5)

* Univariate p refers to log rank test of no difference *vs* any difference between categories.
† Relative risk to other categories of the same factor.
Abbreviation: CI = confidence intervals.
(Courtesy of Lewis JJ, Leung D, Woodruff JM, et al: Retroperitoneal soft-tissue sarcoma: Analysis of 500 patients treated and followed at a single institution. *Ann Surg* 228:355-365, 1998).

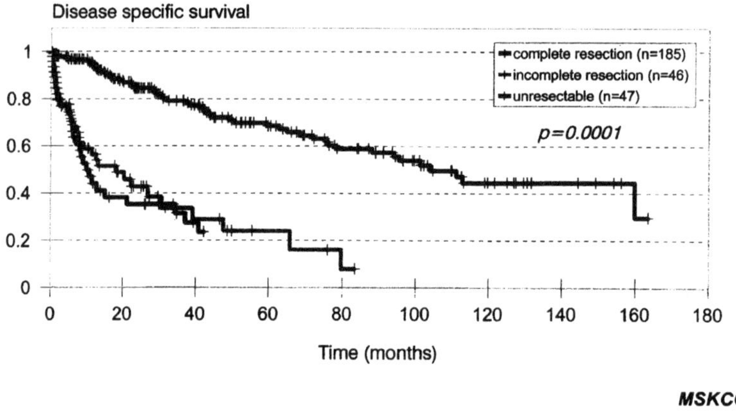

FIGURE 5.—Kaplan-Meier disease-specific survival divided by surgical resection. Of the 231 patients whose disease was resectable, 185 underwent complete resection with gross negative margins. The median survival of this group was 103 months. In contrast, the median survival in those (n = 48) undergoing incomplete resection was 18 months. There was no significant difference in survival between patients whose disease was unresectable and those who underwent incomplete resection (P = 0.4). (Courtesy of Lewis JJ, Leung D, Woodruff JM, et al: Retroperitoneal soft-tissue sarcoma: Analysis of 500 patients treated and followed at a single institution. *Ann Surg* 228:355-365, 1998).

Patients who can be cured should have aggressive surgery. Patients who cannot be cured by surgery should have incomplete resection for symptomatic relief only.

▶ Treatment for retroperitoneal soft-tissue sarcoma remains a dilemma. Often these tumors are very large, involving multiple contiguous organs that make their definitive resection difficult. This study of 500 patients with retroperitoneal soft-tissue sarcoma analyzes treatment and survival. As seen in Figure 3C, complete resection vs. incomplete resection can have a profound impact on survival. In addition, doing an adequate operation the first time is extremely important, because the likelihood of complete resection after the first or second recurrence is dramatically reduced (Figure 3D). With respect to disease-specific survival, these authors showed that grade, size, and surgical margins all were extremely important in multi-varied analysis (see Table 5). As seen in Figure 5, incomplete resection has about the same level of survival as that in patients who were unresectable.

This remains a surgical disease, since adequate systemic treatments are still not available. Therefore, the patient should undergo aggressive attempts at complete surgical resection. These should certainly include a liberal en bloc resection policy to obtain negative pathologic margins. Incomplete resection should be undertaken only for symptom relief.

T.J. Eberlein, M.D.

12 Plastic, Reconstructive, and Head and Neck Surgery

Introduction

This year's section on plastic and reconstructive surgery and head and neck surgery has some distinctly unusual reports. Perhaps more so this year than in the past, a number of articles have been selected to provide the reader with some cutting-edge developments or the advent of new technology. This section is subdivided into wound problems, reconstruction of the trunk (sternum and abdominal wall), breast reconstruction, and head and neck cancer.

More patients receive chemotherapy than in the past and as a result, the clinician must deal more frequently with the issue of intravenous extravasation of chemotherapeutic agents.The first two articles address the nonsurgical and surgical management of these problems. The third article is a preliminary report on the use of the newly developed acrylic glue for wound closures. Added to this section are articles on two highly unusual burn injuries, one about the management of the plastic surgery aspect of lightning injuries and the other on ethylene oxide.

Truncal reconstruction is a challenging situation, and two procedures for closure of sternal wounds are presented, one using muscle flaps and the other using omental transposition. The general surgeon may be asked to harvest the omentum. Following are two articles about closure of large and difficult ventral incisional hernias. The first report is a method that uses local tissues in an innovative fashion and the other uses a transfer of regional tissue, tensor fascia latae flaps.

The section on breast reconstruction contains two important articles, one examining some of the sequelae after lumpectomy and radiation therapy for breast cancer; the other, from M.D. Anderson Cancer Center in Houston, compares resource costs of immediate and delayed breast reconstruction.

The largest section, head and neck cancer, is also subdivided. The first subsection contains another article on the growing concerns about the role of human papillomavirus in the causation of head and neck squamous cell cancer. Also included is a critical appraisal of the role of sentinel node biopsy in oral squamous cell cancer. (A hint: probably not much of a role at present.) Another report emphasizes the importance of routine chest CT as a screening mechanism for patients with a head and neck primary carcinoma. Two articles are included to represent a growing body of literature that examines quality of life and function in head and neck cancer patients. The reconstruction subsection addresses issues of osteoradionecrosis as well as autogenous and alloplastic reconstruction of the mandible.We have also included a novel approach to the treatment of gustatory sweating (Frey's syndrome)—namely, the use of botulinum toxin. The last article has an educational theme: how well do we train general surgery residents in head and neck clinical skills?

I hope the reader finds these selections intriguing and informative. I certainly did.

Edward A. Luce, M.D.

Prevention of Adriamycin-Induced Full-Thickness Skin Loss Using Hyaluronidase Infiltration

Disa JJ, Chang RR, Mucci SJ, et al (State Univ of Maryland, Baltimore)
Plast Reconstr Surg 101:370-374, 1998 12–1

Background.—Extravasation of the cancer chemotherapy drug doxorubicin hydrochloride (Adriamycin) can cause full-thickness skin ulceration. The best way to handle this complication has been debated. One approach is local clysis with hyaluronidase. Although it is used clinically, there are few experimental data on this approach. The authors studied hyaluronidase, heparin, and saline infiltration for the prevention of doxorubicin-induced extravasation ulcers in rats.

Methods.—Experiments were performed in anesthetized Sprague-Dawley rats. Fifteen minutes after subcutaneous injection with doxorubicin, the animals received local infiltration with either saline or heparin, 25 to 100 U, or hyaluronidase, 2.5 to 10.0 U. Control groups received either subcutaneous doxorubicin or subcutaneous saline alone. The rats were killed after 4 weeks for assessment of ulcers at the injection site.

Results.—All rats injected only with doxorubicin alone developed ulcers, average size 33 mm^2. With heparin infiltration, the rate of ulcer development was reduced by 20% to 40%, with up to a 67% reduction in ulcer size. Hyaluronidase infiltration reduced the ulcer rate by 50% to 60%, and it reduced ulcer size by up to 50%.

Conclusions.—These studies in rats show that local infiltration with saline, heparin, or hyaluronidase can reduce the size of doxorubicin-induced extravasation ulcers, perhaps through dilution of the extravasant. The rate of ulcer development can be reduced at least 50% by local hyaluronidase infiltration. This effect may result from the ability of hyaluronidase to reduce the viscosity of the hyaluronic acid component of ground substance, leading to a greater diffusion of doxorubicin into the surrounding tissue, and thus to decreased local concentrations. The authors are conducting further studies to evaluate the impact of time on the efficacy of local antidote therapy for doxorubicin extravasation injury.

▶ We need something. Once ulcerated, the patients have stiffness and pain of the affected extremity. The pain is relieved with excision and coverage, but function is often not significantly improved. All of these problems exist against a background of a clinical picture of metastatic disease.

If we had a local antidote, the patients would certainly benefit. Please note, though, that the hyaluronidase had to be given only *fifteen minutes* after the insult.

E.A. Luce, M.D.

Surgical Management After Doxorubicin and Epirubicin Extravasation

Heitmann C, Durmus C, Ingianni G (Ferdinand Sauerbruch Klinikum, Wuppertal, Germany)

J Hand Surg [Br] 23B:666-668, 1998 12–2

Background.—Doxorubicin and epirubicin are effective intravenous antineoplastic agents, but when they extravasate under the skin, they can cause extensive chemical damage. This damage includes liquefying necrosis in soft tissues and chronic ulcers that, if left untreated, can cause significant disability. These authors describe the surgical treatment and outcomes of 3 patients who experienced doxorubicin or epirubicin extravasation.

Findings.—The 3 patients were a 54-year-old man with chronic lymphatic leukemia, a 62-year-old woman with metastatic carcinoma of the breast, and a 73-year-old woman with metastatic breast cancer. Patients were referred to the authors' service 1 month, 2 days, and 4 weeks, respectively, after extravasation. Patients 1 and 2 experienced pain and swelling, and patient 1 had symptoms of reflex sympathetic dystrophy. The necrotic tissue was repeatedly débrided during 3 or 2 weeks, respectively, with a split-thickness skin graft on days 10 or 4, respectively, to close the wound. Patient 3 experienced sloughing of the skin, subcutaneous tissues, and extensor tendons of the fingers (Fig 3). This patient also underwent repeated débridement, and most of the extensor tendons were resected. The defect was closed with a fascial forearm flap covered by a split-thickness skin graft. Patients 1 and 3 had poor function of the hand after healing, whereas patient 2 had no functional loss.

Conclusions.—Numerous antineoplastic drugs have been shown to extravasate at the site of intravenous administration. The tissue toxicities of these various drugs vary, and the surgeon must know which cytotoxic drug was used and its tissue toxicity to determine whether surgical treatment is

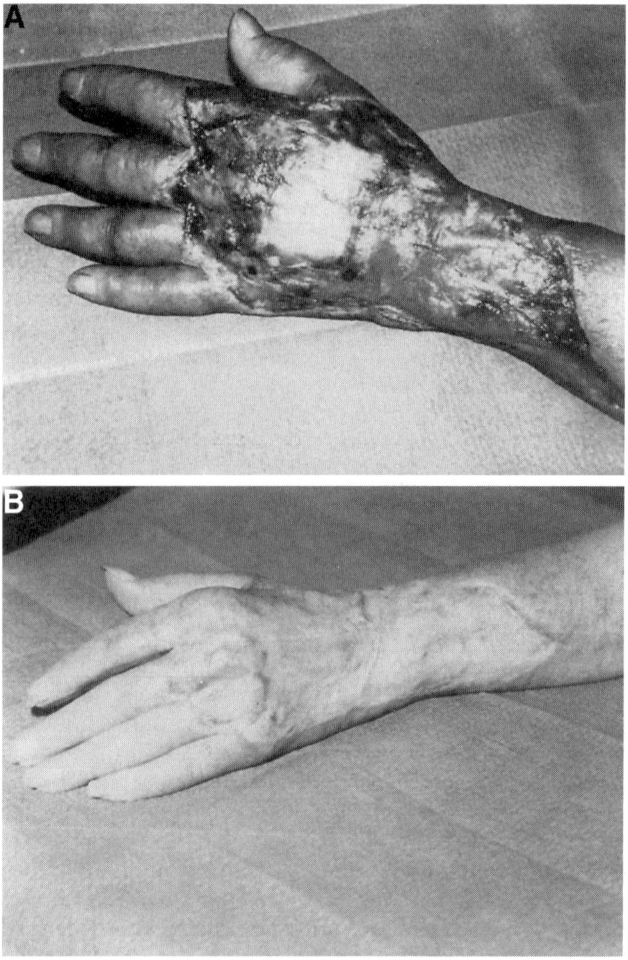

FIGURE 3.—Patient 3. A, skin slough left untreated for 4 weeks. Necrosis of skin, subcutaneous tissue, and extensor tendons can be seen. B, final result with good quality wound cover. The function of the hand remained poor. (Courtesy of Heitmann C, Durmus C, Ingianni G. Surgical management after doxorubicin and epirubicin extravasation. *J Hand Surg [Br]*23B: 666-668, 1998.)

required or a conservative approach is possible. Doxorubicin and epirubicin extravasation produce extensive tissue necrosis by binding to fat. Furthermore, these drugs are not locally metabolized, nor does the lymphatic system remove them. Thus, doxorubicin and epirubicin extravasation always requires extensive surgical débridement to halt the progression of tissue damage. Prompt surgical débridement is also important; in this series, patient 2 was treated shortly after extravasation began (2 days), and she was the only patient to have no functional loss of the hand. Areas closely associated with severe morbidity include extravasations at the dorsum of the hand involving the extensor tendons and the palmar aspect of the wrist involving the flexor tendons, nerves, and arteries.

▶ This succinctly describes the problem. The initial appearance is innocuous. The treating clinician must be aware of the inevitable outcome of delayed tissue necrosis, ulceration, and loss of hand function. Treatment should be prompt, but not necessarily operative. Appropriate splinting combined with active physical therapy and careful monitoring of progress in some patients may permit more accurate delineation of the extent of necrotic tissue and magnitude of débridement. Wound location may be important as well. Palmar-flexor side extravasation with the potential for tendon and nerve function losses should be treated aggressively. Dorsal or extensor injury may be just as extensive and loss of extensor tendon function may occur. A functional hand can be preserved if function of the wrist and the proximal and distal interphalangeal joints are monitored.

E.A. Luce, M.D.

---

n-Butyl Cyanoacrylate Adhesive for Skin Closure of Abdominal Wounds: Preliminary Results

Qureshi A, Drew PJ, Duthie GS, et al (Univ of Hull, Cottingham, North Humberside)

Ann R Coll Surg Engl 79:414-415, 1997 12–3

Purpose.—Tissue adhesives, which achieve rapid and complete closure with little tissue deformation, are widely used for small facial lacerations. However, no previous studies have addressed their use for larger abdominal incisions. A new *n*-butyl 2-cyanoacrylate tissue adhesive was studied for use in closing abdominal surgical wounds.

Methods.—In patients undergoing general or laparoscopic gastrointestinal procedures, the deep fascial layers were closed in the usual way. The skin edges were then approximated, and tissue adhesive was applied sparingly to the edges of the wound. After 10 seconds of light pressure, a second layer of tissue adhesive was applied to the skin edges.

Results.—The *n*-butyl 2-cyanoacrylate tissue adhesive was used to close 240 abdominal wounds in 102 patients. Thirty-nine wounds were larger than 10 cm, 27 measured 5 to 9 cm, and 176 were less than 5 cm. Two long, transverse wounds showed small, superficial skin dehiscence. However, no wound infections occurred, and the overall complication rate was approximately 1%.

Conclusions.—The new *n*-butyl 2-cyanoacrylate tissue adhesive appears to be useful for closing abdominal surgical wounds. After penetrating into the tissue interstices, the cyanoacrylate in this adhesive becomes immobilized by polymerization, with adhesion resulting from attraction between cyanoacrylate molecules. The colorless, sterile adhesive is completely eliminated by enzymatic action in about 1 month. The authors call for a randomized trial to compare *n*-butyl 2-cyanoacrylate tissue adhesive with traditional wound closure.

▶ We need to know a little more about this newest method of skin closure in full-thickness wounds. The early results in facial lacerations are encouraging, but a rigorously controlled prospective trial needs to be carried out to measure results against the traditional methods of wound closure. This trial should include adequate follow-up (1-year) and should also include objective measures of esthetic results. To date, most of the focus has centered on the easily quantifiable indices of wound infection and tissue toxicity only.

E.A. Luce, M.D.

Plastic Surgical Considerations in Lightning Injuries

Matthews MS, Fahey AL (Univ of Medicine and Dentistry of New Jersey, Camden; Cooper Hosp Univ Med Ctr, Camden, NJ)

Ann Plast Surg 39:561-565, 1997 12–4

Background.—Lightning strikes injure up to 1,500 people a year, and as many as 300 victims die annually. Most survivors have neurologic, cutaneous, and/or vascular damage. However, the damage from a lightning strike differs from damage caused by other electrical injuries. These authors discuss the causes and treatments of lightning injuries.

Etiology of Lightning Strike Injury.—Lightning develops in thunderclouds when warm, moist air rises into cold air and the water vapor condenses. As the vapor rises, it loses electrons, and the electrons gather in the lower part of the cloud while the protons gather in the top. Once a critical electrical potential is reached, the negative electrons are discharged toward the positively charged ground. The ground, in turn, discharges protons to meet the negative discharge. An electric burst occurs to normalize the difference in potentials between cloud and ground, and this burst (> 10 million volts) superheats the air, causing the flash of lightning. The extent of injury depends in large part on how much of the electrical load a person is subject to, which itself depends on whether the strike is direct (usually fatal), a ground strike, or a flash discharge. Most lightning injuries are not associated with extensive deep damage, or with death; the greatest risk factor for death is cardiopulmonary arrest.

Treating Lightning Strike Injuries.—The burn injury is influenced by the type of clothing the person is wearing, whether the person has metal close to the skin, and how wet the skin is. Myonecrosis is extremely rare, and most burns are superficial. Local therapy usually resolves the burn, and surgery is typically not needed. Note that myoglobin levels may be elevated because of severe muscle contractions. Other major lightning strike injuries of concern to the surgeon include extreme vasoconstriction and sensation loss in an extremity. Because both of these injuries almost always resolve without intervention, waiting is the rule for at least the first hour after injury. Other types of injuries include cardiopulmonary arrest, central respiratory arrest, hearing impairment, cataracts, and cranial nerve paresis and aphasia.

▶ This article offers an interesting set of observations by the authors. In contrast to classic electrical burns, lightning injuries do not cause deep injury with myonecrosis. So resuscitation at the scene is of paramount importance. Perhaps we need to pass a law that all golfers be certified in CPR.

E.A. Luce, M.D.

Ethylene Oxide Burns From Improperly Sterilized Mammary Implants

Cárdenas-Camarena L (Reconstructive Surgery Inst of Jalisco, México)

Ann Plast Surg 41:361-369, 1998 12–5

Introduction.—Before implantation, breast implants are commonly sterilized with ethylene oxide (ETO) gas. Burns caused by residual ETO on silicone gel implants are reported as a new complication of augmentation mammaplasty.

Patients.—The previously unreported condition occurred in 16 women undergoing augmentation mammaplasty with textured silicone gel prostheses over a 2-month period. All of the prostheses, made by a single manufacturer, were sterilized with ETO gas. The prostheses were ventilated for 24 hours after sterilization and implanted 5 to 15 days later. The condition was unilateral in 14 patients and bilateral in 2. It was characterized by exudation of noninfectious liquid in all patients. Other clinical findings included a rash in 75% of the patients, edema in 61%, pain in 37.5%, and severe cutaneous necrosis in 12.5% (Fig 1). The manifestations occurred within 4 weeks postoperatively; the earlier they appeared, the more severe the involvement. Conservative treatment was tried at first but failed. Definitive management consisted of implant removal, performed at a median of 4 months after the initial surgery.

Discussion.—This is the first study to report burns caused by ETO residues on breast implants. These burns must be recognized and managed promptly; conservative therapy will not be successful and will allow more time for tissue damage to occur. Because of certain characteristics, silicone eliminates ETO very slowly. The authors avoid ETO sterilization of silicone elastomers and other materials capable of dissolving this gas.

► A frightening report. When your reviewer finished reading the article and the accompanying editorial discussion by an "industrial consultant," confusion reigned. The consultant pointed a finger at implants obtained from an international source, yet admitted that in instances of ETO sterilization of biologic implants "aeration time and conditions for ... all implants is not possible to determine" and that aeration times for specific implants "should be established by appropriate studies." The consultant in the editorial discussion reassured the reader that the FDA offers "assurance to surgeons and patients that implants made in the United States are free of cytotoxic levels of sterilent." I am sorry, but, given the performance of the FDA in other areas, perhaps these "appropriate studies" need to be accomplished.

E.A. Luce, M.D.

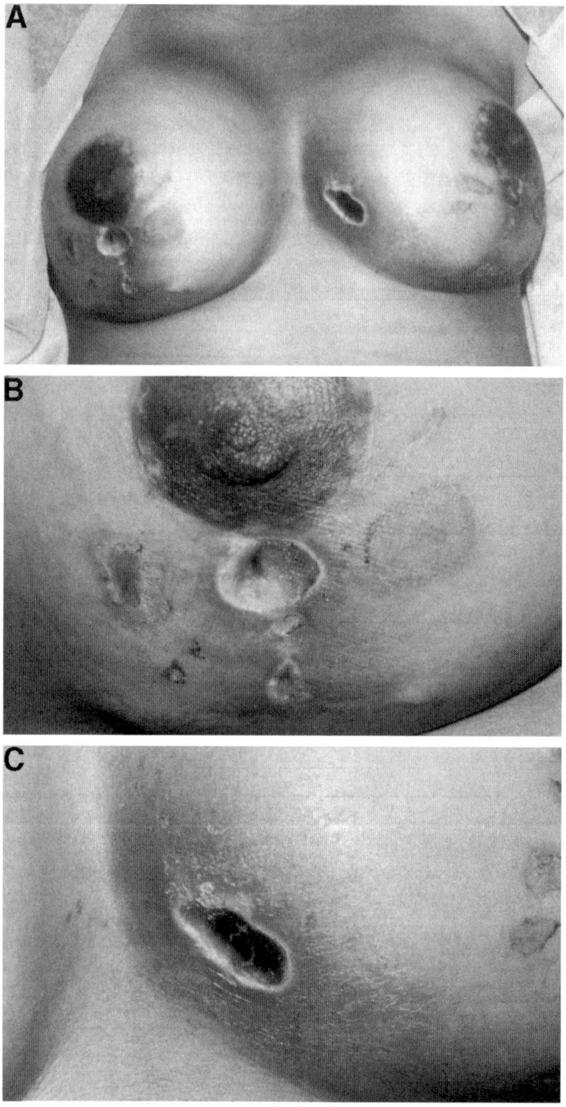

FIGURE 1.—A, A 28-year-old patient underwent breast mastopexy and insertion of implants. This photograph presents the 3-week postsurgical evolution of a condition that first set in 48 hours after surgery. The patient exhibited severe bilateral tissue compromise with cutaneous necrosis. B, Detail of the right breast, showing the principal burn at the level of the incision line. C, Detail of the left breast, where the principal burn can be seen next to the parasternal line, far from the incision. (Courtesy of Cárdenas-Camarena L: Ethylene oxide burns from improperly sterilized mammary implants. *Ann Plast Surg* 41:361-369, 1998.)

Bipedicle Muscle Flaps in Sternal Wound Repair

Solomon MP, Granick MS (Allegheny Univ, Philadelphia)

Plast Reconstr Surg 101:356-360, 1998 12–6

Purpose.—Infection is a serious and potentially life-threatening complication of median sternotomy, and is commonly treated with muscle flaps. The authors have been using a composite pectoralis major muscle and rectus abdominis muscle flap. An experience with this bipedicle muscle flap for sternal wound repair is reported, including long-term results.

Methods.—Forty-two patients, 26 men and 16 women (mean age, 60 years), were treated between 1989 and 1996. The bipedicle repair included a superiorly based pectoralis major muscle flap and an inferiorly based abdominis muscle flap raised in continuity and transposed into the sternal defect. The median sternotomies were performed for a wide range of cardiac operations, most frequently coronary artery bypass grafting. The patients had many associated conditions, including diabetes, chronic hypertension, prolonged postcardiotomy hypotension, previous radiation therapy, pulmonary failure, and steroid use.

Results.—None of the patients died; there were, however, 1 case each of flap failure, persistent infection, pneumothorax, and hernia. There were 3 postoperative hematomas. Nine patients experienced skin sloughing that responded to local wound care. Bleeding or hematoma necessitated reoperation in 3 patients.

Conclusions.—Good results are achieved with the use of a bipedicle pectoralis major–rectus abdominis flap for sternal wound repair (Fig 1). This is a large flap that can obliterate the dead space throughout the entire wound. It is a simple and quick flap to raise, and its complication rate compares favorably with those of other techniques.

▶ The authors correctly point out that one of the problems is the use of the pectoralis major for closure of sternal infection/dehiscence, the inferior third of the wound. The conventional approach to this problem has been the use of a pedicled rectus, usually the right, in cases where the LIMA has been harvested. Actually, I have used this technique for some time, but with 3 important modifications (well, important to me, anyway). The first is to use bilateral flaps and the second is to not undermine the skin from the overlying pectoralis fascia. If the overlying skin is undermined from the pectoralis, the perforators supplying that skin are inevitably divided. (Note that the authors had a substantial incidence of skin slough [20%]. The third is to unnecessarily incise the anterior fascia and roll the rectus out of the fascial compartment, if bilateral flaps are used.

E.A. Luce, M.D.

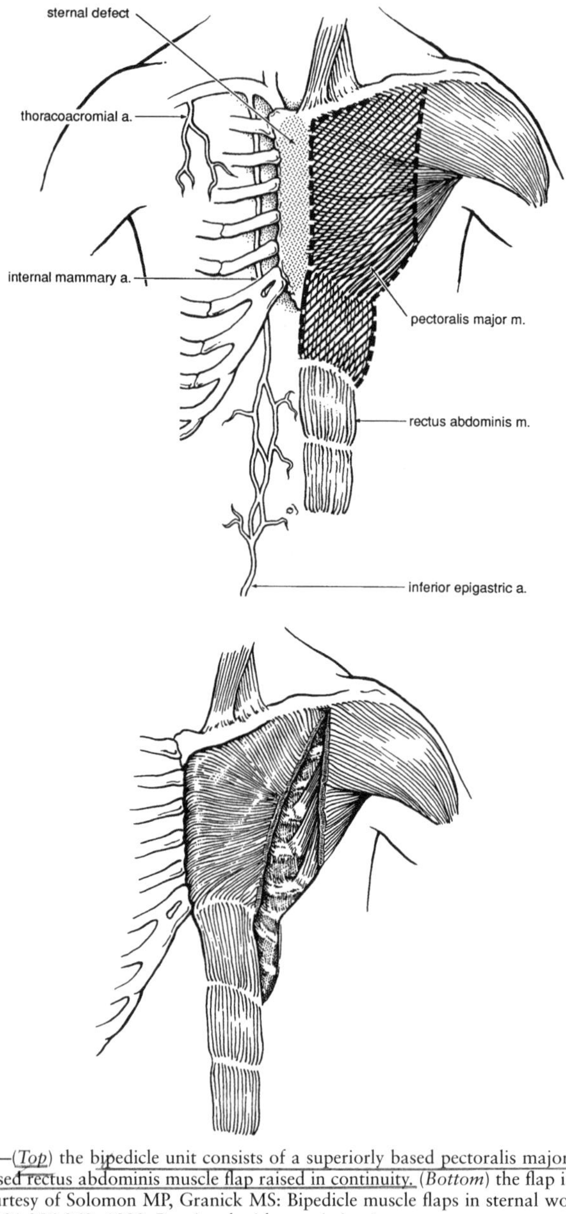

FIGURE 1.—(*Top*) the bipedicle unit consists of a superiorly based pectoralis major muscle flap and an inferiorly based rectus abdominis muscle flap raised in continuity. (*Bottom*) the flap is transposed into the defect. (Courtesy of Solomon MP, Granick MS: Bipedicle muscle flaps in sternal wound repair. *Plast Reconstr Surg* 101:356-360, 1998. Reprinted with permission.)

Results of Omental Flap Transposition for Deep Sternal Wound Infection After Cardiovascular Surgery

Yasuura K, Okamoto H, Morita S, et al (Nagoya Univ, Japan)

Ann Surg 227:455-459, 1998 12–7

Objective.—Aggressive treatment of sternal wound complications after open cardiac surgery decreases in-hospital mortality rates and decreases long-term results. Whereas the omentum, with its ability to repair through cellular proliferation, fibrous tissue formation, and adhesions, has been used to manage these infections, the increase in the number of older, diabetic, and critically ill patients and the prevalence of methicillin-resistant *Staphylococcus aureus* have made treatment difficult. Results of treatment of deep sternal wound infections with transposition of omental flaps are presented.

Methods.—Transposition of omentum was used to treat 47 consecutive patients with deep sternal wound infections. Fourteen patients could not be weaned from the ventilator until the omental flap transposition was performed. Time from the primary surgery to the onset of infection and time from surgery to omental flap transposition were recorded. Whereas early patients were treated with drainage, excision of necrotic tissues, and delayed closure with the omental flap, later patients were treated by a single-stage procedure within 3 days of diagnosis of infection.

Results.—Infection was detected at an average of 17 days after surgery, with flap transposition performed an average of 26 days after surgery. Seven patients (16%) died in the hospital, 6 from uncontrolled infections, sepsis, and multiple organ failure. According to univariate analysis, hemodialysis and ventilatory support were significant predictors of death in the hospital after flap transposition. The closed irrigation technique used 10 years ago resulted in complications from hemorrhage after disruption of the suture line or formation of a pseudoaneurysm. Early diagnosis of infection and muscle or omental flap coverage are imperative. Results are better with omental flaps than with muscle flaps. Flap closure decreases mortality and hospital stay. The timing of surgery for deep sternal wound infections must be individually based.

Conclusion.—Whereas the use of omental flap transposition for deep sternal wound infections improves survival and long-term results, closure should be delayed in patients at high risk until the infection has been mostly eradicated.

► This survey of experience with sternal infections from cardiopulmonary bypass in Japan should be compared with reported series from the USA (for example, at Emory University and the Mayo Clinic). The authors contend that the omentum is the choice of reconstructive procedures and state that their results were superior to those achieved with muscle flaps. Muscle flap closure is the rule in other series and in my experience, with the omentum reserved as a "court of last resort." The rationale for this hierarchy of selection of straightforward: Laparotomy is an additional physiologic insult to these compromised patients.

The authors report a 16% mortality rate, considerably higher than the 2 other institutional series cited, and a significant association with prolonged ventilatory support, perhaps a complication of the requisite laparotomy. Besides, who says that omentum is more resistant to infection of that muscle? Six of the 7 depths were in the single-stage group (débriding and closure) and were due to uncontrolled sepsis. Why not harvest the omentum endoscopically?

E.A. Luce, M.D.

Sliding Door Technique for the Repair of Midline Incisional Hernias

Kuzbari R, Worseg AP, Tairych G, et al (Univ of Vienna, Austria)

Plast Reconstr Surg 101:1235-1242, 1998 12–8

Objective.—The authors describe the sliding door technique that makes it possible to effect a tensionless and autologous repair of large hernias after midline laparotomy.

Methods.—Between 1990 and 1995, 10 patients with an average abdominal musculofascial defect measuring 14 × 11 cm were treated with the operative sliding door technique. Patients were followed up for 14 months to 5.5 years with ultrasound examination to detect recurrent hernias and to establish the contractility of the rectus muscles. Rectus abdominis muscle strength was graded using Janda's system.

> *Technique.*—The medial border of the rectus sheath is identified on both sides of the hernia, and the size of the musculofascial defect is determined. The rectus sheaths are dissected away from the muscles; the anterior layer is dissected particularly carefully. The rectus sheaths, after being incised at the aponeuroses of the external oblique muscles, slide toward the midline. The posterior rectus sheaths are sutured. The rectus muscles are secured with overlapping sutures, and the released anterior layers of the rectus sheaths are sutured.

Results.—There were 2 postoperative complications: 1 necrosis of the skin around the wound that required débridement and grafting. and 1 subcutaneous seroma that required aspiration. No patient had a recurrent herniation or protrusion of the abdominal wall. The strength of the released rectus abdominis muscles provided some functional support to the reconstructed abdominal wall.

Conclusion.—The sliding door technique makes it possible to repair large hernias by releasing the laterally shifted rectus abdominis muscles from their sheaths and allowing them to slide medially. Releasing the rectus sheaths from the pull of the external oblique muscles eliminates the most unyielding pull. Advancement of the rectus abdominis toward the midline en bloc with the anterior layer of their sheaths does not permit tensionless alignment of muscle edges in large, recurrent hernias with considerable fibrosis. Previous abdominal incisions that may have denervated muscles can impair results.

▶ Although this article was included to give readers an exposure to some thoughts about reconstruction of large incisional hernias, I am a little mystified by some technical aspects of this approach. Release of the anterior rectus fascia laterally (relaxing incisions) makes sense and is common to other techniques for closure. But, why dissect the anterior sheath off the rectus? The dissection is tedious, as admitted by the authors, and the anterior fascia is obviously brought to the midline for closure anyway. Why not leave the anterior fascia attached to the underlying rectus? If anything, that would improve the perfusion of the overlying skin. The authors' response ("tension-free repair") is not satisfactory.

E.A. Luce, M.D.

Role of Tensor Fasciae Latae in Abdominal Wall Reconstruction

Williams JK, Carlson GW, deChalain T, et al (Emory Univ, Atlanta, Ga; Univ of Toronto; Indiana Univ, Indianapolis)

Plast Reconstr Surg 101:713-718, 1998 12–9

Background.—The tensor fasciae latae is useful for static reconstruction of abdominal wall defects when closure with local flaps is not possible. The tensor fasciae latae has been used for many types of reconstruction, including repair of joints; reconstruction of the thoracoabdominal wall after tumor excision; closure of rectal fistulas; repair of CSF leaks, bladder exstrophy, and penile chordee; and correction of upper and lower eyelid positioning. In plastic surgery, the tensor fasciae latae is often used for repair of pressure sores, but it has also been used for pharyngoesophageal reconstruction, palatal repair, facial reanimation, and brow-lift suspensions. The efficacy of the tensor fasciae latae in abdominal wall reconstruction was retrospectively analyzed, and guidelines for its use were established.

Methods.—Three common forms of tensor fasciae latae were used for abdominal wall reconstruction in 27 patients: fascial grafts, pedicled musculocutaneous flaps, and microvascular free tissue transfer. Demographics, wound characteristics, and complications were reviewed. The mean follow-up was 23.6 months.

Results.—The average defect size was 14.4 × 13.1 cm. Free grafts were used in 12 patients, pedicled flaps were used in 9 patients, and free flaps were used in 6 patients. Fourteen (51.8%) of the 27 reconstructions were performed in contaminated or infected wounds. There was 1 recurrent enteric fistula. Flap complications occurred in 12 patients, and half of these complications involved partial flap necrosis. Five (18.5%) patients had donor site complications, including a hematoma, seroma, and skin graft dehiscence along the edge of the wound.

Discussion.—Although the complication rate was high in these patients, the repairs adequately restored the integrity of the abdominal wall when an appropriate form of the tensor fasciae latae was used. Tensor fasciae latae free grafts may be considered for repair of abdominal hernias if there is adequate abdominal soft tissue. Pedicled flaps may be considered for defects of soft tissue and fascia, but the arc of rotation and size of the defect limit their use in this context. Tensor fasciae latae free flaps are versatile in orientation and may be useful for repair of supraumbilical defects. In both types of vascularized flaps, tip necrosis is a significant complication.

► I have extremely ambivalent feelings about this flap for abdominal wall reconstruction. The advantages of autogenous tissue are without question. The reliability and consistency of the TFL flap is not (without question, that is). Without a *prior delay*, the necessary length to reach the abdomen is not reliably perfused in the distal portion. Smaller defects should be closed with a "separation-of-parts" approach with local tissue. Larger defects may require a TFL flap, but should have a prior delay if extended beyond midthigh. That prior delay caveat holds for a free flap as much as for a pedicle flap because clearly the perfusion is essentially the same.

E.A. Luce, M.D.

Cosmetic Sequelae After Conservative Treatment for Breast Cancer: Classification and Results of Surgical Correction

Clough KB, Cuminet J, Fitoussi A, et al (Institut Curie, Paris)

Ann Plast Surg 41:471-481, 1998 12–10

Objective.—Conservative treatment, primarily lumpectomy and axillary lymph node dissection, for breast cancer leads to deformity in 20% to 30% of patients. Surgical correction can give unpredictable results. A classification system for these deformities is proposed that allows a better surgical approach.

Methods.—Between 1990 and 1995, 35 patients, aged 29 to 65, had corrective cosmetic surgery at the Institut Curie after conservative treatment for breast cancer. Patients had glandular and cutaneous sequelae. Patients were classified as type I (n = 14) (Fig 2), type II (n = 17) if the treated breast had a deformity, and type III (n = 4) (Fig 4). Type II reconstruction was performed on both breasts and involved reduction mammoplasty, implant reconstruction, and/or defect filling with a single-pedicle transverse rectus abdominus musculocutaneous (TRAM) flap. Type III reconstruction involved mastectomy and immediate reconstruction using a musculocutaneous flap. Patients were followed up for a median of 20 months, with evaluations every 6 months.

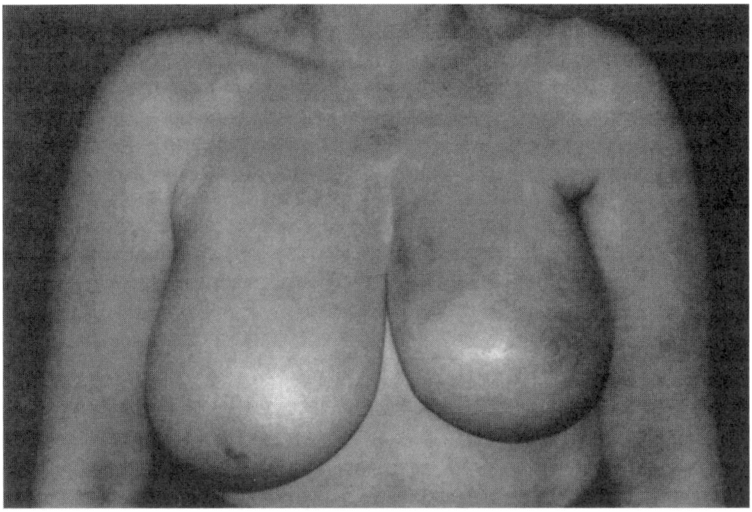

FIGURE 2.—Type I sequelae: breast asymmetry with no deformity of the treated (left) breast. (Courtesy of Clough KB, Cuminet J, Fitoussi A, et al: Cosmetic sequelae after conservative treatment for breast cancer: Classification and results of surgical correction. *Ann Plast Surg* 41:471-481, 1998).

Results.—All but 1 patient received breast reduction or correction of ptosis of the treated breast. The remaining patient received, by request, bilateral breast augmentation. Cosmetic results were very good or good in 71.8% and unsatisfactory in 28.2%. The rate of satisfactory results decreased with time until the 34th month, when satisfaction had dropped to 58.4% primarily because of late poor results in type II patients. Satisfac-

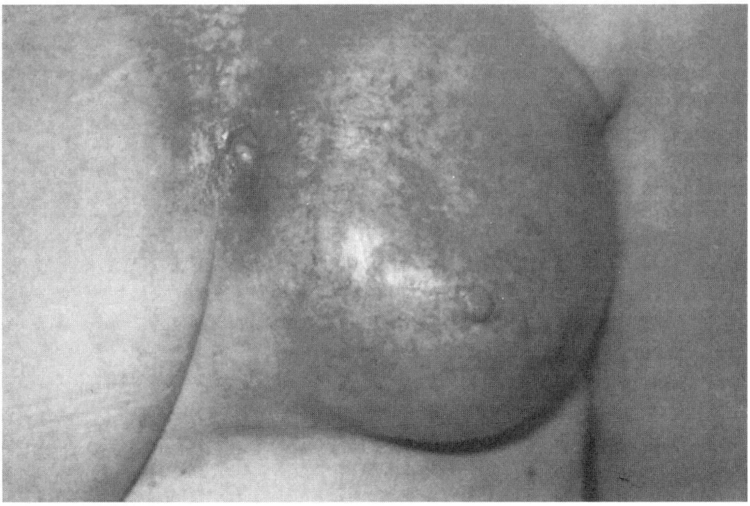

FIGURE 4.—Type III sequelae: "marble breast" with skin necrosis. Reconstruction requires mastectomy. (Courtesy of Clough KB, Cuminet J, Fitoussi A, et al: Cosmetic sequelae after conservative treatment for breast cancer: Classification and results of surgical correction. *Ann Plast Surg* 41:471-481, 1998).

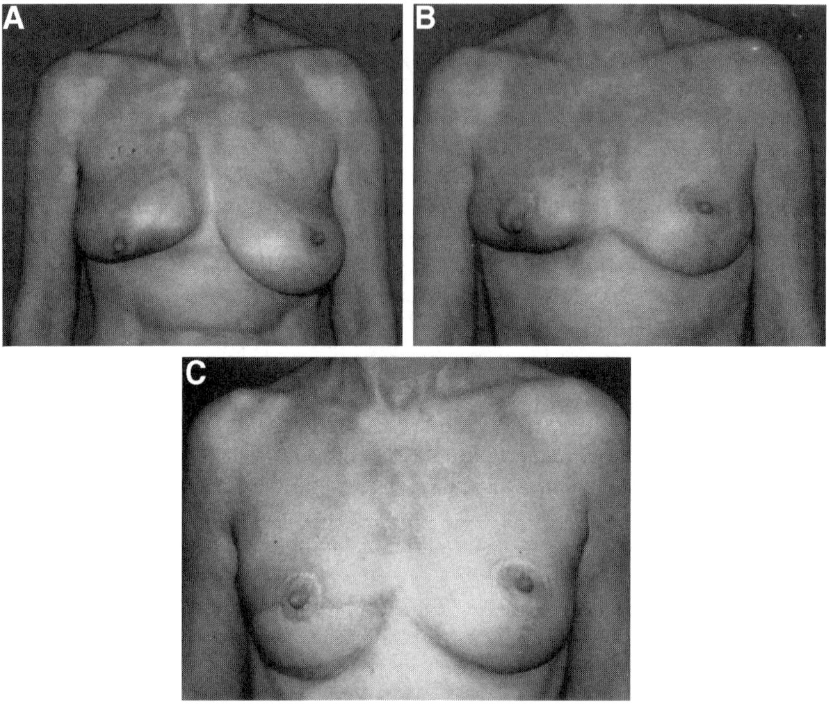

FIGURE 9.—Typical type II deformity after wide resection and radiotherapy of cancer located in the inferior quadrants of the right breast. A, before surgical correction. B, after bilateral mammaplasty. Note retraction of the radiated breast. C, final results after fibrotic resection and low-pole reconstruction with a latissimus dorsi flap. (Courtesy of Clough KB, Cuminet J, Fitoussi A, et al: Cosmetic sequelae after conservative treatment for breast cancer: Classification and results of surgical correction. *Ann Plast Surg* 41:471-481, 1998).

tory results were obtained in 80% of type I patients and in 43.8% of type II patients (at 36 months) (Fig 9). All 4 type III patients had satisfactory results. Approximately 30% of breast cancer patients treated conservatively had a wide variety of sequelae particularly to the irradiated breast. Using a TRAM flap to reconstruct a lumpectomy defect seems extreme. Therefore, the best solution is to prevent type II deformities, which almost always occur postoperatively. For type III patients, the best option is mastectomy followed by immediate reconstruction with a musculocutaneous flap.

Conclusion.—Surgical correction of cosmetic sequelae after conservative treatment for breast cancer is complicated by the variety of sequelae and the problem of sustaining initial satisfactory results.

► A number of salient points arise from this series of patients. The first, also emphasized by the authors, is the necessity in some patients to do an element of glandular remodeling to maintain shape. Clearly, the oncologic surgeon would have to be certain the margins were clear. The second point is that small and large problems (types I & III) are usually treated satisfactorily because they require small solutions (contralateral reduction) or large solutions (TRAM flap for type III). The problem is the results in one half of type II. Many of these patients probably would have benefited more from a "seize the bull by the horns" approach, offering the patient completion mastectomy and TRAM flap reconstruction.

E.A. Luce, M.D.

A Comparison of Resource Costs of Immediate and Delayed Breast Reconstruction

Khoo A, Kroll SS, Reece GP, et al (Univ of Texas MD Anderson Cancer Ctr, Houston)

Plast Reconstr Surg 101:964-968, 1998 12–11

Background.—In breast cancer treatment, performing breast reconstruction at the time of mastectomy is becoming increasingly popular. This is preferable to the patient for many reasons, and charges for this method are lower than those for a separate mastectomy and delayed breast reconstruction. However, there are no data to show whether the costs to the hospital of performing immediate reconstruction are truly lower than those of performing delayed reconstruction. The resource costs of providing immediate vs. delayed breast reconstruction were compared.

Methods.—A total of 276 patients undergoing mastectomies and breast reconstruction were studied. A complete reconstructive procedure, including nipple reconstruction, was performed on each patient. The resource costs of the immediate and delayed approaches to reconstruction were compared. These included such major costs as those for operating room time and days of hospital stay, as well as personnel costs, surgicenter day costs, and the costs of tissue expanders and breast implants, and other costs (Table 1). The surgical fees charged were not considered.

Results.—Of the 276 patients, 194 had transverse rectus abdominus muscle (TRAM) flap reconstructions, and 82 had reconstruction with tissue expanders and implants. Reconstruction was immediate in 219

TABLE 1.—Resource Cost Components in 1993 Dollars

Cost Component	Cost ($)
Operating room hour	548
Hospital day, major surgery	1,216
Hospital day, revision surgery	668
Surgicenter day	530
Staff surgeon hour	156
Surgical assistant hour	43
Anesthesia personnel hour	119
Tissue expander	445
Saline breast implant	950
Tissue expansion session	36

(Courtesy of Khoo A, Kroll SS, Reece GP, et al: A comparison of resource costs of immediate and delayed breast reconstruction. *Plast Reconstr Surg* 101:964-968, 1998.)

patients and delayed in 57. The mean resource cost was nearly $29,000 for patients undergoing delayed reconstruction compared with nearly $18,000 for those undergoing immediate reconstruction. Thus, delayed reconstruction was 62% more costly to perform than immediate reconstruction. The differences were similar when findings were analyzed by type of reconstruction, by unilateral vs. bilateral involvement, and by history of preoperative irradiation.

Conclusions.—It is significantly less expensive to perform a mastectomy with immediate breast reconstruction vs. mastectomy followed by delayed reconstruction. Immediate reconstruction has the potential to conserve substantial health care resources and is the preferred approach when breast reconstruction is performed. At the authors' hospital, immediate reconstruction saves an average of $11,000 per patient.

▶ This article is one of a series published by Kroll and his associates that examine the efficacy and more recently, methods and timing of breast reconstruction. When reading these papers, keep in mind that this group and institution lean heavily toward use of the TRAM flap, rather than alloplastic (implant) reconstruction, favor immediate rather than delayed, and strongly prefer tissue transfer of the TRAM by microvascular means rather than a pedicle flap. But, with data so coherently and succinctly presented, who is to argue? Maybe (just maybe) not even the movers and shakers of managed care.

E.A. Luce, M.D.

Human Papillomavirus in Head and Neck: Squamous Cell Carcinomas in Nonsmokers

Fouret P, Monceaux G, Temam S, et al (Hôpital Tenon, Paris)

Arch Otolaryngol Head Neck Surg 123:513-516, 1997 12–12

Background.—Smoking and alcohol consumption are the most important risk factors for head and neck squamous cell carcinomas (SCCs). Whether infection with oncogenic types of human papillomavirus (HPV) have an independent effect in the head and neck is unknown. The current study determined relationships between smoking and HPV in patients with head and neck SCCs.

Methods and Findings.—One hundred eighty-seven consecutive patients with head and neck SCCs were included in this retrospective study. HPV infection was detected in 20 (10.7%) and was also found in 18.6% of patients with oropharyngeal SCCs, compared with only 6.1% in patients with SCCs in other locations. Only 10 (5%) of the patients were nonsmokers. These 10 patients had an HPV incidence of 50%, which was significantly greater than the 8.5% incidence among smokers. Nonsmokers appeared to have no occupational risk factors. No *p53* gene mutations were noted in cancer cells.

Conclusion.—Human papillomavirus infection may play a role in head and neck SCCs in nonsmoking patients. Though inactivation of the *p53* gene seems to be a common step in the development of HPV-positive and -negative head and neck SCC, it is not known whether the outcomes between these 2 groups differ.

▶ A number of flaws exist in this study (as the authors admit), but this is a highly provocative article. An increasing body of evidence has begun to implicate the tumorigenesis potential of infection with HPV. The mechanism of how this infection would link with tobacco exposure is yet to be determined, but the door is open a sizable crack.

E.A. Luce, M.D.

Gamma Probe–Directed Biopsy of the Sentinel Node in Oral Squamous Cell Carcinoma

Koch WM, Choti MA, Civelek AC, et al (Johns Hopkins Med Inst, Baltimore, Md)

Arch Otolaryngol Head Neck Surg 124:455-459, 1998 12–13

Introduction.—Detection of sentinel nodes (SNs) using radiolabel with technetium Tc 99m sulfur colloid injection for biopsy has been used with increasing frequency to help determine management of malignant melanoma. Inert blue dyes and handheld gamma cameras have been used intraoperatively to locate SNs. The likely location of metastatic disease for a given primary site is best predicted using Lindberg's classic treatise on the pattern of nodal metastases in head and neck squamous cell carcinoma (HNSCC). The feasibility and efficacy of SN biopsy for oral squamous cell carcinoma (SCC) was assessed to enhance applicability of the technique.

Methods.—Five consecutive patients with a T1 or T2 SCC underwent injection with radiolabel with unfiltered technetium Tc 99m sulfur colloid in quadrants around the primary site, followed immediately by dynamic lymphoscintigraphy. Open biopsy of the SN was performed within 2 hours of injection after extirpation of the primary site. Regional or complete neck dissection was undertaken after biopsy of the SN.

Results.—Sentinel node biopsy accurately identified 1 or several nodes in 2 patients, including metastatic nodes in 1 patient. The radiolabel was not able to identify the SN in the remaining 3 patients, despite metastatic disease in the nodes of 2 patients.

Conclusions.—Gamma probe–directed biopsy of the SN in patients with oral SCC was feasible with selected nodal biopsies. It could provide savings of time, cost, and morbidity. Yet, the technique had several limitations: (1) the primary tumor site is typically located near the first echelon nodal basin and obscures the dynamic lymphoscintigram and the independent detection of the radioactive node with the gamma probe; (2) intramucosal injection of the radiolabeled technetium Tc 99m sulfur colloid is technically more tedious than intradermal injection; (3) replacement of a lymph node with metastatic cancer causes diversion of lymphatic flow and radiolabeling of downstream nodes; (4) patients with HNSCC typically receive primary radiation therapy that can change the local lymph channels and make lymphoscintigraphy ineffective; and (5) without general anesthesia, many HNSCC primary sites cannot be reached.

▶ This technique has great promise in the management of melanoma and carcinoma of the breast. A recent innovative modification to sentinel node biopsy in these 2 conditions has been the application of molecular biological concepts for the further analysis of "negative" nodes—negative when assessed with routine histologic means—to determine whether micrometastases are present.

Another carcinoma for which dissection of the lymph node drainage basin is optimal is SCC of the head and neck. A method to identify the sentinel node would be beneficial to limit radical neck dissection. Yet, as the authors outline with the aid of 5 clinical cases, some substantial problems, perhaps even insurmountable problems, exist.

E.A. Luce, M.D.

Role of Chest CT Scanning in the Management of Patients Presenting With Head and Neck Cancer

Houghton DJ, Hughes ML, Garvey C, et al (Royal Liverpool Hosp, England)

Head Neck 20:614-618, 1998 12–14

Objective.—Because the risk of secondary primary tumors in head and neck cancer patients is 7% to 14%, detection of synchronous tumors is important. Although detection typically relies on chest radiographs and upper aerodigestive tract endoscopy, CT has been recommended for its accuracy even though its value in head and neck cancer patients has not been tested. Computed tomography scanning of the chest and ultrasound scanning of the liver were evaluated prospectively at a tertiary-referral center for head and neck cancer patients.

Methods.—Chest CT, ultrasound liver scanning, MRI scanning of the head and neck region, and panendoscopy were performed for staging purposes on 81 consecutive head and neck cancer patients (32 women). Results were compared with those from conventional chest radiographs. Malignant lesions were classified as cavitating within the lung parenchyma, a destructive bony lesion, or mediastinal nodes greater than 1.5 cm in diameter.

Results.—Sixty-seven patients had normal findings on chest CT scans, and 14 (17%) had scans indicating malignancy. Only 3 of these lesions were identified by chest radiographs. Patients with positive scans were much more likely than patients with negative scans to have neck node metastases. There was no correlation between age, sex, Eastern Cooperative Oncology Group (ECOG) status, lesion site, or T stage and the presence of a positive CT scan. Whereas the specificity of chest radiographs compared wih CT scans was 99%, the sensitivity was only 21%.

Conclusions.—Although the cost of CT is higher than that of chest radiography, the accuracy of CT is much higher, thereby reducing the number of patients undergoing unnecessary radical surgery.

▶ A growing body of evidence is strongly suggestive that CT scan, not just chest x-rays, should be the screening tool of choice in head and neck cancer. This study could have been even more elegant if a cost analysis would have been included. Regardless, these findings help to explain the occasional occurrence of the patient who, although successfully treated for the head and neck primary and with negative findings on a chest x-ray, within months develops (manifests) an additional primary carcinoma in the lung.

Some additional questions that could be posed are as follows: What was the tissue diagnosis in those patients with a positive CT scan? What were the chest x-rays results and the panendoscopy results? As far as I could ascertain, only at one point in the discussion did the authors actually mention that 3 chest x-rays demonstrated lesions vs. the 14 positive CT scans.

E.A. Luce, M.D.

Long-term Quality of Life After Treatment of Laryngeal Cancer

Terrell JE, for The Veterans Affairs Laryngeal Cancer Study Group (Univ of Michigan, Ann Arbor; et al)

Arch Otolaryngol Head Neck Surg 124:964-971, 1998 12–15

Objective.—The larynx can be preserved in two thirds of patients with advanced laryngeal cancer. Nonetheless, the effects of chemoradiation, and posttreatment scarring and edema can impair quality of life. There are no well-validated instruments for evaluating laryngeal organ–preservation therapies. Quality of life in patients with advanced laryngeal cancer was assessed with a head and neck cancer–specific quality-of-life instrument (HNQOL).

Methods.—Quality of life was assessed and compared in patients with head and neck cancer. Patients randomly assigned to receive surgery plus radiation therapy were compared with patients randomly assigned to receive induction chemotherapy (CT) plus RT. In addition, patients who had successful organ preservation (CT plus RT with larynx) were compared with patients who underwent laryngectomy (resulting from either planned surgery and RT, or salvage laryngectomy after unsuccessful CT plus RT). Comparisons were made using the SF36 general health status measure, the HNQOL instrument, and the Beck Depression inventory. Smoking status and alcohol use were recorded.

Results.—Surveys were completed by 46 of 65 patients, 25 of whom had surgery and RT, and 21 of whom had CT plus RT. Health status scores of laryngeal cancer patients were significantly lower than U.S. male population norms, especially in the physical functioning (PF), role physical (RP), and role emotional (RE) domains of the SF-36, with a greater than 10-point difference in these domains and a greater than 15-point difference in overall complaints. Patients with organ preservation had better scores on all domains of the SF-36 than did patients who had laryngectomy, suggesting that patients with organ preservation did not have more emotional problems that affected their work, other daily activities, and social activities, or have more nervousness or depression than the U.S. male population aged 55 to 64 years. Six (46%) patients with organ preservation and 2 (6%) patients with laryngectomy continued to smoke. Long-term speech quality studies have demonstrated that patients with laryngectomy do not trade-off a significant quality of life because of decrements in speech loss. One patient (8%) with organ preservation and 9 patients (28%) with laryngectomy had moderate depression scores.

Conclusions.—Although this was a small study, it indicates that increased quality of life in laryngeal cancer patients with organ preservation arises from less pain, improved emotional well-being, and lower depression scores rather than from preservation of speech.

▶ This report addresses the criticism of organ preservation, namely to do so is at the expense of pain, eating, swallowing difficulties, and other quality-of-life issues. The patients with larynx preservation did better than those who had laryngectomy and were much less frequently depressed over the long term. As the authors admit, these anatomical areas are small groups and need further validation. Also, one half of the patients with a preserved larynx continued to smoke vs. about 6% of the patients who had laryngectomy.

E.A. Luce, M.D.

Survival, Function, and Quality of Life After Total Glossectomy

Ruhl CM, Gleich LL, Gluckman JL (Univ of Cinicinnati, Ohio)

Laryngoscope 107:1316-1321, 1997 12–16

Introduction.—Patients with advanced tongue cancer undergo primary surgery with postoperative radiotherapy or radical external beam radiation, with or without brachytherapy and neck dissection. Yet despite aggressive therapy, cure rates remain poor. Reported 5-year cure rates for stage IV cancers average approximately 20%. Total glossectomy may improve survival but is assumed to have a negative effect on quality of life (QOL). Survival rates and QOL after total glossectomy were retrospectively determined in 54 patients.

Methods and Results.—All patients were treated at the study institution between 1970 and 1996. The mean age of the 40 men and 14 women was 57.5 years. Twenty-three patients had T3 primary tumors, and 31 had T4 primary tumors. Neck disease status was N0 in 16, N1 in 17, and N2 in 21. All received postoperative radiation therapy and reconstructive surgery. There were 20 evaluable patients in the group who underwent total glossectomy alone and 15 evaluable patients in the group treated with total glossectomy and total laryngectomy. Seven patients took part in the assessment of QOL and functional status. The 35 evaluable patients had 3- and 5-year Kaplan-Meier corrected actuarial survival rates of 51% and 41%, respectively. Corresponding rates were 57% and 47% in the total glossectomy group, and 48% and 38% in the total glossectomy with total laryngectomy group. Patients who completed QOL questionnaires generally said that they felt well; only 1 complained about the side effects of treatment, and 1 had significant pain. All had received good support from family and friends and were coping well with their illness. Only 1 patient could tolerate a regular diet; 4 received nutrition only by a gastrostomy tube, and 2 required supplementation via the tube. The average score for "understandability of speech" was 46 (range 0-75). Patients also reported problems with socializing and social function.

Conclusions.—Previous studies of patients with advanced tongue cancer have found significant dysfunction after total glossectomy with or without total laryngectomy. Despite functional deficits, some patients in this study had adapted to their illness and felt good about their QOL.

► Some of these conclusions are a stretch. We cannot quibble with the survival results, and the numbers have been duplicated in other reports. There are several important findings:

1. *Most* (not many) total glossectomy patients will not eat.
2. *Most* total glossectomy patients will have severe impairment of speech.
3. *If* the patients are highly motivated and have appropriate resources, a satisfactory quality of life can be obtained. We need confirmation from more comprehensive studies than 7 patients, but the authors deserve congratulations for a solid effort in the right direction.
4. The role of organ preservation in tongue base cancer with chemoradiotherapy needs further study and definition.

E.A. Luce, M.D.

Parotid Mass as First Symptom of a Malignant Lymphoma

von Stritzky M, Wereldsma JCJ, Pegels JG (St Franciscus Gasthuis, Rotterdam, The Netherlands)

J Surg Oncol 67:25-27, 1998 12–17

Introduction.—Primary malignant parotid lymphomas are rarely reported, accounting for fewer than 1% of malignant tumors in the parotid gland. Seven patients with primary malignant parotid lymphomas were retrospectively studied to identify prognostic variables and to assess results of treatment.

Methods.—From 1985 to 1995, 92 patients were treated at the study institution for a parotid mass. Seven (38%) primary malignant lymphomas (an unusually high percentage) were found in 18 malignant tumors. The mean age of these patients was 70 years. Lesions had a mean diameter of

3.1 cm. Minor lymph node swelling in the neck had occurred in 2 patients; no preoperative lesion of the facialis nerve was noted. Five fine-needle aspiration biopsies were performed.

Results.—All patients were treated surgically, with superficial parotidectomy performed in 5 cases. The tumor was locally excised in 1 patient, and another had explorative incision and debulking. Two patients underwent radiotherapy, and 3 (including 1 with radiotherapy) received chemotherapy. Although there was no local recurrence, 3 patients had recurrences in other sites. After a mean follow-up of 66 months, 6 patients (85% overall survival) are still alive. Actual survival duration ranged from 4 to 132 months.

Conclusions.—These primary malignant lymphomas in the parotid gland did not behave differently than lymphomas in the usual sites. Tumor types were Hodgkin's lymphoma, marginal zone B-cell non-Hodgkin's lymphoma, lymphoplasmocytoid non-Hodgkin's lymphoma, and follicular non-Hodgkin's lymphoma. No new prognostic variables were determined. It is difficult to obtain tissue for histologic examination when malignant lymphoma is located in the parotid gland.

▶ This paper was selected because of the unusual nature of the topic, namely, a malignant lymphoma that presents as a parotid mass. Several things need to be mentioned. An unusually high percentage (38%) of parotid malignancies in this series ultimately proved to be malignant lymphoma. Whether this is a referral phenomenon or another explanation exists cannot be deduced from this paper. More importantly, the 7 patients all had the same symptoms and signs as would be present with any other parotid tumor, namely, a painless mass of about 3 cm located in the preauricular or mandibular angle region. Apparently, adenopathy was not detectable either in the neck or elsewhere. The first diagnostic maneuver was a fine-needle aspirate, but all patients (with the exception of one) had a superficial parotidectomy. If the fine-needle aspirate strongly suggested lymphoma, could something less extensive than a parotidectomy be performed? I doubt it; the pathologist will want sufficient tissue to perform the necessary morphological and cellular diagnostic studies to direct the appropriate chemotherapy and radiotherapy. I don't agree with the authors' suggestion that CT scan is of little value. Preoperative CT scan of the head and neck may well detect nonpalpable adenopathy or lymphomatous involvement of Waldeyer's ring.

E.A. Luce, M.D.

Surgical Treatment for Pulmonary Metastases of Squamous Cell Carcinoma of the Head and Neck

Nibu K, Nakagawa K, Kamata S, et al (Univ of Tokyo; Cancer Inst Hosp, Tokyo; Nippon Med College, Tokyo)

Am J Otolaryngol 18:391-395, 1997 12–18

Introduction.—Distant metastases of head and neck cancer are seen more frequently now that local and regional control has improved. The most common site of distant metastases, the lungs, usually indicates wide systemic spread in patients with squamous cell carcinoma (SCC) of the head and neck. In some cases, however, metastases are limited to the lung, and long-term survival may be possible. The role of surgical treatment in such cases was retrospectively reviewed.

Patients and Methods.—Patients were 23 men and 9 women whose average age was 57 years at diagnosis of the head and neck primary tumor. Primary sites were the oral cavity in 13 patients, hypopharynx in 9, larynx in 5, and maxillary sinus in 2; the eyelid, oropharynx, and nasopharynx were each the primary site in 1 patient. When pulmonary metastases were detected, 26 patients had a lobectomy, 4 had a bilobectomy, and 2 had a pneumonectomy. Mediastinal lymph node dissection was performed in all cases. Patients were followed up for 3 years or until death.

Results.—The overall 5-year survival rate in these patients was 32%. Young patients (55 years or younger) had a better 5-year survival rate than older patients (48.6% vs. 10.3%). Patients with SCC of the oral cavity had significantly poorer survival than those with SCC of other head and neck sites. Shorter survival was associated with a shorter disease-free interval between initial treatment and diagnosis of pulmonary metastases. Mediastinal lymph node involvement and pleural invasion were also correlated with survival.

Conclusions.—Patients with pulmonary metastases of SCC of the head and neck should undergo a complete workup to determine the extent of disease and whether metastases are limited to the lung. The distribution or extent of metastatic nodules, as well as their number, appear to affect prognosis. The best candidate for surgery is a patient with a single nodule confined to 1 lobe and without mediastinal involvement.

▶ The first question that should occur to the reader is how big was the universe of patients from which this group of 32 was drawn. One thousand? Ten thousand? If we assume local regional control existed, did the authors set a minimum disease-free interval? (I don't think so.) Moving past those complaints, the results were surprising, perhaps startlingly good: one-third 5-year survival overall and 45% if the oral cavity primaries are eliminated from the calculations.

E.A. Luce, M.D.

Morbidity of Thyroid Surgery

Bergamaschi R, Becouarn G, Ronceray J, et al (Angers Univ, France)
Am J Surg 176:71-75, 1998 12–19

Objective.—Risk factors for morbidity after thyroidectomy were retrospectively assessed in 1,163 patients who underwent 1,192 thyroidectomies.

Methods.—Thyroid ultrasound, thyroid scan, fine-needle aspiration (FNA) cytology, and peripheral basal calcitonin levels were preoperatively assessed in 97.7%, 97.3%, 87.7%, and 84.7% of procedures. Surgical indications were multinodular goiter (n = 539), solitary nodule (n = 452), hyperthyroidism (n = 167, including 33 adenomas, 43 diffuse goiters, and 91 multinodular toxic goiters) medullary thyroid carcinoma (n = 5), and misdiagnosed thyroid neoplasm (n = 29). In patients with solitary nodules, results of FNA cytology were suggestive of malignancy in 84 patients, and medical treatment failed in 368. Surgeons performing thyroidectomies had a patient volume of greater than 100 in 71.3% of cases, 50-100 in 15%, and less than 50 in 13.7%. Permanent recurrent laryngeal nerve (RLN) injury was defined as postsurgical clinical dysphonia lasting 6 months. Permanent hypoparathyroidism was defined as serum parathyroid hormone levels of less than 10 ng/L.

Results.—There were 12 superficial and 7 deep hematomas (1.59%), 3 chyle leaks (0.25%), and 6 abscesses (0.5%). The presence or absence of hematoma or abscess did not affect surgical outcome, presence of hyperthyroidism, or drain use. The incidences of temporary and permanent hypoparathyroidism were 19.9% and 3.8%, respectively. Hypoparathyroidism rates were higher for patients who had total thyroidectomy with neck dissection or completion thyroidectomy, but did not depend on a surgeon's patient volume. There were no patients with hypoparathyroidism after monolateral surgery. The temporary and permanent RLN palsy rates were 2.9% and 0.5%, respectively, with temporary RLN palsy rates significantly higher after total thyroidectomy with neck dissection and completion thyroidectomy. The number of temporary and permanent RLN paralyses were similar after both RLN exposure and nonexposure, and were not affected by a surgeon's patient volume.

Conclusions.—Morbidity after thyroid surgery was not affected by a surgeon's patient volume or by identification of parathyroids and RLNs. Total thyroidectomy with neck dissection or completion thyroidectomy increased the incidence of temporary RLN palsy and permanent hypoparathyroidism.

► Certainly this is a study that raises more questions than it answers despite the wealth of data. This series is *not* one of surgery for neoplastic disease. Also, what does a "completion thyroidectomy" by these authors exactly mean? A prior lobectomy? A prior "subtotal?" Drains didn't decrease the complication rate and, interestingly, no difference in complication rate among surgeons was apparent regardless of the number of cases performed. This outcome may have been the result of supervision by the higher-volume surgeons of surgeons with lower-volume cases.

E.A. Luce, M.D.

Laryngotracheal Reconstruction in the Adult: A Ten Year Experience

Lano CF Jr, Duncavage JA, Reinisch L, et al (Vanderbilt Univ, Nashville, Tenn)
Ann Otol Rhinol Laryngol 107:92-97, 1998 12–20

Objective.—Severe laryngotracheal (LT) stenosis can result from traumatic intubation, patient susceptibility to infection, patient movement while intubated, duration of intubation, history of reintubation, presence of a nasogastric tube, and size of the endotracheal tube. Although endoscopic techniques for treating LT stenosis are the treatments of choice, open LT reconstruction is used for failed endoscopic surgery, failed prior open technique, fixed glottic stenosis, collapse of 1 or more tracheal rings, damage to the integrity of the cricoid cartilage, or stenosis with a scar segment longer than 1 cm. A retrospective review of open surgical techniques for treating LT stenosis is presented.

Methods.—Between July 1986 and July 1996, 41 patients underwent 21 augmentation laryngotracheoplasties, 22 tracheal resections with primary reanastomosis, and 3 tracheal reconstructions with augmentation grafting. Before surgery, all patients had video stroboscopy, and some had pulmonary function tests, computed tomography, magnetic resonance imaging, and tomography. Diagnostic rigid endoscopy was performed under general anesthesia on all patients.

> *Technique.*—The surgical technique has been previously described. The cricoid is split posteriorly being careful not to extend to the posterior commissure or into the esophagus. The fusiform-shaped anterior cartilage graft is sutured in place. For stenoses greater than 3 cm, an appropriately sized Montgomery laryngeal stent is used with a tracheostomy. Four to 6 weeks after surgery, the patient is reoperated to remove the stent. For larger resections, a suprahyoid laryngeal release is performed.

Results.—Success, defined as decannulation within 1 year, was achieved in 63% of patients. Intermediate success, defined as either decannulation after more than 1 year, a repeat open operation, or a major complication, was achieved in 17% of patients. The remaining 20% were tracheostomy dependent. Of the 10 procedures performed on diabetics, 6 failed. Most (76%) of the 41 patients had failed previous endoscopic surgery. Although it was expected that only 40% of McCaffrey stage IV lesions could be decannulated, 57% were actually decannulated, and 100% of McCaffrey stage II lesions were successfully treated. There were no McCaffrey stage I lesions. Patients with diabetes mellitus represented 75% of the failures and tended to have bacterial overgrowth of wounds, which can lead to formation of abundant granulation tissue. Several patients with comorbid conditions eventually may require a tracheostomy.

Conclusion.—The new staging system multiplied by the Cotton grade (a measure of stenosis severity) allows identification of patients likely to succeed. Diabetic patients undergoing LT reconstruction were much less successful then nondiabetic patients.

▶ First, although not stated, since most failures were in the most severe group and most failures were diabetic, the cumulative effect on the success rate might make laryngotracheal reconstruction prohibitively problematic. Second, the diabetic observation is of interest and not previously noted in large series of laryngotracheal reconstruction. The authors have some interesting speculation, but basically the operative factor or factors are unknown. Third, the most provocative aspect for those interested in wound healing is why laryngeal reconstruction by simply incising and releasing the scar posterior and creation of a substantial mucosal deficit should ever work. How does splinting the defect open (with costal or septal cartilage struts) work? Why should it work? Were failures observed in diabetics with severe stenosis, those managed by this technique, rather than resection and primary anastomosis (one suspects that this is the case)? If so, perhaps what is needed is a different conceptual approach, with the provision of epithelial-lined additional tissue. I will leave it to some innovative head and neck surgeon to further develop that concept.

E.A. Luce, M.D.

Alloplastic and Microvascular Restoration of the Mandible: A Comparison Study

Mandpe AH, Singer MI, Kaplan MJ, et al (Univ of California, San Francisco)
Laryngoscope 108:224-227, 1998 12–21

Objective.—Establishment of a continuous rigid mandibular arch soon after oral cavity surgery for carcinomas is necessary for functional and cosmetic rehabilitation. Early reconstruction with cortical bone grafts, Vitallium, or stainless steel trays with cancellous bone had a high failure rate. Alloplastic plating systems failed because of plate exposure and fracture. New microvascular free flap techniques have made free osseocutaneous tissue transfer possible and improved the reliability of mandibular reconstruction. The authors present their experience with alloplastic plates and the microvascular free flap.

Methods.—Over a 6-year period, 22 reconstructions using a fibula free flap and 20 using an alloplastic plating system were performed on 42 patients with oral cavity cancers or osteoradionecrosis of the mandible. In the alloplastic group, 5 patients received an AO plate, and 15 a titanium plate with hollow or solid locking screws. Flap reconstruction used the pectoralis major myocutaneous flap in 19 patients and a radial forearm free flap in 1.

Results.—Sixteen (80%) of 20 reconstructions with the alloplastic plating system were successful. Plate exposure was the cause of the 4 failures. Reconstructions in 3 of 4 patients who lost soft tissue were salvaged with débridement, local wound care, and antibiotics. Duration of hospitalization averaged 13 days for this group. Four patients had complications with the fibula free flap, and 4 patients had medical complications, including an intraoperative hypotensive episode, pulmonary complications, and multisystem failure. Eighteen (82%) of 22 patients receiving a fibula free flap had satisfactory oral intake. Duration of hospitalization averaged 23 days for this group, significantly longer than for the plate group. The plate group had a significantly higher anterior defect failure rate than the fibular group (50% vs. 9%). The lateral defect rates were similar. An osseocutaneous free flap is preferred for reconstruction that fails in the anterior defect because of plate exposure. Soft tissue complications were the most common causes of reconstructive failure in the alloplastic group probably because of the downward pull of the pedicle of the flap against the plate. Other studies reported a 60% success rate with the pectoralis group compared with 100% success rate with the free flap group. Patients in the free flap group had more medical complications and a longer hospital stay than the plate group.

Conclusion.—A fibular free flap is preferred in anterior defects whereas an alloplastic plate provides better results with lateral defects.

▶ The discussion (controversy?) continues on the appropriate method of mandibular reconstruction. The consensus, including this article, is that anterior segmental (central) defects are optimally reconstructed with an osteocutaneous free flap, the fibula. The focus of this paper is mostly for *lateral* defects. The authors selected alloplastic hard tissue reconstruction with a reconstruction plate and soft tissue with a pectoralis major flap in 60% of the cases, the remainder with a vascularized fibula. No information is given with respect to selection criteria, but I suspect age (average age of the reconstruction plate was 10 years older) and coexistent medical conditions. Information is not given about length of follow up in each group, a glaring and not particularly excusable omission. Regardless, the data, particularly length of stay and systemic morbidity, make a good case for plate and pectoralis major flap reconstruction in some patients. In the reviewer's opinion, these would consist of advanced age or significant medical conditions and extremely unfavorable prognosis.

E.A. Luce, M.D.

Fibula Osteoseptocutaneous Flap for Reconstruction of Osteoradionecrosis of the Mandible

Santamaria E, Wei F-C, Chen H-C (Chang Gung Univ, Taipei, Taiwan, ROC)

Plast Reconstr Surg 101:921-929, 1998 12–22

Introduction.—Osteoradionecrosis of the mandible is one of the most devastating and dangerous complications of radiation therapy for head and neck cancer. Preradiation teeth extraction and poor oral hygiene are 2 of the most controversial risk factors in the development of osteoradionecrosis. Exposure of irradiated bone to the intraoral or extraoral environment is the risk factor of greatest concern. Irradiation may cause chronic hypoxia, resulting in hypocellular and hypovascular damage that is responsible for skin atrophy and susceptibility to breakdown and poor or delayed healing response after minor trauma. It may be conservatively managed when superficial. Major bone and soft-tissue necrosis requires a radical approach, with replacement of excised tissue. The use of the fibula osteoseptocutaneous flap for mandibular reconstruction in 12 patients was reported retrospectively.

Methods.—The primary oral tumor was treated with radiation therapy in 3 patients and with tumor resection in the remaining 9 patients. The average time between end of radiation therapy and diagnosis of osteoradionecrosis of the mandible was 8.1 months (range, 2 to 24 months). Extraoral fistula was the most common physical manifestation, alone or combined with cellulitis, pathologic fracture, bone exposure, persistent ulceration, and oral mucosa necrosis. Other findings included sequestration and mottled areas of radiolucency, with sclerotic changes in the margins of affected areas. Most patients were managed conservatively before radical surgery. The major indications for radical treatment were pathologic fracture alone or combined with necrotic bone exposure or persistent fistula. Bony defects after segmental mandibulectomy ranged from 3.0 to 13.0 cm.

Results.—All patients achieved primary bone healing with adequate facial symmetry and improved oral function. No patients had recurrent osteoradionecrosis.

Conclusions.—Two distinct patterns of osteoradionecrosis were observed: posttraumatic (60%) and spontaneous (40%). Spontaneous disease occurred most commonly between 6 and 24 months after irradiation, compared with 3 months after end of radiation in trauma-induced lesions. A second increase in incidence of osteoradionecrosis was observed after 2 years, peaking at 5 years. Key to successful management is adequate debridement with removal of all dead or hypovascular bone and surrounding soft tissue. The most versatile bone stock for reconstructing the mandible is the fibula. Osseointegrated implants have been placed successfully into transplanted fibula as a primary or secondary dental procedure. Primary osseointegrated implants may be useful in patients with osteoradionecrosis because many of them are young and free of tumor.

► Osteoradionecrosis of the mandible is a debilitating problem that severely compromises the success of full rehabilitation of the head and neck patient. The fact that most of these patients are tumor-free further compounds the problem. Although not specifically discussed by the authors, the secondary problems of pain, trismus, and impaired deglutition also affect these patients. Resection of involved mandible, reconstruction with vascularized bone, and importantly, adequate soft tissue replacement are of paramount importance for the optimal result.

E.A. Luce, M.D.

Reconstruction of Total Maxillectomy Defects With Preservation of the Orbital Contents

Cordeiro PG, Santamaria E, Kraus DH, et al (Mem Sloan-Kettering Cancer Ctr, New York)

Plast Reconstr Surg 102:1874-1887, 1998 12–23

Introduction.—In patients undergoing total maxillectomy, it is sometimes possible to preserve the orbital contents. This poses more difficult reconstructive challenges than when maxillectomy is accompanied by orbital exenteration. The reconstruction must support the orbital contents while obliterating any communication between the mouth and nose, reconstructing the palatal surface, and providing facial symmetry. No previous reports have described the use of immediate nonvascularized bone grafts, with a soft tissue free flap or pedicled muscle flap providing a vascularized bed, to address this problem. This approach of immediate reconstruction with preservation of the orbital contents is reported in 14 patients undergoing total maxillectomy.

Methods.—Each patient underwent immediate reconstruction of the orbital floor and maxilla, using nonvascularized bone grafts. The bony reconstruction was done with split ribs in 6 patients, split calvaria in 6, and iliac crest bone in 2. The soft tissue reconstruction, including resurfacing of the palatal and nasal mucosa, was usually achieved with a myocutaneous rectus abdominis free flap. Postoperative radiotherapy was used in 10 patients. The aesthetic and functional results were assessed at least 6 months postoperatively in 13 surviving patients.

Results.—There were no free flap failures. At follow-up, all patients had functional vision, with no need for an eyepatch. Ten patients had ectropion—mild in 4, moderate in 4, and severe in 2. Six patients consented to a secondary procedure to correct lower eyelid ectropion. Speech was rated normal in 6 patients, near normal in 6, and intelligible in 1. All patients but 1 had good chewing function. The aesthetic results were rated good in 9 patients and fair in 4.

Conclusions.—For patients undergoing total maxillectomy with preservation of the globe, a combination of nonvascularized bone grafts with a soft tissue free flap provides a safe and reliable reconstructive approach with good aesthetic and functional results. The rectus abdominis flap is a good choice for soft tissue reconstruction; a temporalis flap with nonvascularized bone graft may be used in patients with smaller orbital floor defects or in those where free flaps cannot be used. The aesthetic results vary, depending on whether the facial muscles and malar eminence are resected. The problem of ectropion may be avoided by using a transconjunctival incision rather than the standard subciliary component of the Weber-Ferguson incision.

► This article is a valuable addition to the literature on head and neck reconstruction. Simply stated, the authors outline a rationale for reconstruction with a contemporary technique of microvascular surgery transfer of soft tissue, combined with a more traditional method of restoration of bony support, nonvascularized rib or calvarial grafts. Preservation of good ocular function in the patients who have had a maxillectomy plus postoperative radiation therapy can be a daunting task, and the authors' results were overall quite good. The singular blemish on the results is the necessity for reoperation for ectropion. Perhaps, the technique of use of a transconjunctival incision may avoid that problem.

I do have a number of niggling criticisms of their study, including no documentation that the bone grafts actually survive. Perhaps their results were obtained with soft tissue augmentation alone. The inclusion of the speech and deglutition result have little to do with reconstitution of the bone and orbital rim and floor would require a more sophisticated evaluation than used in this article.

E.A. Luce, M.D.

Platysma Muscle Cutaneous Flap for Large Defects of the Lower Lip and Mental Region

Moschella F, Cordova A (Univ of Palermo, Italy)

Plast Reconstr Surg 101:1803-1809, 1998 12–24

Objective.—The composite facial muscle cutaneous flap makes it possible to employ the depressor anguli oris flap for covering large defects of the lower lip. With mobilization of an innervated platysma muscle flap, sensation and muscle fibers can restored to the area.

Technique.—A V-shaped defect is created and covered with a V-shaped flap (Fig 1). The flap base is aligned with the labial rim, reorienting the platysma fibers transversely to provide continuity to the oral sphincter. A cheek mucosal flap is raised and rotated to cover the mucosal plane and the vermilion.

Results.—The lower lips of 122 patients with neoplasia of the lower lip were reconstructed between 1988 and 1996. The cases of 3 patients (1 woman), aged 56, 72, and 88, with squamous cell (n = 2) and basal cell

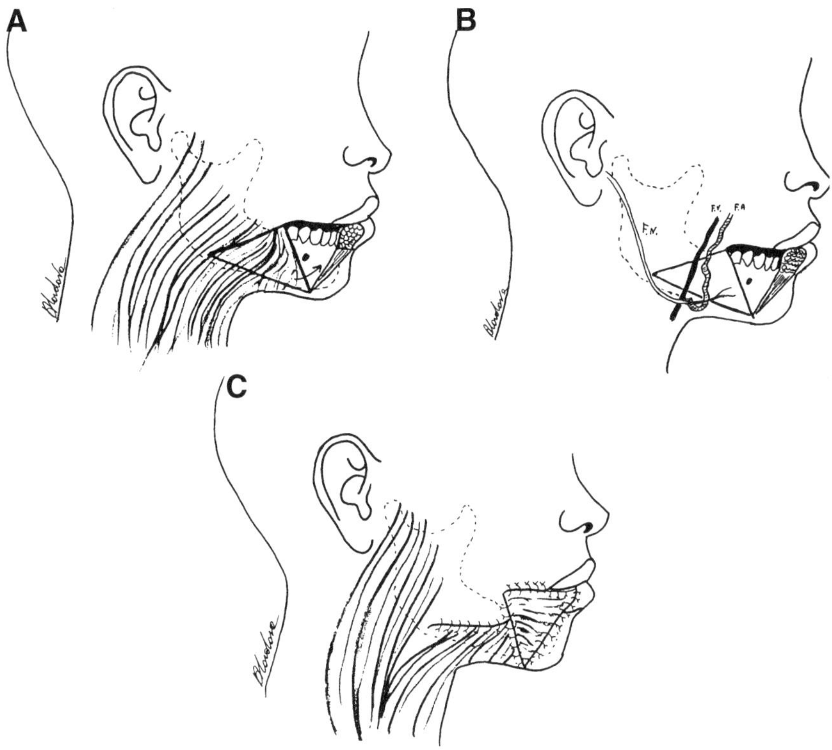

FIGURE 1.—A, Schematic representation of the platysma muscle cutaneous flap. A triangular flap is drawn in the mandibular cheek region. The base coincides with the lateral branch of the V-shaped defect, whereas the tip is oriented toward the anguli of the jaw. B, Neurovascular pedicle of the flap, which is located under the platysma fibers. The mandibular branch of the facial nerve runs above the vascular pedicle. C, The flap, turned 90 degrees, allows reconstruction of a lateral defect of the lower lip and the mental region even if the depressor anguli oris had been demolished. *Abbreviations: FV,* facial vein; *FA,* facial artery; *FN,* facial nerve. (Courtesy of Mosschella F, Cordova A: Platysma muscle cutaneous flap for large defects of the lower lip and mental region. *Plast Reconstr Surg* 101:1803-1809, 1998).

(n = 1) carcinoma, are described. Good to excellent functional and cosmetic results were obtained in all cases.

Discussion.—The platysma muscle cutaneous flap has all the advantages of muscle cutaneous innervated flaps. Motor innervation must be preserved to maintain the muscle tonus and permit acceptable sphincter function. Very careful dissection of the neurovascular pedicle is required, necessitating longer operation times. The perioral sphincter must be reconstructed physiologically, and scars must be hidden within natural folds.

► Right idea, wrong execution. The use of a flap composed of skin and muscle, the latter with retention of its mimetic activity by preservation of the motor innervation, is an elegant rationale and the basis of other attempts at a "like-for-like" reconstruction. Thus, the principles described in this article are worth the review. If the readers also study Fig 1 carefully, all will conclude that this technique does not embody these principles but, rather, uses a local tissue flap only. The platysma is innervated by the cervical, not the marginal mandibular branch of seventh nerve. Dissection to mobilize the flap must be extremely superficial, and a donor site defect scar does not respect the aesthetic subunits of the adjacent cheek, as the author's claim.

E.A. Luce, M.D.

Combining Free Flap Reconstruction and Craniofacial Prosthetic Technique for Orbit, Scalp, and Temporal Defects

Gliklich RE, Rounds MF, Cheney ML, et al (Massachusetts Eye and Ear Infirmary, Boston; Harvard Med School, Boston)

Laryngoscope 108:482-487, 1998 12–25

Objective.—Free flaps have been recommended for large defects of the scalp, temporal bone, and orbit, although the esthetic results may be suboptimal. With advances in osseointegrated implants, implant-borne prostheses are available for patients with complex facial defects. The authors believe that using these 2 techniques in combination can provide good cosmetic results with safe soft tissue coverage. Such an approach mandates presurgical planning, with special attention to the site-specific requirements of prosthetic use (Table 1). The authors report their experience using a site-specific rehabilitation algorithm for patients with scalp, temporal bone, and orbital defects requiring free tissue transfer.

Methods.—Twenty-eight patients who underwent free flap reconstruction for defects of the orbit, scalp, and temporal bone from 1989 to 1996 were analyzed retrospectively. A site-specific reconstruction approach, addressing the goals of free tissue transfer and rehabilitation/ancillary procedures, was initiated in 1994. The numbers of patients who were free of recurrent disease using prostheses, before and after this time were compared.

Results.—Free flap reconstructions included rectus myocutaneous flaps in 12 patients, rectus muscle or myocutaneous flaps in 7, a latissimus dorsi myocutaneous flap in 1, latissimus dorsi muscle flaps in 4, free temporoparietal fascia flaps in 3, and a radial forearm fasciocutaneous flap in 1. The success rate of free tissue transfer was 93%; the perioperative mortality rate was 4%. Since the introduction of the site-specific algorithm,

---

TABLE 1.—Site-Specific Rehabilitation Goals

Site	Goals of Free Tissue Transfer	Rehabilitation/Ancillary Procedures
Scalp	Vascular coverage; smooth contour	Hairpiece
Temporal	Thin, vascular coverage; flat temporal platform	Implant-borne auricular prosthesis ± hairpiece
Orbit	Thin, vascular coverage; maintain orbital cavity depth; preserve brow position	Implant-borne orbital prosthesis; bone grafting to supraorbital rim; brow lift

(Courtesy of Gliklich RE, Rounds MF, Cheney ML, et al: Combining free flap reconstruction and craniofacial prosthetic technique or orbit, scalp, and temporal defects. *Laryngoscope* 108:482-487, 1998.)

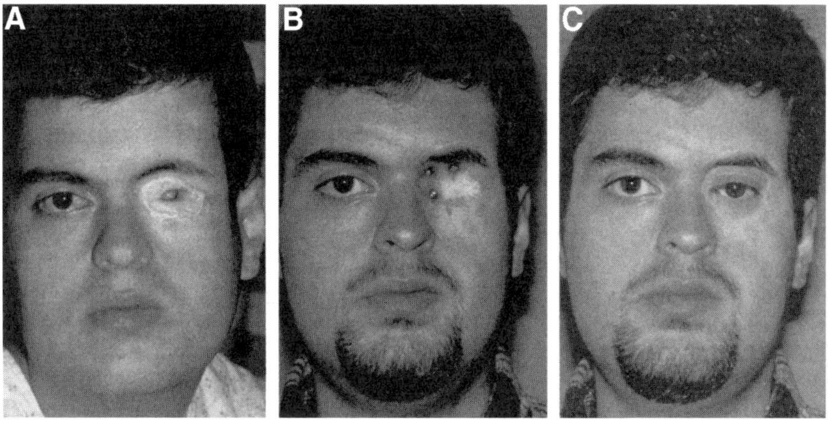

FIGURE 3.—Case 3. A, chronically infected left orbital exenteration cavity in a patient with a history of surgery and radiation for a childhood hemangiopericytoma reconstructed with temporalis muscle and skin grafts. B, after débridement of the cavity and reconstruction with a free rectus muscle flap and split-thickness skin graft, a calvarial bone graft to the supraorbital rim, a direct brow lift, and osseointegrated implants prepare the cavity for a prosthesis. C, patient with orbital prosthesis. (Courtesy of Gliklich RE, Rounds MF, Cheney ML, et al: Combining free flap reconstruction and craniofacial prosthetic technique for orbit, scalp, and temporal defects. *Laryngoscope* 108:482-487, 1998.)

prostheses were actively used by 4 of 7 patients (Fig 3). A total of 9 osseointegrated implants were placed in previously irradiated bone, without hyperbaric oxygen therapy. The implant success rate was 89%.

Conclusions.—For patients with defects of the orbit, scalp, and temporal bone, the use of craniofacial prostheses can significantly enhance the results of free flap reconstruction. The best outcomes are achieved with a site-specific reconstructive approach. The use of osseointegrated implants provides for much better retention of prostheses, thus improving patient tolerance. The patient's life expectancy should be considered in selecting a reconstructive approach that may take an extended period to complete (i.e., osseointegration in irradiated bone).

► The next level in reconstruction of difficult composite defects of the upper two thirds of the face may well be what the authors proposed, namely, a combination of prosthetic technology and our capability to transfer tissue by microvascular means. Certainly, the same conceptual approach could be taken in the middle third of the face for reconstruction of nasal defects, but nasal implants are a little less tolerated psychologically than ear implants. One might take issue with the authors' choice of donor sites, namely, the rectus muscle vs. other donor sites, when less muscle bulk is needed. Consider the use of the serratus anterior, a smaller muscle but large enough to fill some of the defects reconstructed by the authors. Another option would be a fasciocutaneous free flap, such as the radial forearm flap. Clearly, what is crucial in terms of patient acceptance is the willingness of the patient to tolerate a multiple-stage reconstruction.

E.A. Luce, M.D.

Reconstruction of a Large Abdominal Wall Defect Using Combined Free Tensor Fasciae Latae Musculocutaneous Flap and Anterolateral Thigh Flap

Sasaki K, Nozaki M, Nakazawa H, et al (Tokyo Women's Med College)
Plast Reconstr Surg 102:2244-2252, 1998 12–26

Background.—With the development of microvascular techniques of composite tissue transfer, it is now possible to perform full-thickness reconstruction of the abdominal wall. Musculofascial continuity and surface coverage can be achieved through use of a tensor fasciae latae musculocutaneous flap. This flap can be combined in a composite tissue graft with the skin of the anterolateral portion of the upper thigh, which derives its blood supply from the septocutaneous branch of the lateral circumflex femoral artery. The technique and outcomes of this approach are discussed.

> *Technique.*—The composite free tensor fasciae latae musculocutaneous/anterolateral thigh flap may be used for reconstruction of extensive abdominal wall defects after cancer surgery. As part of surgical planning, Doppler flowmetry is performed to map the blood vessels supplying the flaps. The graft includes the areolar tissues adhering to the underside of the tensor fasciae latae, as these may minimize adhesions between the fascia and visceral peritoneum if interposed between the 2. The superior gluteal nerve, which innervates the tensor fasciae latae and is most often found in the posteroinferior aspect of the muscle, is included in the flap dissection. Recipient vessels for the graft are the inferior epigastric or deep circumflex iliac arteries; the greater saphenous vein may also be used as the recipient vein.

Experience.—The investigators have used this composite flap for 4 patients requiring full-thickness abdominal wall reconstruction after cancer extirpation. The smallest flap was 17 × 12 cm and the largest 31 × 20 cm. Blood supply to both the tensor fasciae latae and anterolateral thigh flaps came from the lateral circumflex femoral artery in 3 of the 4 patients (and from the deep femoral artery in 1).

Discussion.—The use of a composite free tensor fasciae latae musculocutaneous/anterolateral thigh flap for reconstruction of extensive abdominal wall defects is discussed. Using the anterolateral thigh flap to enlarge the dimension of the tensor fasciae latae flap helps to overcome many of the disadvantages of the latter flap. The composite flap has provided satisfactory outcomes with low morbidity in 4 patients. It may even partially restore muscular activity to the reconstructed abdominal wall if the neural supply to the muscle component is left undisturbed or is reestablished.

▶ Reconstruction of full thickness massive defects of the abdominal wall can be a daunting challenge. Reconstruction of defects of less magnitude can be accomplished with a shift of a rectus myocutaneous flap or "separation of parts" (component-sharing). Use of tensor fascia lata or tensor fascia lata combined with vastus lateralis or rectus femoris in a pedicle fashion has all those limitations cited by the author, namely, partial necrosis delayed healing and possible secondary intraabdominal complications. The use of free tissue transfer with the combined flap, avoids these problems, but not entirely since the skin territory is not exactly defined. I do have doubts about the reconstitution of the motor innervation as claimed by the authors. Otherwise, this innovative approach could "life-boat" out of a tight spot.

E.A. Luce, M.D.

Up-to-date Report of Botulinum Toxin Type A Treatment in Patients With Gustatory Sweating (Frey's Syndrome)

Laskawi R, Drobik C, Schönebeck C (Univ of Göttingen, Germany)

Laryngoscope 108:381-384, 1998 12–27

Introduction.—Gustatory sweating, or Frey's syndrome, may occur in up to 50% of patients after surgery of the parotid gland. About 15% of patients report severe symptoms. Intracutaneous application of the botulinum toxin has been used successfully in preventing the release of the neurotransmitter acetylcholine at cholinergic synapses. Recent observations of recurrent gustatory sweating after botulinum toxin therapy were reported.

Methods.—Nineteen patients with gustatory sweating after parotidectomy were treated on an outpatient basis with local intracutaneous injections of botulinum toxin type A (BOTOX) into affected skin areas. The iodine-starch test according to Minor was used to determine the exact dimension of affected skin.

Results.—Sweat secretion ceased within 2 days in all treated areas. There were no side effects. One patient was lost to follow-up. Effects of these injections lasted in 10 patients followed for 11-27 months (mean 17.3 months). Gustatory sweating recurred in 8 patients (44.4%) at a mean of 15 months. This was substantiated by Minor's test. Three patients underwent reinjection with cessation of sweat secretion within 2 days. At 2 months after second treatment, all 3 patients were asymptomatic.

Conclusions.—Eight patients reported recurrence of gustatory sweating at a mean of 15 months after injection with BOTOX. This long symptom-free interval was a relief for patients. Three mechanisms may be responsible for delayed or absent regeneration of sweat glands: (1) sweat gland function could be partly or totally abolished; (2) nerve fibers were feebly or not at all regenerated; or (3) regeneration was compromised by scar formation. Intracutaneous injection of BOTOX is an effective and minimally invasive therapy for gustatory sweating that provides long-lasting effect.

► Although Frey's syndrome, or gustatory sweating, is objectively common in parotidectomy patients, it is problematic only for a distinct minority (about 10%). What makes this report about botulinum toxin treatment attractive is the paucity of other successful treatment modalities. The operative options such as sectioning Jacobensen's nerve are not particularly attractive, and nonoperative therapy with scopolamine cream is not particularly acceptable to patients.

E.A. Luce, M.D.

Critical Assessment of the Head and Neck Clinical Skills of General Surgery Residents

Sloan DA, Donnelly MB, Schwartz RW, et al (Univ of Kentucky, Lexington)
World J Surg 22:229-235, 1998 12–28

Introduction.—Multiple-choice tests and subjective evaluations by faculty members do not accurately assess the clinical expertise that should be achieved by general surgery residents. Although head and neck surgery is an important part of general surgery, little is known about the quality of residents' clinical skills in this field. Whether changes in resident education are needed to improve skills in head and neck surgery was determined by using the Objective Structured Clinical Examination (OSCE).

Methods.—Fifty-one general surgery residents from the same residency program examined the same 9 patients with head and neck disease. Both actual (e.g., oral cancer follow-up examination) and simulated (e.g., dysphagia) patients were used in the OSCE. Each clinical interaction was graded by faculty members according to preset objective criteria presented as a checklist, with categories related to history, physical examination, and treatment recommendations. Reliability of the examination was assessed by coefficient α.

Results.—The reliability for the clinical examination, 0.75, was at the lower end of the acceptable range. Performance on the OSCE varied significantly among levels of training and among the residents. Overall performance was best on the dysphagia and anatomy problems and worst on the thyroid and parathyroid problems. The average resident had a score of at least 60%, the lowest level of acceptable performance, on only 2 of the 9 OSCE problems. Junior and senior residents performed better than interns.

Conclusions.—At the study institution, the quality of head and neck teaching was found to be below par. Greater attention needs to be focused on specific outcome assessments of surgical training programs. The OSCE is useful for uncovering weaknesses in surgical curricula and identifying changes that should be made.

▶ This study, done at an institution (University of Kentucky) where general surgery residents are exposed to a considerable volume of head and neck surgical patients and problems, reveals a deficiency in the clinical skills necessary to render care to such patients. One must agree with the authors' conclusion: a specific, structured curriculum is necessary for this core component of general surgery. Based on this central tenet, perhaps a similar type of study needs to be done for other areas of deficiency (the authors apparently have studied the breast) of other critical core components of general surgery, and if such a deficiency exists, similar modular additions to the residency curriculum should be established. All of this emphasizes that we need to start educating by design rather than by chance.

E.A. Luce, M.D.

13 Vascular Surgery

Introduction

The role of various new endovascular procedures in the management of peripheral vascular disease has been the most widely debated topic in peripheral vascular surgery this year. The use of these less-invasive methods of managing peripheral aneurysmal and occlusive disease continues to expand, often outstripping the scientific data that support such use. However, reports from carefully done studies on the use of these new techniques are beginning to be published—particularly the results of stent graft repair of abdominal aortic aneurysms, which to date has largely been done by vascular surgeons. Clearly, the proper use of these new techniques must be defined by a comprehensive understanding of the results and risks associated with the treatment of peripheral vascular problems with these endovascular procedures. These results are then compared to those that can be achieved with modern vascular surgical techniques.

The role of carotid angioplasty and stenting in the treatment of carotid atherosclerosis remains unclear. Evidence continues to accumulate that suggests the risks associated with this procedure, particularly the risk of stroke, may be significantly greater than the risks associated with carotid endarterectomy (Abstract 13–3). Hopefully, this endovascular procedure will remain experimental until these risks are better defined. The investigation of the results of surgical vs. medical therapy in patients with significant carotid atherosclerosis also continues. The publication of the second installment of the results from the NASCET trial (Abstract 13–1) has further clarified the role of carotid endarterectomy in patients with symptomatic carotid atherosclerosis. As expected, a significant stroke risk reduction was demonstrated in patients with symptomatic stenosis between 50% and 69%, although that reduction was only 1% and 2% per year. Furthermore, a number of factors such as symptom type and diabetes mellitus were shown to have a significant impact on the degree of stroke risk reduction in patients with both 50% to 69% carotid stenosis and those with 70% to 99% stenosis.

Clinical trials of several endoluminal aneurysm repair devices continue, and interest in this new technique remains high. However, initial results from clinical use of this technique, as demonstrated by May et al. (Abstract 13–4), are less favorable than expected. Furthermore, the long-term consequence of periprosthetic leak, which appears to occur in 20% to 50% of patients (Abstract 13–5), remains undefined. Because of this, significant work remains to be done to determine the place this new technique will occupy in the management of abdominal aortic aneurysms. Interestingly, the results of the United Kingdom Small Aneurysm Trial (Abstract 13–8) suggest that repair of small aneurysms (< 5 cm in size) is inappropriate, and these small aneurysms are most likely to be technically easy to repair using endoluminal stent grafts. Endovascular techniques have also been suggested as appropriate for management of visceral (renal and mesenteric) artery occlusive disease. Because of the lesser risk associated with angioplasty of these arteries, treatment of both symptomatic and asymptomatic visceral artery disease has been advocated. However, the papers by Williamson et al. and Thomas et al. (Abstracts 13–11 and 13–12) raise the question about whether asymptomatic visceral artery occlusive disease should be treated at all.

The next step in the understanding of the proper management of infrainguinal arterial occlusive disease is beginning. Rather than only focusing on such factors as operative mortality, graft patency, and limb salvage, patient recovery and functional outcome after treatment of lower extremity ischemia are being defined. Nicoloff et al. (Abstract 13–13) demonstrate that, despite excellent operative mortality and graft patency results, functional outcome and freedom from further intervention are limited in such patients. Furthermore, Tarry et al. (Abstract 13–14) demonstrate a fairly high rate of need for revascularization of the contralateral extremity in such patients, meaning that an individual reconstructive procedure must be planned in the context of the likely subsequent need for further reconstructive procedures. Adjuncts such as long-term anticoagulation may decrease the need for subsequent arterial reconstructive procedures and thereby improve the long-term functional outcome in selected patients (Abstract 13–15). In addition, newer methods of evaluating a patient prior to lower extremity arterial reconstruction (Abstracts 13–16 and 13–17) may limit the risk and cost associated with this procedure.

Anticoagulation remains the mainstay in the treatment of venous thromboembolic disease, although endovascular placement of a vena caval filter (Abstract 13–20) is certainly appropriate in properly selected patients. The duration of anticoagulation necessary after an episode of deep venous thrombosis also continues to be evaluated (Abstract 13–21) and new forms of long-term anticoagulation, even orally administered heparin, may be on the horizon (Abstract 13–22). Oral heparin may not be the panacea that some suggest, however, as it will likely be associated with the rare and devastating problem of heparin-associated thrombocytopenia, which fortunately appears to be uncommon in patients undergoing peripheral vascular arterial reconstruction procedures (Abstract 13–24). Regardless, the techniques available to treat patients with peripheral vascular disease continue to evolve and expand, which is fortunate, considering the growing number of patients with these problems.

James M. Seeger, M.D.

Carotid

Benefit of Carotid Endarterectomy in Patients With Symptomatic Moderate or Severe Stenosis

Barnett HJM, for the North American Symptomatic Carotid Endarterectomy Trial Collaborators (John P Robarts Research Inst, London, Ont; et al)

N Engl J Med 339:1415-1425, 1998 13–1

Objective.—Carotid endarterectomy has been shown to be of value in symptomatic patients with significant (70% to 99%) carotid stenosis. Whether carotid endarterectomy is beneficial in patients with lesser degrees of symptomatic carotid stenosis is controversial. Outcomes of carotid endarterectomy in patients with moderate (30% to 69%) stenosis enrolled from December 1987 through December 1996 in the North American Symptomatic Carotid Endarterectomy Trial (NASCET) were compared with patients treated medically.

Methods.—Patients with symptomatic ischemia on the same side as the stenosis within 180 days before study entry were stratified by degree of stenosis (50%-69% or ≤ 50%) and randomly allocated to the endarterectomy group (n = 1,108) or to medical care only (n = 1,118). Neurologic assessments were performed at baseline, at 1, 3, 6, 9, and 12 months, and every 4 months thereafter. Brain imaging studies were obtained after suspected strokes. Duplex ultrasonography was performed at baseline, 1 month later, annually thereafter, and after suspected strokes. Deaths and site, type, severity, and duration of strokes were outcome measures. Patients were studied for an average of 5 years.

Results.—At 5 years, ipsilateral stroke was detected in 22.2% of the high-moderate (50%-60%) stenosis group on medical therapy vs. 15.7% receiving carotid endarterectomy ($P < 0.05$), and in 18.7% of the low-moderate stenosis group on medical therapy vs. 14.9% receiving carotid endarterectomy. Disabling strokes occurred in 7.2% of high-moderate stenosis patients on medical therapy vs. 2.8% of patients receiving surgery ($P = 0.05$) and in 4.7% of the low-moderate stenosis group on medical therapy vs. 4.6% receiving surgery. Cox regression analysis demonstrated surgery to be most beneficial in men, those with recent strokes, those with recent hemispheric symptoms, and those taking 650 mg aspirin daily. Furthermore, patients with severe (70%-99%) stenosis carotid endarterectomy had only a 6.7% incidence of ipsilateral stroke at 8 years' follow-up.

Conclusion.—Carotid endarterectomy in patients with symptomatic stenosis of 50% to 69% reduces stroke risk by a modest but significant degree. In contrast, carotid endarterectomy in patients with less than 50% symptomatic stenosis is of little value. Furthermore, in patients with severe symptomatic carotid stenosis, the stroke risk reduction from carotid endarterectomy is very durable.

▶ This second installment of results from the NASCET trial further clarifies the role of carotid endarterectomy in patients with symptomatic carotid atherosclerosis. Patients with symptomatic stenoses greater than 50% are confirmed to benefit from carotid endarterectomy although the benefit is modest, whereas those with stenoses less than 50% do not. Furthermore, the results of the post-hoc analyses of the influence of various risk factors on the benefit of carotid endarterectomy are very intriguing, but must be viewed with caution. It is not surprising that the risk of stroke, and thereby the benefit of carotid endarterectomy, increases with the severity of the indicated symptom (stroke > hemispheric transient ischemic attack > amaurosis fugax). It is also intuitive that factors such as diabetes, contralateral occlusion, and hypertension would increase the risk of postoperative stroke, thereby limiting the stroke-risk reduction of carotid endarterectomy. In contrast, it remains unclear why left-sided disease should increase the risk of postoperative stroke and why women have a lower overall stroke risk than men, although this later finding was also seen in the Asymptomatic Carotid Atherosclerosis Study. Regardless, the results of this and other carotid endarterectomy trials continue to make appropriate selection of patients for carotid endarterectomy easier.

J.M. Seeger, M.D.

Comparison of North American Symptomatic Carotid Endarterectomy Trial and Population-based Outcomes for Carotid Endarterectomy

Hallett JW Jr, Pietropaoli JA Jr, Ilstrup DM, et al (Mayo Found, Rochester, Minn)

J Vasc Surg 27:845-851, 1998 13–2

Background.—The North American Symptomatic Carotid Endarterectomy Trial (NASCET) has recommended carotid endarterectomy (CEA) for treatment of transient ischemic attacks, nondisabling strokes, and ipsilateral high-grade stenosis in highly selected patients. It is not known whether the results of the NASCET can be achieved in an entire geographically defined population, but it is important to determine whether the NASCET recommendations are to be applied to community-dwelling patients.

Methods.—The medical records of all patients living in Olmsted County, Minnesota, who had undergone CEA for transient ischemic attacks or nondisabling stroke between 1970 and 1995 were reviewed. Survival rates to ipsilateral stroke after CEA were determined for all patients with symptoms. Results were compared with the results of the NASCET.

Results.—Two hundred ninety-seven patients (189 men and 108 women) underwent 322 CEAs during the study period. For 254 patients, transient ischemic attacks or nondisabling strokes were the indications for CEA. Survival without ipsilateral stroke was 97% at 2 years compared with 91% at 2 years in the NASCET. Furthermore, survival rates without an ipsilateral stroke were 93% at 5 years and 92% at 10 years after CEA for symptomatic lesions, and the rate of survival free of any stroke was 90% at 5 years and 80% at 10 years. The rate of perioperative stroke was 19.2% in patients older than 80 (vs. 2.2% in patients younger than 80 years), and the survival at 8 years in patients with diabetes mellitus was only 27% (vs. 67% in patients without diabetes).

Discussion.—Early outcome in patients with symptoms after CEA in this population-based study was similar to the early outcome of patients in the NASCET. Furthermore, results from this study demonstrate the long-term effectiveness of CEA in preventing stroke when the operation is performed by expert surgeons.

▶ Further documentation of the immediate and long-term benefit of CEA in symptomatic patients with greater than 70% carotid stenosis is presented in this population-based study from the Mayo Clinic. Most interesting are the high perioperative stroke risk in patients older than age 80 years of age (who were excluded in the NASCET trial) and the poor long-term survival of patients with diabetes mellitus. Thus, results similar to those reported in NASCET can be achieved by expert surgeons in community-dwelling patients but, as always, results from a specific group of patients (NASCET) cannot be assumed to apply to others such as symptomatic patients older than age 80.

J.M. Seeger, M.D.

Randomized Study of Carotid Angioplasty and Stenting Versus Carotid Endarterectomy: A Stopped Trial

Naylor AR, Bolia A, Abbott RJ, et al (Leicester Royal Infirmary, England)
J Vasc Surg 28:326-334, 1998 13–3

Objective.—The cost-effectiveness and safety of carotid endarterectomy (CEA) for symptomatic severe internal carotid artery disease has been called into question, and the use of the purportedly less expensive and safer carotid angioplasty (CA) procedure has been advocated. Results of a prospective, consecutive, randomized trial of CEA compared with CA for treatment of severe internal carotid artery disease are presented.

Methods.—Patients (aged 54-76 years) with ipsilateral 70% to 99% ICA stenosis were randomly allocated to receive CEA (n = 12), or CA (n = 11). Deaths or strokes (disabling or nondisabling) within 30 days were recorded.

Results.—Only 10 CEA patients and 7 CA patients were treated before the trial was suspended. Patients randomized to CEA experienced no short-term adverse events. In contrast, five of 7 patients randomized to CA had CA-related strokes.

Conclusion.—Compared with CEA, CA posed a significant risk of stroke. As a result, the study was stopped.

▶ The stroke risk associated with CA and stenting remains unclear. However, the results from case trials of highly selected patients treated by the developers of the procedure may significantly underestimate that stroke risk. Although this report of a randomized trial that was stopped because of strokes in 5 of the 7 patients undergoing CA could be an aberration, these results cannot entirely be discounted. At present, I find it difficult to recommend CA to any patient with carotid atherosclerosis who is not at very high risk for CEA.

J.M. Seeger, M.D.

Aneurysm

Concurrent Comparison of Endoluminal Versus Open Repair in the Treatment of Abdominal Aortic Aneurysms: Analysis of 303 Patients by Life Table Method

May J, White GH, Yu W, et al (Univ of Sydney, Australia)
J Vasc Surg 27:213-221, 1998 13–4

Objective.—The long-term outcome after endoluminal repair (ER) of abdominal aortic aneurysm (AAA) is not known, and concurrent comparison studies of ER and open repair (OR) have not been conducted. Results of a concurrent comparison of ER and OR in consecutive patients with AAA using life table analysis are presented.

Methods.—Primary elective ER (108 patients; 8 women; average age, 70) or OR (195 patients; 44 women; average age, 69) repair of AAA was performed on 303 patients between May 1992 and May 1996. ER patients were followed up with contrast-enhanced CT within the first 10 days, at 6 and 12 months, and annually thereafter. Outcomes were survival and successful AAA repair, which was defined for ER as continuing endograft function without leak or conversion to OR.

Results.—ER was initially successful in 95 patients (88%), whereas the remaining 13 in whom ER was attempted were converted to OR. There were 6 perioperative deaths (5.6%, 3 after initially successful ER procedures and 3 after conversion to OR) and 18 patients (26%) had significant postoperative complications. There were 10 late deaths, and 13 patients had ER repair failure due to endoleak (7 perioperative and 6 late). In the OR group, there were 11 perioperative deaths (5.6%) and 38 patients (20%) had significant postoperative complications. There were 10 late deaths, and one patient had a late OR repair failure due to an aortoenteric fistula. ER resulted in significantly shorter ICU stays and less blood loss than OR, but mortality and complications rates associated with the two procedures were equivalent. Furthermore, the incidence of long-term repair failure was significantly higher in the ER group (23% vs. 0.5%), and the probability of ER success at 3 years was only 71% by Kaplan-Meir analysis.

Conclusion.—ER of AAA is safe and potentially associated with less perioperative morbidity. However, OR remains the most reliable method of successfully managing AAA, and patients should be made aware of the higher failure rate associated with ER of AAA.

► This report presents the most complete picture of ER of AAA to date. From these data, it is clear that this procedure, even when those patients who require conversion to OR are included, is associated with less morbidity; the hospital length of stay, ICU stay, and blood loss were less in the ER group. Furthermore, although the operative mortality was equal between the 2 groups, approximately one half of the patients who underwent ER were at high risk for OR. However, it is also clear that aneurysm repair using the endoluminal approach is less secure and more prone to late failure because of endoleaks. Therefore, not unexpected with this new technique, "what you make on the popcorn, you lose on the peanuts." ER likely will find a place in the treatment of patients with AAA, but that place remains unclear to me at present. I hope that, before ER is made widely available, more careful studies with good long-term follow-up such as this one will be done to define the risks and benefits of this new procedure.

J.M. Seeger, M.D.

Clinical Consequences of Periprosthetic Leak After Endovascular Repair of Abdominal Aortic Aneurysm

Matsumura JS, for the Endovascular Technologies Investigators (Northwestern Univ, Chicago; et al)

J Vasc Surg 27:606-613, 1998 13–5

Objective.—One of the complications observed with endovascular repair of abdominal aortic aneurysm (AAA) is periprosthetic leak, no matter which device is used to effect repair. The risk factors, natural history, and clinical consequences for patients with such leaks were reviewed.

Methods.—Initial and follow-up angiograms, contrast-enhanced CT scans, abdominal duplex scans, and plain abdominal films were reviewed from 68 patients who underwent attempted tube endograft AAA repair between February 10, 1993 and January 24, 1995. Risk factors for periprosthetic endoleak were assessed.

Results.—Nine patients were converted to open repair, and the mean follow-up for the remaining 59 (who were successfully treated with the tube endograft device) was 27 months. Endoleaks were detected by the first postoperative CT scan in 28 patients (47%). Fourteen of these early endoleaks sealed spontaneously, 12 during the first year of follow-up and 2 during the second. Two additional endoleaks were sealed using endoluminal techniques. Late endoleaks developed in 4 patients, including 1 that had spontaneously sealed an early leak and 1 that had a persistent early leak. Spontaneous closure did not occur in any of the late leaks, and the patient with the late leak after spontaneous closure of an early leak suffered nonfatal aneurysm rupture. Five patients with persistent early endoleaks and the 2 patients with late endoleaks who did not have an early leak underwent graft explantation and surgical repairs, and one patient with a persistent early leak had a successful second endograft repair. All patients with persistent leaks had aneurysm enlargement unless the leak was repaired or the endograft was explanted. Migration of the device attachment system was significantly correlated with endoleak. Clinical outcome was not different for patients with persistent endoleaks compared with those who did not have endoleaks, except for the patient who suffered aneurysm rupture. However, 5 patients died of non–graft-related causes during follow-up (3 with persistent leaks), and 1 patient without a leak underwent endograft explanation and surgical aneurysm repair.

Conclusion.—Although initial endoleaks were common, half of them sealed spontaneously. In addition, patients with persistent leaks fared as well as patients without leaks. However, 1 patient with a persistent leak had a nonfatal aneurysm rupture, and aneurysm enlargement occurred in all patients with a persistent endoleak. Therefore, at a minimum, routine CT evaluation is necessary in patients with endoleaks after endovascular AAA repair.

► Endoleaks appear to develop in up to 40% of patients after endoluminal aneurysm repair and, if persistent or untreated, are associated with aneurysm enlargement and occasionally aneurysm rupture. Endoleaks that appear late are of greatest concern because these appear unlikely to seal spontaneously. These late leaks may occur in up to 20% of patients, and at present, it is not known whether there is a point after which late endoleaks will not occur. For now, endoluminal aneurysm repair is clearly less secure than open repair, and lifetime surveillance with contrast CT (or possibly color flow Doppler) is necessary after endoluminal repair of an AAA.

J.M. Seeger, M.D.

Continued Expansion of Aortic Necks After Endovascular Repair of Abdominal Aortic Aneurysms

Matsumura JS, for the EVT Investigators (Northwestern Univ, Chicago; et al)
J Vasc Surg 28:422-431, 1998 13–6

Objective.—Aortic neck dilation sometimes occurs after repair of an infrarenal abdominal aortic aneurysm (AAA) and continued dilation could lead to endoleak or catastrophic device failure after endoluminal aneurysm repair. However, this phenomenon and its progression have not been well studied. The rate of neck size enlargement after AAA repair with a tube endograft system, the duration of this phenomenon and its relationship to endoleak, endograft size, device migration, change in aneurysm size, attachment system failure, and preoperative neck diameter were investigated as part of a multi-institutional study of endoluminal repair of infrarenal aortic aneurysms.

Methods.—Between February 10, 1993 and January 24, 1995, 59 patients in 13 institutions received endovascular tube grafts for AAA repair. Endograft use was halted in January 1995 because of fractures detected in the metallic attachment system. Patients were followed up for an average of 27 months. Preoperative and postoperative CT scans were reviewed to determine proximal and distal aortic neck size. Annual neck expansion rates were calculated and related to endoleak rate, endograft size, device migration, aneurysm size change, attachment system failure, and preoperative neck diameter.

Results.—Aortic neck enlargement continued for at least 24 months after surgery and continues into the third year of follow-up. Mean neck dilations during the first and second years were 0.7 and 0.9 mm for the proximal neck and 1.7 and 1.9 mm for the distal neck. In 5 patients, distal neck size increased more than 6 mm over the pre-repair size, and in 3 there was also migration of the distal attachment system. Neck expansion rates were not correlated with neck dimension and initial neck size, endograft diameter, endograft sizing, and change in aneurysm size.

Conclusion.—Aortic neck expansion after AAA repair continues for at least 2 years, raising the likelihood of late failure after endoluminal AAA repair.

▶ The concern about long-term successful exclusion of aortic aneurysms with stent grafts remains real. This article, based on the EVT data, demonstrates significant expansion of the proximal and distal stent graft attachment sites over only a 2-year period. In 14% of the patients there was at least a 6-mm or more expansion of an attachment site, resulting in endoleaks, aneurysm enlargement, and even aneurysm rupture in 1 patient. At present, if I had an AAA, and was in good health, I would proceed with standard surgical repair so I would know that my aneurysm would be permanently repaired.

J.M. Seeger, M.D.

Impact of Transrenal Aortic Endograft Placement on Endovascular Graft Repair of Abdominal Aortic Aneurysms

Marin ML, Parsons RE, Hollier LH, et al (Mount Sinai School of Medicine, New York)

J Vasc Surg 28:638-646, 1998 13–7

Objective.—Many infrarenal abdominal aortic aneurysms (AAAs) do not have enough normal aorta immediately below the renal vessels to allow a secure, long-term attachment of the graft. Animal studies have demonstrated the feasibility of transrenal endograft attachment. Results of using a transrenal endograft attachment for repair of AAA with a Palmaz balloon expandable system in high-risk patients are reported.

Methods.—Fifty-three patients undergoing AAA repair with an endograft placed entirely below the renal artery (n = 16) or with a porous portion of an endograft attachment system placed across the renal arteries (n = 37)were reviewed. All repairs were done using a balloon expandable system similar to the Parodi device that consisted of a Palmaz balloon expandable stent sutured to a tapered 28 to 8 mm expandable polytetrafluoroethylene graft implanted in an aortofemoral, femoral/femoral configuration. Patients were followed up at 1 week, and at 3, 6, and 12 months with duplex ultrasonography and CT scans. Average length of follow-up was 10.3 months.

Results.—Significantly more proximal aortic endoleaks occurred in infrarenal endografts compared with the transrenal endografts. In addition, median serum creatinine levels before and after endografting were equivalent between the 2 groups except for 2 patients in whom the right renal artery was covered with a malpositioned transrenal endograft and a right kidney infarction occurred. Although these 2 patients had a significant rise in serum creatinine level, neither developed hypertension. Furthermore, significant renal compromise was not seen in any other patient despite symmetrical renal infarction (< 20%) demonstrated in 2 patients undergoing transrenal endograft placement by follow-up CT scan.

Conclusion.—Transrenal aortic endograft placement can reduce the risk of endoleaks in patients with AAAs and a short infrarenal aortic neck. However, inadvertent renal artery occlusion is a risk unless careful attention is paid to placement of the balloon expandable device. In addition, long-term follow-up will be necessary to determine whether late sequalae of this technique will affect renal function.

▶ Endograft fixation in the juxtarenal or even the suprarenal aorta would clearly allow expanded use of endoluminal aneurysm repair. This study demonstrates that placing a Palmaz stent across the renal orifices is usually (but not always) associated with minimal renal compromise. However, renal artery occlusion occurred in 2 patients in this study and follow-up is very short (< 1 year). For now, this approach may be useful in high-risk patients with short life expectancies. However, it must remain experimental and be used in only very selective patients until the risk of long-term renal compromise is clearly defined.

J.M. Seeger, M.D.

Mortality Results for Randomised Controlled Trial of Early Elective Surgery or Ultrasonographic Surveillance for Small Abdominal Aortic Aneurysms

Powell JT, for the UK Small Aneurysm Trial Participants (Charing Cross Hosp, London; et al)

Lancet 352:1649-1655, 1998 13–8

Purpose.—To avoid potentially fatal rupture of abdominal aortic aneurysms (AAAs), prophylactic surgical repair is recommended for aneurysms measuring more than 6.0 cm in diameter, which is about 3 times larger than the normal diameter. However, it remains unclear whether surgery is the best approach for smaller aneurysms. The risk of rupture is low for such aneurysms but may be decreased further by elective surgery; however, surgery carries a mortality of 5% to 6%. The impact of prophylactic repair of small AAAs on long-term mortality was assessed.

Methods.—The randomized, multicenter trial included 1,090 patients with asymptomatic AAAs measuring 4.0 to 5.5 cm in diameter. The patients were aged between 60 and 76 years and were fit for elective surgery. They were randomized to either early elective open surgery or ultrasound surveillance. In the ultrasound group, surgery was recommended if the AAA grew to exceed 5.5 cm in diameter, grew at a rate of more than 1 cm/yr, or became tender, or if iliac or thoracic aneurysm repair was required. Patients were followed-up for a mean of 4.6 years or to death, with mortality analyzed by intention to treat.

Results.—Cardiovascular risk factors were similar between groups. Surgery was performed according to protocol in 92% of patients assigned to early elective surgery and in 54% of those assigned to ultrasound surveillance. Median time to surgery was 2 months in the elective surgery group and 3 years in the ultrasound group. No significant difference was observed in mortality at 2, 4, or 6 years, or in overall mortality, which was about 33% in both groups by 6 years. Early elective surgery was associated with a 30-day operative mortality of nearly 6%. Though survival was initially worse in the early surgery group, it was later worse in the ultrasound surveillance group, with survival curves crossing over at about 3 years. Risk of death was not significantly affected by age, sex, or initial aneurysm size. For patients assigned to surveillance, the median aneurysm growth rate was 0.33 cm/yr.

Conclusions.—For patients with small, asymptomatic AAAs, early elective surgery does not improve the chances of long-term survival. Ultrasound surveillance is a safe alternative for aneurysms measuring 4.0 to 5.5 cm in diameter, with surgery suggested by an increase in diameter to 5.5 cm or by a rapid rate of growth. With either approach, about two thirds of patients will still be alive after 6 years. The results have important implications for aneurysm screening programs.

▶ In this carefully done randomized study, early surgery for AAAs between 4.0 and 5.5. cm in diameter was not shown to improve survival at 5 years compared with careful follow-up alone. However, most patients in the study had aneurysms less than 5.0 cm in size, and the follow-up in the surveillance group was rigorous (and unlikely to be duplicated in everyday practice). Furthermore, there was a trend toward improved survival in those patients with aneurysms more than 5.0 cm in size, and most patients in the surveillance group who survived had undergone aneurysm repair by the end of the study. Regardless, this study does confirm a low rupture rate for aneurysms less than 5 cm in size and raises serious questions about the benefit of surgical repair of very small (less than 5 cm) AAAs.

J.M. Seeger, M.D.

Oxygen Delivery Is an Important Predictor of Outcome in Patients With Ruptured Abdominal Aortic Aneurysms

Peerless JR, Alexander JJ, Pinchak AC, et al (Case Western Reserve Univ, Cleveland, Ohio)

Ann Surg 227:726-734, 1998 13–9

Introduction.—Previous studies have demonstrated higher levels of oxygen delivery (DO_2) to predict a lower risk of multiple organ dysfunction (MOD) and improved survival in high risk for septic general surgical patients. Patients with ruptured abdominal aortic aneurysms (AAAs) have blood loss without associated injury and do not have the same metabolic derangements that are associated with infection. However, they are also at high risk of development of MOD and death. The association between postoperative hemodynamic function, oxygen transport, and the occurrence of MOD were assessed and the usefulness of DO_2 was compared with previously identified predictors of outcome in patients with ruptured AAAs.

Methods.—Hemodynamic data were prospectively collected at 4-hour intervals in 57 consecutive patients (mean age, 70.5 years) who survived 24 hours after undergoing repair of infrarenal ruptured AAA. Patients were resuscitated to standard parameters of perfusion; MOD was based on assessment of failure in 6 organ systems. Patients with and without MOD were compared in measures of hemodynamic data, red blood cell requirements, colon ischemia, and organ failure.

Results.—Compared with patients without MOD, those in whom MOD developed had a significantly lower cardiac index and DO_2 for the first 12 hours after ruptured AAA repair; the difference was most notable at 8 hours. Furthermore, by regression analysis, the strongest predictors of MOD were DO_2, early onset of renal failure, and total number of red blood cells transfused.

Conclusion.—Compared with risk factors identified in earlier reports, DO_2 was an earlier and better predicator of MOD after a ruptured AAA. The inability to achieve a normal DO_2 in the first 8 hours after repair was strongly correlated with the development of MOD and a high mortality rate. Strategies focused on restoration of normal DO_2 may be beneficial in improving outcome in patients at high risk of MOD.

► Mortality after ruptured AAA is most commonly caused by MOD and DO_2 appears to be an early predictor of outcome after ruptured AAA. Unfortunately, DO_2 is likely a manifestation of the underlying cellular injury rather than an important mechanism in the development of MOD, as efforts to improve DO_2 do not appear to improve survival. Thus, prevention of AAA rupture by elective repair remains the only effective method of reducing the mortality associated with aneurysm disease of the aorta.

J.M. Seeger, M.D.

Renal/Mesenteric

Treatment of Ostial Renal-Artery Stenoses With Vascular Endoprostheses After Unsuccessful Balloon Angioplasty

Blum U, Krumme B, Flügel P, et al (Univ Hosp Freiburg, Germany)

N Engl J Med 336:459-465, 1997 13–10

Objective.—Results of balloon angioplasty for treatment of ostial renal artery stenosis have been unsatisfactory, with rates of stenosis recurrence ranging from 15% to 42%. Therefore, treatment of the obstruction with various stents has been recommended. Long-term clinical, duplex sonographic and angiographic results of treatment of ostial renal artery atheroma with stents were reported.

Methods.—After technical failure of conventional balloon angioplasty for ostial renal artery atherosclerotic lesions in 82 arteries in 75 patients with sustained hypertension, short Palmaz stents were implanted in 74 arteries in 68 patients (24 women), aged 31 to 80 years. Indications for stent placement were arteries with immediate elastic recoil after angioplasty, residual stenosis greater than 50%, and a trans-stenotic gradient greater than 20 mm Hg (63 arteries); re-stenosis (10 arteries); or dissection (1 artery). Patients were followed for an average of 27 months with duplex sonography, intra-arterial angiography, and blood pressure and serum creatinine measurements.

Results.—Initially, all stent placements were successful, with only minor hematomas occurring in 3 patients. Hypertension was reversed in 11 patients, improved in 42, and unchanged in 15. Serum creatinine levels stabilized and creatinine levels remained unchanged in a subgroup of patients with severe renal impairment. Duplex sonography diagnosed re-stenosis greater than 50% in 2 patients after 3 months, in 3 patients after 6 months, in 2 patients after 12 months, and in 1 patient after 24 months. Angiography demonstrated restenosis greater than 50% in 1 patient at 24 months. By Kaplan-Meier analysis, 57 patients were free of primary occlusion at 6 months.

Conclusion.—The use of endoluminal stents for ostial renal artery stenosis is a safe and effective treatment. A prospective comparative study of stent placement vs. surgery is recommended.

► It is clear that balloon angioplasty alone is inadequate for the treatment of patients with renovascular hypertension who have ostial renal artery lesions. Placement of short endoluminal stents at the time of angioplasty appears to improve the results in such patients, suggesting that this may be an appropriate alternative to surgical bypass. However, restenosis occurs in 20% to 40% of patients at a mean follow-up of approximately 2 years (10% by arteriography and 20% renal duplex in this study), and only 71% of patients had hypertensive improvement, so that the effectiveness and durability of balloon angioplasty and stenting remains inferior to surgical renal artery repair. Thus, once again, endovascular treatment of arterial disease is a trade-off between decreased initial morbidity and decreased effectiveness and long-term durability of treatment.

J.M. Seeger, M.D.

Prophylactic Repair of Renal Artery Stenosis Is Not Justified in Patients Who Require Infrarenal Aortic Reconstruction

Williamson WK, Abou-Zamzam AM Jr, Moneta GL, et al (Oregon Health Sciences Univ, Portland)

J Vasc Surg 28:14-22, 1998 13–11

Objective.—It is controversial whether prophylactic revascularization of incidentally discovered asymptomatic renal artery stenosis (ARAS) is of value in patients who undergo infrarenal aortic reconstruction. The long-term functional outcome of ARAS was evaluated in patients who underwent reconstruction of the infrarenal aorta for occlusive or aneurysmal disease.

Methods.—Preoperative aortograms were available for evaluation in 171 of 200 consecutive patients who required infrarenal aortic reconstruction between 1985 and 1990 at the Portland Veterans Affairs Hospital. The patients had an average age of 63, and 99% were men. Patients were stratified according to degree of renal artery stenosis into 5 groups: group A, 0%; group B, 1% to 29%; group C, 30% to 69%; group D, 70% to 99% (unilateral and bilateral); and group E, occluded. No patient had evidence of renovascular hypertension or ischemic nephropathy. Blood pressure, antihypertensive medications, and creatinine level were recorded at baseline and assessed during the follow-up period, which averaged 6.3 years. Baseline and follow-up angiograms were reviewed by someone blinded to all preoperative and follow-up data.

Results.—There were 32 patients in group D, 24 with unilateral and 8 with bilateral ARAS of 70% to 99% and 3 patients in group E, each with occlusion of 1 artery and 50% to 70% stenosis in the contralateral artery. According to multiple regression analysis, older age, preoperative hypertension, and coronary artery disease were significantly associated with a stenosis of more than 70%. At follow-up, mean systolic blood pressure and the number of antihypertensive medications being used were higher for patients with 70% or more ARAS, but diastolic blood pressure and serum creatinine levels were not significantly different. In addition, patients with 70% or more ARAS did not have decreased survival at 7 years, and none required dialysis.

Conclusion.—Although patients with high grade renal artery stenosis undergoing aortic reconstruction require increased antihypertensive medication for blood pressure control during follow-up, survival and renal function are unaffected. Thus, prophylactic renal revascularization in asymptomatic patients confers no additional benefit in patients who need infrarenal aortic reconstruction.

► I have always felt that modification of the natural history of an ARAS was the weakest indication for renal revascularization. This is because it is clear that addition of a renal artery bypass to aortic reconstruction increases the risk of the procedure, whereas the risk of leaving an ARAS alone is largely unknown. This study suggests that the clinical significance (progression to renal failure, mortality) of an ARAS is minimal, although the retrospective nature of this study and the small number of patients with significant renal stenosis evaluated precluded any definitive conclusions. Balloon angioplasty of asymptomatic renal artery lesions, does reduce the risk of treatment of these lesions which could change the risk benefit ratio in favor of treatment of ARAS. However, only carefully controlled prospective studies of this problem will determine whether treatment of these lesions in any manner is indicated.

J.M. Seeger, M.D.

The Clinical Course of Asymptomatic Mesenteric Arterial Stenosis

Thomas JH, Blake K, Pierce GE, et al (Univ of Kansas Med Ctr, Kansas City)

J Vasc Surg 27:840-844, 1998 13–12

Objective.—The incidence of subsequent symptom development in patients with asymptomatic significant mesenteric artrial occlusive disease remains unclear. The purpose of this study was to identify angiographic findings and clinical factors that may contribute to the development of acute or chronic mesenteric ischemia in patients with asymptomatic mesenteric artery stenosis.

Methods.—Between 1989 and 1996, 980 consecutive aortograms were reviewed within 1 week of being obtained to identify patients with more than 50% stenosis in at least 1 mesenteric artery. Eighty-two such patients who had no current symptoms of mesenteric ischemia then completed questionnaires about symptoms of acute or chronic mesenteric ischemia at 6-month intervals. Follow-up ranged from 1 to 6 years with an average of 2.6 years.

Results.—Ten patients were lost to follow-up and 12 were subsequently excluded because they had mild (< 50%) disease. Of the remaining 60 patients, 4 developed symptoms of acute or chronic mesenteric ischemia and one died from bowel necrosis. All of these patients had severe disease (> 75% stenosis or occlusion) of all the mesenteric vessels so that acute or chronic mesenteric ischemia developed in 27% of the 15 patients with severe disease developed during follow-up. Furthermore, of the 15 patients with this degree of disease, 13 (87%) died, had mesenteric ischemia, or experienced other abdominal symptoms during follow-up. The overall mortality in the entire group during follow-up was 40%.

Conclusion.—Patients with significant 3-vessel disease should be considered for prophylactic mesenteric arterial reconstruction, especially when other aortic procedures are planned. In contrast, those with 1- or 2-vessel disease should be managed expectantly.

▶ Management of asymptomatic mesenteric arterial occlusive disease remains controversial. This study demonstrates that patients with severe stenosis in all 3 mesenteric vessels have a significant risk of developing mesenteric ischemia (27% over 2.5 years). The authors recommend that such patients should undergo prophylactic mesenteric reconstruction. I would agree and even would consider prophylactic mesenteric reconstruction as an isolated procedure in selected good risk patients because symptoms of chronic mesenteric ischemia are not always specific and do not always develop prior to acute bowel infarction.

J.M. Seeger, M.D.

Peripheral Vascular

Patient Recovery After Infrainguinal Bypass Grafting for Limb Salvage
Nicoloff AD, Taylor LM Jr, McLafferty RB, et al (Oregon Health Sciences Univ, Portland)
J Vasc Surg 27:256-266, 1998 13–13

Background.—The results of infrainguinal bypass surgery for limb salvage are typically analyzed in terms of graft patency, limb salvage, and patient survival rates, with little attention given to functional outcomes. Ideally, such surgery should culminate in restoration of premorbid functional status, including ambulation and independent living, with no recurrence of limb ischemia or repeat surgery. A retrospective analysis was performed to determine the frequency of such ideal results in patients undergoing infrainguinal bypass surgery for limb salvage.

Patients.—The review included 112 consecutive patients undergoing initial infrainguinal bypass for limb salvage. The patients were 56 men and 56 women with a mean age of 66 years. The mean follow-up after surgery was 42 months.

Outcomes.—Perioperative mortality rate was 6%, and the wound complication rate was 24%. Five-year graft patency rate by life table analysis was 77%, limb salvage rate was 87%, and patient survival was 49%. After surgery, 88% of patients were living independently at home, and 92% were ambulatory. At last follow-up or at death, 73% of patients who had been living independently at home before their limb salvage operation continued to live at home, and 70% of patients who were ambulatory before the procedure were still ambulatory. The mean wound healing time was 4 months; however, 22% of patients had not reached complete wound healing at last follow-up or at death. Fifty-four percent of patients required additional operations to maintain graft patency, to treat wound complications, or to treat recurrent or contralateral ischemia, with a mean of 1.6 operations per patient. Twenty-three percent of patients underwent amputation of the index or contralateral extremity. The rate of ideal results—including long-term symptom relief, maintenance of functional status, and no recurrences or repeat surgeries—was only 14%.

Conclusions.—Despite low perioperative mortality and good long-term graft patency and limb salvage rates the results of infrainguinal bypass grafting for limb salvage are rarely ideal. Most of these patients require additional treatment as time goes on, and they often experience persistent or recurrent symptoms until death. Even if the initial bypass operation is successful, patients also remain at risk of major amputation. Regardless, infrainguinal bypass procedures do achieve clinically important palliation in patients with limb-threatening ischemia, despite the low rate of ideal results.

▶ This interesting article confirms what we all know from experience, that infrainguinal bypass for limb salvage is seldom associated with an ideal outcome, and that recurrent ischemia (in either lower extremity) and repeat reconstructive procedures are common. Furthermore, in this study, only 68% of patients who were ambulatory and living at home prior to surgery maintained that status. This occurred despite very acceptable results for operative mortality, bypass graft patency, and limb salvage. Most patients clearly prefer attempted limb salvage to primary amputation. However, faced with these sobering results, we clearly must carefully select patients for infrainguinal bypass for limb salvage and fully inform them of the expected results.

J.M. Seeger, M.D.

Fate of the Contralateral Leg After Infrainguinal Bypass

Tarry WC, Walsh DB, Birkmeyer NJO, et al (Dartmouth-Hitchcock Med Ctr, Lebanon, NH)
J Vasc Surg 27:1039-1048, 1998 13–14

Objective.—About 25% of patients undergoing infrainguinal bypass eventually require vascular intervention in the other leg. The natural course of the contralateral leg was delineated, and factors predictive of intervention in that leg were identified in a prospective review.

Methods.—Records of 450 patients who underwent infrainguinal bypass for occlusive disease between January 1987 and August 1996 were reviewed. Patients with bilateral disease or contralateral limb-threatening ischemia were excluded. A total of 383 patients (60% men), aged 33 to 95, were studied for an average of 38 months. Outcome measures were survival and subsequent interventions in the contralateral leg.

Results.—Comorbid conditions included diabetes in 54% and coronary artery disease (CAD) in 50%. The initial operation was performed because of limb threat in 90% of the patients. Intervention in the other leg was necessary in 77 patients (20%) at an average follow-up of 31 months for a rate of 13% at 2 years and 30% at 5 years after the initial surgery by life table analysis. Intervention consisted of amputation in 13 patients (17%), and infrainguinal bypass in 64 patients (83%). Risk factors for intervention in the other leg were younger age (relative risk [RR], 2.2), diabetes (RR, 2.4), CAD (RR, 1.8), and lower ankle brachial index (ABI) in the other leg at initial surgery (RR, 2.1). According to the Cox regression model, 8% of the patients without risk factors and 67% of the patients with risk factors would require contralateral intervention at 5 years. There were 167 deaths during the follow-up period, and the overall survival rate after the initial bypass was 76% at 2 years and 51% at 5 years. Survival free of intervention in the contralateral leg was 68% at 2 years and 37% at 5 years, and survival after intervention in the contralateral leg was 64% at 2 years and 33% at 5 years. Lower survival was predicted by diabetes, older age, lower initial ABI, and dialysis-dependent renal failure.

Conclusion.—Diabetes, lower ABI, CAD, and older age were predictive of subsequent intervention in the contralateral leg after infrainguinal bypass and risk factors are additive. This information is helpful in determining instances in which preservation of the contralateral saphenous vein is important and in identifying patients who need careful follow-up.

▶ Several factors are changing the dictum of using the "best" available conduit for infrainguinal bypass when the ipsilateral saphenous vein is absent. Studies such as this have shown a high rate of subsequent need for contralateral bypass, particularly in patients with diabetes mellitus. Furthermore, studies of bypasses done with the use of an alternative vein (arm vein, lesser saphenous vein, superficial femoral vein) have demonstrated good long-term graft function. As suggested by the authors of this study and by Dr. Frank LoGerfo in a discussion of this paper, when faced with a patient with diabetes mellitus, especially one who also has symptomatic CAD, I use alternative veins for conduit for an infrainguinal bypass when the ipsilateral saphenous vein is inadequate.

J.M. Seeger, M.D.

Warfarin Improves the Outcome of Infrainguinal Vein Bypass Grafting at High Risk for Failure

Sarac TP, Huber TS, Back MR, et al (Univ of Florida, Gainesville)
J Vasc Surg 28:446-457, 1998 13–15

Objective.—The effect of long-term anticoagulation therapy after autogenous vein infrainguinal revascularization on patency and limb salvage rates is not known. Results of postoperative anticoagulation therapy in patients at high risk of graft failure were prospectively evaluated in a randomized study.

Methods.—Patients at high risk for graft occlusion (n = 56) were allocated to long-term anticoagulation therapy with warfarin plus aspirin (WAR) (n = 32, 37 grafts) or aspirin alone (n = 24, 27 grafts). All patients received 325 mg aspirin daily, and patients randomized to WAR were

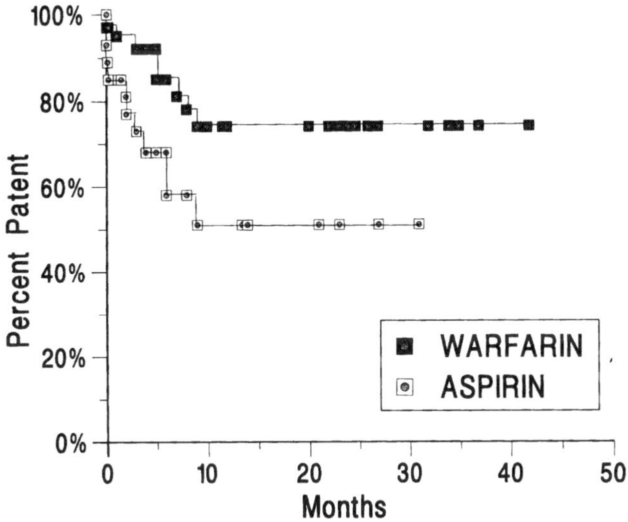

FIGURE 1.—Primary patency rate with Kaplan-Meier method (log-rank test = 0.04). *Dashed lines* indicate standard error greater than 10%. (Courtesy of Sarac TP, Huber TS, Back MR, et al: Warfarin improves the outcome of infrainguinal vein bypass grafting at high risk for failure. *J Vasc Surg* 28:446-457, 1998.)

given standard heparin therapy immediately after surgery followed by warfarin therapy to maintain the international normalizing ratio between 2 and 3. Perioperative blood transfusions, complications, graft patency rates, limb salvage rates, and survival rates were compared statistically.

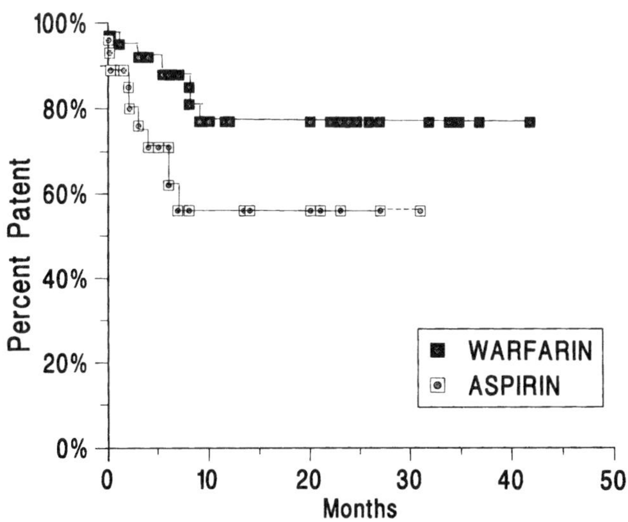

FIGURE 2.—Primary assisted patency rate with Kaplan-Meier method (log-rank test = 0.05). (Courtesy of Sarac TP, Huber TS, Back MR, et al: Warfarin improves the outcome of infrainguinal vein bypass grafting at high risk for failure. *J Vasc Surg* 28:446-457, 1998.)

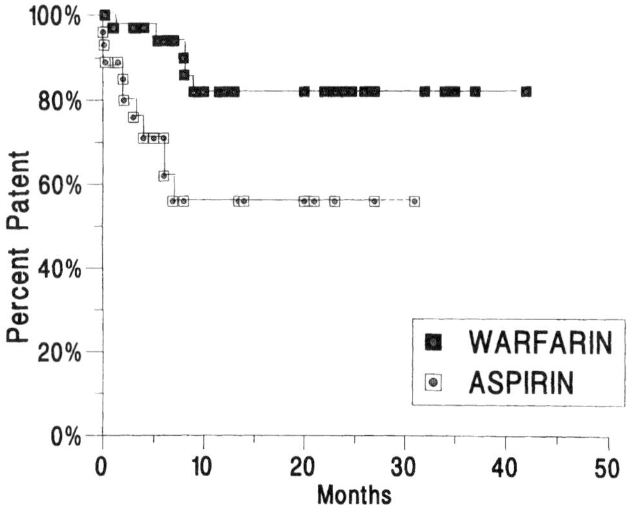

FIGURE 3.—Secondary patency rate with Kaplan-Meier method (log-rank test = 0.01). (Courtesy of Sarac TP, Huber TS, Back MR, et al: Warfarin improves the outcome of infrainguinal vein bypass grafting at high risk for failure. *J Vasc Surg* 28:446-457, 1998.)

Results.—Before discharge, there was 1 death (in the WAR group), 5 graft occlusions (4 in the aspirin group and 1 in the WAR group), and 3 amputations (all in the aspirin group), so that immediate (7-day) primary graft patency and limb salvage rates were higher in the WAR group. Patients in the WAR group also had a significantly higher incidence of

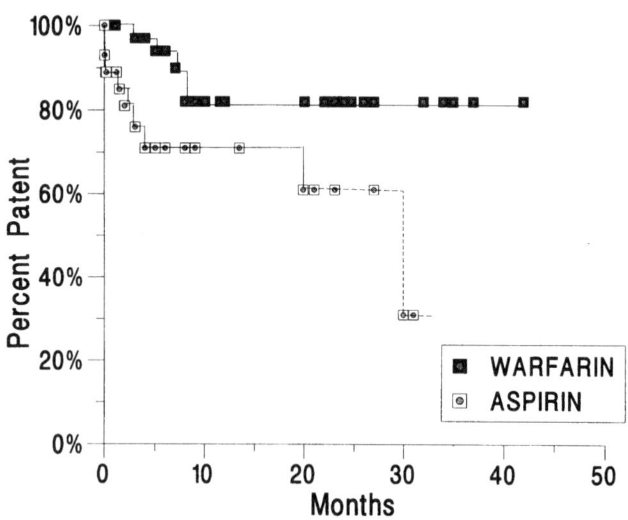

FIGURE 4.—Limb salvage rate with Kaplan-Meier method (log-rank test = 0.02). *Dashed lines* indicate standard error greater than 10%. (Courtesy of Sarac TP, Huber TS, Back MR, et al: Warfarin improves the outcome of infrainguinal vein bypass grafting at high risk for failure. *J Vasc Surg* 28:446-457, 1998.)

postoperative wound hematoma, but numbers of both groups had similar packed red-cell use, nonhemorrhagic wound complication rates, and overall complication rates. Both groups had similar cumulative 5-year survival rates and long-term hemorrhagic complication rates as well. Furthermore, the 3-year primary graft patency rate, assisted graft patency rate, secondary graft patency rate, and limb salvage rate were significantly higher in the WAR group than in the aspirin group (Figs 1 through 4).

Conclusion.—Compared with aspirin alone, anticoagulation therapy with warfarin improves the 3-year graft patency and limb salvage rates for patients at high risk for graft failure undergoing infrainguinal vein bypass grafts.

▶ This study from our group confirms that long-term anticoagulation with warfarin improves both graft patency and limb salvage in the subset of patients at high risk of graft failure. Although this may not have been surprising, these data and the finding that long-term hemorrhagic complications were limited strengthen the recommendation for routine use of this therapy in such patients.

J.M. Seeger, M.D.

Duplex Ultrasound Scanning Defines Operative Strategies for Patients With Limb-threatening Ischemia

Ligush J Jr, Reavis SW, Preisser JS, et al (Wake Forest Univ, Winston-Salem, NC)

J Vasc Surg 28:482-491, 1998 13–16

Introduction.—Conventional arteriography (CA) remains the standard preoperative imaging study for planning lower-extremity arterial reconstructive procedures. Color flow duplex ultrasound arterial scanning (DUSAS) has been proposed as an alternative to CA, and several studies have compared the accuracy of the 2 techniques with one another in terms of their accuracy in defining infrainguinal arterial occlusive disease. However, the role of DUSAS in planning lower extremity arterial reconstruction remains unclear. This prospective study compared DUSAS with CA for preoperative planning in patients undergoing infrainguinal reconstruction for critical lower-extremity ischemia.

Methods.—The study included 36 patients undergoing a total of 40 vascular reconstructions for SVS/ISCVS grade II or III chronic lower-extremity ischemia. All but 2 patients were initially evaluated using DUSAS, from the aorta to the pedal vessels. Based on this study, the adequacy of arterial inflow was assessed, and a distal target vessel for bypass was determined. The patients then underwent conventional lower-extremity angiography, and an independent surgical plan was made without knowledge of the DUSAS findings. These 2 preoperative revascularization strategies were compared with the actual operation performed, and the ability of DUSAS and CA to predict the correct operation was determined.

Results.—Eighty-three percent of the actual operations performed were correctly predicted by DUSAS vs. 90% by CA. The difference between correct operations predicted by these 2 studies was not significant by the McNemar test. Six of the 7 incorrect predictions by DUSAS were correctly predicted by CA, and 3 of the 4 incorrect predictions by CA were predicted by DUSAS. Furthermore, only 1 artery identified as an adequate target for bypass by DUSAS was found to be inadequate, and this artery was identified as adequate by CA as well.

Conclusions.—DUSAS is a reliable technique for predicting operative revascularization strategy in patients with critical lower-limb ischemia, and vessels judged adequate on the basis of DUSAS are almost always suitable for bypass at operation. The authors call for a prospective study of lower-extremity revascularization performed solely on the basis of DUSAS or with adjuvant intraoperative angiography.

▶ Although CA is familiar and comforting, it is becoming increasingly clear that, in many patients requiring intervention for peripheral vascular disease, it is unnecessary. It is also expensive, associated with risks, and not always accurate. Many of us have given up CA in most patients prior to carotid endarterectomy and aneurysm repair. Likely, in the next few years, we will do the same for patients with occlusive disease, thus saving our patients time, discomfort, and money.

J.M. Seeger, M.D.

Distal Lower Extremity Arteries: Evaluation With Two-dimensional MR Digital Subtraction Angiography

Lee HM, Wang Y, Sostman HD, et al (Cornell Univ, New York)
Radiology 207:505-512, 1998 13–17

Background.—Two-dimensional time-of-flight (TOF) MR angiography allows imaging of the tibial run-off vessels of the calf and foot. However, various artifacts lead to reduced image quality and diagnostic accuracy. Two-dimensional MR digital subtraction angiography potentially avoids these limitations. MR digital subtraction angiography was compared with TOF MR angiography for imaging of distal lower-extremity arteries.

Methods.—Twenty-three consecutive patients undergoing MR angiography of the foot and ankle for clinical indications were studied prospectively. Thirty-seven extremities were imaged with both 2-dimensional TOF MR angiography and MR digital subtraction angiography. The scans were read in a randomized, blinded fashion, with attention to 7 potential arterial segments and the number of digital arteries visualized. The 2 studies were compared for overall image quality and for the capability to demonstrate patent arterial segments.

Results.—Both patent arterial segments and digital arteries were better imaged by MR digital subtraction angiography than by TOF MR angiography. The image quality was also higher with MR digital subtraction angiography.

Conclusions.—Two-dimensional MR digital subtraction angiography is more effective than TOF MR angiography in demonstrating patent arterial segments in the tibial run-off vessels. The authors call for larger studies using conventional angiography to establish the diagnostic accuracy of MR digital subtraction angiography.

▶ The evaluation of lower-extremity arterial occlusive disease using MR arteriography is also improving. I suspect that in a few years standard contrast arteriography will be used to evaluate very few patients before vascular reconstructive procedures.

J.M. Seeger, M.D.

Effect of Cilostazol on Walking Distances in Patients With Intermittent Claudication Caused by Peripheral Vascular Disease

Money SR, Herd JA, Isaacsohn JL, et al (Ochsner Clinic, New Orleans, La; Methodist Hosp, Houston; Metabolic & Atherosclerosis Research Ctr, Cincinnati, Ohio; et al)

J Vasc Surg 27:267-275, 1998 13–18

Objective.—There are few effective medical treatments for the severe functional impairment experienced by patients with intermittent claudication (IC) caused by peripheral arterial occlusive disease. Whether treatment with cilostazol (a drug with vasodilator, antiplatelet, antiproliferative, and prostacyclin-enhancing properties), would increase walking distance in patients with IC was evaluated in a double-blind, randomized multicenter study.

Methods.—Cilostazol (100 mg twice daily) (n = 119) or placebo (n = 120) was administered for 16 weeks to patients (33% female), aged 41 to 91, with IC. Safety assessments were performed at weeks 2, 4, 8, 12, and 16, and variable-grade, constant-speed treadmill testing was performed at 2 screening visits and at weeks 8, 12, and 16. Functional status assessments were also made with use of the Medical Outcomes Questionnaire (SF-36) and the Walking Impairment Questionnaire (WIQ). Claudication symptoms were assessed by physicians and patients at week 16.

Results.—Patients in the treatment group walked significantly farther than patients in the placebo group at all time points (96.4 vs. 31.4 meters at 16 weeks). Furthermore, walking difficulty was decreased in the treatment group and unchanged in the placebo group. SF-36 and WIQ scores for the treatment group were significantly higher than for the placebo group and investigator and patient assessments also favored the treatment group. Ankle brachial index improved in the treatment group from 0.64 at baseline to 0.70 at 16 weeks, but was essentially unchanged in the placebo group (0.68 at baseline vs. 0.69 at 16 weeks).

Conclusion.—Cilostazol significantly improved walking speed, distance, and comfort in patients with IC.

► I fully expect a salesman for cilostazol to appear in my office soon with a copy of this study in hand. However, I remain unconvinced that cilostazol will not be the pentoxifylline of the '90s. As seen in similar trials of other treatments of patients with IC, both the placebo and treatment groups improved during the study with the improvement in the cilostazol group being only marginally, although statistically, significantly greater. Ankle brachial indices in the cilostazol group also increased, which could not be explained and suggested that the groups may not have been well matched. Although this new drug may eventually be shown to have benefit in patients with IC, for now I will continue to use risk factor modification and exercise as my first line of treatment for these patients.

J.M. Seeger, M.D.

Venous

Superior Maturation and Patency of Primary Brachiocephalic and Transposed Basilic Vein Arteriovenous Fistulae in Patients With Diabetes

Hakaim AG, Nalbandian M, Scott T (Boston Univ)

J Vasc Surg 27:154-157, 1998 13–19

Objective.—The classic approach to establishing vascular access for chronic hemodialysis has been the creation of a primary radial artery–to–cephalic vein arteriovenous fistula (RCAVF), if a suitable forearm cephalic vein can be identified. However, although RCAVFs remain patent in patients with diabetes mellitus, they usually do not mature sufficiently to provide adequate vascular access. Other options include upper-arm brachiocephalic arteriovenous fistulae (BCAVFs) and transposed basilic vein arteriovenous fistulae (TBAVFs). These 3 fistula types in 2 vascular access sites (forearm and arm) were compared for primary patency rate and degree of maturation in patients with a history of diabetes mellitus.

Methods.—The study included 40 men and 18 women (mean age, 61 years) with type I or type II diabetes who underwent creation of an autogenous arteriovenous fistula as initial access for hemodialysis. An RCAVF was created in 10 patients, a BCAVF in 22 patients, and a TBAVF in 26 patients. The initial approach to locating a suitable vein was by physical examination under tourniquet compression. If no forearm or upper-cephalic veins with a diameter of 2 mm could be identified, venography was performed to identify a vein for use in creating a TBAVF. Fistula maturation and patency rates were compared between groups.

Results.—Seventy percent of RCAVFs failed to mature, compared with 27% of BCAVFs and 0% of TBAVFs. The 18-month cumulative primary patency rate was 33% for RCAVFs, 78% for BCAVFs, and 79% for TBAVFs. The 3 groups were similar in age, sex, mortality, aspirin use, erythropoietin use, hematocrit levels, history of congestive heart failure, and of peripheral vascular disease.

Conclusions.—For diabetic patients requiring vascular access for hemodialysis, RCAVFs have low maturation and cumulative patency rates compared with BCAVFs and RBAVFs. With their greater maturation and improved patency, BCAVFs and TBAVFs are the preferred autogenous conduits in diabetic patients with renal failure. More study is needed to determine why RCAVFs fail to mature in patients with diabetes.

▶ We too have tended to use autogenous upper arm arteriovenous fistulas for dialysis access in patients with diabetes mellitus, and the superior patency and maturation rates described in this paper confirm that approach. Why forearm arteriovenous fistulas fail to mature in patents with diabetes mellitus remains unclear, but may be related to forearm arterial disease, as suggested by the authors.

J.M. Seeger, M.D.

Suprarenal Filter Placement

Greenfield LJ, Proctor MC (Univ of Michigan, Ann Arbor)

J Vasc Surg 28:432-438, 1998 13–20

Objective.—The location of vena caval filter placement may influence the complications associated with the procedure. The clinical outcomes of patients with Greenfield filters placed in the suprarenal (SR) and infrarenal (IR) inferior vena cava (IVC) were prospectively determined.

Methods.—Outcome data were prospectively collected from 1,932 patients undergoing IVC filters. Data included results of color flow Doppler scans of the IVC and lower extremities, anteroposterior and later abdominal radiographs, and history and physical examination to determine lower extremity edema, coloration, and need for support hose. Filters were placed in the IR location in 1,784 patients (92.4%) and in the SR location in 148 (7.6%). Outcome data were available in 749 patients (42%) with IR placement and 73 patients (49%) with SR.

Results.—The rate of pulmonary embolism was 8% after SR placement and 4% after IR placement. The short-term caval occlusion rate was 5% after SR placement (vs. 4% for IR), and the long-term occlusion rate was 2.7% after SR placement. Complication rates for SR and IR placement were similar. The mean survival for patients undergoing SR placement was 56 months, slightly longer than the 53 months survival for patients undergoing IR placement. Survival was significantly related to underlying diagnosis and indication for placement. There was no significant association between survival and recurrent pulmonary embolism. Only 1 patient developed new evidence of venous disease after SR placement.

Conclusion.—SR placement is safe and effective for treatment of caval thrombosis, with morbidity and mortality rates similar to those for IR placement.

▶ This study of a relatively large number of patients assures us that SR placement of a Greenfield filter is safe and effective. The risks of SR filter placement, including renal or hepatic vein thrombosis, were minimal. The incidence of recurrent pulmonary embolism was somewhat higher after SR filter placement, but this appears to be due to inclusion of results from placement of a SR filter in patients who had recurrent pulmonary embolism after placement of an IR filter.

J.M. Seeger, M.D.

A Prospective Controlled Study of the Efficacy of Short-term Anticoagulation Therapy in Patients With Deep Vein Thrombosis of the Lower Extremity

AbuRahma AF, Stickler DL, Robinson PA (West Virginia Univ, Charleston; Boehringer Ingelheim Pharmaceuticals Inc, Ridgefield, Conn)

J Vasc Surg 28:630-637, 1998 13–21

Objective.—There is no general agreement about the duration of anticoagulant therapy for patients with deep vein thrombosis (DVT). The results of a prospective controlled study of short-term vs. conventional long-term anticoagulant therapy in patients with DVT of the leg are presented.

Methods.—Between January 1987 and January 1995, 105 symptomatic patients with unilateral DVT of the leg were treated initially with anticoagulant therapy consisting of intravenous standard heparin followed by warfarin on days 3 to 5 to obtain an international normalizing ratio (INR) of 2 to 3. Warfarin was then continued for either 3 months (group A, n = 54), or 6 weeks (group B, n = 51). Clinical examinations and duplex imaging studies were performed at 6 weeks, 3 and 6 months, and every 6 months thereafter. Patients were followed up for an average of 59 months. Risk factors for DVT were determined, and complications were recorded. Post-thrombotic syndrome (PTS), and the presence of chronic postphlebitic changes on duplex ultrasonography with or without the clinical signs, were recorded.

Results.—Eleven group A (long-term warfarin) patients and 7 group B (short-term warfarin) patients were excluded from the analysis. Immediate complications occurred in 4 group A patients (2 with pulmonary embolism and 2 with significant bleeding) and in 3 group B patients (1 with pulmonary embolism and 2 with bleeding). Duration of hospitalization was significantly shorter for group B patients than for group A patients (5 vs. 8 days, respectively). There were 3 late deaths in group A and 2 in group B. PTS developed in 18 of the group A patients (42%) and in 20 of the group B patients (46%). Similar numbers of group A and B patients also had recurrent venous thromboembolic events (23% and 20%, respectively). Two group A patients had late complications (1 with hemorrhage and 1 with Coumadin necrosis) as a result of warfarin therapy. Recurrent DVT or PTS was significantly more common in patients with cancer than in those without cancer, and the incidence of these problems in such patients was lower in group A compared with group B patients.

Conclusion.—Short-term and long-term anticoagulant therapy for DVT are equally effective, except for patients with cancer. Because of the complications and higher costs seen with longer-term anticoagulation therapy, short-term therapy may be less risky.

▶ Although the conclusions of this study must be viewed in light of its small size, its results are intriguing. With the exception of patients with cancer, the risk of recurrent DVT was low and was unaffected by the length of warfarin anticoagulation (6 weeks vs. 3 months). Furthermore, the risks of postthrombotic syndrome symptoms were also unaffected by the length of anticoagulation. If these results can be confirmed, it would certainly simplify treatment of DVT and reduce its risk and cost.

J.M. Seeger, M.D.

Orally Administered Heparin for Preventing Deep Venous Thrombosis

Gonze MD, Manord JD, Leone-Bay A, et al (Ochsner Med Institutions, New Orleans, La; Emisphere Technologies Inc, Tarrytown, NY)

Am J Surg 176:176-178, 1998 13–22

Objective.—Heparin has a large molecular size that compromises absorption after oral administration. The synthetic acetylated amino acid molecule sodium *N*-(8-[2-hydroxybenzoyl]amino) caprylate (SNAC) facilitates gastrointestinal absorption of heparin. Oral heparin administration could have major advantages over other therapeutics options for anticoagulation. A rat model was used to evaluate an oral combination of SNAC and heparin for the prevention of venous thrombosis.

Methods.—Sprague-Dawley rats were assigned to receive either oral saline, oral SNAC, oral heparin, oral SNAC with heparin, or IV heparin. Thirty minutes after this treatment, the exposed internal jugular vein was bathed in a sclerosant mixture for 2 minutes. Two hours later, the vein was examined for the presence or absence of thrombus, and, if thrombus was present, the vein was excised and the thrombus weighed. The incidence of deep venous thrombosis and the thrombus weights were then compared among groups. In addition, activated partial thromboplastin times at 30 minutes after treatment were compared for animals receiving oral SNAC, oral heparin, and SNAC with heparin.

Results.—Venous thrombosis developed in 89% of the control group vs. 25% of the SNAC-with-heparin group and 11% of the IV heparin group ($P < 0.01$) (Fig 1). Furthermore, the mean thrombus weight was reduced in both the SNAC-with-heparin and IV heparin groups (Fig 2) compared

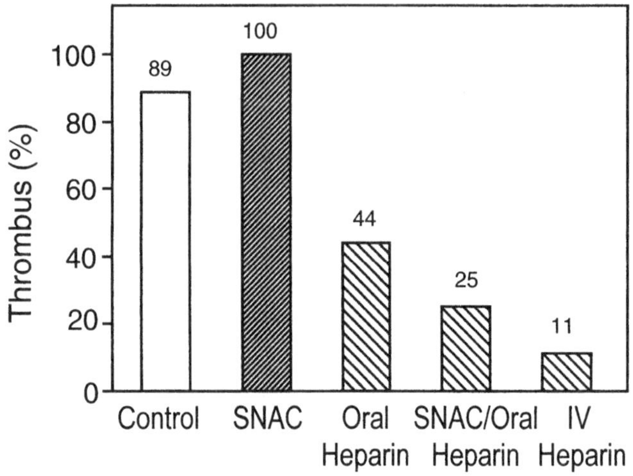

FIGURE 1.—Administration of combination SNAC and heparin significantly reduced the incidence of deep venous thrombosis compared with controls, and SNAC-only and oral heparin–only groups. The combination of SNAC and heparin was as effective as the IV heparin. (Reprinted from Gonze MD, Manord JD, Leone-Bay A, et al: Orally administered heparin for preventing deep venous thrombosis. *Am J Surg* 176:176-178. Copyright 1998, with permission from Excerpta Medica Inc.)

with controls. Activated partial prothrombin times were also significantly increased with oral SNAC and heparin but unaffected by oral SNAC and oral heparin alone.

Conclusions.—Experiments in rats suggest that oral treatment with a combination of SNAC and heparin may be as effective as IV heparin in preventing venous thrombosis. Further study is needed to define the

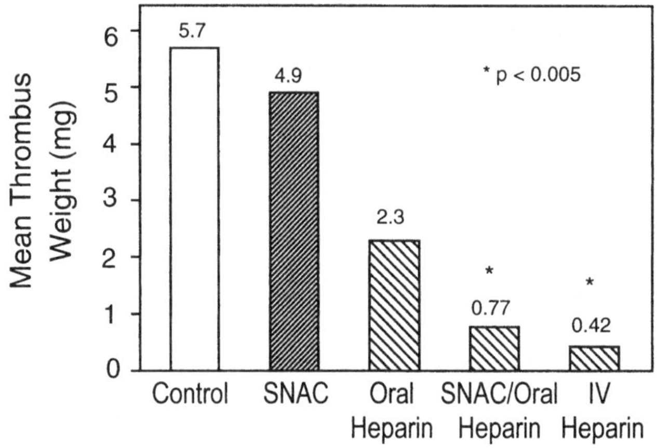

FIGURE 2.—Administration of combination SNAC and heparin significantly reduced the mean thrombus weight compared with controls, and SNAC-only and oral heparin–only groups. The combination of SNAC and heparin was as effective as the IV heparin. (Reprinted from Gonze MD, Manord JD, Leone-Bay A, et al: Orally administered heparin for preventing deep venous thrombosis. *Am J Surg* 176:176-178. Copyright 1998, with permission from Excerpta Medica Inc.)

mechanisms of this action and the potential clinical role of oral administration of SNAC with heparin.

▶ This interesting work bares watching. If adequate anticoagulation can be achieved using oral heparin, treatment of deep venous thrombosis and management of patients at high risk for graft failure will likely be simpler and possibly safer.

J.M. Seeger, M.D.

Trauma/Miscellaneous

Management of Severe Proximal Vascular and Neural Injury of the Upper Extremity

Manord JD, Garrard CL, Kline DG, et al (Ochsner Clinic and Alton Ochsner Med Found, New Orleans, La; Louisiana State Univ, New Orleans)

J Vasc Surg 27:43-49, 1998 13–23

Background.—Traumatic injuries of the proximal upper extremity can be treated aggressively or conservatively. Aggressive measures include vascular and nerve repair, with the goal of restoring some function, and conservative measures include control of hemorrhage alone without nerve repair, and in some cases amputation, with the belief that the extremity will no longer be functional. These authors report their experience with revascularization and delayed treatment of neural trauma in patients with traumatic proximal upper extremity injury.

Methods.—Forty-six patients (40 men and 6 women; mean age, 27 years) had unilateral traumatic injury of the brachial plexus and at least 1 vessel of the upper extremity or ipsilateral neck. The vascular injuries were treated by primary repair, interposition bypass grafting, or ligation (of selected venous injuries). Delayed nerve repair was then done if there was a potentially reversible nerve injury that was unlikely to recover spontaneously. Disability before and after any treatment was graded on a 100-point functional disability scoring system developed by the American Medical Association (100 points = total limb disability). Patients were studied for a mean of 43 months after injury.

Findings.—Most patients initially had altered pulses (38 patients, or 83%). Of the 44 patients who underwent urgent vascular exploration, 43 (93%) had arterial injuries, 37 (86%) had involvement of the subclavian or axillary artery, and 3 (7%) had venous injuries. Vascular repair procedures included intraposition or bypass grafting in 25 and primary repair in 17. The most common neurologic disturbance was flail arm (22 patients, or 48%). Of the 44 patients who underwent delayed nerve exploration (30-358 days after injury), all had injuries to the brachial plexus or its terminal components. Nerve repair procedures included nerve grafts in 29, end-to-end repair in 4, a combination of these in 3, and neurolysis only in 6. Overall, 40 of 46 patients (86%) experienced objective improvement and the mean disability score for all patients improved significantly from 83% initially after recovery from injury to 52% at the end of follow-up.

(52% represents stabilizing functions, gross manipulations, and a light load capacity.) Furthermore, patients with neurologic injuries other than nerve root avulsion at the spinal cord had improved disability scores during follow-up, whereas those with nerve root avulsions did not improve.

Conclusions.—Aggressive treatment of proximal upper extremity injuries can be associated with at least limited function in most patients with vascular and neural injuries. Amputations should be reserved for patients who have extensive nerve avulsions at the level of the spinal cord, for those who have massive soft-tissue loss, or for those who might not survive an attempted limb salvage.

▶ Combined neural and vascular injuries of the proximal upper extremities can be devastating. However, this report demonstrates that the long-term outcome does not appear to be uniformly dismal. Although most patients did not regain fine hand movements, the injured extremity was rarely painful and was at least as functional as a prosthesis. These data strengthen the concept of repairing the vascular injuries in all but those few patients in whom the neural injury is obviously irreversible.

J.M. Seeger, M.D.

The Incidence of Heparin-induced Antibodies in Patients Undergoing Vascular Surgery: A Prospective Study

Jackson MR, Gillespie DL, Chang AS, et al (Walter Reed Army Med Ctr and Inst of Research, Washington, DC)

J Vasc Surg 28:439-445, 1998 13–24

Background.—Heparin-induced thrombocytopenia is associated with the formation of antibodies against a complex of heparin and platelet factor 4 (PF4). Patients undergoing intraoperative anticoagulation for peripheral vascular disease may have increased rates of heparin-induced antibodies. This possibility was studied using a highly sensitive heparin/PF4 enzyme-linked immunosorbent assay (ELISA).

Methods.—Fifty-four patients received unfractionated porcine heparin for anticoagulation during peripheral vascular surgery. No heparin was given after the end of surgery. The patients were 36 men and 18 women, with a mean age of 67 years. The surgical procedure performed was carotid endarterectomy in 36 patients, aortic reconstruction in 11, and infrainguinal bypass in 7. Before and at a mean of 2 weeks after surgery, the ELISA was used to evaluate the patients' serum for heparin/PF4 complex immunoglobulin G antibodies. An optical density ratio of patient plasma to normal plasma was considered a positive result if it was 1.8 or greater.

Results.—The patients received a mean intraoperative heparin dose of 9,089 U. Two patients (3.7%) were antibody-positive before surgery and both remained positive after surgery. Only 1 patient went from antibody-negative to antibody-positive status after surgery. The mean change in ELISA optical density ratio after surgery was not significantly different between patients with and patients without previous heparin exposure. Intraoperative anticoagulation was associated with a reduction in platelet count from 227,620 to 185,706 per µL. Similar reductions in the platelet count were seen in patients with and without previous heparin exposure (−23% and −18%, respectively). One antibody-negative patient experienced graft occlusion after femorotibial bypass; this was the only thrombotic complication.

Conclusions.—Heparin associated antibodies are uncommon in patients undergoing peripheral vascular surgery. Mild postoperative thrombocytopenia appears to be unrelated to heparin/PF4 antibody formation, and standard heparin anticoagulation for vascular surgical procedures does not appear to carry a significant risk of heparin-induced thrombocytopenia and thrombosis.

► Although this article is reassuring, it does not mean that patients undergoing vascular surgical procedures are not at risk for this potentially devastating complication. However, the risk appears to be low, and more widespread use of ELISA for heparin antibodies (such as in the study described here) may allow rapid differentiation of heparin-induced thrombocytopenia from other types of thrombocytopenia. That would allow patients who need anticoagulation with heparin to continue to receive it despite thrombocytopenia they might be experiencing from other causes.

J.M. Seeger, M.D.

14 Noncardiac Thoracic Surgery

Introduction

This year's review of the thoracic surgical literature provides an overview of the three most vibrant and progressive areas in the field. Specifically, lung volume reduction surgery is still inching its way toward becoming a standard procedure. Although the Health Care Financing Authority has not approved funding to the Medicare population, many insurers nevertheless have continued to fund the procedure. Recent results from the NIH in reviewing 17 centers revealed a 30% mortality at 18 months following the procedure. This, along with the questions regarding the durability of the palliative response seen in patients undergoing volume reduction surgery, has led many to question its efficacy compared with the best medical therapy. Because many of these emphysema patients have for years been neglected medically, not receiving pulmonary rehabilitation or appropriate medical care (not funded by Medicare), the mere fact that they have become the focus of intense study may benefit them from the medical therapy that they now receive. Nevertheless, it is a vibrant time for this new procedure. This procedure has been a focus of this YEAR BOOK review for the last several years. This is because the potential number of patients that would require this procedure is phenomenal. It is estimated that more than 160,000 Americans every year would be candidates for this procedure should its efficacy be proved. Of course, efficacy of a surgical procedure is the result of appropriate patient selection, appropriate surgical technique, and a reduction of operative mortality and sound physiologic impact. This YEAR BOOK reviews each of these areas in terms of progress made in our understanding as to which patients should be operated on using volume reduction surgery, the best surgical technique, minimizing surgical complications, and studying the physiologic effects of the procedure on patients. We will then look at some unique situations where volume reduction surgery seems to have found a place in the therapeutic armamentarium of thoracic surgeons.

Not surprisingly, the next area reviewed is surgery for non–small-cell lung cancer. This disease will have occurred in approximately 190,000 patients in 1998. Nearly 155,000 to 170,000 of these patients will ultimately succumb to the disease. While surgery remains the foundation of therapy for non–small-cell lung cancer, conventional treatments in the new arrangements seem to be making some improvement in the outlook, particularly in locally advanced disease. Specifically, we will be looking at a number of articles that seek to further define the appropriate staging and markers of extensive disease. This particular area marks one of increasing enthusiasm and excitement for the thoracic surgeon. Due to the large number of patients being diagnosed with this disease on an annual basis, advances in staging, therapy, and basic understanding will provide patients in large numbers with an enhanced chance at long-term survival.

The third area is a review of surgical pulmonary metastasectomy, its applications and approaches. This particular field continues to move forward based on historical understanding of the biology of pulmonary metastases for a variety of malignancies. Specifically, we will look at the role of median sternotomy and the resection of lung metastases, as well as the treatment of hepatic and pulmonary metastases from colorectal cancer. Due to the reduction in morbidity and mortality of the surgical approaches, it appears that surgical metastasectomy is finding its way into more advanced metastatic disease in the chest. The long-term results after repeated surgical removal of pulmonary metastases is also evaluated. Once again, the surgeon is confronting new frontiers, as repeat pulmonary metastasectomy is becoming standard practice in a variety of centers across the country.

Following this, a concluding section consists of a variety of abstracts on articles looking at interesting clinical challenges, ones where the thoracic surgeon may find specific reviews of great interest. The review will cover large-cell neuroendocrine tumors, intraoperative intrapleural hypertonic platinum treatment of carcinoma pleuritis, as well as some basic problems such as chest tube insertion, experience with the video-assisted approach to mediastinal tumors and primary sarcomas of the mediastinum. The review will be looking at the aggressive approach to this extremely rare entity.

This YEAR BOOK review presents practicing thoracic surgeons, whether trained in cardiothoracic surgery or well-versed general surgeons extending their practice to the chest, with a variety of new information. We keep our eye on the rising indications for volume reduction surgery by reviewing papers that enhance our understanding of which patients should undergo the procedure, as well as the physiologic effects on these patients. We review advances in treatment of the most significant thoracic malignancy facing the thoracic surgeon, non–small-cell cancer. We follow that with discussion of a surgical approach to metastasectomy of pulmonary malignancies and our enhanced understanding about its application and its increasingly aggressive nature. We conclude with a review of some unique clinical challenges based on some interesting reports that have highlighted these in specifics.

David J. Sugarbaker, M.D.

Lung Volume Reduction Surgery: Progress and Pitfalls

INTRODUCTION

The appropriate technique for performing volume reduction surgery has been a discussion in evolution. The technique of open volume reduction surgery via median sternotomy, while the initial procedure performed, has given way in the majority of centers to a minimally invasive aproach. The comfort of having the open sternotomy to surgeons less willing or able to perform minimally invasive techniques makes it a gold standard against which all other results of volume reduction surgery are to be compared. Nevertheless, this very high risk group of patients, with significant and multiple medical co-morbidities, appear to be the group that will benefit most from a minimally invasive approach with minimal surgical trauma.

David J. Sugarbaker, M.D.

Patient Selection Criteria for Lung Volume Reduction Surgery

McKenna RJ Jr, Brenner M, Fischel RJ, et al (Chapman Med Ctr, Orange, Calif; Lakewood Regional Med Ctr, Calif; Univ of California at Los Angeles)
J Thorac Cardiovasc Surg 114:957-967, 1997 14–1

Background.—Patient selection criteria for lung volume reduction surgery (LVRS) vary widely in the literature. The results of LVRS in patients with emphysema were analyzed to refine the patient selection criteria for LVRS.

Methods.—Bilateral staple LVRS was performed in 154 patients (98 men, 56 women; mean age, 67 years) with heterogeneous, severe emphysema. Data were gathered on potential selection criteria including findings on history and physical examination, arterial blood gas levels (room air), prednisone dose, imaging results (including CT and lung perfusion), and results of pulmonary function tests. The main outcomes of interest were the change in forced expiratory volume in 1 second (FEV_1) and the dyspnea score (measured by the Modified Medical Research Council scale). Analysis of variance was used to determine relationships between potential selection criteria and the outcome measures.

Findings.—Of the 154 patients, 7 died (4.5%), and pulmonary function data were available for 138 of the 147 survivors. The pattern of emphysema on chest radiography was strongly associated with differences in outcome. Patients with a bilateral upper lobe pattern had a mean 73.2% improvement in FEV_1 (from 0.64 to 1.07 L), which was significantly better than the improvement seen with a diffuse or lower lobe pattern (38% improvement, from 0.7 to 0.93 L). The dyspnea scale, however, did not differ significantly depending on the pattern of emphysema. Age was also associated with differences in outcome. Patients younger than 70 years had a significantly better improvement in FEV_1 (76% improvement, from 0.64 to 1.08 L) than did patients aged 70 years or older (48% improvement, from 0.69 to 0.97 L). Again, the dyspnea score did not differ significantly between age groups. The preoperative prednisone dose had no significant association with the outcome measures, nor did the preoperative FEV_1, residual volume, total lung capacity, severe hypoxemia, hypercarbia, or diaphragmatic excursion. However, the preoperative use of 4 L or more of supplemental oxygen was associated with significantly worse outcomes compared with patients using less than 4 L of supplemental oxygen. All patients using 4 L or more of oxygen required continued supplementation after surgery, whereas only 68% of patients using less than 4 L did so.

Conclusions.—A bilateral upper lobe pattern was the best selection criterion for LVRS in these patients with heterogeneous, severe emphysema. Although differences in outcomes were seen in patients of different ages, even the older patients benefited from the procedure, and thus age is not a contraindication to the procedure. Patients who required 4 L or more of supplemental oxygen preoperatively had poorer outcomes and thus may not be good candidates for the procedure. The other criteria examined had no significant effect on outcomes and thus should not be considered selection criteria for LVRS in this population.

▶ This article from a group who does a high volume of volume reduction surgery is interesting in that it sheds light on the indications for selection of patients who would benefit most from volume reduction surgery. Dr. McKenna and his group are known nationally as pioneers in the field of thoracoscopic volume reduction. From this article, it is clear that there are some patients who, if selected appropriately, will benefit significantly from this procedure. Specifically, those patients with radiographic upper lobe disease whose age is less than 70 years were noted to have a significant improvement in FEV_1. Conversely, those patients on more than 4 liters of oxygen did not appear to benefit from the procedure. Those patients who had elevated CO_2, had been on prednisone, or had very poor residual volumes were not at adverse selection for the procedure.

It appears that there is a continuum between patients with panacinar emphysema and those patients who have a giant bullous lesion in the lung. It has been known for a long time that patients with giant bullous disease will benefit significantly from the resection of the bullous lesion allowing normal lung to re-expand. As we are seeing in LVRS in this article, those patients whose disease mimics a giant bullous lesion benefit the most physiologically from volume reduction surgery. Therefore, patients in the future who have heterogeneous disease are to be among the surgeon's most desirable patients to undergo LVRS.

D.J. Sugarbaker, M.D.

Morphologic Grading of the Emphysematous Lung and Its Relation to Improvement After Lung Volume Reduction Surgery

Wisser W, Klepetko W, Kontrus M, et al (Univ of Vienna; Lainz Hosp, Vienna)

Ann Thorac Surg 65:793-799, 1998 14–2

Background.—Lung volume reduction surgery is used to treat "heterogeneous" severe emphysema. However, different authors have reported different degrees of heterogeneity, and in fact, these authors have successfully operated on lungs with homogeneous patterns. To better define the different morphological forms of emphysema, a morphological grading scale was created based on imaging studies, and the grades were related to outcomes after lung volume reduction surgery.

Methods.—A total of 47 patients (27 men, 20 women; mean age, 55.9 years) with emphysema who underwent bilateral lung volume reduction surgery were studied. Pulmonary function tests and other functional parameters were measured before and 3 months after the operation. The morphological grading scale was based on standard chest radiographs and CT scans. Four variables were used to quantify the morphology of emphysema: the degree of hyperinflation (DHI), the degree of impairment in diaphragmatic mechanics (DIDM), the degree of heterogeneity (DH6), and the severity of parenchymal destruction (SPD). The DHI was measured on a 5-point scale (0 = normal, 4 = severe). The DIDM was measured in centimeters and represented the maximum difference between full inspiration and expiration on lateral chest radiographs. The DHG was determined by dividing the lungs into 12 segments based on 3 levels (upper border of aortic arch, 2 cm below carina, and 2 cm above highest diaphragmatic dome) and 2 extra-anatomic segments at each level per lung. The DHG was determined from the amount of destroyed lung parenchyma in the 12 segments and was graded on a 5-point scale (0 = normal, 4 = no normal lung). The SPD score was a composite of the individual extent of parenchymal destruction in the 12 segments (range 0-48).

Findings.—Lung volume reduction surgery significantly improved the forced expiratory volume in 1 second FEV_1, from 25.3% of predicted before surgery to 42.5% after surgery. Interobserver agreement was good for all 4 variables of the morphological grading system. Overall, neither DHI, DIDM, nor SPD correlated significantly with the degree of improvement in FEV_1. However, DHG was significantly associated with functional improvement. A DHG score of 1 was associated with an improvement in FEV_1 of 60.5%, whereas a DHG score of 4 was associated with 160.3% improvement. When the 4 patients who died within 30 days of surgery (8.5% mortality rate) were analyzed separately, SPD was found to have a significant correlation with survival; patients who died had a mean SPD score of 28.4, whereas the SPD score of survivors was 21.3.

Conclusions.—This morphological grading system is easy to use and reproducible. Furthermore, some of these patients had homogeneous patterns (DHG = 0 or 1), and they, too, benefited from lung volume reduction surgery. Future research to define the morphology of emphysema will allow better comparison between centers and perhaps improve selection criteria for lung volume reduction surgery.

▶ This interesting article seeks to find a radiologic correlate to those patients with heterogeneous disease that will benefit most from lung volume reduction surgery. Specifically, these authors looked at four parameters that would signify radiographically the severity of hyperexpansion of the lung and chest wall due to diffuse emphysema. While those parameters signifying only hyperexpansion were not significant in their ability to predict improvement following lung volume reduction surgery, the diffuse heterogeneity quotient was the one that was the most important. Specifically the DHG demonstrated that those patients with heterogeneous disease benefited most in their forced expiratory volume in 1 second following volume reduction surgery. This supports Dr. McKenna's observation (Abstract 14–1) that patients with heterogeneous disease appear to benefit most from volume reduction surgery probably because there is significant improvement in the more normal lung function as the space occupying diseased lung is removed. These authors have made an important contribution in that they suggest a means whereby a CT scan could be used to quantitate the heterogeneity of the disease and, therefore, predict which patients will benefit most from volume reduction surgery. As many of these patients have significant co-morbid medical problems, the surgeons need to know which patients may benefit most as they seek to complete the equation of risk benefit in recommending which patients should indeed undergo the surgery where the risks may be high, but the benefits may be significant. Undoubtedly, one of the most important suggestions that these authors have made is the need to standardize the grading and description of the emphysema in patients undergoing volume reduction surgery. Indeed one of the major obstacles to comparing data has been the ability to match patients in terms of the extent of their emphysema, the type of their emphysema, and their degree of impairment.

D.J. Sugarbaker, M.D.

MR Analysis of Lung Volume and Thoracic Dimensions in Patients With Emphysema Before and After Lung Volume Reduction Surgery

Gierada DS, Hakimian S, Slone RM, et al (Washington Univ, St Louis)

AJR 170:707-714, 1998 14–3

Purpose.—Lung volume reduction surgery can reduce symptoms and improve pulmonary function for some patients with severe emphysema. The mechanism of this benefit is unclear but probably involves changes in diaphragmatic and chest wall mechanics. Studying thoracic volume and dimensions after lung volume reduction surgery may help to explain its effects. The accuracy of MRI for measuring lung volume and thoracic dimensions before and after lung volume reduction surgery was studied.

Methods.—Baseline studies were performed in 21 patients and postoperative studies in 9 patients. At each investigation, the patients underwent fast gradient-echo breath-hold MRI of the chest at full inspiration and expiration. A semiautomated computer program was used to delineate the lungs and measure cross-sectional areas, thus deriving lung volumes. The results were compared with plethysmographic and CT measurements. Comparison of anteroposterior and transverse lung dimensions and lung height before and after surgery was performed to assess postoperative changes in thoracic structure.

Results.—The correlation coefficient for MRI vs. plethysmographic measurements of inspiratory lung volume was $r = 0.77$. The SEM was −12%, with MRI measurements being lower. For CT vs. plethysmography, the correlation coefficient was $r = 0.86$ with an SEM of −13, CT showing the lesser volume. Comparison of MRI vs. CT showed a correlation coefficient of $r = 0.87$ with an SEM of 4%, MRI showing the greater volume. For expiratory volume measurements by MRI vs. plethysmography, the correlation coefficient was $r = 0.77$. The SEM was 6%, with MRI showing the greater volume. All thoracic volumes were reduced after lung volume reduction surgery, particularly when measured at expiration.

Conclusion.—In patients with severe emphysema, MRI and CT provide similar measurements of lung volume. However, these results are significantly different from those of plethysmography. Lung volume reduction surgery alters thoracic dimensions in a way consistent with improved respiratory mechanics. The results suggest a role for MRI in studying the effects of changes in thoracic structure on pulmonary function.

▶ This article is an extremely important one in that it provides specific anatomic correlations of the changes in chest wall configuration following volume reduction surgery. It has been known to surgeons performing lung transplantation for emphysema over the years that the chest wall can reconfigure rather dramatically and rather quickly following the implantation of a normal lung where a hyperexpanded emphysematous lung had been. We had not been aware of the changes that are capable in the patient with volume reduction surgery to the degree that these authors have informed us using both MRI and CT. This important physiologic, anatomic correlation to the performance of volume reduction surgery tells us specifically that the rather static and, in some cases, chronic, changes in chest wall configuration can be altered rather dramatically in the postoperative period by the successful performance of volume reduction surgery. This fundamental principle that the chest wall will reconfigure almost immediately following volume reduction surgery lends significant support to the concept that this procedure has a sound physiologic basis whereby it will improve the functional performance of patients following volume reduction surgery by restoring the normal anatomic, physiologic function of the chest wall, performing as the means of improving the mechanical ventilation of the lung in these patients. However, the use of MRI in the routine clinical assessment of patients appears to still be somewhat limited. The CT scan appears to have a superior ability to characterize the parenchymal abnormalities in patients with emphysema. However, the chest wall may be better characterized by the use of MRI, which appears at this point to be restricted to investigational use only.

D.J. Sugarbaker, M.D.

Relation Between Preoperative Inspiratory Lung Resistance and the Outcome of Lung-Volume–Reduction Surgery for Emphysema

Ingenito EP, Evans RB, Loring SH, et al (Brigham and Women's Hosp, Boston; Beth Israel Deaconess Med Ctr, Boston)

N Engl J Med 338:1181-1185, 1998 14–4

Introduction.—Lung volume reduction surgery is increasingly used in an attempt to relieve dyspnea and improve exercise tolerance in patients with emphysema. However, the procedure is not effective in all patients. It has been suggested that this surgery improves lung function by increasing elastic recoil and airway tethering. If so, lung resistance during inspiration might be a useful test for evaluating the appropriateness of lung volume reduction surgery. This study assessed the relationship of inspiratory lung resistance and other physiologic parameters to the results of lung volume reduction surgery.

Methods.—The study included 29 patients with severe end-stage chronic obstructive pulmonary disease who were scheduled for lung volume reduction surgery. Each patient underwent measurement of lung resistance during inspiration, static recoil pressure at total lung capacity, static lung compliance, expiratory flow rate, and lung volume. These measurements were evaluated for their relationship to changes in forced expiratory volume in 1 second (FEV_1) at 6 months postoperatively. Patients in whom FEV_1 increased by at least 0.2 L and 12% above baseline were considered to have had a positive response to surgery.

Results.—Twenty-three of the 29 patients had some improvement in FEV_1 after surgery, and 15 were considered responders. The only preoperative physiologic variable that predicted surgical outcome was lung resistance during inspiration, which was inversely correlated with postoperative improvement in FEV_1. As a preoperative test for predicting a response to surgery, inspiratory lung resistance of 10 cm H_2O/L/sec had a sensitivity of 88% and a specificity of 92%.

Conclusion.—Preoperative measurements of inspiratory lung resistance may help to select those patients with emphysema who are most likely to benefit from lung volume reducing surgery. In patients without high elevations in inspiratory resistance, obstruction probably results from dynamic airway collapse related to loss of airway tethering by the lung parenchyma. These findings need to be confirmed in a larger group of patients with a more heterogeneous distribution of emphysema.

▶ This important article has identified a single test that appears in this small group of patients to significantly predict those who will benefit most from volume reduction surgery. Specifically, the measurement of inspiratory lung airway resistance is identified as an important predictor of a positive response to surgery. Specifically, the authors point out that a loss of tethering is thought to be the principal reason that patients benefit from volume reduction surgery. This restoration of the tethering appears to be an important factor in the improvement of patients postsurgery. These observations are more or less in compliance with the concept that patients with intrinsic small airway disease are not the ones who will benefit most from volume reduction surgery. Specifically, it is these patients with small airway disease who have a high inspiratory resistance and therefore these patients derive less benefit from volume reduction surgery. This may be a very important and simple test that will help predict a positive response to volume reduction surgery and help select patients for this new and innovative surgical procedure.

D.J. Sugarbaker, M.D.

Lung Volume Reduction Surgery and Airflow Limitation

Fessler HE, Permutt S (Johns Hopkins Med Institutions, Baltimore, Md)
Am J Respir Crit Care Med 157:715-722, 1998 14–5

Introduction.—Increased vital capacity (VC) is usually observed after lung volume reduction surgery (LVRS). The mechanism leading to the increase in VC is not understood. A mathematical analysis and graphic depiction of the mechanism of improvement in expiratory airflow and VC after LVRS for end-stage emphysema were reported.

Methods.—The analysis of LVRS is based on the relationship between lung function and respiratory muscle function. Previously published reports of pulmonary mechanics in patients with α_1-antitrypsin deficiency, chronic obstructive pulmonary disease, and asthma were reviewed.

Results.—A major determinant of airflow limitation typical of these diseases was found to be the ratio of residual volume to total lung capacity (RV/TLC). The ratio of RV to TLC was the most influential determinant of improvement in pulmonary function after LVRS. Regardless of underlying lung disease, impairment of airflow usually occurred because of mismatch between the sizes of the lungs and the chest wall. The effects of LVRS were almost always attributed to improvement of that match.

Conclusions.—When airflow is improved by LVRS, it does so mainly by improving the fit between the lungs and chest wall, decreasing RV more than TLC. The greatest utility of this analysis is in hypothesis generation. This information needs to undergo retrospective and prospective validation.

► This important article provides a sound mathematical and physiologic basis for the results of volume reduction surgery. Specifically, the authors' theoretical model of emphysema allows us to estimate the benefit to the emphysema patient by the resection of heterogeneously diseased lung, as well as lung which is diseased in a homogeneous or panacinar manner. The most important conclusion that these authors make is that lung volume reduction surgery works by improving the "fit" of the lung with the chest wall in a physiologic, anatomic fashion. Specifically, the hypothetical case of emphysema that is reviewed notes that while the removal of blebs or bullae would theoretically improve the postoperative forced expiratory volume in 1 second, right through resection of 80% of the existing diseased lung, homogeneous lung will plateau in its improvement after approximately 60% of the lung has been removed. Certainly, this remains a theoretical approach, as practically speaking, more than 30% resection clinically is fraught with increased complications, space problems, infection, and mortality. Nevertheless, the important point is that the more diseased the lung that is resected is, the more theoretical, as is pointed out in this article, as well as real, benefit is enjoyed by patients undergoing the procedure. This article enlightens the surgeon to understand that the more diseased lung is the target of surgical resection. Therefore, as has been previously discussed, techniques for determining the level and heterogeneity of the disease are important in targeting that area of lung in patients so that the result of surgical intervention will be maximal.

D.J. Sugarbaker, M.D.

Effect of Lung Volume Reduction Surgery on Diaphragm Strength

Criner G, Cordova FC, Leyenson V, et al (Temple Univ, Philadelphia)

Am J Respir Crit Care Med 157:1578-1585, 1998 — 14–6

Introduction.—Earlier reports conflict regarding the effect of lung volume reduction surgery (LVRS) on respiratory muscle function. The effects of LVRS vs. pulmonary rehabilitation on lung function, exercise capacity, and respiratory muscle strength were assessed in 37 patients with severe, nonbullous diffuse emphysema.

Methods.—Before and after 8 weeks of pulmonary rehabilitation, 24 patients underwent a variety of pulmonary function studies, an incremental symptom-limited maximum exercise test, a 6-minute walk test, and measurement of volitional maximum static inspiratory and expiratory mouth pressures, and transdiaphragmatic pressures during maximum static inspiratory efforts and bilateral supramaximal electrophrenic twitch stimulation. Thirteen patients underwent similar physiologic measurements before and 3 months after LVRS. Seven patients in the pulmonary rehabilitation group underwent LVRS and were assessed 3 months after LVRS.

Results.—Patients who underwent rehabilitation had no changes in spirometry or carbon monoxide–diffusing capacity per unit of alveolar volume (DL_{CO}/V_A), and lung volumes demonstrated a slight worsening in hyperinflation. There were no changes in gas exchange, 6-minute walk distance, maximum oxygen uptake, or breathing pattern during maximum exercise after rehabilitation. There was a significant increase in exercise time after rehabilitation. Inspiratory muscle strength (PI_{max}, $Pdi_{max\ combined}$, $Pdi_{max\ sniff}$, Pdi_{max}, and Pdi_{twitch}) were similar before and after rehabilitation. After LVRS, forced vital capacity (FVC) increased 21%, forced expiratory volume in 1 second (FEV_1) increased 34%, total lung capacity (TLC) decreased 13%, functional residual capacity (FRC) was reduced 23%, $FRC_{trapped\ gas}$ decreased 57%, residual volume (RV) decreased 28%, PCO_2 was significantly lower, 6-minute walk and total exercise time during maximum exercise increased significantly, minute ventilation and tidal volume during maximum exercise increased significantly, respiratory rate decreased significantly, inspiratory muscle workload as measured by Pdi TTI was significantly lower, and all measurements of respiratory muscle strength were significantly greater. There was a significant correlation between increases in PI_{max} and reductions in RV and $FRC_{trapped\ gas}$ after LVRS.

Conclusions.—Lung volume reduction surgery significantly enhances diaphragmatic strength that is associated with a decrease in lung volumes and an improved exercise performance. Further investigation is required to determine the relationship and stability of these changes over time.

▶ This article is interesting and provides an important insight into the physiologic effects of volume reduction surgery as contrasted to pulmonary rehabilitation. As noted by the authors, in the group of patients who underwent only pulmonary rehabilitation, there is no change in the measurement of diaphragmatic strength. On the other hand, in patients undergoing volume reduction surgery, there was a significant improvement in diaphragmatic strength as measured by the authors. This insight provides a sound physiologic reason why volume reduction surgery may lead to prolonged improved functional status of patients undergoing the procedure. This is precisely the type of information needed to establish the credibility of this procedure in patients suffering from chronic hyperinflation as a result of their emphysema. Further studies of diaphragmatic strength will be important in elucidating the mechanisms for sustained effects. Specifically, the durability of volume reduction surgery has been called into question recently. Therefore, measurements in diaphragmatic strength and its sustained improvement will provide important insight into the reasons behind some patients continuing to maintain an improved functional status, whereas other patients appear to slip back into their preoperative state of significant pulmonary dysfunction.

D.J. Sugarbaker, M.D.

Improved Exercise Performance Following Lung Volume Reduction Surgery for Emphysema

Ferguson GT, Fernandez E, Zamora MR, et al (Univ of Colorado, Denver; Wayne State Univ, Detroit)

Am J Respir Crit Care Med 157:1195-1203, 1998 14–7

Introduction.—Until recently, the effects of lung volume reduction surgery (LVRS) on exercise performance have been limited to simple measures of walk distance. Two recent trials indicate that exercise performance, as assessed by maximal exercise testing, does produce improvement shortly after LVRS. The short-term effects of LVRS on exercise performance (using maximal and submaximal steady-state exercise testing), patient function, dyspnea, and quality of life were assessed in 27 patients with severe hypoxemic chronic obstructive pulmonary disease (COPD).

Findings.—Of the 27 patients, 18 completed preoperative and postoperative exercise performance and pulmonary function testing at a median of 4 months after LVRS. Exercise performance, ventilatory capacity/ceiling, and resting ventilatory reserve were significantly improved after LVRS. Improvements were also observed in resting $Pa{CO_2}$ and pH. There were no changes in any other resting exercise/metabolism parameters. Improvements in dyspnea, walk distances, and quality of life were associated with improvements in exercise performance after LVRS. Surgical mortality from LVRS was 4%. Short-term all-cause mortality was 19%. Short-term mortality was correlated with decreased expiratory muscle strength and markedly elevated dead space ventilation.

Conclusions.—In selected patients with severe emphysema, LVRS can produce significant improvements in measures of exercise performance, dyspnea, and quality of life. All-cause short-term mortality in this series of patients with end-stage COPD who underwent LVRS may be somewhat higher than expected, based on earlier trials.

▶ This is an important article that highlights the difficulty assessing the postoperative morbidity and mortality in patients undergoing lung volume reduction surgery. Specifically, the use of the term postoperative mortality vs. "all-cause" mortality is an important distinction to make. While the patients in this study enjoyed a 4% postoperative mortality, an all-cause mortality of 19% was noted in the same group of patients. This is in keeping with the pretrial 30% 18-month mortality recently quoted at the National Emphysema Treatment Trial (NETT) steering committee meeting (Washington, DC); these data came from the patients submitted by the participating centers.

It is a critical question to assess whether or not the all cause mortality of 20% in this series and 30% as quoted in the NETT patients submitted represents a negative criterion for performing volume reduction surgery.[1] Specifically, while patients may be improved in their forced expiratory volume in 1 second and overall functional status, patients need to know what their all cause mortality will be over an 18 to 24 month period, and, more specifically, whether or not this all cause mortality will be lower than those patients undergoing medical therapy alone. Indeed, the use of the term all cause mortality in a more protracted sense is the critical question in lung volume reduction surgery vs. maximal medical management. Without a control arm of patients receiving only maximal medical management for a protracted period of time, there will be no way to determine whether volume reduction surgery enhances not only the quality of life, but also the extent of life. Therefore, trials that have a 6 month or 8 month crossover arm allowing all patients at 6 to 8 months to receive surgery are devoid of the critical information required to answer the question that is presented by this particular discussion.

D.J. Sugarbaker, M.D.

Improved Lung Function and Quality of Life Following Increased Elastic Recoil After Lung Volume Reduction Surgery in Emphysema

Norman M, Hillerdal G, Orre L, et al (Karolinska Hosp, Stockholm)

Respir Med 92:653-658, 1998 14–8

Purpose.—For patients with severe emphysema, lung volume reduction surgery—in which the most severely damaged parts of the lung parenchyma are resected—can significantly improve forced expiratory volume, maximal ventilation, and quality of life. The mechanism by which this benefit arises has been unclear. The authors have been performing a protocol of physiologic tests in their patients undergoing lung volume reduction surgery. Their findings suggest that increased elastic recoil may play a role in the postoperative improvement.

Methods.—The analysis included 14 patients—7 men and 7 women with a mean age of 62 years—undergoing bilateral lung volume reduction surgery. All submitted to a protocol of tests before and 3 months after surgery, including radiographs; spirometry and measurement of diffusion capacity; tests of elastic recoil and working capacity; rest and exercise blood gas measurement; perfusion scintigraphy; radiospirometry; and a quality-of-life questionnaire.

Findings.—After lung volume reduction surgery, forced expiratory volume in 1 second increased by a mean of 26%, whereas mean total lung capacity decreased by 16%. The ratio of residual volume to total lung capacity decreased, suggesting a reduced level of hyperinflation. Transpulmonary pressure at maximal inspiration increased from 0.95 to 1.35 kPa as the coefficient of retraction increased from 0.12 to 0.19 kPa/L, demonstrating improved pulmonary elastic recoil. The patients' mean testing partial pressure of arterial oxygen increased from 8.7 to 9.8 kPa. The patients registered considerable improvement on the respiratory-related quality-of-life questionnaire, as well as a 26% increase in work capacity on a bicycle exercise test.

Conclusion.—The mechanism of improvement after lung volume reduction surgery appears to involve improved pulmonary elastic recoil. Significant short-term improvements are noted in symptoms, quality of life, work capacity, blood gases, and lung function.

► This is an important article because it, for the first time, reports on the measurements of quality of life in patients undergoing volume reduction surgery. While the improvements in elastic recoil, as documented in this paper, have been previously described by the Pittsburgh group,[1] this important investigation in this small group of patients has looked very carefully at the quality of life measurements, both before and after volume reduction surgery. There is a strong correlation, as presented in this article, between the overall physiologic improvements in forced expiratory volume in 1 second and elastic recoil with the patient's overall sense of well being. This important documentation allows us to suggest that patients undergoing volume reduction surgery who are likely to show physiological benefit have a significant chance at improving their quality of life. These types of objective measurements are very important in understanding when and how to apply volume reduction surgery. Further studies in larger groups of patients will be required to establish the overall efficacy of volume reduction surgery in improving quality of life. Specifically, in addition, as we saw in Abstract 14–7, these improvements in quality of life will need to be balanced and weighed against the overall "all-cause mortality" that appears to accompany this procedure.

D.J. Sugarbaker, M.D.

Reference

1. Sciurba FC, Rogers RM, Keenan RJ, et al: Improvement in pulmonary function and elastic recoil after lung-reduction surgery for diffuse emphysema. *N Engl J Med* 334:1095-1099, 1996.

Bilateral Lung Volume Reduction Surgery via Median Sternotomy for Severe Pulmonary Emphysema

Date H, Goto K, Souda R, et al (Okayama Univ, Japan; Minami-Okayama Hosp, Japan)

Ann Thorac Surg 65:939-942, 1998 14–9

Introduction.—Recent reports from North America and Europe have shown that lung volume reduction surgery, using either sternotomy or thoracoscopy, produces significant short-term improvement in respiratory status in carefully selected patients with emphysema. Nearly 55% of Japanese males are current smokers; more than 10,000 patients presently receive home oxygen therapy for chronic obstructive lung disease. The results of 39 lung volume reduction surgeries performed by medial sternotomy in patients with severe diffuse emphysema were reported.

Methods.—The mean age of 35 males and 4 females was 65 years (range, 54 to 74 years). All patients were former heavy smokers; none had α_1-antitrypsin deficiency. Nine patients (23%) had a bilateral upper lobe pattern of emphysema. The most emphysematous portions of lungs were excised bilaterally through a median sternotomy using a linear stapling device fitted with strips of bovine pericardium to prevent air leakage.

Results.—There were no operative deaths. Prolonged air leak was the most common complication; 5 patients required reoperation for air leak. There were no pleural infections. Follow-up was 1 to 20 months. The mean forced expiratory volume in 1 second improved by 41% from 735 mL to 1,037 mL in 33 patients who completed 3-months' follow-up. Significant improvements were also observed in other measures of pulmonary function tests, arterial blood gas analysis, 6-minute walking distance, and dyspnea. These improvements were observed for at least 1 year.

Conclusions.—Bilateral lung volume reduction surgery by median sternotomy is safe and effective in carefully selected patients with severe emphysema. Findings in Japanese patients were similar to those reported earlier for patients with severe emphysema from North America and Europe.

▶ This article is important because it demonstrates the use of volume reduction surgery in a different subset of patients with emphysema caused by heavy smoking. Specifically, 55% of the male Japanese population, as noted in this article, is comprised of smokers. This unbelievable prevalence of smoking in a moderate industrial country should cause a sense of alarm for all surgeons treating patients suffering from the disease as resulting from tobacco. Nevertheless, this study has shown that in this group of patients, volume reduction surgery with a similar approach utilizing a median sternotomy appears to have a positive effect on the physiologic parameters as previously described in western studies. It is important to duplicate these results in different racial groups so that the physiologic underpinnings of the procedure can be validated in a variety of different cultural and racial situations.

D.J. Sugarbaker, M.D.

Lung Volume Reduction Surgery: A Cost and Outcomes Comparison of Sternotomy Versus Thoracoscopy

Ko CY, Waters PF (Univ of California, Los Angeles)

Am Surg 64:1010-1013, 1998 14–10

Objective.—Most patients with chronic obstructive pulmonary disease improve after lung volume reduction surgery (LVRS). The outcomes and costs of video-assisted thoracoscopy (VATS) were compared with those of sternotomy.

Methods.—Between 1995 and 1997, 42 patients with severe emphysema underwent bilateral LVRS by sternotomy (n=19) or thoracoscopy (n=23) at the University of California at Los Angeles. Follow-up was identical for both groups. Outcome analysis included number of operating-room hours, length of hospital stay, number of days in intensive care, number of days on a ventilator, oxygen dependence, morbidity, mortality, pulmonary function tests, arterial blood gases, and patient self-assessments.

Results.—Patient groups had similar preoperative data. Operative time was significantly less for sternotomy than for VATS (118 vs. 168 minutes). VATS patients spent significantly fewer days in ICU than did sternotomy patients (1.2 vs. 8.9), significantly fewer days on a ventilator (1.1 vs. 7.1), fewer days with an air leak (6.7 vs. 10.7 days), and significantly fewer days in hospital (9.7 vs. 13.8 days). Postoperative oxygen dependence was lower in both the VATS and sternotomy groups (40% and 25%). Total lung capacity improved by 11% in the VATS group and 7% in the sternotomy group. Forced expiratory volume in 1 second improved by 62% in the VATS group and 28% in the sternotomy group. The 30-day mortality was 4% in the VATS group and 15% in the sternotomy group, and long-term mortality was 4% and 10%, respectively. Inpatient costs were $27,178 for the VATS group and $37,299 for the sternotomy group.

Conclusion.—Although LVRS is beneficial to most patients regardless of the procedure used, VATS is less expensive, and results in a shorter hospital stay and less postoperative morbidity and mortality.

▶ This article looks carefully at the outcomes of volume reduction surgery via sternotomy and thoracoscopy. The authors are extremely skilled surgeons with significant experience in both approaches. Of interest is the fact that not only from the standpoint of cost did thoracoscopy appear better than median sternotomy, but also from the standpoint of morbidity, mortality, and length of stay. Specifically, there were fewer days on the ventilator, fewer days with air leak, and significantly fewer days in the hospital for those patients undergoing the video-assisted approaches vs. the median sternotomy. In addition, apparently there was an increase in the forced expirate volume in 1 second in the video-assisted thoracic surgery group that was significantly greater than in the sternotomy group.

It is of interest that this article, carefully done by a highly skilled group of surgeons, so conclusively proves the superiority of the video-assisted thoracic surgery approach over the patients undergoing sternotomy. This article has, I think, captured the spirit of the movement across the country that has at most of the major centers embraced a minimally invasive approach in this high-risk group of patients. The current National Emphysema Treatment Trial has a significant cost study associated with it, which should give us prospective data that hopefully will confirm the data from the group at UCLA.

D.J. Sugarbaker, M.D.

Bovine Pericardium Versus Bovine Collagen to Buttress Staples for Lung Reduction Operations

Fischel RJ, McKenna RJ Jr (Chapman Med Ctr, Orange, Calif)

Ann Thorac Surg 65:217-219, 1998 14–11

Introduction.—Prolonged air leak is the most common complication after surgery for emphysema. The bovine pericardium patch was developed to decrease air leak. Use of the Peri-Strip patch increases cost of a bilateral staple operation by $3,000 to $4,000. The efficacy (ability to reduce postoperative air leaks) and handling characteristics of a less expensive product (INSTAT; bovine collagen) were compared with those of Peri-Strips (bovine pericardium).

Methods.—Fifty-seven consecutive patients underwent bilateral thoracoscopic stapled lung volume reduction procedures for heterogeneous bullous emphysema. Bovine pericardium (Peri-Strips) were used on one side and bovine collagen (INSTAT) were used on the ipsilateral side to buttress the staples.

Results.—The average time to chest tube removal was 8.6 and 10.7 days, respectively, for Peri-Strips and INSTAT. There were no significant differences observed in right- or left-sided applications. Air leaks lasting more than 7 days occurred in 20 patients with Peri-Strips and 25 patients with INSTAT. No complications were noted that could be attributed to the collagen or pericardium.

Conclusions.—Peri-Strips and INSTAT were equally effective in buttressing staple lines in thoracoscopic stapled bilateral lung volume reduction surgeries. Cost savings in materials of as much as 80% can be realized when using INSTAT instead of Peri-Strips for buttressing staple lines in patients undergoing lung reduction surgeries.

► The use of pericardial strips with the original descriptions of volume reduction surgery was thought to be the reason why this procedure could now be safely performed. Specifically, the St. Louis group suggested that without the use of bovine strips, Dr. Brantigan's work could not have been reproduced in their institution.[1] However, Dr. Brantigan[2] did not use staplers, and it appears that the primary improvement in the morbidity and mortality of volume reduction surgery over the initial series by Dr. Brantigan comes from the use of staplers made by several companies. Indeed, the use of the bovine pericardial strips as a superior method of buttressing has not held up in a number of studies. This study simply confirms my own experience that bovine pericardium adds a tremendous amount of expense to this procedure, without any significant improvement in air leak. In my own institution, autologous buttresses or "plications" have been used to try to circumvent the tremendous cost of pericardial strips. Alternative methods such as the use of collagen as well as polytetrafluoroethylene are currently under development and evaluation as a means of avoiding this unconscionable cost that is added to the lung volume reduction surgery procedure. Again, it is not clear that buttressing a staple line is required or is advantageous over stapling alone. In addition, there appears to be a variety of new techniques to buttress staple lines that are far less costly and potentially much more efficacious than the use of the bovine strip.

D.J. Sugarbaker, M.D.

References

1. Cooper JD: Technique to reduce air leaks after resection of emphysematous lung. *Ann Thorac Surg* 57:1038-1039, 1994.
2. Brantigan OC, Mueller E: Surgical treatment of pulmonary emphysema. *Am Surg* 23:789-804, 1957.

Lung Reduction Operation and Resection of Pulmonary Nodules in Patients With Severe Emphysema

DeRose JJ Jr, Argenziano M, El-Amir N, et al (Columbia Univ, New York)
Ann Thorac Surg 65:314-318, 1998 14–12

Purpose.—Most patients with lung cancer also have evidence of chronic obstructive pulmonary disease, and 20% or more have severe pulmonary dysfunction. Even with early-stage tumors, these patients may not be considered candidates for surgery because of inadequate pulmonary reserve. Lung volume reduction surgery has become a useful surgical treatment for severe emphysema. The use of combined resection of pulmonary nodules and lung volume reduction surgery was evaluated in patients with severe emphysema.

Methods.—Evaluation for lung volume reduction surgery revealed suspicious pulmonary nodules in 21 of 327 patients (6%). Fourteen of these patients were managed with combined lung volume reduction and pulmonary nodule resection. The patients were 8 men and 6 women whose mean age was 69 years. Before surgery, 71% of the patients were dependent on oxygen, 36% had a partial pressure of carbon dioxide of 45 mmHg or greater while breathing room air, and 36% were dependent on steroids. Mean forced expiratory volume in 1 second (FEV_1) was 680 mL. Forced vital capacity was 54% of the predicted value, and the ratio of FEV_1 to vital capacity was 37% of predicted. The surgical approach to lung volume reduction was adjusted according to the area of concomitant tumor resection.

Results.—A total of 16 lung lesions were resected, 9 of which proved to be non–small-cell cancers. The mean nodule size was 1.7 cm. One patient with previous thoracic surgery died during the postoperative period. Of the remaining patients, all were alive and well at a mean follow-up of 23 months. At 6 months, the dyspnea index had improved from 3.6 to 1.9, FEV_1 from 27% to 35% predicted, forced vital capacity from 54% to 69% predicted, and 6-minute walk distance from 817 to 1,100 feet. There was 1 case of mediastinal recurrence at 12 months; this patient had had 2 separate bronchioalveolar carcinomas.

Conclusions.—For patients with suspicious pulmonary nodules and severe pulmonary dysfunction, the combination of lung volume reduction surgery and tumor resection offers a chance of tumor cure with improved quality of life. Even if the nodule is benign or infectious, this approach permits definitive diagnosis and treatment of the nodule. The need for new criteria to assess operability and resectability among patients with severe emphysema and pulmonary nodules was emphasized.

▶ This article highlights an interesting finding that has come as the result of volume reduction surgery and the enhanced study of patients with late stage emphysema. In the community of epidemiologists looking for patients at higher risk for lung cancer, where screening may be the most advantageous, it is clear now that patients who have alterations in pulmonary function suggestive of chronic obstructive pulmonary disease are at increased risk for the development of carcinoma of the lung. Specifically, Harvey Pass (personal communication) has noted in his publication that patients with altered pulmonary function studies suggesting emphysema are indeed a high-risk subset of patients who smoke. Therefore, in addition to the highest risk group of patients who have already had a previous lung cancer, we can add this new large population of patients that have demonstrable spirometric findings of emphysema. This is important as the surgeon approaches patients for lung volume reduction surgery, as the nodule that may be ignored in the population at large cannot be ignored in a patient with severe emphysema. This article suggests that 5% of all patients presenting for volume reduction surgery may indeed have a bronchogenic carcinoma. This is an astounding figure. We all need to be on our guard for the detection of primary bronchogenic carcinoma in this newly recognized high-risk group of patients. This article further suggests that adequate resection can be performed simultaneously with volume reduction surgery. Indeed, given the small size of these lesions, they would seem to support a generous wedge excision in this subgroup.

D.J. Sugarbaker, M.D.

Incidental Lung Carcinoma Detected at CT in Patients Selected for Lung Volume Reduction Surgery to Treat Severe Pulmonary Emphysema

Rozenshtein A, White CS, Austin JHM, et al (Columbia-Presbyterian Med Ctr, New York; Univ of Maryland, Baltimore)

Radiology 207:487-490, 1998 14–13

Background.—Lung volume reduction appears to reduce dyspnea and improve pulmonary function in patients with severe pulmonary emphysema. The authors routinely perform chest CT in patients being considered for lung volume reduction surgery. This imaging study has identified a number of patients with previously unsuspected primary lung tumors. An experience with incidentally detected lung cancer in patients undergoing lung volume reduction surgery for severe emphysema was presented.

Methods.—During an 18-month period, 148 patients at 2 hospitals underwent preoperative chest CT before lung volume reduction surgery for severe pulmonary emphysema. The patients were 84 men and 64 women; mean age, 65 years. Lung nodules identified on CT were preoperatively selected for excision, but their presence did not affect the decision to perform lung volume reduction surgery. All suspicious lesions were excised as completely as possible at surgery.

Findings.—Seventeen patients (11%) had a total of 18 suspicious pulmonary nodules detected at CT. Sixteen of the nodules were resected; 1 could not be found at surgery; and 1 patient had intraoperative complications. Nine (56%) of the resected nodules were non–small-cell carcinomas. Thus, 5% of the 148 patients had incidentally detected lung cancers. There were 4 adenocarcinomas, 3 of which showed bronchiolar differentiation; 3 poorly differentiated tumors; and 2 squamous cell carcinomas. All the carcinomas were peripheral, with maximum diameters of 1.0 to 3.8 cm. Eight carcinomas were graded stage I; the other was not surgically staged. The remaining 7 resected nodules were benign.

Conclusions.—Five percent of patients undergoing lung volume reduction surgery for severe pulmonary emphysema had stage I primary lung cancers. These findings underscore the importance of preoperative chest CT in patients who are candidates for this procedure. Chest CT will not only identify patterns of lung destruction, but will also detect many cases of potentially curable cancer. About half the nodules detected by CT will be malignant.

▶ This article is of interest because it begins to develop a new therapeutic procedure for the treatment of patients with severe emphysema and accompanying lung nodule. The concept of performing a therapeutic volume reduction surgery in the setting of bronchogenic carcinoma is an interesting one. Previous reports and the literature would suggest that patients with extremely limited pulmonary function would not be candidates for primary resection of lung carcinomas. This interesting approach utilizes the therapeutic benefit of volume reduction surgery as it may be applied to this subgroup of patients when combined with primary resection of the lung nodule. It will be important for the surgeon approaching a patient with severe emphysema and a primary carcinoma of the lung to ascertain the geographic distribution of the emphysema. Indeed, the markers of patient selection and of improvement with volume reduction surgery will be even more important as the surgeon approaches a patient with primary bronchogenic carcinoma and severe emphysema. Nevertheless, this article suggests that when combined, primary resection of bronchogenic carcinoma and lung volume reduction surgery can be performed safely with a therapeutic benefit to the patient, both in terms of the resection of their carcinoma, as well as in terms of improved pulmonary function postoperatively. This unique procedure will apply to a large number of patients as is suggested by Abstract 14–12, comprising almost 6% to 10% of patients presenting for volume reduction surgery. This new combined procedure will require additional study as we seek to further evaluate the biologic course of carcinoma in this subgroup of patients, as well as the overall effect on their pulmonary function in the postoperative period. It appears that one cannot assume that the biology of lung tumors in this subgroup of patients will mirror the biologic behavior of tumors in patients with more normal anatomic and physiologic lung function.

D.J. Sugarbaker, M.D.

Effect of Volume Reduction on Lung Transplant Timing and Selection for Chronic Obstructive Pulmonary Disease

Bavaria JE, Pochettino A, Kotloff RM, et al (Univ of Pennsylvania Med Ctr, Philadelphia)

J Thorac Cardiovasc Surg 115:9-18, 1998 14–14

Background.—Lung transplantation has been the traditional treatment for end-stage chronic obstructive pulmonary disease. The results of a pilot program of lung volume reduction offered as a bridge to extend time to transplantation were reported.

Methods.—Thirty-one patients assessed for lung transplantation between 1993 and 1997 met physiologic criteria for volume reduction: forced expiratory volume in 1 second of 25% or less, residual volume exceeding 200%, and significant ventilation/perfusion heterogeneity. The patients completed 6 weeks of pulmonary rehabilitation, then underwent baseline pulmonary function and 6-minute walk testing. These patients were offered lung volume reduction and were listed simultaneously for transplantation. Volume reduction was achieved by a video-assisted thoracic approach in 87% and by bilateral median sternotomy in 13%. After surgery, the patients were divided into 2 groups: those with satisfactory outcomes 4 to 6 months after volume reduction and those with unsatisfactory results.

Findings.—Seventy-seven percent of the patients had satisfactory outcomes 4 to 6 months after lung reduction. The 7 patients with unsatisfactory outcomes included 1 who died in the perioperative period. Four patients with successful results experienced significant deterioration in pulmonary function during intermediate-term follow-up and were reconsidered for lung transplantation. Two of these patients have subsequently had transplantation with good postoperative pulmonary function outcomes. Three patients had α_1-antitrypsin deficiency; 2 of these had poor volume reduction outcomes.

Conclusions.—Lung volume reduction has greatly affected the practice, timing, and selection of patients for lung transplantation at the authors' institution. Lung volume reduction in the current series was a safe option, although its value may be limited in patients with α_1-antitrypsin deficiency.

▶ The observation that patients with emphysema awaiting lung transplantation may be better served with volume reduction surgery is an interesting and provocative one. At my institution, volume reduction surgery has now become the preliminary procedure of choice before listing patients for lung transplantation. Indeed, when one looks at the registry and finds that roughly 43% of the patients undergoing lung transplantation are dead within five years,[1] indeed the alternatives such as volume reduction surgery gain a significant advantage in my mind. For many years there have been theoretical problems with the applications of lung transplantation to patients with severe bilateral emphysema. These problems theoretically were to arise out of the differential compliance between the donor and recipient lungs. Indeed, many patients do develop problems based on this differential ventilation and compliance. In addition, the problems with infection and underlying rejection that are responsible for the majority of deaths in these patients are not seen in patients undergoing volume reduction surgery. Therefore, it appears clear that in the years ahead patients will not be considered for lung transplantation unless they have contraindications to volume reduction surgery as pointed out by these authors, such as α_1-antitrypsin or some other contraindication. However, it is difficult to imagine what contraindications to volume reduction surgery would not also be profound contraindications to transplantation. It may be in the years ahead that in patients with severe emphysema, volume reduction surgery will become the treatment of choice prior to lung transplantation. Indeed, the results of the National Emphysema Treatment Trial will be extremely important in evaluating the efficacy of this approach in the transplant population.

D.J. Sugarbaker, M.D.

References

1. Arcasoy SM, Kotloff RM: Lung transplantation. *N Engl J Med* 340:1081-1091, 1999.

Thoracoscopic Volume Reduction of the Native Lung After Single Lung Transplantation for Emphysema

Venuta F, De Giacomo T, Rendina EA, et al (Univ of Rome "La Sapienza")
Am J Respir Crit Care Med 156:292-293, 1997 14–15

Background.—After single lung transplantation in emphysema, the remaining native lung is predisposed to late hyperinflation. This may result because of decreased compliance in the transplant (as occurs with obliterative bronchiolitis) or in the native lung itself (as occurs with chronic obstructive pulmonary disease). A patient was described who had late hyperinflation in the native lung after single lung transplantation for emphysema, and was successfully treated by volume reduction via thoracoscopy.

Case Report.—Woman, 44, with panlobular emphysema underwent right single lung transplantation. After surgery her PaO_2 was 90 mm Hg and $PaCO_2$ was 35 mm Hg. Three years after transplantation, her PaO_2 and $PaCO_2$ were still good (86 and 39 mm Hg, respectively), but her forced expiratory volume in 1 second (FEV_1) had fallen to 0.53 L (18% of predicted). The native left lung was hyperinflated as revealed by chest radiography, with displacement of the mediastinum and depression of the left hemidiaphragm. Lung biopsy and culture results were negative, and the patient did not respond to empirical treatment for obliterative bronchiolitis. The posterior and apical segments of the upper lobe and the apical segment of the lower lobe showed significantly decreased perfusion on single photon emission CT. Thus a video-assisted thoracoscopic stapling procedure was performed with the patient under general anesthesia and with 1-lung ventilation. Unperfused areas of the native lung were resected and volume was reduced by approximately 25%. Mechanical ventilation was discontinued at the end of the procedure. The patient received oxygen for 48 hours and had a pleural drain for 34 days because of a low-volume air leak. The patient noted immediate improvement after the procedure, and FEV_1 was 1.8 L (60% of predicted). Postoperative radiography indicated that the mediastinal shift was no longer present, and the diaphragm had a normal contour. Eight months after surgery, results of pulmonary function tests are stable.

Conclusions.—Early after surgery, hyperinflation is usually transient and decompression is not required. However, with late hyperinflation, volume reduction may be indicated. Before volume reduction, infections and obliterative bronchiolitis should be ruled out. If volume reduction of the native lung is required, a video-assisted thoracoscopic procedure can provide good results.

▶ The differential compliance between the native lung and the transplanted lung in patients undergoing lung transplantation for severe emphysema is the source of significant clinical problems postoperatively. Indeed, the application of volume reduction surgery in this subset of patients at the time of transplantation or subsequent to transplantation would appear to be an intuitive, straightforward application of this surgical procedure. In my own institution, the use of volume reduction surgery has been applied in several situations in the post transplant period when hyperinflation of the native lung is accompanied by compression and dysfunction of the transplant graft. The question that I would raise at this point is whether prophylactic simultaneous volume reduction surgery should be carried out at the time of single lung transplantation in all patients undergoing transplantation for severe bilateral emphysema. It may be that the avoidance of even incremental compression of the transplanted lung would lead to improved graft function in the long-term. This case report is of interest because it demonstrates clearly the efficacy of a lung volume reduction procedure in patients undergoing contralateral single lung transplantation. The authors are to be congratulated for demonstrating this so clearly in this article. We await a prospective randomized trial of volume reduction surgery at the time of transplantation vs. subsequent to transplantation, as clinical problems would demand.

D.J. Sugarbaker, M.D.

Lung Volume Reduction Surgery as an Emergency and Life-saving Procedure

Hansson B, Jorens PG, van Schil P, et al (Univ Hosp Antwerp, Edegem, Belgium; St-Augustinus Hosp, Antwerp, Belgium)

Eur Respir J 10:2650-2652, 1997 14–16

Introduction.—Lung volume reduction surgery (LVRS) is emerging as a promising and unique therapeutic approach for carefully selected patients with severe emphysema. A patient with severe chronic obstructive pulmonary disease (COPD) was described who underwent LVRS while ventilator dependent, a condition in which LVRS has been considered to be contraindicated.

> *Case Report.*—Man, 51, with severe COPD and a predominant emphysema component from nicotine abuse was admitted while on holiday in a southern European country with fever, dyspnea, and bilateral pneumothorax. Two chest tubes were inserted. Intubation and mechanical ventilation were needed for respiratory insufficiency and sepsis. He received CPR for cardiac arrest. An additional 4 chest tubes were inserted with separate suction systems. He was transferred to Belgium where bilateral LVRS was performed through a median sternotomy as a last resort. The most diseased areas of the upper lobes containing air leaks were resected bilaterally using a linear stapler with strips of bovine pericardium. A pleurectomy was also performed. He was treated with intravenous fluconazole for a respiratory infection with *Candida albicans*. He was extubated 14 days after surgery. He was discharged on postoperative day 28 and ceased smoking. At 3 months after surgery, he had a remarkable improvement in spirometric values, with an increase in forced expiratory volume in 1 second of about 100%. These findings were sustained at 18 months' follow-up.

Conclusions.—Lung volume reduction surgery may be used in carefully selected patients with COPD who are ventilator dependent, even in situations where the surgery is a lifesaving measure.

► Lung volume reduction surgery has been traditionally thought of as a procedure applied in an elective setting to a well-characterized group of patients with careful preoperative study. Indeed authors have suggested that the emergency application of volume reduction surgery has no place in a patient with life-threatening complications of emphysema. This study is of interest in that it demonstrates that in such an emergency, life-threatening situation, volume reduction surgery can be applied with very positive results. Indeed, the application of volume reduction surgery to the ventilator-dependent patient in the appropriate clinical setting may be of some value. The reader is directed to this interesting article with the thought that a broader application of volume reduction surgery to ventilator patients may be completed in the future.

D.J. Sugarbaker, M.D.

Non–Small-Cell Lung Cancer: Progress in Understanding

INTRODUCTION

The most common malignancy in the United States, and the principal killer of men and women, remains non–small-cell lung cancer. New and effective therapies continue to be the primary goal, but we await their arrival. Energy is therefore directed at an enhanced understanding of tumor biology. The following articles were selected on the basis of their ability to enhance the surgeon's understanding of the tumor stage of individual patients, which therefore may enhance our ability to develop new strategies in their care.

David J. Sugarbaker, M.D.

Lymph Node Staging in Non–Small-Cell Lung Cancer With FDG-PET Scan: A Prospective Study on 690 Lymph Node Stations From 68 Patients

Vansteenkiste JF, Stroobants SG, De Leyn PR, et al (Catholic Univ Leuven, Belgium)

J Clin Oncol 16:2142-2149, 1998 14–17

Purpose.—In patients who have non–small-cell lung cancer (NSCLC) without distant metastases, the presence of lymph node metastases has a major impact on prognosis. Preoperative imaging techniques have been studied, but have given unsatisfactory results; thus, invasive surgical staging by mediastinoscopy remains standard practice. Positron emission tomography (PET) with the radiolabeled glucose analog ^{18}F-fluoro-2-deoxy-D-glucose (FDG) is highly accurate in differentiating between benign and malignant pulmonary nodules. This procedure was compared with CT scanning for effectiveness in locoregional lymph-node scanning in patients with NSCLC.

Methods.—The study included 68 patients undergoing evaluation for potentially operable NSCLC. In addition to cervical mediastinoscopy, thoracic CT and FDG-PET were performed in each patient. All imaging studies were interpreted without knowledge of the surgical-pathologic findings; the PET scans were graded on a 5-point scale. With knowledge of the pathologic results, a receiver operating characteristic analysis was performed to assess the relationship between standardized uptake values

(SUVs) and the presence of metastatic nodes. With these data, the likelihood ratios of node metastases according to SUV were established.

Results.—Invasive staging data were available on a total of 690 lymph-node stations. Fifty-nine percent of patients were correctly staged by chest CT; 18% were understaged and 28% were overstaged. The combination of FDG-PET and CT improved the accuracy of staging to 87%, with the remainder approximately equally split between understaging and overstaging. The sensitivity of CT in detected N2/N3 disease was 75%, with a specificity of 63% and accuracy of 68%. The combination of PET and CT had a sensitivity of 93%, specificity of 95%, and accuracy of 94%.

Receiver operating characteristic analysis suggested the an SUV threshold of 4.40 best distinguished between benign and malignant nodes. However, this SUV threshold was no more effective than the 5-point visual scale. Likelihood ratios were 0.152 for an SUV of 3.5, 3.157 for an SUV of 3.5 to 4.5, and 253.096 for an SUV of greater than 4.5.

Conclusions.—For patients with NSCLC, noninvasive lymph-node staging is more accurately achieved with a combination of PET and CT scanning than with CT alone. The study establishes an SUV threshold for distinguishing between benign and malignant lymph nodes, though its performance is no better than that of a simple visual scale. Mediastinal FDG-PET scanning offers a very high negative predictive value of 99%, which could reduce the number of NSCLC patients undergoing invasive surgical staging.

► This article highlights the increasing importance of PET scanning in the evaluation of patients with lung cancer. Specifically, this study demonstrates the inadequacy of CT scanning in the preresectional radiographic staging of the mediastinum. Moreover, the need for mediastinoscopy in this group of patients as has been previously the case, may not be indicated in situations where the CT scan in conjunction with the PET scan are, where the mediastinum is determined to be negative. This study is of interest in that it is at odds with previous studies, which suggested that PET scanning for the mediastinum is not as accurate as mediastinoscopy. This article is included in this year's YEAR BOOK review because of the extraordinary negative predictive value of the CT scan in the Belgian group when combined with FDG-PET of 99% negative predictive value. This would have profound implications on the number of mediastinoscopies that need to be done. This report bears watching and comparison with subsequent studies from the United States and Europe. Nevertheless, FDG-PET scanning is becoming an important and potentially very useful modality, particularly in patients with N2 disease, who are then treated with subsequent induction therapy. The recent data suggest that those patients who are successfully downstaged to either N1 or N0 disease from N2 disease will benefit most from therapeutic surgical resection. Conversely, those patients with persistent N2 disease despite induction therapy are to suffer a very poor prognosis and may not be a group in which therapeutic pulmonary resection is justified. The ability of the PET to predict the successful downstaging of patients would be an important application of this new technology.

D.J. Sugarbaker, M.D.

Lymph Node Metastasis in Small Peripheral Adenocarcinoma of the Lung

Takizawa T, Terashima M, Koike T, et al (Niigata Cancer Hosp, Japan)

J Thorac Cardiovasc Surg 116:276-280, 1998 14–18

Objective.—Whether all patients with lymph-node metastases from small peripheral carcinomas of the lung can be identified before or during resection is not known. The clinical and pathologic features of small peripheral adenocarcinoma of the lung were retrospectively investigated, with special emphasis on lymph-node metastasis.

Methods.—Between January 1980 and December 1996, 157 of 789 patients (75 men), aged 29 to 85, who were undergoing lobectomy for clinical stage I peripheral lung cancer had small-cell adenocarcinomas. Nodal status was assessed, and the histopathologic characteristics of the tumor were determined.

Results.—Postoperatively, 11 patients were found to have N1 metastases and 16 to have N2 metastases. Lymph-node metastases were observed during surgery in 8 patients. Metastases were located in single nodes in 10 patients, a segmental node in 1, a lobar node in 5, an interlobar node in 2, a pretracheal node in 1, and a highest mediastinal node in 1. Whereas 13 (11%) of 120 patients without pleural involvement had lymph-node metastases, 14 (38%) of 27 with pleural involvement had lymph-node metastases. Female sex, degree of differentiation, and pleural involvement were significantly associated with metastases, according to multiple regression analysis. Estimated 5-year survival was 91% for patients with N0 tumors, and 28% for patients with N1 or N2 tumors ($P=0.0000$).

Conclusion.—Nodal assessment during surgery is not sufficient for identifying lymph-node metastases in patients with small peripheral adenocarcinoma of the lung. Lobectomy and complete hilar mediastinal lymphadenectomy are necessary to determine N stage. Female sex, degree of differentiation, and pleural involvement are significantly associated with lymph-node metastases.

▶ This article is interesting in that the small peripheral adenocarcinomas studied by this group demonstrated a significant number of N1 and N2 nodal metastases. These metastases were noted only at the time of lobectomy with complete hilar node dissection. Of interest is the fact that pleural involvement correlated with a 38% incidence of nodal metastases, whereas tumors less than 2 cm did not have pleural involvement and had only an 11% nodal involvement. However, although the authors' statement that lobectomy is therefore required for accurate staging may be true, the estimated 5-year survival for the N0 patients was 91%, but was only 28% for patients with N1 or N2 disease. This suggests that the lobectomy had a sustained therapeutic value in only 28% of the patients noted to have N1 or N2 involvement. Given the fact that most conservative resections are done in patients with extremely poor lung function, it is not clear that the additional perioperative morbidity and mortality of a full thoracotomy and lobectomy would be justified in this high risk group of patients. It is of interest that the N1 survival is so low at 28%. This is roughly half of the previous reported series on N1 nodal disease and long-term survival. Nevertheless, the importance of complete nodal sampling via lobectomy is underlined, as is the importance of pleural involvement in predicting the presence of nodal disease in adenocarcinomas of the lung.

D.J. Sugarbaker, M.D.

Systematic Lymph Node Dissection for Clinically Diagnosed Peripheral Non–Small-Cell Lung Cancer Less Than 2 cm in Diameter

Sugi K, Nawata K, Fujita N, et al (Yamaguchi Univ, Japan)

World J Surg 22:290-295, 1998 14–19

Objective.—For patients with peripheral non–small-cell lung cancers (NSCLCs) measuring less that 2 cm, standard treatment is lobectomy with systemic mediastinal and hilar lymph node dissection. However, some surgeons prefer to just perform nodal sampling to avoid the morbidity of extensive lymph node dissection. The relative therapeutic benefits of these competing approaches are unknown. A randomized trial was performed to compare radical systematic lymph node dissection with lymph node sampling in patients with small NSCLCs.

Methods.—The study included 115 patients with peripheral NSCLCs measuring less than 2 cm in diameter. All underwent lobectomy with either lymph node sampling or radical systematic lymph node dissection. The patients were entered into the study on the basis of preoperative clinical studies only. The 2 groups were compared for recurrence rate and prognosis.

Results.—At surgery, 4 patients were found to have tumors larger than 2 cm, 1 to have disseminated disease, 2 to have intrapulmonary metastases, and 2 to have small-cell carcinoma. Systemic lymphadenectomy was associated with a longer duration of operation and higher morbidity. Lymph node metastases were discovered in 19% of patients in the dissection group (N1 disease in 7% and N2 disease in 12%). The rate of metastases in the sampling group was 20% (N1 in 5% and N2 in 14%). The recurrence rates were 10% in the dissection group and 13% in the sampling group, with most of the recurrences being distant. The 5-year survival rate was similar as well: 81% in the dissection group and 84% in the sampling group.

Conclusion.—In patients undergoing lobectomy for clinically diagnosed peripheral NSCLCs measuring less than 2 cm in diameter, systematic lymph node dissection does not appear to be necessary. Lymph node sampling offers similar recurrence and survival rates and reduced morbidity. Most recurrences in this group of patients are distant and include synchronous distant and local recurrences.

▶ This article looks at a subgroup of patients with small peripheral non–small-cell lung cancers measuring less than 2 cm, where a standard lobectomy is done with or without mediastinal node dissection. Indeed, radical node dissection is compared with nodal sampling. This question has been asked by a large number of surgeons worldwide as they approach patients with non–small-cell lung cancer. Indeed, in most other malignancies, including breast cancer, the role of systematic lymph node dissection as a therapeutic endeavor has been discarded. Nevertheless, data in non–small-cell lung cancers suggest that N1 patients do better than patients with N2 disease, and therefore that there is a therapeutic role for systematic lymph node removal. However, when disease is present in N2 nodes, it is not clear that therapeutic lymphadenectomy is of value. This study suggests that, indeed, in small tumors, lymph node sampling for staging accuracy is as valuable as radical lymphadenectomy. Given the attendant increased morbidity and length of operative time for radical lymphadenectomy in this group of patients with small tumors, one can only conclude from this article that it is not of sufficient value to be practiced in a systematic way. However, I underscore the importance of complete nodal sampling prior to surgical resection in all peripheral adenocarcinomas of the lung and any other tumors where there is a higher incidence of occult nodal metastases. The importance of preresection identification of nodal disease is highlighted by the fact that the only data that suggests that their survival can be altered are data from studies utilizing induction chemoradiotherapy prior to surgical resection. The flip side is that adjuvant or postoperative chemotherapy or radiotherapy has not been demonstrated to be of any value in prolonging survival. Therefore, if one does not detect lymph node metastases in the mediastinum prior to resection, there appear to be no data at the present time to support the probability of altering the rather dismal outlook of this subgroup of patients.

D.J. Sugarbaker, M.D.

Prognostic Assessment of 1310 Patients With Non–Small-Cell Lung Cancer Who Underwent Complete Resection From 1980 to 1993

Inoue K, Sato M, Fujimura S, et al (Tohoku Univ, Sendai, Japan; Sendai Kosei Hosp, Japan; Natl Sendai Hosp, Japan)

J Thorac Cardiovasc Surg 116:407-411, 1998 14–20

Objective.—The revised stage grouping adopted by the International Union Against Cancer (UICC) and the American Joint Committee on Cancer has not been validated. The prognoses of 1,310 patients with completely resected non–small-cell lung cancer, as predicted by the International Union Against Cancer-revised TNM staging system, were investigated.

Methods.—Survivals of 1,310 patients (342 female) were calculated, using the Kaplan-Meier method, after lobectomy or pneumonectomy with lymph node dissection.

Results.—Using the revised system, 5-year survivals for patients with T1 N0 M0, T2 N0 M0, T1 N1 M0, and T2 N1 M0 diseases were 80%, 65%, 57%, and 42%, respectively. There were significant survival differences between patients with T1 N0 M0 disease and those with T2 N0 M0 disease and between patients with T1 N1 M0 disease and those with T2 N1 M0 disease, but not between patients with T2 N0 M0 disease and those with T1 N1 M0 disease. There was no significant 5-year survival difference between patients with T2 N1 M0 disease (42%), patients with T3 N0 M0 disease (34%), and those with T3 N1 M0 disease (38%). Patients with T3 organ invasion had 5-year survivals of 35% for pleural invasion, 26% for chest-wall invasion, and 43% for pericardial invasion. Three-year survival for diaphragmatic invasion was 0%. Five-year survivals for patients with completely resected T3 N2 M0 disease and completely resected stage IIIB disease were 11% and 36%, respectively. Patients with T3 N2 M0 disease and stage IIIB disease had similar 5-year survivals.

Conclusion.—Survival calculations support most of the revisions. The authors suggest, however, that stages T3 N2 M0 and IIIB, T3 N1 M0 and IIB, and T2 N0 M0 and T1 N1 M0 be combined because survivals are similar, and they also recommend including diaphragmatic invasion in stage T4.

▶ This interesting, well-studied group of patients who have undergone surgical resection for non–small-cell lung cancer tends to support the UICC's staging revision published last year in I *Chest.*[1] Some interesting points are emphasized by Inove et al. The first is that patients with T2N0 lesions do significantly worse than patients with T1N0 lesions. Indeed, it is this subgroup of 80% vs. 65% long-term survival that seems to justify current national and North American trials looking at the role of adjuvant chemotherapy in patients with T2N0 disease. In addition, there are current studies under way looking at the efficacy of induction chemotherapy in patients with clinical T2N0 disease given the rather poor overall five year survival (65%) as noted in this study. In addition, the study emphasizes the relatively poor prognosis of patients with T3N2 tumors. Indeed, this subset of patients with N2 disease appears to do significantly worse than patients with T1 or T2N2 lesions. Indeed, I suggest that these patients should be characterized as 3B, given their dismal survival in this manuscript. Indeed this subgroup of patients would appear to be one that could significantly benefit from innovative induction chemoradiotherapy strategies prior to surgery.

Nevertheless, the revised UICC and American Joint Committee on Cancer staging system appears to be validated in large part by this very important, well-characterized, and well-studied group of patients.

D.J. Sugarbaker, M.D.

Reference

1. Mountain CF: Revisions in the international system for staging lung cancer. *Chest* 111:1710-1717, 1997.

"Incomplete Resection" in Non–Small Cell Lung Cancer: Need for a New Definition

Guyatt GH, for the Canadian Lung Oncology Group (McMaster Univ, Hamilton, Ont, Canada; et al)

Ann Thorac Surg 65:220-226, 1998 14–21

Introduction.—The prognosis and management of an incompletely resected non–small-cell lung cancer (NSCLC) is uncertain. This is partly the result of controversy in the current literature regarding the definition of "incomplete resection." The prognostic value of positive surgical resection margin or highest nodal station sampled at thoracotomy was retrospectively assessed in 399 patients with NSCLC.

Methods.—Surgical records and pathologic reports from a randomized trial comparing CT with mediastinoscopy for staging of lung cancer were reviewed for data regarding pathologic findings at the surgical resection margin, the highest mediastinal nodal station sampled at thoracotomy, histologic type, tumor size, N status, and evidence of vascular or lymphatic invasion. These variables were used as independent variables in logistic regression models to predict recurrence.

Results.—Complete data were available at 3-year follow-up for all except 1 of 399 patients. There were 2 significant predictors of recurrence: tumor size and N2 disease. No other variables predicted early recurrence or death.

Conclusions.—In this large series of patients with NSCLC, surgical resection margin and highest nodal station sampled at thoracotomy that were involved by carcinoma were not predictive of recurrence. Rather, tumor size and N2 disease were significant predictors of recurrence. This data strongly suggest that traditional definitions of incomplete resection should be reexamined.

► This interesting study by the Canadian Lung Oncology Group is important in lending some data to the question of what is an incomplete resection. By convention, previous national trials have designated patients whose highest lymph node removed in the chest is positive as being incompletely resected. This is based on the concept that the next lymph node may well be involved, which is, of course, out of the surgeon's operating field and therefore not resectable. While this appeared to have intuitive basis, there have been no data to suggest that highest lymph node positive does indeed reflect negatively on survival. This well-studied group of patients suggests just the opposite. Indeed highest node positive did not predict for early recurrence or death. As noted in the Abstract 14–20, tumor size and the presence of N2 disease were the two most important predictors of early recurrence and death. Therefore, it appears from this article that patients with highest lymph node positive should be considered completely resected. Other definitions of incomplete resection would appear to still stand, such as tumor at resection margins.

The authors, however, do not make a specific recommendation as to whether postoperative radiation can indeed sterilize a positive margin. Their recommendation that radiation therapy was of no value is based on an extremely small sample, and it does not appear to support any definitive conclusion in the negative. Certainly, radiation therapy can achieve local control on a variety of settings, and its application to the patient who has a positive margin appears to be sound, based on the knowledge of the effects of radiation in its mechanism of action. Surgical re-resection appears to have been of somewhat limited value, particularly in those patients who have the peribronchiolar persistent disease.

D.J. Sugarbaker, M.D.

Survival in Resected Stage I Lung Cancer With Residual Tumor at the Bronchial Resection Margin

Snijder RJ, Brutel de la Rivière AB, Elbers HJJ, et al (Sint Antonius Hosp, Nieuwegein, The Netherlands)

Ann Thorac Surg 65:212-216, 1998 14–22

Introduction.—Complete resection offers excellent survival results for patients with stage I non–small-cell lung cancer (NSCLC). However, in some apparently complete resections, examination of the bronchial resection margin will show microscopic residual tumor. It is unclear whether this microscopic residual tumor affects survival. The survival of patients with microscopic residual tumor at the bronchial resection margin after surgery for stage I NSCLC was retrospectively examined.

Patients.—A total of 834 patients who had pulmonary resection of stage I NSCLC during a 16-year period were studied. Eight hundred two patients were considered to have complete resection; 23 had residual tumor at the bronchial resection margin. These patients were 22 men and 1 woman whose mean age was 66 years. The pattern of residual tumor was carcinoma in situ in 12 patients, mucosal residual disease in 8, and peribronchial residual disease in 3. Follow-up data on local and distant recurrence and survival were analyzed to assess the impact of the microscopic residual tumor.

Outcomes.—Five-year survival was 54% for patients with complete resection vs. 43% in those with residual tumor. However, within the residual tumor group, 5-year survival was 58% for patients with residual carcinoma in situ vs. 27% for those with invasive disease, i.e., mucosal or peribronchial residual disease. For patients with residual tumor, adjuvant radiotherapy did not improve survival. Five patients underwent revision surgery, and their 5-year survival was 40%.

Conclusions.—The survival of patients with residual tumor at the bronchial resection margin after surgery for stage I lung cancer depends on the pattern of microscopic residual disease. If the residual disease is carcinoma in situ, 5-year survival is similar to that of patients with complete resection. If the residual disease is invasive, than survival is reduced. These patients may benefit from revision surgery or, if the patient cannot tolerate another operation, follow-up bronchoscopy.

▶ The clinical problem of microscopic residual tumor often confronts the practicing thoracic surgeon. It is my routine practice, as well as the routine practice of many thoracic surgeons, to always assess the bronchial resection margin prior to closure of the chest and completion of the surgery. This practice is routine in most centers as occult disease at the bronchial margin is thought to lead to subsequent disease recurrence. This study does provide rationale for this practice. Indeed, those patients who had disease at the resection margin did significantly worse than those patients who had a complete resection did. Of further interest is the question as to why these patients do not do as well. Is the invasive presence of tumor at the margin simply a marker of more aggressive biology or an indication of the inadequacy of the surgical resection completed? Certainly, the principal of complete surgical resection and adequate local control appears to be an important one that is validated by this study. It has been my thought through the years that patients in whom there is disease noted outside the bronchial mucosa in the peribronchial tissues clinically behave more like patients with N2 disease than patients with endobronchial tumor along the bronchial mucosa where additional surgical resection appears to be justified. Indeed, patients who have disease in peribronchial lymphatics would appear to have disease in transit to the N2 stations and, therefore, should be categorized in the clinician's mind as a potentially poor outcome mimicking patients with documented N2 disease.

D.J. Sugarbaker, M.D.

Do Molecular Markers Predict Survival in Non–Small-Cell Lung Cancer?

Greatens TM, Niehans GA, Rubins JB, et al (Veterans Affairs Med Ctr, Minneapolis; Univ of Minnesota, Minneapolis)

Am J Respir Crit Care Med 157:1093-1097, 1998 14–23

Background.—Survival from non–small-cell lung cancer (NSCLC) is variable, even after adjustment for pathologic disease stage. Various tumor cell markers have been suggested as useful predictors of postoperative survival. However, some studies have given conflicting results, and the clinical value of the markers is questionable. A combination of markers might provide greater ability to predict survival. Seven putative biological markers of survival in patients with resected NSCLC were tested.

Methods.—The analysis included 101 consecutive patients with NSCLC who had exploratory thoracotomy with curative intent over a 5-year period. All were followed for at least 2 years. Polymerase chain reaction with single-strand conformation polymorphism was performed to evaluate mutations in the *p53* tumor suppressor gene and the *K-ras* oncogene. Immunocytochemical tests for p53 protein, bcl-2 protein, c-erbB-1 protein, c-erbB-2 protein, and MIA-15-5 antigen were performed as well. Independent associations between the variables and patient survival were assessed in a Cox proportional hazards model, with tumor pathologic stage and molecular markers as covariates.

Results.—Nineteen patients had K-ras mutations, all but 2 of whom had adenocarcinoma. Forty patients had p53 mutations. Expression of the other antigens varied. Survival was strongly and inversely related to surgical tumor stage. The only molecular marker to be strongly related to survival was MIA-15-5, which was significant on both univariate and multivariate analysis. However, this study found that overexpression of MIA-15-5 antigen was related to improved survival, whereas a previous report suggested that it was related to poorer survival.

Conclusion.—These molecular markers do not appear to be useful predictors of survival in patients undergoing surgery for NSCLC. Although these markers may still have prognostic significance, it is likely to be small and would require a much larger study for confirmation.

▶ This study does not support the use of *p53* or *K-ras* as a predictive molecular marker in non–small-cell lung cancer. This is of interest as most major studies with large numbers of patients have shown both *K-ras* and *p53* to be significant markers of poor prognosis. This is of particular importance in patients with Stage I disease that has been surgically resected. If one could construct a molecular substaging system for Stage I disease, one might be able to identify patients at high risk for distant recurrence and, therefore, treat them in the adjuvant setting with conventional chemotherapy. This article does identify MIA-15-5 as a potential marker of good prognosis. Indeed, antigenic markers of improved survival have been rare. Most markers studied, including those from our own laboratory, have been markers of poor prognostic value. Nevertheless, this is a carefully and well-done study that bears mention because of the negative predictive value of the *K-ras* and *p53* mutations noted.

D.J. Sugarbaker, M.D.

Prognostic Value of Loss of Heterozygosity and KRAS2 Mutations in Lung Adenocarcinoma

De Gregorio L, Manenti G, Incarbone M, et al (Istituto Nazionale Tumori, Milan, Italy)

Int J Cancer 79:269-272, 1998 14–24

Objective.—Because approximately one third of non–small-cell lung cancer patients with adenocarcinoma have point mutations at codon 12 of the K-*ras*-2 gene, loss of heterozygosity (LOH) on the most commonly affected chromosomal regions and mutation at codon 12 of the K-*ras*-2 gene were investigated for their prognostic value.

Methods.—Samples of tumor tissue and normal parenchyma from 125 patients were investigated, using PCR amplification techniques, for LOH and K-*ras*-2 gene mutations.

Results.—Loss of heterozygosity ranged from 24% at 10p to 55% at 17p13. There were 47 (26%) patients with a point mutation at codon 12 of the K-*ras*-2 gene. More males than females and significantly more smokers than nonsmokers had point mutations (29% vs. 11%). Five-year survival rate was significantly associated with aspartic and valine mutations but not with the most common cysteine mutations. There was no association between LOH and survival.

Conclusion.—K-*ras*-2 gene mutations were significant predictors of survival in patients with lung adenocarcinoma.

▶ This article is of importance as it notes that the K-ras mutation may have subtypes that are of increased significance in predicting a poor survival. In addition, the prognostic value of the LOH/loss of satellite instability has been studied by some investigators and noted to be of prognostic significance. The LOHs were relatively common in this study, but were not significant prognostic factors. However, the K-ras tube mutations were noted in 26% of cases more common in male than female, and a trend was clearly observed between the type of K-ras mutation and poor survival. This suggests that while molecular substaging of Stage I patients will be important, there may be additional value at looking at specific types of mutations such as the wild type K-ras vs. the GAT and Val GTT mutations. Indeed, there are a variety of genetic aberrations in non–small-cell lung cancer that may lead us to a firmer platform to predict patients who will suffer early recurrence. These patients, therefore, would be the ideal ones in whom adjuvant therapy could be applied in a routine fashion similar to what is done in breast cancer and colon cancer.

D.J. Sugarbaker, M.D.

Detection of Occult Micrometastases in Non–Small Cell Lung Carcinoma by Reverse Transcriptase-Polymerase Chain Reaction

Salerno CT, Frizelle S, Niehans GA, et al (Univ of Minnesota, Minneapolis; Minneapolis VA. Med Ctr)

Chest 113:1526-1532, 1998 14–25

Purpose.—Immunohistochemical approaches have been used to detect the presence of occult micrometastases (OMs) in regional lymph nodes from patients with non–small-cell lung cancer (NSCLC). Recent studies have examined the use of reverse transcriptase-polymerase chain reaction (RT-PCR) to detect OMs at the molecular level. The cell surface glycoprotein MUC1 is expressed in most epithelial tissues and in normal lung tissue, but not in normal lymph node tissue. This study used an RT-PCR for MUC1 to detect OMs in histologically negative lymph nodes from patients with NSCLC.

Methods.—The study included 28 patients with benign or malignant thoracic disease. Primary tumors and lymph nodes were tested for the presence of MUC1 mRNA by an RT-PCR. The DNA-based assay was specific and sensitive, detecting MUC1 mRNA concentrations as low as a single cancer cell. The results were compared with those of immunohistochemical staining.

Results.—None of 11 mediastinal lymph nodes from patients without malignant disease expressed detectable MUC1 transcripts. Of 18 primary NSCLCs studied, 16 expressed MUC1 mRNA. The RT-PCR was also positive for MUC1 mRNA in 34% of lymph nodes from patients with stage I NSCLC, in 33% of nodes from patients with stage II disease, and in 44% of nodes from patients with stage IIIa disease. A total of 88 nodes were tumor free on histologic examination. MUC1 mRNA was detected in 38% of these nodes, as well as in 87% of histologically positive nodes.

Seventy percent of patients had detectable OMs. Twenty histologically negative, RT-PCR–positive nodes were studied by immunohistochemistry, which showed OMs in 9 cases. The RT-PCR would result in upstaging in 11 of 23 patients: from stage Ia to stage IIIa in 5 patients; from stage Ib to IIb, 2 patients; from stage IIb to IIIa, 1 patient; from stage IIb to IIIa, 2 patients; and from stage IIIa to IIIb, 2 patients.

Conclusions.—The RT-PCR assay can detect MUC1 mRNA in histologically negative lymph nodes from patients with NSCLC. The RT-PCR may be more sensitive in detecting MUC1 than immunohistochemical studies used for the detection of OMs. It remains to be seen whether the detection of MUC1 mRNA is related to survival. To evaluate the clinical relevance of the RT-PCR, the investigators plan to use the assay in an ongoing Cancer and Leukemia Group B study.

▶ The detection of occult micrometastatic disease has been the focus of several investigative studies recently published. The concept that small numbers of malignant metastatic cells can be detected, and, therefore, more advanced clinical stages be elucidated at the time of therapy, would could lead to altered therapeutic strategies. Indeed, the fact that roughly 30% to 40% of resected Stage I patients will recur distally suggests that micrometastatic disease is present at the time of surgical resection. The authors in this particular study have been pioneers in elucidating the value of reverse transcriptase polymerase chain reaction and detecting the MUC1 type antigens in non–small-cell lung cancer. This is extremely important as one could perform these studies routinely in a very efficient fashion on lymph nodes and, therefore, detect micrometastatic disease. In a strategy similar to the one utilizing molecular markers of a poor prognosis, this strategy attempts to document micrometastatic disease that is nondetectable by current histopathologic methods. This would appear to be an extremely sound strategy to identify patients who are at high risk for recurrence based on their tumor biology at the time of surgical resection. The authors are to be congratulated for an innovative approach to non–small-cell lung cancer that has the potential of impacting the therapy for a larger number of patients succumbing to this disease.

D.J. Sugarbaker, M.D.

Serum Carcinoembryonic Antigen as an Adjunct to Preoperative Staging of Lung Cancer

Rubins JB, Dunitz J, Rubins HB, et al (Univ of Minnesota, Minneapolis)

J Thorac Cardiovasc Surg 116:412-416, 1998 14–26

Objective.—There are indications that elevated preoperative levels of carcinoembryonic antigen (CEA) are predictive of poor survival after curative resection of lung cancer. To determine if CEA levels would be a useful prognostic indicator, the biologic plausibility of CEA was evaluated by correlating elevations in serum CEA with tumor size, histologic type, and stage.

Methods.—Between July 1991 and January 1993, serum CEA levels were determined before bronchoscopy in 130 patients with suspected lung cancer. CEA levels were correlated with histologic tumor type, surgical stage, tumor size, and liver function tests.

Results.—Malignant disease was diagnosed in 111 patients (2 females) by bronchoscopy, needle biopsy, mediastinoscope, or resection. Fifty patients with limited lung cancer underwent resection which included 8 pneumonectomies, 39 lobectomies, and 3 wedge resections. All margins were histologically free of tumor. CEA was a significant and independent predictor of survival, with a risk ratio of 1.086 or an 8.6% increase in risk of death for every 1 ng/mL increase in CEA. The estimated 3-year survival for patients with stage I or II squamous cell carcinoma was 60% of those with preoperative CEA levels less than 2 ng/mL, 40% of those with CEA levels of 7 ng/mL, and 20% of those with CEA levels of 14 ng/mL. The 3-year survivals for patients with stage I or II adenocarcinoma, with these 3 levels of CEA, were 45%, 30%, and 10%, respectively.

Conclusion.—Patients with elevated preoperative levels of CEA have a poor prognosis independent of other predictors. Elevated levels of CEA can be used as an additional staging tool.

► This is an alternative strategy for identifying patients who are at high risk for local recurrence. As we have seen in previous studies listed in this YEAR BOOK, the goal of identifying patients who are at increased risk for distant and local recurrence at the time of surgical resection is the primary objective of a large number of investigators. This is because no matter which malignancy has been studied previously, the efficacy of chemotherapy is thought to be enhanced in situations where tumor bulk is minimal. Indeed, the ideal patient to receive chemotherapy is one who has only micrometastatic disease that is clinically nondetectable. The use of the CEA in this study had a strong predictive value for poor outcome depending upon its serum blood level. This study bears repeating. Indeed, larger series need to be completed looking at the level of CEA in patients undergoing surgical resection for non–small-cell lung cancer. The authors have made a significant contribution to the literature by demonstrating the efficacy of measuring CEA in patients with resected Stage I and II disease. Of note is the fact that in patients with Stage I and II disease their survival was independently predicted by their level of CEA. This is a very important observation that will, I'm sure, become clinically relevant as additional data is assimilated by other centers.

D.J. Sugarbaker, M.D.

Operative Approach for Multiple Primary Lung Carcinomas

Okada M, Tsubota N, Yoshimura M, et al (Hyogo Med Ctr for Adults, Akashi City, Japan)

J Thorac Cardiovasc Surg 115:836-840, 1998 14–27

Introduction.—The reported prevalence of multiple primary lung cancers—including synchronous and metachronous cancers—ranges from 1% to 10%. These rates would probably be higher if previous studies had used advanced imaging techniques such as CT. An 11-year experience with the management of patients with multiple primary lung cancers was reported.

Patients.—A second cancer was found in 57 of 908 patients undergoing primary lung cancer surgery, for a rate of 6.3%. Synchronous cancers occurred in 3.1% of patients and metachronous tumors in 3.2%. The average ages were 64 and 63 years, respectively. The patients were followed for a median of 51 months.

Outcomes.—From the time of initial treatment, the 5-year survival rate was 70% for patients with synchronous tumors and 66% for those with metachronous tumors. From the time of development of a metachronous tumor, 5-year survival was 33%. Preoperative radiography or bronchoscopy detected 57% of synchronous tumors; 39% were found at surgery. Patients with stage I or II disease had significantly better survival than those with stage III or IV disease.

Conclusion.—Multiple primary lung cancers have a better prognosis than locally recurrent or metastatic disease, so prompt identification is essential. Synchronous lesions should be carefully evaluated during primary surgery, and patients should receive close follow-up for metachronous lesions. Patients with multiple primary lung cancers should have precise staging, aggressive surgery if the disease is in an early stage, and tissue-sparing resection, if possible.

▶ This study is of interest in that it demonstrates that patients who develop a second lung cancer can enjoy a survival similar to patient's survival after initial resection. Specifically, patients in this study who developed either a metachronous or synchronous primary had an approximately 70% overall survival, which is comparable to a reported series of resected Stage I patients. This is important because the implications for following patients postsurgery are profound. Indeed, many HMOs are restricting the use of chest x-rays in the postoperative assessment and follow-up of long-term patients following lung cancer surgery. Indeed, this follow-up is not for the detection of recurrent metastatic disease, but is primarily aimed at detecting early new metachronous primary lesions. This approach appears to be justified by this report, given the excellent long-term survival of these patients developing either simultaneous or second primaries. Indeed, the nihilistic approach towards patients with lung cancer in general needs to be addressed in a systematic fashion by physicians, including surgeons, medical oncologists and radiation therapists who deal with lung cancer on a regular basis. This study is getting the news out that not only do patients who have a primary diagnosis of lung cancer benefit from aggressive therapy, but patients who develop a second lung tumor can also be expected to have an excellent long-term outlook if their disease is detected at an early stage.

D.J. Sugarbaker, M.D.

Metastasectomy Applications and Approaches

INTRODUCTION

Pulmonary metastasectomy is a common surgical intervention performed by the practicing thoracic surgeon. It remains, however, without prospective evidence of its efficacy. It is performed on the intuitive basis that the resection of small lung metastases can be performed with less destruction to the lung, and therefore early resection is favored over a watch-and-wait policy. The following articles illustrate the surgeon's approach to the biology of tumor metastases with surgical intervention.

David J. Sugarbaker, M.D.

Median Sternotomy: The Preferred Incision for Resection of Lung Metastases

van der Veen AH, van Geel AN, Hop WCJ, et al (Univ Hosp Rotterdam, The Netherlands)

Eur J Surg 164:507-512, 1998 14–28

Objective.—For most types of cancer, the lungs are the major site of metastases. Resection of pulmonary metastases is increasingly accepted, and may be performed through a unilateral or bilateral approach. For several years, the authors have used median sternotomy as the first choice for all patients with resectable lung metastases. Experience with this approach is analyzed, including the accuracy of preoperative CT.

Methods.—Over 10 years, 78 patients with pulmonary metastases from various types of cancers underwent attempted resection via a median sternotomy. All patients were operated on with intent to cure; if disease was found to be extensive, the incision was extended. The results were reviewed to assess the feasibility and morbidity of the median sternotomy approach. In addition, the accuracy of preoperative CT in predicting the number and extent of metastases was analyzed.

Results.—A total of 82 median sternotomies were performed. In 49% of patients, preoperative CT failed to demonstrate the extent of disease accurately. Resection of metastases was performed in 72 patients. On histologic examination, tumor-free margins were detected in 81% of patients. Thirty-six patients proved to have unilateral disease and 36 to have bilateral disease; many cases of bilateral involvement were missed on preoperative CT. Lobectomy was required in 2 patients, and 2 underwent anterolateral extension of the sternotomy. The rate of minor complications, such as partial pneumothorax or pulmonary infection, was 14%. There were no operative deaths. The patients stayed in the hospital a median of 9 days. Overall 5-year survival in this series was 38%.

Conclusions.—The authors report good results with median sternotomy for patients undergoing surgical resection of pulmonary metastases. Advantages of this approach include bilateral staging and demonstration of occult metastases, complete clearance in a single procedure, and reduced morbidity. Preoperative CT cannot accurately predict the extent of pulmonary metastases and should not be used alone when deciding on the surgical approach.

▶ This particular report is of some interest as it highlights some of the misconceptions noted by those who propose to approach the patient with pulmonary metastases with only surgical bimanual manipulation as the final common way of determining whether micrometastases are present. Specifically, this article suggests that all patients with metastatic disease should undergo median sternotomy because in this cohort of patients 49% failed to have the preoperative CT scan demonstrate accurately the extent of disease. As noted in the article, many cases of bilateral involvement were missed on the preoperative CT scan. Of interest also is that 36 out of 72 patients had unilateral disease, yet these patients received a median sternotomy.

The primary problem with this report is that the type of CT scan used is, unfortunately, out of date. High resolution spiral CT scanning has been noted in recent series to detect nodules at the 2 mm level or less. The detection of disease at this level allows for minimally invasive approaches that resect CT detected disease with a very high degree of accuracy. In addition, it is not clear whether the authors feel a repeat sternotomy in situations is indicated, particularly when unilateral disease is detected even by the outdated CT scans used here.

It appears that the best approach to metastatic disease in the chest is to first characterize it with state of the art radiographic means—that is to say a spiral high resolution CT scan. Following this, the method of choice would appear to be directed by the surgeon's own clinical competence in particular surgical procedures. It is my personal bias that median sternotomy is left as long as possible as the last resort. This allows the surgeon the luxury of performing a median sternotomy when repeat metastasectomy is required in the presence of more central bilateral disease.

D.J. Sugarbaker, M.D.

Surgical Treatment of Hepatic and Pulmonary Metastases From Colorectal Cancers

Regnard J-F, Grunenwald D, Spaggiari L, et al (Institut Mutualiste Montsouris, Paris)

Ann Thorac Surg 66:214-219, 1998 14–29

Introduction.—For patients with colorectal cancer, hepatic and pulmonary metastases often occur together. Chemotherapy has given poor results in such patients, and the metastases are resectable only rarely. However, as resection of colorectal metastases becomes more accepted, there is evidence that some patients with double hepatic and pulmonary metastases may benefit. Data from 2 French studies were pooled to assess the results of resection for hepatic and pulmonary metastases of colorectal cancer, and to identify prognostic factors for patient selection.

Methods.—The analysis included 239 patients undergoing surgical resection of pulmonary metastases of colorectal cancer at 2 centers over a 25-year period. Forty-three of these patients (18%) had previously had complete resection of hepatic metastases. Intermediate and long-term outcomes were analyzed, and factors associated with prognosis were determined.

Results.—The pulmonary metastases were resected a median of 18 months after the hepatic metastases. The 43 patients underwent a total of 27 metastasectomies, 6 wedge resections, 5 lobectomies, 3 segmentectomies, and 2 pneumonectomies. There were no postoperative deaths, but 2 major postoperative complications. Resection for recurrent pulmonary metastases was performed in 16% of patients. At follow-up, 21 patients were alive and 14 of these were disease free. Median survival after pulmonary resection was 19 months, with a 5-year probability of survival of 11%. Prognosis was significantly associated with the patients' carcinoembryonic antigen blood levels before thoracotomy, and with the number of pulmonary resections performed. Outcomes tended to be better for patients who waited more than 36 months between the hepatic and pulmonary resections.

Conclusions.—Some patients with double hepatic and pulmonary metastases from colorectal cancer can benefit from surgical resection of their metastases. The results appear to be best for patients with normal levels of carcinoembryonic antigen before thoracotomy and for patients with late metachronous pulmonary metastases. However, the relative merits of chemotherapy and resection must be considered on an individual basis.

▶ This interesting report notes that in a small subset of patients developing both hepatic and pulmonary metastases an aggressive surgical approach may be indicated. Of interest is the note that patients who had normal carcinoembryonic antigen (CEA) levels were those who benefited most from this aggressive approach. It has been my experience that patients with pneumotrophic colorectal metastases usually do not have elevated CEA levels. Specifically, those patients who develop pulmonary metastases only, without evidence of other visceral disease, in many situations have a normal CEA level. This undoubtedly highlights a biologic subset of patients' colorectal cancer whose biology would favor aggressive surgical resection of their pulmonary metastases. This would bear further study and, therefore, CEA levels should be considered prior to instituting such an aggressive approach in patients with both hepatic and pulmonary metastases. The other interesting fact was that patients with more than 36 months between the development of pulmonary and hepatic metastases appeared to do best, again indicating that those patients with indolent tumor biology would appear to benefit most from an aggressive surgical approach.

D.J. Sugarbaker, M.D.

Long-term Results After Repeated Surgical Removal of Pulmonary Metastases

Kandioler D, Krömer E, Tüchler H, et al (Univ of Vienna; Ludwig Boltzmann Inst, Vienna)

Ann Thorac Surg 65:909-912, 1998 14–30

Background.—Surgical resection of isolated pulmonary metastases is standard therapy, but few data exist on whether resection is useful for recurrent pulmonary metastases. Data from patients undergoing second, third, and even fourth resections for recurrent pulmonary metastases were retrospectively examined.

Methods.—Thirty-five patients (mean age, 44 years) underwent a total of 82 metastasectomies for epithelial carcinoma (n = 20), osteosarcoma (n = 10), or soft tissue sarcoma (n = 5). Fourteen patients with epithelial carcinoma underwent 2 metastasectomies, 3 patients had 3 operations, and 3 patients had 4 operations. Four patients with osteosarcoma had 2 metastasectomies and 6 had 3 operations. Three patients with soft tissue sarcoma had 2 metastasectomies and 2 patients had 3 operations. Disease-free intervals (DFIs) were calculated for 2 different intervals. The DFI1 was the interval between the resection of the primary tumor and the first metastasectomy. The DFI1 was divided into periods of less than 20 months, 20 to 50 months, and greater than 50 months. The DFI2 was the interval between the first metastasectomy and the second one. The DFI2 was divided into periods of less than 10 months, 10 to 40 months, and greater than 40 months. Survival rates were then calculated for the various intervals and periods.

Findings.—The 5-year survival rate for DFI1 was 48%, and 28% of patients lived for more than 10 years. Patients with the longest DFIs had significantly improved survival rates; a DFI1 of greater than 20 months and a DFI2 of greater than 40 months were associated with significantly improved survival. Furthermore, patients with a long DFI1 tended to have a long DFI2. Survival was not significantly influenced by the nature of the primary tumor or by the size, number, or viability of the metastatic tumors.

Nor did the number of subsequent metastasectomies have a significant influence on survival.

Conclusions.—Almost half of the patients were alive 5 years after a first metastasectomy, and 28% survived to 10 years. These results confirm the utility of repeat surgical removal of metastatic tumors. The prognosis is best for patients with the longest disease-free interval. Neither the size, number, nor viability of the metastases had an effect on survival. Thus these tumor characteristics should not be a consideration in performing repeat metastasectomy; all patients with recurrent metastases should be considered for repeat resections.

▶ This study's most important contribution is that it highlights the following facts. Patients who have recurrent pulmonary metastatic disease should continue to be considered for operative intervention as long as there is no evidence of metastatic disease at other sites and as long as their primary remains controlled. It has been the practice of many thoracic surgeons through the years to continue to "cherry pick" pulmonary metastases in a sequential fashion as they appear. In other centers, however, the presence of a second pulmonary metastases well after the initial resection has doomed patients to nonoperative therapy. This study simply points out that tumor biology should dictate the surgeon's approach. Patients who continue to develop pulmonary metastases in a sequential fashion without evidence of other visceral disease should continue to be considered for surgical resection with parenchymal sparing procedures in order to maximize their longevity, which is often brought to a close by the lack of additional functioning pulmonary parenchyma. This is an important concept that needs to be considered. In my experience, renal cell carcinoma can notoriously develop sequential metastases over a 5- to 7-year period. Many patients have been referred to me after having been declared to be inoperable elsewhere because of the development of these recurrent pulmonary lesions. The reader should be fully aware, however, that for the majority of patients, repeat pulmonary metastasectomy will not result in long-term survival. Nevertheless, the surgeon must be aware of tumor biology as the primary driving factor behind his or her decision to operate or withhold operative therapy.

D.J. Sugarbaker, M.D.

Interesting Clinical Challenges

Introduction

The last group of articles were selected because they addressed common surgical problems or because they provided new information on rare clinical situations.

David J. Sugarbaker, M.D.

Large Cell Neuroendocrine Carcinoma of the Lung: A Histologic and Immunohistochemical Study of 22 Cases

Jiang S-X, Kameya T, Shoji M, et al (Kitasato Univ, Sagamihara, Kanagawa, Japan)

Am J Surg Pathol 22:526-537, 1998 14–31

Background.—The term "large-cell neuroendocrine carcinoma" (LCNEC) refers to a poorly differentiated, high-grade neuroendocrine tumor. On a morphologic and biologic basis, it is between atypical carcinoid and small-cell lung cancer (SCLC). A recent study of bcl-2 protein expression in various types of lung cancer identified 2 cancers, previously diagnosed as non-SCLCs, which fulfilled the criteria for LCNEC. This led to a review of previous neuroendocrine tumors to seek possibly missed cases of LCNEC.

Methods.—The review, performed without knowledge of the original pathologic diagnoses, included 766 primary lung cancers resected between 1982 and 1995. Cancers histologically diagnosed as LCNEC were confirmed by immunohistochemistry, using a large panel of neuroendocrine markers, including amine-peptide neuroendocrine hormones.

Results.—The review identified 22 LCNECs, a rate of 2.87%. Each case was subsequently confirmed by immunohistochemistry, staining positive for 3 or more general neuroendocrine markers. In addition, 12 of the 22 tumors tested positive for neuroendocrine hormones. The histologic findings of the LCNECs included markedly decreased or absent organoid architecture, raising the possibility that the tumor could be mistaken for poorly differentiated adenocarcinoma or squamous cell carcinoma. Eighteen of the tumors had been previously diagnosed as non-SCLCs. The clinical outcomes of the patients with LCNEC were significantly worse than those of non-SCLC patients of similar stage.

Conclusions.—This is the first large review of a series of lung cancers to seek cases of LCNEC. The light microscopic neuroendocrine features of LCNEC may be difficult to recognize: this tumor must be differentiated from non-SCLC, as well as from atypical carcinoid or SCLC. In cancers with a subtle or absent organoid architecture, the best indicator of neuroendocrine differentiation is a rosettelike structure.

► Large-cell neuroendocrine carcinoma is often mistaken for non–small-cell lung cancer. This particular report highlights the poor overall prognosis suffered by patients with large-cell neuroendocrine tumors. Specifically, the authors found that large-cell neuroendocrine carcinomas were present at a rate of approximately 3% of all non–small-cell lung cancers. Specifically, they noted that 12 of the 22 tumors tested positive for neuroendocrine hormones. Eighteen of these 22 tumors had been misdiagnosed as non–small-cell lung cancer. Given the fact that the clinical outcome is significantly less, the authors put forth the concept of improved diagnosis at the time of pathologic inspection with the use of the light microscopic findings as an unreliable way of differentiating this tumor from non–small-cell lung cancer.

Subtle changes were absent; organoid architecture along with the differentiation in a rosette-like structure appear to be the two best indicators that large-cell neuroendocrine tumors may be present. Many authors have suggested that this particular tumor should be treated as a small-cell lung-cancer variant with adjuvant chemotherapy following surgical resection. The practicing thoracic surgeon should be aware of the presence of large-cell neuroendocrine tumors, and, when they are discovered, understand their significance in terms of the need for postoperative therapy.

D.J. Sugarbaker, M.D.

Intraoperative Intrapleural Hypotonic Cisplatin Treatment for Carcinomatous Pleuritis

Ichinose Y, Yano T, Asoh H, et al (Natl Kyushu Cancer Ctr, Fukuoka, Japan)
J Surg Oncol 66:196-200, 1997 14–32

Introduction.—In some cases, carcinomatous pleuritis—which may include carcinomatous effusion and/or pleural dissemination—may not be recognized until the chest has been opened for surgery. When this occurs, the chest is usually just closed, because surgery is not appropriate for patients with this condition. The authors have developed a new approach to this problem, involving intraoperative, intrapleural administration of distilled water combined with cisplatin. The results of this approach in 21 patients were studied, including examination of the adverse effects of treatment and the pharmacokinetics of cisplatin in the blood.

Methods.—The patients all had carcinomatous pleuritis of non–small-cell lung cancer discovered at thoracotomy. Intraoperative intrapleural hypotonic cisplatin was administered for 15 minutes after the completion of intrathoracic surgical procedures. Cisplatin was given in a solution of 50 μg/mL in distilled water that had been prewarmed to 38°C to 40°C. After removal of the cisplatin solution and saline washing of the thoracic cavity, the chest was closed with chest tube drainage.

Survival and pleural disease control were compared for the 21 patients undergoing intraoperative intrapleural hypotonic cisplatin treatment and 29 historical controls not receiving this treatment. Measurements of total and free blood platinum levels were performed in 5 of the treated patients.

Results.—At a median follow-up of 41 months, 6 of 21 patients receiving hypotonic cisplatin were still alive. Although survival was not significantly different from that in the untreated group, hypotonic cisplatin did improve pleural disease-fee survival. Just 14% of treated patients had observable pleural disease after operation, whereas 90% of untreated patients had pleural effusion and/or growth of pleural disseminated tumors a mean of 9 months postoperatively. Treated patients had increased postoperative drainage volume but still recovered uneventfully. Hypotonic cisplatin treatment produced very low blood platinum levels that would be unlikely to cause systemic adverse effects.

Conclusion.—For patients with non–small-cell lung cancer who have carcinomatous pleuritis discovered at thoracotomy, intraoperative intrapleural hypotonic cisplatin appears to have a significant antitumor effect. The authors' experience suggests that this treatment may retard the development of pleural disease with no adverse effects. The antitumor effect of hypotonic cisplatin is believed to be synergistic, producing a high local control rate and the elimination of cancer cells in drainage fluid.

▶ This is a very provocative article in that it suggests that the local treatment of disseminated intrapleural disease may result in long-term survival in a certain subset of patients. Specifically, the author is to be congratulated on an innovative approach to a dreadful problem. The finding of pleural implants at the time of planned therapeutic pulmonary resection is a disappointing clinical finding that usually results in closure of the chest without a therapeutic pulmonary resection being performed. Nevertheless, in a certain subset of patients, where distant disease is not present and nodal disease in the mediastinum is absent, aggressive local treatment of pleural disease may be indicated. The use of hypotonic platinum is an interesting approach, and the use of heat through the warming of the platinum would also appear to enhance its antineoplastic effects. This is an important article suggesting that local approaches to extensive disease in the chest may result in improved survival. Continuous lavage with heated intraoperative chemotherapy may be indicated in a certain subset of patients presenting with carcinomatous pleuritis. The dismal overall outlook of patients presenting with malignant pleural effusions would seem to suggest that innovative new approaches are required to move this particular stage of non–small-cell lung cancer off the dime.

D.J. Sugarbaker, M.D.

Chest Tube Insertion: A Prospective Evaluation of Pain Management

Luketich JD, Kiss M, Hershey J, et al (Mem Sloan-Kettering Cancer Ctr, New York; Univ of Pittsburgh, Pa)

Clin J Pain 14:152-154, 1998 14–33

Purpose.—Chest tube insertion is a common bedside procedure that can cause substantial patient discomfort and morbidity. At the authors' hospital, a review suggested that this procedure was not being performed in a standardized and pain-free manner. A prospective study of pain associated with chest tube insertion, including the effects of a new chest tube insertion protocol, is reported.

Methods.—The prospective case series included 52 patients undergoing chest tube insertion for symptomatic malignant pleural effusions. Interim analysis of the first 26 patients suggested unacceptably high levels of pain and anxiety during this procedure. Analysis led to a revised protocol, including specific guidelines for premedication and proper technique, with the goal of achieving painless chest tube insertion. This protocol was followed for the subsequent 26 patients. Pain and anxiety ratings—assessed on a verbal self-report score of 1–10—were compared for the 2 groups.

Results.—Mean pain rating decreased from 6.2 for patients managed by the conventional approach to chest tube insertion to 3.7 for those managed under the new protocol. In the first part of the study, 46% of patients had a pain or anxiety rating of 9 or 10; this number of patients dropped to 8% in the latter part. The new protocol decreased the mean anxiety rating from 4.5 to 1.5.

Conclusions.—A conventional approach to chest tube insertion may be associated with unacceptably high levels of patient pain and anxiety. Through a multidisciplinary approach to this common procedure—emphasizing staff education, premedication, and close attention to local anesthetic dosage and delivery—a truly painless chest tube insertion can be achieved. Pain reduction is not correlated with premedication alone, which suggests that a comprehensive approach is needed.

▶ This article addressed one of the most common complaints of thoracic surgical patients about their hospital stay. Specifically, the insertion of a chest tube can vary from being a painless procedure to one of the most uncomfortable procedures performed in modern hospitals. These authors have demonstrated nicely that attention to detail and allowing adequate time for local anesthesia and intravenous anxiolytics and analgesics to take effect prior to inserting the chest tube will lead to improved patient satisfaction and reduced anxiety. I applaud the authors' systematic approach to a very difficult but very common problem. This approach can be applied to a variety of surgical interventions. The authors have demonstrated that a systematic approach will yield improved results. The authors have stated clearly that resident and patient education are the keys to achieving the type of success that they have documented here. All thoracic surgeons could be reminded again of the pain and discomfort associated with the insertion of chest tubes. All could benefit from a quick review of this article and its application to our everyday practice.

D.J. Sugarbaker, M.D.

Multicenter VATS Experience With Mediastinal Tumors

Demmy TL, Krasna MJ, Detterbeck FC, et al (Univ of Missouri Hosp, Columbia; Univ of Maryland Hosp, Baltimore; Univ of North Carolina, Chapel Hill; et al)

Ann Thorac Surg 66:187-192, 1998 14–34

Objective.—The utility and safety of video-assisted thoracic surgery (VATS) in the diagnosis and treatment of thoracic tumors were retrospectively reviewed.

Methods.—Between August 1992 and July 1997, 48 patients (21 men), average age 41, of the Cancer and Leukemia Group B thoracic surgeons underwent thoracoscopic tumor excisions or incisional biopsies using the VATS technique. Patients were studied for an average of 20 months.

Results.—There were 22 patients who were asymptomatic at diagnosis. Seventy percent of patients with malignancy were symptomatic. Symptomatic patients had significantly larger lesions than asymptomatic patients (6.4 vs. 3.6 cm), had a longer hospital stay (4.3 vs. 2.6 days), and longer chest tube duration (2.3 vs. 1.5 days). Attachment was vascular in 11 patients and spinal in 10. Tumors were located in the anterosuperior compartment in 10% of patients, in the middle compartment in 40%, and in the posterior compartment in 50%. Conversion to thoracotomy was necessary for 6 patients. Patients undergoing conversion had significantly longer postoperative stays than nonconverted patients (5.5 vs. 3.2 days) and significantly longer chest tube duration (3.2 vs. 1.9 days). There were no perioperative deaths or major complications. Minor complications included 1 patient with a 4-day pleural air leak, 1 patient with ileus, 1 with superficial wound infection, 1 with severe postoperative pain, 1 with pneumothorax, 1 with pleural effusion, and 1 with Homer syndrome for 3 months. Two patients were treated for histoplasmosis-related mediastinal cysts. One bronchogenic cyst and 1 liposarcoma recurred during the follow-up.

Conclusion.—VATS is a safe and effective technique for diagnosing and treating benign mediastinal tumors, particularly those occurring in the middle and posterior compartments.

► The authors, who are from several large institutions performing a large variety of video-assisted thoracic surgical procedures, report on their results with VATS in the removal of benign mediastinal tumors. It appears that the VATS approach is to be considered standard, particularly for posterior mediastinal tumors. This is primarily because of the straightforward resection afforded most posterior mediastinal tumors and their benign nature. While anterior mediastinal tumors can also be resected as is demonstrated by this particular report, it is my belief that, many times, the proximity of large vascular structures to intermediastinal masses precludes their safe removal. In addition, the need to perform more extended resections with malignant tumors, which are more common in the anterior mediastinum, makes the VATS approach to this subgroup of patients less appealing. Nevertheless, there are certain patients, particularly the elderly patients with a small benign thymoma, where a video assisted approach does have some appeal. Nevertheless, the authors should be congratulated for putting together an excellent series from a variety of institutions suggesting that the overall approach is a sound one with broad application to a large number of surgeons.

D.J. Sugarbaker, M.D.

Primary Sarcomas of the Mediastinum: Results of Therapy

Burt M, Ihde JK, Hajdu SI, et al (Mem Sloan-Kettering Cancer Ctr, New York)
J Thorac Cardiovasc Surg 115:671-680, 1998 14–35

Objective.—There is little information about the diagnosis and treatment of rare primary mediastinal sarcomas. The presentation, treatment, and outcome in patients with primary sarcomas of the mediastinum at Memorial Sloan-Kettering Cancer Center are reviewed.

Methods.—Records of 47 patients (18 female), aged 2.5 to 69, who received a diagnosis of primary mediastinal sarcoma between 1940 and 1992, were retrospectively reviewed. Recurrence was recorded, and actuarial survival was calculated using the Kaplan-Meier method.

Results.—At diagnosis, 42 patients had had symptoms, including chest or shoulder pain (38%), dyspnea (23%) and weight loss (19%), for 0 to 16 months. Thirteen percent of patients had a history of radiation therapy. Most tumors were diagnosed initially by chest radiograph, and later by CT and MR in addition to plain chest radiographs. Histologically, sarcomas were malignant peripheral nerve tumors in 12 patients, spindle cell sarcomas in 7, leiomyosarcoma in 5, embryonal rhabdomyosarcomas in 4, and liposarcomas in 4. Tumors were high-grade in 25 patients, low-grade in 12, and indeterminate in 10. Surgery was performed in 34 (72%) patients, with 15 also receiving radiotherapy, and 13 receiving chemotherapy in addition to radiotherapy. Two patients refused treatment. Twelve patients had more than 1 surgery for the primary tumor or recurrent tumor. Twelve patients had serious complications, including pulmonary emboli (n = 3), upper extremity phlebitis (n = 2), and pulmonary infection and sepsis (n = 2). Four patients died after surgery. Resection was complete in 22 (47%) patients; 14 (64%) patients, 7 of whom were treated with both radiation and chemotherapy, had a local recurrence. Metastatic disease developed in 20 patients, 7 of whom had completed resected tumors. Patients with high-grade tumors had a significantly lower 5-year survival than patients with low-grade tumors. Patients with complete resection had a significantly longer survival than patients with incomplete or no resection.

Conclusion.—Patients with primary sarcomas of the mediastinum have a 5-year survival of 32% and a high recurrence rate (64%). The biggest influence on survival is complete resection of the tumor.

▶ This group of authors has provided another excellent contribution to the literature on an extremely rare problem. Only an institution the size of Memorial Sloan-Kettering Cancer Center could report on such a large number of very rare primary sarcomas of the mediastinum. The authors provide excellent insight into the need for extensive local resection. Indeed, long-term survival in this series was directly related to the ability of the surgeon to obtain a complete resection. Given the aggressive nature of primary sarcomas of the mediastinum, this is all too often an unachievable goal. The variety of sarcomas presented here demonstrates that these tumors must be individualized in their treatment. The concomitant use of induction radiochemotherapy may be of value, in my experience, in reducing the size of some primary sarcomas of the mediastinum and, therefore, enhancing the surgeon's chances of achieving a complete resection. Nevertheless, in this group of patients, complete surgical resection remains the gold standard of therapy.

D.J. Sugarbaker, M.D.

Subject Index

A

C

D

E

F

G

H

I

J

K

L

M

N

O

Q

R

T

U

W

X

Author Index